Natural
Detoxification

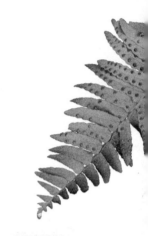

Jacqueline Krohn MD

Frances Taylor MA

Hartley
&Marks
PUBLISHERS

Published by

HARTLEY & MARKS PUBLISHERS INC.
Post Office Box 147   3661 W. Broadway
Pt. Roberts, WA   Vancouver, BC
98281   V6R 2B8

LIBRARY OF CONGRESS CATALOGING-IN-PUBLICATION DATA

Krohn, Jacqueline, 1950–
    The whole way to natural detoxification : clearing your body of
toxins / Jacqueline Krohn, Frances Taylor.
        p.   cm.
    Includes bibliographical references and index.
    ISBN 0-88179-187-3
        1. Toxicology—Popular works.   2. Health.   3. Alternative medicine.
I. Taylor, Frances A., 1938–   . II. Title.
    RA1213.K76 1996   96-22512
    615.9—dc20   CIP

Design and Composition by The Typeworks.
Cover design by Diane McIntosh.
Set in Scala.

Natural Detoxification

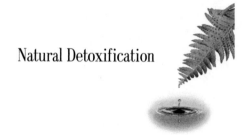

DEDICATION

To those healthcare practitioners in all medical disciplines who:
- Have shed the shackles of dogma
- Have the courage to look beyond the "accepted and standard" treatment
- Think independently
- Treat on the cutting edge of medicine
- Hold the good of their patients as their foremost concern

ACKNOWLEDGMENTS

Our thanks and gratitude to:

- The many healthcare practitioners, both past and present, whose genius and courage enabled the development of the techniques presented in this book.
- Our office staff who gave us support and encouragement and who, as always, stepped in to do the extra work necessary to enable us to continue seeing patients in addition to writing this book.
- Cheryl Sedlacek for her talent and industry at the computer.
- Alice Kernodle and Susan Deininger for their many fact-finding phone calls made on our behalf.
- Melissa Schneider for all of her information gathering errands.
- Jinger Prosser for her participation in the first edition
- Erla Mae Larson for her contributions and suggestions, as well as for sharing her knowledge of nutrition over the years.
- Sue Tauber, in whose mind the original idea for this book originated.
- Elizabeth McLean, our editor, with whom it has again been our privilege to work. Her wisdom, skill, and attention to detail assure appropriate and logical organization, as well as ease of reading.
- Susan Juby and the staff of Hartley & Marks whose talents produced this final presentation of our book.
- Our families, who again have allowed us the hours it took to write this book.

Contents

CONTENTS

Foreword

ALMOST EVERY DAY the news brings reports of yet another environmental catastrophe that results in overt injury to and dysfunction of the multiple complex organs and systems of those people affected. But it isn't just environmental disasters that influence people's health. Rene Dubose once said that "exposures to toxic materials may be so low as to have only nuisance effects and so go unnoticed." However, low level exposures may be even more dangerous than critical exposures if they fail to mobilize the body's natural detoxification systems. The lack of adequate response can result in subtle or serious diseases.

In this book, Dr. Jacqueline Krohn and Frances Taylor alert us to the presence and sources of daily toxic exposures and tell us how to protect ourselves. I can think of no greater contribution to the health of our threatened population than a readable and easy-to-understand book on simple, yet effective, techniques to reduce our body's burdens of toxic materials.

Since 1985 the Center for Occupational and Environmental Medicine has treated hundreds of patients with multiple problems arising from chemical injury and intoxication, using many of the techniques outlined in this book. Our center is one of several environmental programs in the nation, and there are many more patients who could benefit from detoxification treatments than can be treated in these few centers.

If we adhere to the principles outlined by the authors, we can undoubtedly reduce the chances of major organ and system injury due to toxic exposure of all kinds.

The subject of environmental medicine in general and detoxification in particular are inadequately taught in medical schools and post graduate training programs. The book will be helpful to both professionals and lay readers. *Natural Detoxification* will be a great resource for all who want and need to learn about this important subject.

Allan Lieberman MD
Medical Director
Center for Occupational and
Environmental Medicine
North Charleston, SC

Preface

IN WORKING WITH our patients, we discovered that nearly every one of them had toxins of some sort in their bodies. Some had numerous toxins and were laboring under such an overwhelming load that their health would be permanently damaged without some type of cleansing. Others were mildly affected by only a few toxins.

In May of 2000, the Cerro Grande forest fire burned over 48,000 acres in and around Los Alamos, leaving 402 families homeless. Since the fire, the urgent need for detoxification has become even clearer to us. Because of the many toxins to which people were exposed, symptoms among the entire population have increased dramatically. Breathing difficulties, headaches, muscle aches, fatigue, sinus problems, insomnia, nightmares, irritability, and other symptoms plague many of the people living in Los Alamos.

Most people are not exposed to a forest fire, but there are numerous substances and situations in everyday life that can be toxic to an individual. We have attempted to discuss all of those that most people might encounter, not in an effort to frighten you, but in order to present a comprehensive reference. Readers should be able to identify those toxins that might be affecting them.

The methods of achieving cleansing, detoxification, and balance are many and varied. We have endeavored to present a broad spectrum of possibilities and methods, including some that are considered alternative by standard medicine. Every discipline of medicine and healing has some techniques that are of merit. The discerning individual will examine these techniques and incorporate those that are appropriate into an overall health program.

Cleansing toxins from the body can dramatically increase quality of life. It is our hope that readers of this book who suffer from toxic overload will find ideas, information, and inspiration for improving their health.

Jacqueline Krohn, MD, MPH, C.Hom.
Frances A. Taylor, MA, C.Hom.
Los Alamos, New Mexico
2000

xiii

Introduction

UNTIL RECENT YEARS, the concept of toxic overload and its effect on health has not been a common one. Even now, the treatments for this problem—detoxification procedures—are not familiar to most people. Many people are laboring under a heavy body burden of toxins, and their health is suffering because of it. They usually have no idea why they are experiencing difficulty or that there is something they can do about it.

The purpose of this book is to explain:

- what toxins are and how they can affect us
- where we encounter toxins
- how to identify health problems connected with toxicity
- methods of cleansing, balancing, and detoxification
- which problems require professional help
- which problems you may be able to solve on your own
- methods of preventing toxic overload

Because people with widely varying backgrounds and health challenges will be reading this book, we have tried to make it comprehensive. We are not endeavoring to use "scare tactics," but to make people aware of their exposure possibilities. Exposures may range from very few and mild to numerous and dangerous. In addition, each person will have a different response to the toxins he or she encounters. People may not seem to be affected at all by their exposures, they may be mildly affected, they may be severely affected, or they may be permanently damaged by them.

We want to help readers identify their exposures and become aware of how they may be affected by them. Each reader will have a very individual range of toxic exposures, and their response to them will also be individual.

We want to help readers understand who needs detoxification procedures and why, and to show how they can go about cleansing and balancing their bodies. We discuss many different detoxification procedures, some that are self-help, and others that require professional help. Some people will have to utilize a number of different methods and the time required to detoxify their bodies will be lengthy. Others will need little help to regain their health. If you have multiple problems, it is essential that you have professional guidance, preferably from a health care professional who is proficient in several techniques. Such a person will be able to outline and help you follow a comprehensive detoxification program.

Often, people initially feel worse as they begin to detoxify. However, this is a small price to pay, because people who need detoxification will not regain their health until they cleanse and balance their bodies.

A wide range of contemporary cleansing and balancing techniques are discussed in this book, as outlined below.

- *Saunas:* Private saunas and saunas in a detoxification unit are important to many detoxification programs.
- *Detoxification baths:* Can be taken in your own bathtub to remove toxins.
- *Hydrotherapy:* Hot and cold water administered with baths, compresses, packs, and sprays help to relax the body and relieve pain, or to stimulate.
- *Nutrients:* Help cleanse the body and supply building blocks for tissue repair and enzymes needed for detoxification.
- *Diet:* Specialized diets cleanse the body and supply energy for detoxification.
- *Fasting and juicing:* Accelerate the detoxification process and cleanse metabolic wastes and toxins.
- *Exercise:* Imperative for detoxifying the body, even at low levels. Toxins are released from the fat cells during exercise and eliminated from the body.
- *Bodywork:* Facilitates the release of toxins, as well as the cellular memory of toxic events.
- *Allergy extracts:* Control reactions and protect the immune system. Special types help the body release stored toxins and prevent subsequent accumulations.
- *Chelation:* Removes heavy metals and atherosclerotic plaque.
- *Homeopathic remedies:* Treat and balance many conditions.
- *Bach flower remedies:* Help cleanse internal toxins that affect the emotions.
- *Herbs:* Cleanse and treat many health problems.
- *Aromatherapy:* Helps the body to detoxify and rebalance.
- *Breathing:* Helps cleanse the body using various breathing techniques.
- *Oxygen:* Increased oxygen levels help the body detoxify.
- *Compresses, packs, and poultices:* Draw out many types of toxins.
- *Medicated soaks:* Draw out toxins, and have antimicrobial action.
- *Organ cleansing:* Helps restore full organ function and further enables detoxification.
- *Color therapy:* Restores "missing" color from the body to help restore balance.
- *Gem therapy:* Energy within crystals can help balance the body physically, mentally, and emotionally.
- *Light therapy:* Light energy is capable of influencing the healing process and can provide therapeutic benefits that aid detoxification.
- *Sound therapy:* Sound affects many body systems and helps restore inner rhythms, to regain balance.

- *Electromagnetic therapy:* Balances the body electromagnetically.
- *Mind and spirit techniques:* Counseling, Neuro Emotional Technique (NET), journaling, laugh therapy, hug therapy, meditation and prayer, and forgiveness can all help cleanse toxins of the mind and spirit.

In addition to covering detoxification methods in detail, we have prepared charts for some specific conditions to guide you and your healthcare professional as you prepare an individual program.

Once balance and health have been regained, it is essential that they are maintained. People who have been ill do not want to return to that state; healthy people do not want to become sick. We have included prevention guidelines to help the reader avoid toxic exposures and to maintain a clean, healthy lifestyle.

PART I

Approaches

to

Detoxification

THE EXPRESSION "everything old is new again" from a popular song can be applied to many things, including detoxification. The idea of detoxification, cleansing, and balancing is new to many people today, but it is actually a very old concept. When you consider that most ancient treatments were really detoxification and cleansing procedures, it becomes obvious that detoxification has been practiced for a very long time. In addition, the first theories of pathology (disease) revolved around the imbalance of various components in the body.

Our detoxification needs and the reasons for them are considerably changed from those of ancient people. Medical treatment that was not available to them is common-

place to us, but we have many more and different exposures to toxins in our lives. At the same time, we have many more detoxification techniques to help us. However, we have lost the realization of the necessity for detoxification and balancing.

Part I examines evolving detoxification needs and principles. A historical overview looks at the "old" methods and applications of detoxification and cleansing. A contemporary discussion clarifies the "new" ways and how they may apply to you. A broader understanding of detoxification will enable you to identify and understand your needs. You will also learn the various types of professional help available to you.

CHAPTER I

Detoxification Demystified

IN OUR SOCIETY TODAY, the majority of disease is blamed on stress, poor diet, genetics, physical and chemical agents, biological organisms, degeneration, inflammation, autoimmunity, lack of exercise, and abnormal growths. While these factors do indeed cause disease, there is an underlying factor that contributes to all health problems. Toxicity is the common component. Exposure to toxins and subsequent toxic accumulation cause untold health problems, both immediate and long term.

Despite our exposures to toxins, however, it is possible to enjoy good health. We do not have to live in fear, nor do we have to be obsessed by "our poisonous world" or to succumb to "germaphobia." Most people do not have to create or escape to a remote, sterile environment. By using simple treatments we can improve our current state of health. Detoxification techniques and balancing methods make it possible for us to rebuild our bodies and immune systems. Common sense protective measures allow us to maintain our health, resulting in longer lives, with a significantly lower risk of degenerative diseases and other illnesses.

What Is a Toxin?

A toxin is often defined as a poisonous substance produced by plants, some animals, and disease-causing bacteria. Another, but rather narrow, definition for a toxin is a xenobiotic, which means a foreign chemical not produced by the human body. Dr. Elson Haas of the Preventive Medical Center of Marin in San Rafael, California, defines a toxin more broadly as "any substance that creates irritating and/or harmful effects in the body, undermining our health or stressing our biochemical or organ functions."

In this book, the term toxin will refer to anything that can be harmful or hazardous to the body, or that affects the balance of the body.

How Are We Exposed to Toxins?

Since the beginning of human history, people have been exposed to toxins that have affected their health. Over many thousands

Toxins may come from many sources, including:

- food
- water
- air
- plants
- organisms
- chemicals
- toxic metals
- noise
- weather
- altitude
- radiation
- electromagnetic fields
- geopathic stress
- excess of body chemicals
- emotional trauma
- loss of spirituality and faith

of years, our bodies have evolved to tolerate most naturally occurring substances. However, the "Chemical Revolution" that has occurred since World War II and ever increasing industrialization in all parts of the world have multiplied our exposures to harmful substances to incalculable levels. Our bodies have been exposed to over two million new synthetic substances with no time to adapt. Chemical exposures for most people do not occur from a toxic waste spill or from mass pesticide spraying. They come from small-scale exposures that occur day after day, contributing to a buildup of chemicals in our bodies. Because our bodies have had no previous experience with these chemicals, they have no efficient mechanism to metabolize or eliminate them.

Today the health of people is affected adversely on a daily basis. While industry and science have made incredible progress, we have paid a high price for it. Our air is no longer clean; the soil is contaminated; our water supply contains high levels of toxic chemicals and microorganisms; the purity

of our food cannot be guaranteed, and its quality is dangerously low.

We are all exposed to toxins as we go through our daily schedules—even by something as simple as taking a shower. Performing our daily toiletries, such as putting on makeup or shaving, exposes us to chemicals unless we have selected these products with care. Going to the beauty salon or barbershop can mean a massive exposure. The grocery store provides a wide variety of exposures, including laundry and cleaning products; pesticides, both from produce and treatment of the store premises; and personal care products. Shopping in malls and large discount stores results in formaldehyde exposures. Even going to work or school can subject our bodies to toxins.

Regardless of their occupation, all people are exposed to toxins. Mechanics who generally work with no skin protection are exposed to gasoline, greases, oils, and solvents. Numerous building materials cause toxic exposures for contractors, carpenters, and house painters. Office workers are exposed to chemicals emitted by computers, copy machines, paper, correction fluid, and the personal care products of their coworkers. Like office workers, teachers are exposed to office supplies and others' personal care products, but may also be subjected to other toxins. Science teachers use many toxic chemicals in the laboratory, and shop, auto mechanics, and industrial arts teachers work with a variety of toxic materials. Medical supplies, laundry and cleaning products, and pesticides can adversely affect the health of people involved in the healthcare field.

Typical Daily Exposures for a Female Office Worker

- *Morning shower: chlorine and other contaminants in water; chemicals in soap, shampoo, and hair conditioner*
- *Clothes: fabric softener and dry-cleaning chemicals*
- *Toiletries: deodorant, makeup, hair spray, perfume*
- *Eating meals: various chemical and biological contaminants*
- *Traveling to and from work: exhaust fumes from vehicles, air pollution*
- *Workplace: cleaning supplies, office furnishings, outgasing from building materials, indoor air pollution*

- *Work activities: computers, copiers, fax machines, office supplies, personal care products of coworkers*
- *Shopping: formaldehyde in stores, pesticides on produce, chemicals from cleaning supplies used and sold in store*
- *Drinking and cooking with water: various chemical and biological contaminants*
- *General exposures: tobacco smoke; animal hair and danders at home or on the clothes of coworkers; dust and dust mites; mold in bathrooms and kitchens; plant pollens and terpenes*

Homemakers are exposed to cleaning and laundry products, the family's personal care products, pesticides, dust, and mold. Children are subjected to numerous exposures, at home, at school, and in their recreational activities.

■■ EXTERNAL TOXINS

Our exposures to toxins are classified as external and internal. External toxins are those to which we are exposed in our daily lives. Sources of external toxins include foods, water, air, plants, microorganisms, solvents, pesticides, herbicides, agricultural and industrial chemicals, toxic metals, noise, weather, temperature, altitude, and radiation. The exposures may be from serious contamination, such as industrial pollution, or from everyday toxins, such as cleaning supplies, perfume, or cigarette smoke.

Any of these exposures can cause a variety of symptoms in the sensitive person. Symptoms can include headaches, muscle pain, fatigue, mental confusion, emotional upset, poor coordination, skin rashes, neurological problems, and vision disturbances. Toxic chemicals have been associated with decreased immune function, autoimmune disease, enzyme dysfunction, hormonal imbalance, psychological abnormalities, nutritional deficiencies, and cancer.

■■ INTERNAL TOXINS

Internal toxins are those which are stored or produced in our bodies. Our bodies act like sponges, absorbing the chemicals to which we are exposed. Water-soluble chemicals are absorbed and then excreted. However, fat-soluble chemicals accumulate in our fat cells and cell membranes, becoming internal toxins. When the body is under stress, it releases these chemicals from the fat to circulate in the bloodstream. Later, these chemicals will return to the fat cells and cell membranes, to be released another time. The release and return cycle of these chemicals continues indefinitely unless we help our bodies rid themselves of toxins.

Internal toxins can include normal metabolic products. The improper formation or metabolism of normal body chemicals, such as hormones and neurotransmitters, can cause a harmful imbalance. Internal toxins also include substances that our bodies create in response to various conditions, and which become toxic in excess amounts. For example, injury, anesthesia, and pollution cause the body to produce free radicals that are toxic to all tissues. Exercise can cause an excess of lactic acid in the muscles, resulting in stiffness and pain in people who cannot properly process it.

Stress, emotional trauma, and cumulative life experiences can also become internal toxins. People who are experiencing emotional or spiritual challenges will benefit from special detoxification methods.

Symptoms caused by internal toxins include headaches, fatigue, memory loss, mental confusion, "flulike" symptoms, mucous membrane irritation, skin problems, iritis (inflammation of the iris), and musculoskeletal pains. Internal toxins can also cause gastrointestinal symptoms such as nausea, vomiting, and diarrhea.

What Is Detoxification?

The term "detoxification" means to diminish or remove the toxic quality of a compound, and the body contains mechanisms that do just that. Toxic compounds are changed through chemical reactions into less toxic compounds that can be excreted from the body.

The term "depuration"—which means to cleanse or purify—may be more accurate for describing the methods we use to cleanse the body. In this book, we use the term detoxification for all cleansing processes discussed because it is more commonly used, both by the lay person and in the medical world. The terms cleansing, balancing, and detoxification are often used interchangeably. Balancing, which means to achieve homeostasis or equilibrium in the body, enables detoxification; detoxification cleanses; cleansing leads to balance. This interaction in the body helps to restore and maintain health.

Who Needs to Detoxify?

Our bodies detoxify naturally every day, which allows some people to stay balanced. For many others, a slow detoxification system and a multitude of exposures cause their bodies to gradually become overloaded. The detoxification mechanisms of the body become unable to completely cleanse the tissues and the organs, and the body is unable to maintain balance. In these cases, detoxification procedures will help the body to cleanse and balance itself, removing the cause of disease before illness manifests.

Almost everyone would benefit from some detoxification measures, although some people are affected more seriously by toxic exposures. Biochemical individuality and genetic differences partially determine the effects of toxins.

In 1987, medical experts participating in

6

The Rainbarrel Effect

People are subjected to a wide range of physical, emotional, and environmental stresses that contribute to their toxic burden. The body burden can be viewed as "rain," which gradually fills the "rainbarrel" of our bodies. We can adjust to a few stressors, but as the rainbarrel level rises, our metabolism loses its adaptability and we begin to experience toxic overload. Our detoxification mechanisms no longer function adequately and the body cannot maintain its balance. We develop symptoms because our toxin levels are too high. Eventually, the body cannot cope with its toxic burden and our rainbarrel overflows, resulting in disease.

If we periodically empty our rainbarrel with detoxification procedures, we can withstand the stresses of moderate exposures. However, if our rainbarrel continues to fill, additional stressors will cause it to overflow, with resulting symptoms. This is why some exposures can cause us distressing symptoms, while others do not. Our reaction depends in part on how full our rainbarrel is at the time of the stress.

a workshop by the Board on Environmental Studies and Toxicology of the National Academy of Sciences estimated that approximately 15 percent of the U.S. population is sensitive to chemicals found in common household products. In 1993, studies by Dr. Iris Bell of the University of Arizona on healthy college students and adults aged 60 to 90 demonstrated that 15 to 17 percent felt ill after exposure to chemicals contained in pesticides, auto exhaust, paint, new carpet, and perfume. Such sensitive people are often called human canaries. Their symptoms signal the presence of toxic chemicals in the environment, just as the death of canaries formerly used in mines signaled the presence of deadly gases.

People who are burdened by a toxic overload will demonstrate numerous symptoms; however, many people are not aware that their symptoms may be a warning sign from their body. Signals that you may need to undergo detoxification include chronic respiratory problems, asthma, or sinus problems; abnormal body odor, bad breath, or coated tongue; frequent unexplained headaches, back or joint pain, or arthritis; environmental sensitivities, food allergies, or multiple allergies; poor memory, mental confusion, insomnia, depression, irritability, or chronic fatigue; brittle nails and hair, psoriasis, or adult acne; and being underweight or overweight.

Even if we lived in a pollution-free environment, ate organic foods from soils that had no pesticide residue, drank pure water, and breathed clean air, many people would still need detoxification from internal toxins, or metabolic products. People who have minor health problems often carry a toxic load in their bodies. Without proper cleansing and balancing, toxins stored in the body will continue to cause health problems and can lead to degenerative diseases later in life.

It's a Question of Balance

Early civilizations looked on disease as a matter of imbalance or disequilibrium in the body. Today, this philosophical approach is still valid; health can be viewed as a question of balance. A healthy body is a remarkable instrument, maintaining harmony among many elements in order to maintain health.

To have good health, we must be balanced:

- *Allergically:* Allergic reactions imbalance the body by causing an increase in antibodies, an activation of immune system cells, and tissue inflammation as the body releases chemicals in an attempt to heal itself.

- *Biochemically:* Life is possible because hundreds of biochemical reactions take place in our bodies each second. Acid-alkaline balance in the body must stay within an optimal range for the detoxification pathways to function properly.

- *Electrically:* An electrical imbalance in the body causes sleep problems, acute sensitivity to weather changes, and symptoms when exposed to electrical equipment or appliances.

- *Emotionally:* Emotional health depends on balance. Love must be given and received. Anger, grief, and anxiety must be expressed and relieved.

- *Energetically:* The breakdown of organic molecules releases energy that is used by cells. An imbalance in this energy makes it impossible for the body to perform its work and maintain body temperature.

- *Environmentally:* A safe home and workplace that has minimal environmental stresses and toxins is necessary to maintain health.

- *Enzymatically:* Enzymes are essential for biochemical reactions. A deficiency or excess of any enzyme affects the efficiency, speed, and balance of these reactions. Detoxification reactions in the body are enzyme controlled.

- *Hormonally:* Hormones play a major role in metabolism, circulation, water and electrolyte balance, reproduction, and stress. An imbalance can greatly reduce or even stop these processes in the body.

- *Magnetically:* Our brains produce a steady magnetic field, and we project a magnetic field into the space around our bodies. An imbalance affects our biological cycles, such as the sleep cycle.

- *Microbiologically:* Our bodies contain normal microbiological flora that aid in body functions, such as digestion. A deficiency or an overgrowth of these organisms, or an infection by pathogenic organisms, can cause imbalance and illness.

- *Nutritionally:* The body must have a certain balanced amount of nutrients for proper functioning, repair, and good health. A continued deficiency of any vitamin, mineral, essential fatty acid, or amino acid can lead to serious health problems.

- *Psychologically:* Psychological health depends on the proper balance between emotions and the mind. An imbalance of any of the other health factors can affect psychological health.

- *Spiritually:* Spiritual balance is necessary for health. The sense of our higher self must be nurtured by prayer, worship, or meditation, depending upon a person's beliefs. Neglecting this aspect can cause a serious imbalance, resulting in illness.

• *Structurally:* The skeleton must be aligned properly to keep the body healthy and balanced. In addition, all of the cells of the body must be structurally correct and in balance.

The human body is in a constant process of biological change, subject to both internal and external stimuli. It may help to picture a well-balanced mobile formed from all of the above elements. The slightest touch on one part of the mobile causes all of the remaining elements to move. They re-establish balance by conforming to a different but stable position. Larger changes to one part of the mobile cause more active movement of the other elements and more time is needed to achieve a balance. Some changes to our balance occur rapidly, in seconds or minutes, while others may take days or years to occur.

If the tension created by an imbalance remains, the healing process is impeded. When our functions become rigid, unadaptable, and unable to change, disease usually results. Unraveling the imbalance and finding the causative factors can be a difficult and slow process.

Benefits of Detoxification

The benefits of detoxification are many, and can improve every aspect of your health. As your body detoxifies, you can expect digestion to improve, sinus congestion to clear, blood pressure to normalize, mental clarity and memory to improve, and emotional and hormonal fluctuations to stabilize. Once your body achieves balance, your energy level will rise.

With the removal of its toxic burden, the body's immune system will be strengthened, enabling it to cope more effectively with common illnesses. Chronic health problems can be expected to improve or disappear entirely.

In addition to helping restore the body and mind to full health, detoxification increases the effectiveness of any subsequent healing treatment. Over the long term, people who maintain the balance of their body can expect to live longer in better health, to experience fewer degenerative diseases such as diabetes, arthritis, and cancer, and to recover from illness and injury more quickly.

The Way to Health

There are many ways of detoxification but, for complete health, the whole person must be addressed: body, mind, emotions, and spirit. Healing is a comprehensive process of cleansing and rebalancing. People with a low toxic burden will need only a few detoxification methods, and their health will be restored quickly. Those with more serious health problems will have to follow a more complete detoxification program, and their recovery will take longer. If you have serious health problems, consult a qualified practitioner to help you detoxify. Choose a person who is proficient in more than one method of detoxification, who can help you cleanse, rebalance, and rebuild your body.

Once you have taken steps to cleanse and balance your body, you will want to maintain your new level of wellness; thus, methods of prevention are also important. Preventive techniques help to ensure continued good health.

We are the guardians of our own health—it is our most precious gift. Without it, our adaptability declines, our quality of life suffers, and our enjoyment of life is mediocre. Cleansing and balancing the body to restore health becomes a learning experience, even an adventure, when we accept the challenge to pursue the best health possible and therefore the highest quality of life.

CHAPTER 2

Historical Approaches

HUMANS HAVE ALWAYS interacted extensively with their physical world. The relationship of ancient peoples with their earth was a clean and nurturing one. It provided them with air to breathe, water to drink, food for nourishment, materials for shelter, substances for maintaining their well-being, and beauty for their enjoyment. Except in extreme circumstances, the earth was not toxic, and they were not damaged by their world. Unfortunately, these people sometimes damaged their world. They over-hunted and stripped the land of its vegetation, cutting down trees for shelter and firewood. When the land was depleted and would no longer support them, however, they were able to move to another area.

As civilizations developed and populations increased, people began to congregate in cities. The problem of pollution began in these ancient cities. Garbage was thrown into city streets, and drainage water and sewage ran down the middle of the streets. Drinking water became contaminated. People contracted diseases from the unsanitary conditions. Indoor fires and poor ventilation in the small dwellings of the masses fouled the air in many homes. Houses were shared with domestic animals that ate the scraps thrown on the floor. Rodents were rampant, spreading infectious diseases.

Because early humans often did not understand the physical origin of their illnesses, they developed the philosophy that disease was a spiritual matter caused by supernatural forces. For many centuries, medicine was a mixture of practical treatments, magic, superstition, and religion. Medicine men and women were the first physicians.

The ancient Greeks separated medicine from religion and formulated the earliest principles of scientific medicine. By the end of the sixth century they had developed the doctrine of the humors, which formed the basis of ancient medical pathology. For centuries, it was believed that an equilibrium between the four humors—blood, phlegm, yellow bile, and black bile—must be achieved to maintain health.

Early Detox Methods

Early medical treatment of illness sought to re-establish humoral harmony through diet, internal medicine, purging, vomiting, bleeding, cupping, and other techniques. All of these were early cleansing and balancing methods.

Cleansing and Balancing Methods

As time went by, it might be expected that each culture would develop its own unique program of medical treatment. This was not the case. The recorded history of all cultures and countries shows almost identical techniques, with some local variations. Many of these treatments evolved concurrently.

■■ BLOODLETTING

Bloodletting was perhaps the favorite of the ancient treatments, but it was not used on the very young or old. The purpose of bloodletting was to cleanse and balance the humors by removing "bad blood." Bleeding was used as a cleansing technique in the case of abscesses; swelling of the spleen; fever; diseases of the mouth, eye, and head; headaches; and gynecological disorders. In the case of hemorrhage, whether from a ruptured blood vessel, wound, or childbirth, bleeding was used as a "balancing" treatment.

The most common method of bleeding was to open a vein to divert the blood from the problem area or to use freshwater leeches, a milder method of bloodletting. At first, ancient physicians performed all of the bloodletting. When the university schools of medicine were organized around 1000 A.D., bloodletting became the task of the barber-surgeons. Both bloodletting and surgery were considered beneath the dignity of the university-trained physicians, and surgeons and barber-surgeons were below them in status. Below them were the apothecaries and bathhouse keepers who frequently rented the leeches to their clients.

Cupping was another favorite bloodletting method. A small piece of hemp (tow) was burned in a cup. As soon as it had burned out, the cup was placed over a cut on lightly greased skin. Suction from the cup caused it to fill with blood. If the skin had not been cut, the cup was left in place until it fell off, producing a blood blister. A cupping glass over the stomach was considered to be an infallible cure for seasickness.

Bloodletting began centuries before the birth of Christ and remained popular into the 19th century. Every civilization in the world has practiced bleeding. It is still practiced today, even in North America, but on a very reduced scale, and for more practical reasons. Leeches are valuable for removing blood from bruises and black eyes, and for removing the congestion from around a reattached amputated limb.

■■ COUNTER-IRRITATION

Another method of balancing the humors by drainage was to cause a chronic inflammatory reaction in the form of a running sore. This sore could be maintained for long periods of time, and the humors could be continuously released from the body. For treatment of asthma and paralysis, counter-irritation was as popular as bloodletting. The blister was the simplest method of counter-irritation and was commonly produced by applying a poultice of a cantheride (blistering agent). The poultice was left in place until a blister of the appropriate size was formed.

Counter-irritation was sometimes produced by direct application of a cautery, a hot instrument manufactured in a variety of shapes. Different numbers of blisters were called for to treat different diseases, and the design in which these blisters were placed on the skin was thought to be of great importance. In addition to the use of the solid cautery, boiling liquids such as honey, oil, syrup, or wax were used for cauterization. The physician applied the cautery until a sizzling noise, noxious smell, and shriveling of the skin were obtained.

Cauterization is used on a limited basis today to treat nosebleeds. However, a chemical or electric cautery is used to cauterize the skin and vessels in the nose rather than a hot instrument.

■■ ENEMAS

Enemas have been used without exception by all cultures. Not only were enemas employed as a cleansing procedure, but also as a standard beginning treatment for almost every illness, injury, or health problem, including diarrhea. The Egyptians and Greeks routinely gave enemas to treat wounds received in battle. At one time, only physicians administered the enemas, and many early physicians required that an enema be ad-ministered before bleeding. Medication and nutrients were sometimes administered in the enemas.

Many cultures used ritual and routine cleansing with enemas to help maintain health. Even today, some cultures still use the enema as a vital part of treatment for all conditions. Enemas can be a valuable part of a detoxification program and are still used to relieve extreme constipation.

■■ CATHARTICS

A cathartic, sometimes called a purgative, is a substance taken orally that causes an active movement of the bowels. Because constipation was considered a disease rather than a symptom, cathartics were used even more frequently than enemas to cleanse the digestive tract.

Cathartics have been used for centuries, but because of their toxicity several of the favorites used by the ancients are now obsolete. Calomel was dangerous because it disturbed the mineral balance of the body and could result in mercury poisoning. Croton oil blistered the skin and deaths were reported from as few as 20 drops.

Cathartics were often considered an essential part of treatment, helping to remove and cleanse morbid humors. Each humor had its specific purgative, which was supposed to act on it and it alone. As with bleeding, purgatives were not used with the very young or very old. This routine use of cathartics for all medical conditions has long been abandoned. However, laxatives—a mild form of cathartic—are still sometimes prescribed by physicians and used by many people.

■■ EMETICS

An emetic is a substance that induces vomiting. Nearly all the ancient civilizations routinely used emetics as cleansing treatments, in addition to cathartics and enemas. An active emetic, such as white hellebore, was supposed to recall the humors from the innermost recesses of the body. Until this century, it was felt that emetics and cathartics cleansed the body of harmful accumulations, increased the appetite, promoted digestion, cooled the system, and destroyed wind.

Emetics were standard treatment for gastric disturbances, and they were used as routine treatment for many medical conditions. Emetics were kept ready for the "ease, comfort, and happiness" of the patient. With our better understanding of physiology and digestion, we now realize that these measures are too harsh, and in some instances can be fatal. Proper diet and nutrition better aid digestion, and cleansing can be accomplished by milder methods. However, emetics are still used today to induce vomiting in some poisoning cases.

■■ TREPHINATION

Trephination involves cutting a section of bone out of the skull. Evidence of trephined skulls dates to around 10,000 B.C. Over the years, many ancient trephined skulls with round or oval pieces of bone removed have been found all over the world. The holes vary in size, and some skulls found in North America contain multiple holes.

For 2,000 years, surgeons have used trephination to relieve brain compression caused by fractures. However, many ancient trephined skulls show no evidence of frac-

ture. It is believed that trephination was also performed as a purification or cleansing treatment, and that the bones removed were worn as protective amulets. As late as the 17th century, surgeons trephined skulls as treatment for epilepsy and other nervous and convulsive diseases, to "allow evil air to breathe out." Until recent years, some tribal societies used trephination for treatment of chronic headaches.

■■ BATHS

Numerous types of baths have been used by all civilizations to wash away illness and to purify and cleanse the body. Sickness was considered an unclean state, and purification of both the sick person and the home was required. The original baths were taken in rivers, seas, lakes, and pools. Springs were considered to be divine, with special powers for healing, and enhancing fertility.

The temperature of the medicinal bath varied with its medical purpose and the disease involved. For centuries, cold baths and cooling compresses have been used to treat fevers and help reduce pain. Tepid or warm baths were used to calm hysterical and agitated, mentally ill patients, because warm water has a sedative effect that tends to induce both relaxation and sleep.

The most popular was the hot bath, dating back as far as ancient Egypt. A hot bath is clinically analgesic, but is also stimulating to the nervous system. The Greeks and Romans frequented bathhouses in which both hot and cold baths were available. In medieval Europe, there were no baths in private homes and the general public went to bathhouses, not just for cleanliness, but for their health. Bleeding, cupping, and massage were available at bathhouses, along with various tonics and herbal remedies.

The hot bath caused sweating, which was considered therapeutic as well as cleansing. According to ancient tradition, there were three kinds of sweat: the sweat of illness, of toil, and of bathing. Steam baths and wet saunas are used today to help respiratory diseases and relieve rheumatic pain. They are also helpful for skin tone and texture.

■■ MASSAGE

Humans have practiced some form of massage throughout their history. Some massages were no more than an oil rub. Others involved deeper bodywork to relieve muscle tension and help eliminate waste matter from the muscles. Massage also served as a mechanical cleanser, pushing out waste products, particularly in those suffering from constipation.

Massage has been described with many different terms, such as passive exercise, therapeutic manipulation, stroking and kneading, rubbing, and mechanotherapy. As medical theory and practice have expanded, bodywork has kept pace. During this century, there has been an explosion of techniques, practitioners, and discoveries of new ways in which the hands can be used to affect human physiology. Regardless of the technique used, massage helps to cleanse and balance the body.

■■ ACUPUNCTURE

Organized medicine began in China in the first millennium B.C. Although the origin of acupuncture in China is not clear, the first

written reference to it dates to 90 B.C. It is probable that the technique is older.

Acupuncture involves inserting, into the skin, fine metal needles one-half to several inches in length. Some needles are inserted gently and others are inserted with force to different depths. The needles may then be heated, twirled, or vibrated. They are left in place for varying amounts of time, depending on the condition being treated.

The points where the needles are inserted are called acupuncture points, which are located on meridians that run the length of the body. These meridians are called energy pathways and are believed to control certain physical conditions. Traditional Chinese physicians believe that all disease or pain is the result of imbalance in the energy flow along these meridians. Inserting acupuncture needles at the appropriate points restores and balances the energy by diminishing an excess and replenishing a deficiency. Order and harmonious balance are thus restored in the chi, or life force, that circulates through all the organs of the body.

■■ FASTING

True fasting means complete abstinence from food and beverage, including water. Early humans began to fast in an attempt to placate divine powers they believed to be displeased with them. As time went by, fasting became part of religious and purification rituals. Hippocrates and other early physicians felt that fasting dried the body and balanced the humors, but it was not used with infants or the elderly. Although fasting was occasionally prescribed as a cleansing treatment, most early physicians preferred the emetic, cathartic, and bleeding approaches to cleanse and balance the body.

Today many people use periodic fasting as a cleansing procedure and in religious observances. Very few people follow true fasting, but consume some type of juice or broth in addition to water.

■■ EARLY MEDICATIONS

Early medications in most cultures were prepared from plants. Flowers, fruits, roots, barks, leaves, juices, oils, and resins were used. Many plants were believed to have specific applications for balancing a particular humor or element. The Chinese claim to have used herbal remedies for over 10,000 years, to balance their five elements of fire, metal, earth, water, and wood. Ancient literature in India listed 760 plants as having medicinal properties. They, too, were used to balance their five elements of wind, fire, water, earth, and space. However, history points to the Egyptians as the first people to use plant remedies in an organized way.

Resinous materials were used as remedies for their antiseptic properties, while wine and other alcoholic preparations were widely used for their anesthetic properties. Mineral remedies were also used, particularly in Egyptian and Hindu pharmacies. In most cultures, mercury was considered the "king of metals" and was given both externally and internally.

Many cultures, especially in the ancient East, felt that water had cleansing and cooling properties, and purified both body and soul. Water was employed for its own medicinal properties and also as a vehicle for other remedies.

Several ancient civilizations classified medicines according to their function, such as emetic, purgative, laxative, tonic, and aphrodisiac, for a total of 35 different classifications. Medications were prescribed in several forms, including infusions, decoctions, mixtures, pills, salves, syrups, pastes, plasters, poultices, powders, ointments, suppositories, tinctures, and fumigations. Preparation of these various forms of medication was governed largely by astrology. A particular phase of the moon or positions of the planets and stars were considered an important prerequisite in preparation procedures.

Treatment with all medications was an attempt to cleanse, purify, or balance the humors or elements of the body. Although most ancient remedies are not in use today, some medicinal herbs are still given for the same conditions. Modern scientific research into the medicinal actions of these herbs continues to verify the effectiveness of many of these "folk remedies." Many modern prescription medicines have been derived from plants.

CHAPTER 3

Contemporary Approaches

MANY DIFFERENT CLEANSING, detoxification, and balancing techniques are discussed in later chapters. In order to better understand these therapy modalities, it is necessary to understand the philosophy of the medical discipline offering that therapy.

Current Medical Disciplines

As the practice of medicine evolved over the centuries, many different schools of thought and methods of treatment developed. Several medical ideologies exist today. In some instances, these ideologies work in harmony but, sadly, there is often conflict and competition among them.

Most people are unaware of the differences in medical disciplines and what each has to offer. Every person should have enough knowledge to be able to make an informed decision about the type of practitioner with whom the responsibility for health care will be shared.

■■ ALLOPATHY

In North America, the most common medical practice is allopathy, sometimes called orthodox or modern medicine. Although medicine is often described as the art of healing, allopathy is based on a belief in medicine as a science. Physicians with an MD degree are allopaths, and most of the medical schools in North America are allopathic.

There are two general divisions in allopathy: medicine and surgery. The medical division is descended from the European university system, established over 900 years ago. Surgery's historical roots come from the barber-surgeons who practiced minor surgeries for hundreds of years. Although a medical doctor may choose to be a general practitioner (GP), both medicine and surgery have many different types of specialties:

Medicine	Surgery
Internal medicine	Surgery
Cardiology	Orthopedics
Gastroenterology	Urology
Pediatrics	Ear, nose, and throat
Geriatrics	Obstetrics and
Dermatology	gynecology
Immunology	Anesthesiology
Epidemiology	Ophthalmology
Allergy	
Neurology	
Psychiatry	
Radiology	
Pathology	

Detoxification and Allopathy

Few detoxification treatments are offered in allopathic medicine. It does not generally acknowledge the effects of chemicals on the body except in cases of poisoning and death. The allopathic use of drugs for most treatments introduces more chemicals to bodies that are already laboring under a toxic load.

Practitioners do use chelation therapy—a method of removing chemicals from the body—for lead poisoning, but most do not acknowledge its value for ath- *erosclerosis. Some physical therapy treatments, such as soaks and whirlpools, offer minimal detoxification possibilities.*

While some allopaths suggest special diets and exercise, which can be cleansing, these are not primary constituents of allopathic practice. Most allopaths seldom recommend nutritional supplements or acknowledge their role in detoxification, repair, and maintenance of health. Some practitioners even feel that nutritional supplements are injurious to health.

Because of these specialties, allopathic practices often tend to be rather compartmentalized, focusing on parts of the body or particular body systems, frequently without considering the emotional and psychological aspects that are always involved in both health and illness. For traumas, acute bacterial infections, and medical emergencies, allopathic medicine is very effective, but it does not handle viral infections, degenerative diseases, serious cancers, mental illness, or functional illness nearly as well.

Allopathic medicine defines health primarily as the maintenance of a certain level of measurable values and vital signs. These include normal values for blood pressure, body temperature, pulse, respiratory rate, visual acuity, auditory threshold, electrolyte balance, height, and weight. Many of these values are determined by lab tests, and in general, allopathic medicine relies on technology for diagnosis and treatment. The body and its functions must display no ab-

normalities; dysfunctions in the life processes are considered to be disease.

Allopaths treat disease with medications that produce different effects from those that the disease produces. Many allopaths use only pharmaceuticals; if they use nutritional therapy, it is usually as a minor secondary treatment. They only receive approximately 10 to 20 hours of nutritional instruction in medical school. However, it is becoming more common for allopaths to ask patients about their dietary habits or to attempt to correct some health problems with changes in diet.

There are allopaths who have augmented their practices with techniques that are not part of traditional allopathic procedure. For example, environmental medicine physicians receive additional hours of training in nutritional, homeopathic, herbal, and many other therapies. They treat environmentally ill patients and patients in need of detoxification, using contemporary cleansing and balancing methods. Other physicians have added basic "hands-on" modalities developed by chiropractors that allow them to both balance and treat the body (see Chiropractic, below).

■ OSTEOPATHY

The basic theory of osteopathy has altered little since its inception in the mid-19th century. Osteopathy accepts the interrelationship of all parts of the body, as well as the body's inherent capacity to resist disease and to repair itself. The osteopathic philosophy of disease considers that strains or dislocations in the skeletal system affect the body's structural integrity and can result in disease. Osteopaths use physical manipulation to correct skeletal and other problems.

Osteopaths are often primary care physicians, who prescribe drugs and perform surgery. They combine broad medical knowledge with their manipulation techniques. Nineteen osteopathic medical colleges in the United States grant DO degrees. Osteopathic pharmacology and medical specialties are the same as allopathic pharmacology and medical specialties. Osteopaths and allopaths take the same medical licensing exams.

Osteopathic manipulations balance the skeleton, restore nerves, increase lymph and blood circulation, and relieve muscle spasms. These are valuable balancing and cleansing techniques. Although it depends on the practitioner, osteopathy generally places more emphasis on diet and exercise than does allopathy. Many osteopathic physicians also have additional training in alternative methods of treatment.

■ CHIROPRACTIC

Chiropractic derives from the Greek words *kheir,* meaning hand, and *praktikos,* meaning practical. It was developed by D.D. Palmer in 1895 and was conceived as a natural approach to healing, drawing upon the recuperative powers of the body. From 17 chiropractic colleges in North America, chiropractors receive a DC degree, which permits them to use spinal manipulation to correct spinal imbalances. They believe such imbalances can cause many diseases and other health problems.

Chiropractic was negatively affected by the Flexner Report (1910), which consolidated allopathic medical education and strengthened its position (see Homeopathy, below). With time, government support and financing became available to allopathic medical education, while chiropractic education remained tuition driven and received no external support for research. Organized medicine also promoted licensing regulations, believing that chiropractic graduates would be unable to pass the exams. However, chiropractic schools upgraded their curriculum and their graduates began to pass the Basic Science Board exams. In 1974, the Council of Chiropractic Education (CCE), which received recognition from the Department of Education, was established and set up standards for the chiropractic profession. All North American chiropractic colleges are now accredited by the CCE.

Modern chiropractic treatment has added diagnostic techniques, including X-ray and applied kinesiology, but chiropractors cannot prescribe drugs or perform surgery. Much emphasis is placed on exercise, diet, and nutritional supplementation. Chiropractors incorporate treatments with heat and ice, massage, electrical stimulation, traction, ultrasound, and trigger-point therapy (locating and working with the specific points on the body that cause the tension or pain).

Chiropractic offers several cleansing modalities. Manipulation treatments both balance and cleanse. Their knowledge of nutrition enables chiropractors to recommend many cleansing and balancing nutrients. Trigger-point therapy and electrical stimulation also cause the release of toxins.

Chiropractic practitioners have developed many new hands-on techniques that are useful in balancing the body. These include Contact Reflex Analysis (CRA) and Nutrional Reflex Technique (NRT). These two techniques utilize the body's reflexes to analyze the structural, metabolic, and nutritional needs of the body, allowing determination of the root cause of a health problem. Bio Set, Nambudripad's Allergy Elimination Technique (NAET), and Total Body Modification (TBM) are techniques that combine kinesiology, acupressure, and other methods to treat allergies and other health problems. They are discussed in detail in chapter 27, Allergy Treatment and Chelation.

❚❚ HOMEOPATHY

Homeopathy is a medical system developed 200 years ago by German physician Samuel Hahnemann (1755–1843). Hahnemann was critical of the harsh, suppressive, conventional medical therapies of the day. He developed the Law of Similars, based on his experiences and the writings of Hippocrates and Paracelsus, which states that a substance that causes symptoms in healthy persons can help cure a sick person who has similar symptoms. Hahnemann chose the word homeopathy to describe this medical system. The Greek root *homoios* means similar, and the root *pathos* means suffering or disease.

Hahnemann discovered that the body's responses to illness are an effort to heal itself. He realized that these efforts to heal were not always strong enough to complete the healing process, and he concluded that treatment should stimulate the symptoms developed by the body in response to illness.

To cure a patient, Hahnemann found he had to choose the homeopathic remedy that most closely fit the patient's main symptoms, as well as the way in which the symptom is affected by qualities such as heat, cold, and motion. Emotional symptoms may be as important or even more important than physical symptoms. An important principle of homeopathy is the individualization of the remedy to the person's physical and emotional characteristics.

Hahnemann treated the "vital force"—a person's overall, interconnected energetic and defense processes that aid in self-healing. The vital force guides the homeopath to determine whether or not a remedy is working. Hahnemann realized that he was practicing "energy medicine," as the body seemed to "resonate" with the remedy used.

Homeopathy spread throughout Europe and then the United States. The first national medical association in the United States was the American Institute of Homeopathy, founded in 1844. The survival rate of

Flexner Report

The Flexner Report described the "unscientific basis" of some medical schools. It placed the highest value on those medical schools with a full-time teaching faculty who taught a more "scientific" analysis of the human body. Only graduates of the schools that received a high rating were allowed to take the medical licensing exams.

patients treated with homeopathic remedies in 1900 was two to eight times that of patients given the conventional medical care of that era. Homeopathy was used successfully during cholera, typhoid, scarlet fever, and yellow fever epidemics.

Homeopathy offered an integrated, coherent, systematic basis for its practice, and it threatened orthodox medicine of the day. Partly in response to the growth of homeopathy, a rival medical group, known as the American Medical Association (AMA), formed in 1847 to slow the development of homeopathy. In 1855, the AMA ruled that orthodox physicians would lose their membership in the AMA if they consulted with a homeopathic physician or other "nonregular" practitioner.

By the early 1900s, there were 22 homeopathic medical schools and more than 100 homeopathic hospitals in the United States. Education at the homeopathic medical schools was of similar quality to that offered at the orthodox medical schools of the day. However, in 1910 Abraham Flexner prepared a report for the Carnegie Endowment for the Advancement of Teaching in cooperation with leading members of the AMA.

The Flexner Report gave the homeopathic colleges poor ratings. As a result, the homeopathic schools converted to a more orthodox medical program based on "pure science" and the theory that germs (microorganisms) cause disease. Less time was spent studying homeopathic principles and remedies. With this change in curricula, graduates of homeopathic schools were not as skilled at homeopathic prescribing as were earlier graduates.

Pain-killing drugs and antibiotics that seemed to work magically soon became the most used medicines in North America. Orthodox physicians were able to see and treat patients in a shorter period of time because their approach was less comprehensive than that of homepaths. Drug companies, which controlled the major medical journals, were antagonistic toward homeopathy. By 1950, all homeopathic medical schools in the United States had closed or were no longer teaching homeopathy.

In the last 20 years, however, homeopathy has regained popularity because of people's desire for more natural treatments without the serious side effects that can accompany pharmaceuticals. (See chapter 28, Homeopathy and Bach Flower Remedies, for further discussion of remedies.) Homeopathy is used widely in Europe, India, and Britain. In Britain, 42 percent of physicians refer patients to homeopaths, and India has more than 100 homeopathic medical colleges. There are now several academies in the United States where a homeopathic education may be obtained.

▌▌ HOMOTOXICOLOGY

In an attempt to synthesize medicine, the German physician Hans-Heinrich Reckeweg proposed the concept of homotoxicology in 1955. It is considered by some to be a "marriage" between allopathy and homeopathy, and is based on the assumption that the body is a dynamic system that constantly adjusts to the environment to remain in a state of balance. Reckeweg considered disease to be the body's struggle against endogenous (internal) and exogenous (external) homotoxins—substances that are toxic to humans—and the attempt to compensate for homotoxically related damage.

Reckeweg described five interlinked subsystems of the body's defense that combat and render toxins harmless:
• production of antibodies
• use of neuronal adaptation hormones
• toxin defense by the nervous system
• detoxification by the liver
• detoxification by the connective tissue
Homotoxicological remedies stimulate and regulate the self-healing capabilities of the body, and avoid any damage resulting from the therapy. Reckeweg felt that treatment should involve as few side effects as possible because the body is already under stress. His treatments were designed to give rapid, optimum relief with no inhibition or suppression of symptoms, which prevents the body from eliminating the homotoxins.

For simple treatments, Reckeweg prescribed individual homeopathic remedies, organ and tissue preparations, sarcodes (remedies made from healthy tissue), nosodes (remedies made from diseased tissue or microorganisms), trace elements, catalysts, and homeopathically prepared allopathic drugs. For syndromes, in which a group of symptoms occur that characterize a particular disease, Reckeweg used combination homeopathic remedies. These remedies cover a broad range of possible causes of the health problems and functional disorders, including constitutional circumstances and environmental influences.

There are no homotoxicological medical schools in the world, but some practitioners from other medical disciplines have adopted homotoxicological principles in their practices. Homotoxicology offers many of the same cleansing and balancing techniques as homeopathy.

▌▌ NATUROPATHY

Naturopathy had its beginnings in treatments that included clean air, food, and water. It was first brought to the United States from Germany in 1892. In 1902, a group of German homeopathic physicians enlarged the treatment methods to include herbs, homeopathy, and physical therapy. The name naturopathy is a combination of the words nature and homeopathy.

The philosophy of naturopathy includes the following principles of healing:
• To first do no harm
• To recognize the healing power of nature
• To treat the whole person
• To identify and treat the cause of illness
• To realize that prevention is the best cure
• To teach the principles of healthy living and preventive medicine
Naturopathic physicians receive training in clinical nutrition, physical medicine, homeopathic medicine, botanical medicine,

naturopathic manipulations, psychological medicine, cleansing protocols, and minor surgery. They may elect to do further training in naturopathic obstetrics, acupuncture and Oriental medicine, and Ayurvedic medicine.

In the early 1900s, there were as many as 45 naturopathic medical schools in the U.S. These schools were affected by the 1910 Flexner Report, as were homeopathic and chiropractic schools. By 1955 there were only two schools left, and by 1978, just one.

Today there are five accredited naturopathic medical colleges in North America: the National College of Naturopathic Medicine in Portland, Oregon; Bastyr University of Natural Health Sciences in Seattle, Washington; the Southwest College of Naturopathic Medicine in Scottsdale, Arizona; Bridgeport University in Bridgeport, Connecticut; and the Canadian College of Naturopathic Medicine in Toronto, Ontario. Graduates of these schools are trained to be primary care physicians and are granted an ND degree. Several states currently provide licensing for naturopathic physicians.

▌▌ AYURVEDIC MEDICINE

Ayurvedic medicine is more than 5,000 years old, and is the oldest medical system known. This Indian system of preventive medicine and health care is still practiced today, in India and around the world. The Ayurvedic practitioner concentrates on the constitutional type of the patient rather than the presence of disease.

In Ayurvedic medicine, treatment is based on *doshas,* which are metabolic body types. Doshas influence physique, and have

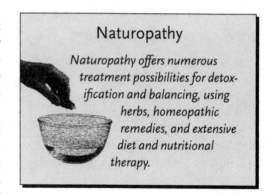

Naturopathy

Naturopathy offers numerous treatment possibilities for detoxification and balancing, using herbs, homeopathic remedies, and extensive diet and nutritional therapy.

a great influence on a person's health and well-being. Body type dictates appropriate diet, physical activity, and the correct choice of medical treatments, as well as specific prevention techniques. The dosha is like a blueprint that maps the innate tendencies in a person's system, including both physical and mental attributes.

The three basic doshas are Vata, Pitta, and Kapha. Most people are a combination of two dosha types, with one dosha more prominent. Vata is the most active dosha and causes the majority of problems, especially if the disorders relate to stress. A balance between all three doshas is essential for optimum health.

Ayurvedic medicine teaches that when the doshas are balanced a person will have good health and energy. If the balance is disturbed, the body will be susceptible to stressors such as microorganisms, overwork, or poor nutrition. Balancing the body prevents disease and promotes emotional and spiritual growth. Diet, exercise, daily routine, and seasonal routine all work to balance the body.

There are two approaches to Ayurvedic treatment, constitutional and clinical. Their

Ayurvedic Medicine

The Ayurvedic physician considers every aspect of life, including physical, mental, emotional, and spiritual. This medical system can treat chronic illnesses connected to lifestyle, as well as acute and traumatic conditions. Its techniques emphasize balancing and detoxification.

use depends on the type and severity of the disorder. Balancing the doshas is the goal of both types of treatment. Constitutional treatment utilizes diet, mild herbs, specially prepared mineral substances, and lifestyle adjustments to balance the body and return it to harmony. Clinical treatment employs strong herbs and medications, purification and cleansing methods (including medicated enemas), therapeutic vomiting, nasal medications, and therapeutic bloodletting.

The herbs used in both types of Ayurvedic treatment are selected according to their taste or essence, which indicate their properties. For example, herbs that are pungent, sour, and salty cause heat and increase Pitta. Sweet, bitter, and astringent herbs cool the body and decrease Pitta. All plants are categorized by these properties, which the Ayurvedic herbalist utilizes in determining the correct prescription.

There are 108 medical colleges in India that grant degrees in Ayurvedic medicine upon completion of a five-year course and a hospital residency. In North America, there is no state or provincial licensing for practitioners of Ayurvedic medicine, although there are several private colleges. Ayurvedic medical care is available from some Indian practitioners who have come to North America. In addition, some non-Indian practitioners (including naturopaths, chiropractors, osteopaths, and allopaths) have added Ayurvedic medical treatments to their practices after receiving training through Ayurvedic seminars and institutes.

▐▐ CHINESE MEDICINE

Chinese medicine is another ancient system of health maintenance and healing that is still available today. It has been practiced for over 3,000 years in China and is now utilized by many Western practitioners. In Chinese medicine, a balance between *yin* and *yang* determines health. These are two complementary qualities that co-exist in all of nature, including the body. Yin is negative, feminine, contractive, small, dark, and associated with water and metal. Yang is positive, masculine, expansive, big, light, and associated with fire and wood.

All substances, places, and times are either yin, yang, or a combination of the two. Organs of the body are classified as either yin or yang. Yin organs function in partnership with a corresponding yang organ, with hollow organs considered to be yang, and solid organs yin.

Chinese medicine also classifies all substances and objects by five elements: fire, wood, earth, water, and metal. Organs of the body, foods, and drugs are all designated by their elemental content.

Organs in Chinese medicine are actually considered as "spheres of function." When a Chinese physician speaks of an organ, he is considering not only the organ, but the functions related to that organ. There are twelve organs (tsang) in Chinese medicine, although two—the "circulation-sex" and "triple warmer"—have no exact anatomical equivalent. The "circulation-sex" or peri-cardium (sac around the heart) is known as the "gate of life." The "triple warmer" assim-ilates and transports energy and maintains body temperature. Some people feel it corre-lates with the endocrine system.

Beyond the qualities of yin and yang, and the five elements, a universal, vital energy called *chi* (spelled in many different ways) flows both into and throughout the human body. Some of our chi is inherited from our parents and the rest comes from the air we breathe and the food we eat. Chinese medi-cine directs that chi must be balanced; each organ must have the optimum amount of chi for the body to function properly. A defi-ciency or an excess of chi is considered to constitute disease. Diagnosis requires locat-ing the chi imbalance, and treatment cor-rects the chi balance in the organs.

Chi flows along invisible energy meridi-ans throughout the body. Each meridian is named for the organ through which it flows. Meridians transport chi, serve as the com-munications system for the body, regulate organ systems, and connect the interior and exterior of the body. Exterior flows mirror the deep, internal flows of energy in the body. All treatment is done on the surface, exterior flows, leading to the correction of in-ternal chi.

Chinese doctors make a diagnosis though looking, listening and smelling (these two words are identical in Chinese), asking, and touching. The Chinese physi-

Chinese Medicine

Chinese medicine is best known for treating chronic illnesses and any condition that does not require surgery. Its balancing treatments and lifestyle recommendations are valuable detox-ification methods.

cian also examines the tongue, palpates parts of the body, and takes the pulse. There are 28 different pulse qualities that are diag-nostic of distinct imbalances.

After examination of the patient, imbal-ances are identified, including whether they represent a deficiency or an excess. Treat-ment may include acupuncture, herbal remedies, massage, exercise, diet, or a com-bination of these and other treatments.

Training in Chinese medicine is avail-able in North America, with over 30 schools of acupuncture in the United States alone. Programs vary in length, depending on the school. Licensing laws vary from state to state and province to province. Schools that teach only acupuncture techniques grant de-grees for licensed acupuncturists (L.Ac.). Schools that teach a full Chinese medicine curriculum in addition to acupuncture grant either an OMD (Oriental Medical Doctor) or a DOM (Doctor of Oriental Medicine) degree. The two degrees are equivalent.

■■ VIBRATIONAL MEDICINE

Vibrational medicine is energy medicine. Dr. Richard Gerber of Livonia, Michigan, the author of *Vibrational Medicine,* defines it as a healing philosophy that treats the whole person—the mind, body, and spirit—by delivering measured amounts of frequency-specific energy to the human multi-dimensional system. It seeks to heal the physical body by balancing the higher energetic systems.

Modern medicine is based on the Newtonian concept of the human body as a complex machine. Vibrational medicine, based on the Einsteinian viewpoint, considers the human body to be a multidimensional organism made up of physical systems that are interrelated with complex regulatory energetic fields. Vibrational medicine techniques direct healing energy into these energy fields.

Although alternative medicine more commonly uses vibrational healing methods, modern medicine does use some energy techniques. The use of electromagnetic

Vibrational Healing

Vibrational healing methods include homeopathy, acupuncture, some types of bodywork, Reiki, flower essences, gem therapy, sound therapy, color therapy, and other techniques. All of these therapies affect and heal the body on an energetic level. Vibrational medicine cleanses and balances the body at the deepest cellular level.

fields to stimulate fracture healing, radiation to treat cancer, and electricity to alleviate pain are all energy modalities. (See chapter 32, Energy Balancing, for a detailed discussion.)

PART II

The Body

OUR BODIES ARE MIRACULOUS, marvelous creations. They function day in and day out, and unless they are causing a problem, we seldom think of them or give them any special consideration. We use our bodies 24 hours each day and do not often consider allowing them to rest and regenerate, other than when we sleep. We push them to the limits of their tolerance and capabilities. We tend to take better care of and pay more attention to the needs of our automobiles than we do to the condition and needs of our bodies. We "feed" our vehicles the best fuel, but we do not feed our bodies well. We give our automobiles regular checkups, but we do not do the same for our bodies. We make sure we change the oil in our vehicles, check the spark plugs, and fix rust spots, while ignoring signs of "wear and tear" in our bodies.

Our bodies continue to function even when we need detoxification, sometimes laboring under a very large toxic burden. They signal us with symptoms when the toxic load is exceeding their detoxification capabilities. It seems incredible, if not miraculous, that our bodies continue to function as well as they do, when you consider their many toxic exposures, and the little care we give them.

Part II is designed to enable you to better understand your body and its role in detoxification. Our bodies are equipped with the means to accommodate and eliminate many different types of toxins. These mechanisms, which are part of our normal body metabolism, demonstrate how very special our bodies are. It is only when they become overwhelmed that we must step in and help them with detoxification procedures.

CHAPTER 4

Responses to Toxins

ANY SUBSTANCE OR CONDITION that is harmful to the body can be considered a toxin. The response of the body to toxins depends on both the susceptibility of the person and the nature of the toxin. Responses to toxins vary widely from person to person, and the factors involved are discussed below. The nature of toxins also varies widely and, while the general variances are introduced in this chapter, specific toxins are discussed in detail in subsequent chapters.

Susceptibility to Toxins

People are not equally susceptible to the adverse effects of toxins. A person's susceptibility and response to toxins varies with age, gender, health status, genetic factors, enzyme metabolism, nutritional status, and lifestyle factors. These factors can cause a wide variation in responses to toxins.

Studies of lead poisoning dramatically demonstrate susceptibility differences and the effects of exposure patterns. An article in the May 1994 *Journal of Occupational Medi-*

cine by Janet L. Gittleman reported that lead levels in the children of parents who lived near and worked at a battery reclamation operation were higher than those of other children living in the same area. Another study in the July 1991 *Journal of Occupational Medicine* by Douglas G. Hodgkins found that seniority, corresponding to the length of the exposure, yielded the most significant air lead/blood lead association among lead acid battery workers. Lead levels in workers removed from exposure were dependent on the length of job tenure and renal function of the individual worker.

▪▪ AGE AND HEALTH STATUS

Although infants have detoxification enzymes at birth, their detoxification rate is slower than that of adults, causing them to be easily affected by toxins. Children and elderly people are more susceptible to toxins than healthy adults are.

People who have lowered immune defenses or impaired body defense mecha-

Genetic Factors
in Lead Poisoning

Genetic factors have been shown to affect the severity of lead poisoning. The December 1987 issue of Discover *magazine reported on fraternal 10-month-old twin girls from Washington, D.C. who had high lead levels in their blood, but exhibited completely different symptoms. One twin exhibited many symptoms of lead poisoning, including constipation, insomnia, crankiness, and failure to thrive, and the other, whose lead levels were the same, appeared to be healthy.*

nisms (such as the skin, the lungs, and the gastrointestinal tract) are particularly affected by toxins. Because the majority of detoxification takes place in the liver, people with liver disease will be easily affected by toxins.

❚❚ GENDER

Females are more sensitive to toxins than are males. They are generally smaller than men, and their lower weight causes them to become ill from chemicals more quickly. Women have more adipose (fatty) tissue and thus more fat cells in which fat-soluble toxins are deposited.

Women have lower levels of the enzyme alcohol dehydrogenase, and are less able to detoxify alcohol. Women have higher levels of estrogen and progesterone, which causes them to sensitize more easily, as some detoxification enzymes are particularly sensitive

to hormones. Hormonal changes during pregnancy also affect detoxification enzyme activity, increasing the ability to eliminate some drugs.

❚❚ GENETIC FACTORS

Genetically determined differences in susceptibility to toxins is called ecogenetics. Genetics determine which enzymes are available for the body's detoxification processes, and some people do not have enough specific detoxification enzymes.

Geneticists theorize that as people are exposed to more chemicals, more individuals with chemical susceptibility will be identified. More abnormal enzymes will be demonstrated. The current observed genetic variations probably represent only a small fraction of the diversity that will be identified.

❚❚ GENETIC ENZYMATIC DEFECTS

One or more of about 50 inherited enzymatic defects can determine a person's susceptibility to chemicals. For example, the enzyme alpha-1-antitrypsin continuously protects the lungs from the proteolytic enzymes released from white blood cells. People with an alpha-1-antitrypsin deficiency may be more sensitive to and suffer more adverse effects from air pollution than other people. People with a homozygous deficiency (a defect in two genes) are at increased risk to develop emphysema.

Enzymatic defects are rare and most have been identified from studying the metabolism of pharmaceutical drugs; they have not been studied in relation to environmental pollutants. The metabolism of some drugs has been found to be controlled by a single gene. Further investigation is expected to show that one gene can control the metabolism of many drugs.

ENZYME METABOLISM

The efficiency of detoxification enzymes directly affects the rate of detoxification. One of the enzymes that metabolizes drugs and chemicals is debrisoquine hydroxylase. It is controlled by a single gene, which has different forms (polymorphism). Individuals with slow rates of debrisoquine hydroxylation (poor metabolizers) are found more frequently in European populations than in Asian populations.

Parkinson's disease and lung cancer in smokers have been associated with the slow metabolism of chemicals by this enzyme. In several epidemiological studies, Parkinson's disease has been associated with pesticide use. Patients who cannot metabolize and rid their bodies of pesticides may be more susceptible to Parkinson's disease.

Another detoxification enzyme metabolizes S-carboxymethyl cysteine. Many people with food sensitivities are poor metabolizers of this chemical, but vitamin C supplementation has sometimes been found to increase the activity of this enzyme. This may partially explain why large doses of vitamin C are helpful for some allergy patients.

The slow metabolic action of another group of enzymes has caused peripheral neuritis (inflamed nerves in hands and feet) and increased risk of bladder cancer in some people. Many of these enzymes are part of the cytochrome P-450 family, which constitute a major detoxification system (see Phase I Detoxification in chapter 5).

■■ NUTRITIONAL STATUS

Nutrient levels determine which vitamins, minerals, amino acids, and fatty acids are available to the body. Many enzymes require a particular vitamin and/or mineral in order to function. If the nutrients are not present, the enzyme becomes paralyzed or inactive, and detoxification cannot take place, causing increased susceptibility to new toxins. Diet is very important for replenishing the needed nutrients.

■■ LIFESTYLE FACTORS

Susceptibility to toxins also depends on the total chemical burden of the body—the quantity of chemicals competing for detoxification. Lifestyle directly determines the total burden. People who eat a nutrient-deficient diet and food contaminated with additives, hormones, and preservatives will add to their toxic load. Drugs, including prescription drugs, smoking, and alcohol consumption also contribute to toxic burdens. Personal care, cleaning, and laundry products are toxic exposures for many people. Lack of exercise and a sedentary lifestyle further contribute to the problem, as exercise is necessary for the elimination of toxins.

People who are exposed to a myriad of toxins and who do not take steps to detoxify their bodies will become overloaded. Chemicals and toxins are stored in the fat, brain, and other lipid tissues, such as cell membranes. New chemicals entering the body cannot be metabolized because of the existing chemical overload. The backlogged chemicals can damage the detoxification system as well as the endocrine, nervous, and immune systems.

Nature of Toxins

Responses to toxins also vary with the nature of the toxin. Many toxins, particularly external toxins, are chemicals. There is more documented information regarding the effects of chemicals that are foreign to the body (xenobiotics) than for other toxins. The Environmental Protection Agency (EPA) estimates that approximately 500,000 chemicals are in use today, and each year more than 5,000 new chemicals are added. Our bodies are exposed to many of these chemicals daily.

The response of the body to chemicals can differ according to the structure of the chemical. Some responses to toxins are immunological in nature, while others are not. For example, many people develop asthma in response to plicatic acid found in cedar. This asthma is caused by an antigen-antibody response initiated by the immune system. The plicatic acid acts as an antigen, and the body produces antibodies in response. Other people experience an asthma attack when exposed to formaldehyde, but do not have an antigen-antibody response. Their response is caused by a different mechanism.

Many chemicals that the body absorbs tend to remain in the tissues for long periods of time. Most of these chemicals are lipophilic, which means they dissolve readily in fat, one of the main components of cell membranes. Lipophilic, or lipid-soluble, chemicals are complex and difficult for the body to break down and excrete, whereas water-soluble chemicals can be excreted unchanged or after undergoing simple metabolic changes. If a chemical is lipid-soluble and nonpolar (uncharged), it has to undergo two chemical steps or phases to become a polar (charged), water-soluble chemical. Specific enzymes are required for these conversions. (See chapter 5, Phases of Detoxification, for a detailed discussion.)

The exposure dose of the chemical and the length of the exposure can also affect the response of the body to a particular toxin. Large, overwhelming doses can be more toxic immediately than smaller doses over a long period of time. The efficiency of the detoxification mechanisms, individual tissue sensitivities to the chemical, and efficiency of the excretion systems of the body also affect the toxicity of a chemical.

The body processes or detoxifies substances produced by the body, such as hormones, vitamins, cholesterol, and fatty acids, in the same way that it detoxifies xenobiotics. Even though they are endproducts of metabolism and natural substances, they would become toxic (internal toxins) if allowed to build up. The same detoxification mechanisms that detoxify xenobiotics detoxify these internal toxins.

There are many toxins that are not chemicals, including weather, altitude, noise, radiation, geopathic stress, electromagnetic fields, emotional trauma, loss of spirituality and faith, and cumulative life experiences. These non-chemical toxins are removed from the body by various mechanisms, depending on the toxin. Some are removed by mechanisms within the body; others are cleansed by external processes and techniques. For example, techniques needed to detoxify mind and spirit toxins are very different from those necessary to remove chemical toxins.

Phases of Detoxification

THE DETOXIFICATION PROCESS in the body is composed of two phases, known as Phase I and Phase II. These phases are two different biochemical processes that enable the body to eliminate xenobiotics and other chemicals.

Phase I Detoxification

This phase of detoxification changes non-polar, nonwater-soluble chemicals into relatively polar (electrically charged) compounds with the help of enzymes that add a polar or reactive group. Phase I detoxification prepares the chemical so that a small molecule can be added or modified during Phase II, which will make the chemical water-soluble, allowing it to be excreted naturally by the body. The changes in Phase I constitute a type of chemical reaction known as biotransformation. Typical changes that occur to most chemicals include:

1. Oxidation reactions (electrons are lost)
   - *Dehalogenation:* Eliminates a halogen group (containing fluorine, chlorine, bromine, or iodine) and adds an oxygen group
   - *Desulfuration:* Eliminates a sulfur group
   - *Hydroxylation:* Adds a hydroxyl (oxygen and hydrogen) group
   - *Deamination:* Removes an amino group (nitrogen and hydrogen combined as NH_3)
   - *Sulfoxidation:* Adds an oxygen to a sulfur group
2. Reduction reactions (electrons are gained)
   - *Azo reduction:* splits a nitrogen-to-nitrogen (N_2) bond
   - *Reductive halogenation:* Replaces a halogen group with hydrogen
   - *Aromatic nitro reduction:* Converts nitrogen dioxide (NO_2) to an amide (NH_2)
   - *Aldehyde and ketone reduction:* Converts aldehydes and ketones (organic chemical compounds) to an alcohol

At least 50 enzymes in 10 families governed by 35 different genes allow Phase I to take place. The major enzymes required

Biotransformation

Because of the possibility of toxic compounds forming when there is an imbalance between Phase I and Phase II, it has been suggested that biotransformation is a more appropriate term than detoxification when describing Phase I and Phase II. However, we use the term detoxification because it is more frequently used in the literature describing the Phase I and Phase II reactions.

during Phase I are known as the cytochrome P-450 monooxygenase system and the mixed-function amine oxidase system. The primary system is the cytochrome P-450 monooxygenase system, which catalyzes and initiates the Phase I processes. The mixed-function amine oxidase system detoxifies chemical groups called amines, which contain nitrogen and hydrogen.

Many forms of cytochrome P-450 enzymes are involved in Phase I reactions. The highest concentration of cytochrome P-450 occurs in the liver, which is the most active site of metabolism. The lungs and the kidneys are secondary organs of biotransformation, with about one-third of the liver's detoxification capacity. Cytochrome P-450 has also been found in the intestines, adrenal cortex, testes, spleen, heart, muscles, brain, and skin.

The action of detoxification enzymes depends on the presence of various minerals. For example, alcohol dehydrogenase, an enzyme that converts alcohols (such as ethanol) to aldehydes in an oxidation reaction, depends on an adequate supply of zinc to function properly. In the next metabolic step, the enzyme aldehyde oxidase changes the aldehyde into an acid that can be excreted in the urine. Aldehyde oxidase depends on an adequate supply of molybdenum and iron. Other minerals that are required by enzymes include manganese, magnesium, sulfur, selenium, and copper.

Usually, the enzymatic reactions in Phase I decrease chemical toxicity. However, toxic or reactive chemicals can form during Phase I that are more toxic than the original compound. This is known as bioactivation. When Phase II detoxification proceeds normally, these chemicals are then rendered harmless and excreted. However, if there is an imbalance in the active levels of Phase I and II detoxification, these toxins will remain in the body. Imbalance between Phase I and Phase II is associated with increased symptoms of nervous, immune, and endocrine system toxicity.

Toxic chemicals produced during Phase I include teratogens (causing fetus malformation), mutagens (causing cell mutation), and carcinogens (causing cancer). For example, benzo[a]pyrene, a chemical found in coal tar and cigarette sidestream smoke, is biologically inert until it is converted by the mixed-function amine oxidase system into a metabolite that can then initiate cancer-causing activity. During Phase I, many compounds also form dangerous reactive free radicals—chemicals with an unpaired electron that can cause tissue damage. A buildup of free radicals can increase the risk of cancer. (See Free Radicals in chapter 20, Toxins Produced in the Body, for further discussion.)

The level of functioning of Phase I can be measured with a simple caffeine metabolism test. A known quantity of caffeine is ingested, and saliva samples are taken twice at specified intervals. The efficiency of caffeine clearance is directly related to the efficiency of Phase I detoxification. Rapid clearance of caffeine shows enzyme induction (increased production), either from xenobiotic exposure or toxins within the body. A slow rate of caffeine clearance indicates that cytochrome P-450 activity in the liver is abnormal. Patients with slow caffeine clearance have difficulty eliminating xenobiotics and other toxins.

Phase II Detoxification

In Phase II detoxification, chemical groups are added, or conjugated, to the chemical. The chemical becomes water-soluble and can be excreted through the kidneys, or, if the chemical is of high molecular weight, through the bile. If a xenobiotic already has a chemical group on the molecule that is suitable for a Phase II reaction, Phase I is not required. The xenobiotic is detoxified directly by Phase II conjugation.

Major conjugation reactions include:

- *Acetylation:* Acetyl Co-A (coenzyme A and acetic acid) is added to form a mercapturic acid conjugate; this is the chief detoxification/transformation pathway for amines and amides (organic compounds containing nitrogen). Needs B_5 to function. Can be adversely affected by pollutant overload and enzyme deficiency, either acquired or genetic.

- *Amino acid conjugation (acylation):* Peptide (compound formed by two amino acids linked by a special bond) conjugation using acyl Co-A (coenzyme A and carboxylic acid) and the amino acids taurine, glycine, glutamine, and to a lesser extent, arginine and ornithine. Glycine is the most commonly used amino acid. Glutamine is important in ammonia detoxification. This conjugation forms hippuric acid, which is excreted in the kidneys and can be measured.

- *Glucuronidation (gluconation):* Addition of a sugar group, using glucuronic acid; the major conjugation reaction for xenobiotics and internally produced chemicals converting them to water-soluble metabolites. Acts on certain pharmaceuticals; coal tar derivatives; dyes; phenols; excess vitamins D, E, and K; melatonin hormones; bile salts; bilirubin; steroid hormones; and estrogen.

- *Glutathione conjugation:* Reduced glutathione combines with xenobiotics to form less toxic compounds. Plays a major role in conjugating reactive metabolites formed during cytochrome P-450 biotransformation. Predominant defense against free radicals. Results in formation of mercapturic acid.

- *Methylation:* Addition of a methyl (CH_3) group, using the amino acid methionine to supply the methyl group. Detoxifies many synthetics and endogenous toxic compounds; the neurotransmitters epinephrine, norepinephrine, and serotonin; and

Metabolic Factors in Chronic Fatigue

In 1994 at the 29th annual meeting of the American Academy of Environmental Medicine, Dr. Jeffrey Bland, of HealthComm in Washington state, presented a study of patients with chronic fatigue. He measured the metabolic rates of 76 patients for Phase I and Phase II respectively, as fast/fast, slow/slow, or fast/slow. Dr. Bland found that 55 percent of patients were fast/fast metabolizers (normal), 30 percent were slow/slow metabolizers, and 15 percent were fast/slow metabolizers.

Patients with fast/slow metabolic rates are most at risk for problems, including a risk for cancer from a buildup of free radicals formed during Phase I detoxification. (See Free Radicals in chapter 20 for further discussion.)

nutrients. This reaction is B_6 dependent.

- *Sulfur conjugation (sulfation):* Includes several processes including sulfonation, which adds inorganic sulfate to hydroxyl groups for detoxification, and reduction of cyanides by adding sulfur. Is involved in detoxification of drugs, food additives, certain environmental pollutants, steroid and thyroid hormones, heavy metals, and monoamine neurotransmitters. Requires more energy than other conjugation reactions and will not take place when energy is low.

The function of Phase II can be evaluated through the ingestion of both acetaminophen and aspirin. This test measures the recovery of the products of glutathione conjugation, sulfur conjugation, glucuronidation, and glycine conjugation (acylation) in the urine. Comparison to normal values allows evaluation of the efficiency of Phase II. A high ratio between Phase I and any of the Phase II pathways implies imbalanced detoxification in the body.

Rates of Detoxification

The efficiency of Phase I and Phase II is adversely affected by deficiencies of vitamins, minerals, amino acids, and fatty acids. Inadequate protein intake specifically reduces Phase I clearance, and insufficient calories decreases overall detoxification function. In addition, these processes can be affected by foreign chemicals for which the body has no detoxifying mechanisms, poisoning of detoxification enzymes by heavy metals, toxic overload from overwhelming exposures, and a deficiency of detoxification enzymes due to genetic inheritance.

The detoxification process requires large amounts of caloric energy, which comes mainly from the food we eat. If we do not eat enough protein, the body breaks down vital tissue protein to produce the energy it needs. This decreases the available amounts of Phase I and Phase II enzymes, amino acids, and peptides, because the body breaks down protein to amino acids and peptides. The greater the toxic burden of the body, the higher the need for protein, carbohydrate, fat, and micronutrient intake.

Nutrients Required for Phase I Detoxification

VITAMINS	ACTION
Beta-carotene: yellow, red, and green vegetables	Converted in body to vitamin A, which helps to protect lipid portion of cell membrane. Promotes healthy intestinal mucosa necessary for absorption of other nutrients. Vitamin A is also necessary for conversion of alcohols to aldehydes. Deficiency decreases cytochrome P-450 activity.
Vitamin B_1 (thiamine): dairy, meats, legumes, whole grains, nuts	Thiamine pyrophosphate (the form of thiamine most easily utilized by the body) is necessary for moving an aldehyde group from one molecule to another. Also needed by the enzyme necessary for glutathione formation.
Vitamin C: fruits, green vegetables, tomatoes	Needed for cytochrome P-450 function and electron transport. Also increases antioxidant protection.
Vitamin E: vegetable oils, green leafy vegetables, milk, eggs, nuts, whole grains	Prevents formation of free radical form of vitamins A and K and fat-soluble hormones. Helps prevent an overactive cytochrome P-450 system, which can be a source of free radicals.

MINERALS	ACTION
Copper: meat, seafoods, nuts	Activates several enzymes. In superoxide dismutase (SOD) and other enzymes. SOD is the major antipollutant and detoxification enzyme.
Iron: beans, meats, dark green vegetables	Contained in cytochrome P-450.
Magnesium: nuts, legumes, dark green vegetables, beans	Needed for glutathione synthesis, ammonia detoxification, and production of the main source of energy for the body.
Manganese: leafy vegetables, whole grains, nuts, bananas, beans	In enzymes superoxide dismutase (SOD) and glutathione synthetase, and other enzymes. SOD is a major detoxification enzyme and glutathione synthetase is necessary for glutathione synthesis.

MINERALS	ACTION
Molybdenum: whole grains, legumes, seeds	In aldehyde oxidase, an enzyme that helps change aldehydes to acids, which are excreted in the urine.
Sulfur: garlic, eggs, onions, meats, beans	All glutathione enzymes contain sulfur. Glutathione is a free radical quencher and necessary compound for oxidation reduction reactions.
Zinc: shellfish, meats, dairy, pumpkin seeds, beans, spinach	In alcohol dehydrogenase, an enzyme that breaks down alcohols.

OTHER NUTRIENTS	ACTION
Alpha-ketoglutaric acid: supplement required	Helps detoxify ammonia. Addition of an ammonia group to this acid forms glutamic acid, which is transformed to glutamine, providing the major pathway for removing ammonia from the body.
Choline: whole grains, cheese, legumes, meats	Cytochrome P-450 enzymes are dependent on choline. Also combines with an acetyl group to help increase intestinal peristalsis (contraction during digestion), which aids in elimination of toxins.
Fatty acids: flaxseed, soybeans, fish oils	Speeds up transit time of the stool, averting buildup of toxins and reducing toxic load for the liver.
Lecithin: legumes, grains, eggs, fish	Allows for safe transport of fats through the bloodstream.
Methionine: meat, eggs, whole grains	Adds a methyl group to xenobiotics that aids in their excretion from the body; precursor for cysteine and other sulfur amino acids.
Oils: flaxseed, evening primrose, black currant seed	The body exchanges these oils for contaminated fat, which is eliminated through bile excretion and feces.
Silymarin: milk thistle	Helps detoxify the liver of alcohol and various pollutants. Has both protective and restorative effect on the liver. Prevents depletion of glutathione. Flavonoids in silymarin protect against oxidant stress.

Nutrients Required for Phase II Detoxification

VITAMINS	ACTION
Folic acid: dark green leafy vegetables, cabbage family, organ meats	Coenzyme form is an intermediate carrier for methylation conjugation.
Vitamin B_1 (thiamine): dairy, meats, legumes, whole grains, nuts	Needed for glutathione production. Provides energy for Phase II conjugation.
Vitamin B_2 (riboflavin): milk, meat, dark green leafy vegetables	Needed for the enzyme glutathione reductose.
Vitamin B_3 (niacin): meat, eggs, poultry, fish, whole grains	Needed for recycling glutathione, a Phase II conjugate.
Vitamin B_5 (pantothenic acid): nuts, meats, whole grains, green vegetables, potatoes	Bound to coenzyme A, a carrier of acetyl groups. Essential in acetylation conjugations of several classes of chemicals. Also important in deamination processes, which detoxify organic compounds containing nitrogen.
Vitamin B_6 (pyridoxine) : meats, vegetables, whole grains, green leafy vegetables, potatoes	Required for metabolism of methionine to glutathione. A deficiency of B_6 slows methylation conjugation.
Vitamin B_{12} (cobalamin): meat, dairy products, eggs, spirulina, chlorella	Coenzyme form participates in methylation reaction.
Vitamin C: fruits, green vegetables, tomatoes	Quenches free radicals produced by Phase I.

MINERALS	ACTION
Germanium: garlic, shiitake mushrooms, onions	Raises glutathione levels for Phase II detoxification, increases oxygen utilization at cell levels, and is a free radical scavenger. Helps with toxic metal detoxification.

MINERALS	ACTION
Magnesium: nuts, legumes, dark green vegetables, beans	Needed for glutathione production and activates many detoxification enzymes. The enzyme methyl transferase requires magnesium.
Manganese: leafy vegetables, whole grains, nuts, bananas, beans	Required for glutathione production, as well as by many different enzymes.
Molybdenum: whole grains, legumes, seeds	Helps in synthesis and use of sulfur amino acids, is a component of detoxification enzymes, and is necessary for utilization of vitamin C at cell level.
Selenium: brewer's yeast, garlic, liver, eggs	Is in the enzyme glutathione peroxide, necessary for detoxification.
Sulfur: garlic, eggs, onions, meats, beans, cheese, peanuts	Necessary for sulfur conjugation. Because of its high sulfur content, garlic is very helpful in removing heavy metals.
Zinc: shellfish, meats, dairy, pumpkin seeds	In enzymes necessary for conjugation.

OTHER NUTRIENTS	ACTION
Cysteine: eggs, meats, onion family	Detoxifies pesticides, plastics, hydrocarbons, and other chemicals.
D-glucarate: vegetables	Helps convert xenobiotics to water-soluble compounds.
Glycine: whole grains, meats, dairy	Stimulates production of glutathione. Also aids in detoxification of benzoic acid and phenol.
L-glutathione (reduced form): produced in the body from cysteine, glutamic acid, and glycine	Increases water solubility of xenobiotics, enabling excretion through urine.
N-acetyl-cysteine (precursor to glutathione): supplement required	Converted by the body to cysteine.
Taurine: meats, seafood	Needed for acylation reaction.

CHAPTER 6

Organs of Protection and Detoxification

Toxins can enter the body in three ways: by absorption through the skin; by inhalation through the respiratory tract into the lungs; or by ingestion through the mouth into the gastrointestinal tract. The skin, lungs, intestines, and kidneys have all developed some protective mechanisms and methods of detoxification, although the liver is the body's major organ of detoxification.

The Skin

The skin consists of two major layers. The outer layer, the epidermis, is made of four thin layers of epithelial cells. The inner layer, the dermis, is composed of connective tissue.

∎ THE EPIDERMIS

This outer layer of protective skin is approximately 1 millimeter thick and is composed of tightly packed cells. The top layer of the epidermis is pigmented and varies in thickness in different areas of the body, determining how easily chemicals can penetrate the skin and how rapidly they are absorbed. An exception is the palm of the hand, where this layer is thicker than in other areas of the body, yet absorbs chemicals more readily.

New skin cells form in the basal cell layer, replacing the entire epidermis approximately once a month. Melanocyte cells, which form part of the epidermis, produce melanin pigment. Melanin determines skin color, and also protects against ultraviolet injury, sunburn, and skin cancer. Melanin absorbs ultraviolet and visible light, and quenches free radicals.

Epidermal cells produce lipids and a protein called keratin. Lipids, which include cholesterol and free fatty acids, help protect the skin against water loss and cracking. With the aid of sunlight, the epidermis also produces vitamin D, an essential nutrient for maintaining calcium and phosphate levels in the body (needed for the growth and repair of bones).

∎ THE DERMIS

The thicker dermis lies under the epidermis and is composed of the proteins collagen and elastin. These proteins make the skin elastic and give it strength. Unlike the epidermis, it is well supplied with blood, lymph vessels, and nerves.

The dermis also contains the eccrine and apocrine sweat glands, sebaceous glands, and hair follicles. Eccrine sweat glands are distributed over the body's surface, helping to regulate its temperature. Apocrine sweat glands open into hair follicles and lose cells as they release secretions. Sebaceous glands are located near hair follicles. They secrete sebum, a lipid mixture that has some antibacterial and antifungal properties. Sebum also helps the body excrete lipid-soluble toxins, but only in small amounts.

■ HOW TOXINS ENTER THE SKIN

Toxins vary in their ability to enter the skin, and several factors affect their absorption. To be absorbed, a toxin must also be somewhat water-soluble. Toxins that are only lipid-soluble or only water-soluble are poorly absorbed. Oily solutions usually penetrate the skin easily, as it readily absorbs lipids. When the skin is wet, water-soluble chemicals penetrate more easily. At higher environmental temperatures, the skin is more absorbent. In addition, chemicals penetrate cracked or injured skin more easily than intact skin. Some toxins are absorbed directly through hair follicles in the skin.

Solvents can easily penetrate the skin because of their lipid (fat) solubility. Caustic chemicals, such as acids and alkaline solutions, can also penetrate the skin. Once a chemical has penetrated the epidermis, it moves into the dermis. The rich blood supply of the dermis readily transports the chemical into the bloodstream.

■ PROTECTIVE DEVICES

The normal microbial flora of the skin is a major barrier to infection, as is the sebum. Although sebum helps to prevent the invasion of substances from the external environment, such as bacteria, it cannot block the absorption of toxins through the skin. The epidermal cells are also capable of producing a variety of lipids that afford protection similar to that of sebum, but cannot stop toxins. Hair on the skin can be protective if it prevents a toxic substance from reaching the skin.

Some people use physical barriers in an attempt to protect against toxic skin exposures. Barrier creams are one method, although they cannot usually block toxin absorption. Rubber gloves may be useful, but some chemicals and microorganisms can penetrate the gloves. Thin plastic gloves prevent toxins from contacting the skin. However, if a chemical gets inside the glove, it will actually be absorbed more readily.

■ DETOXIFICATION

Because it contains the enzyme cytochrome P-450, the skin can metabolize drugs, steroid hormones, and some xenobiotics. It converts these chemicals into more water-soluble forms, which can then be excreted from the body. Small amounts of toxins are eliminated in the sweat excreted from the pores and through the sebaceous glands of the skin.

The Lungs

The lungs are part of the respiratory tract. The upper air passage of the respiratory tract consists of the nose, the pharynx, the hypopharynx, and the larynx, which houses the vocal cords. The lower air passage stretches from the vocal cords through the trachea and into the lungs.

As we breathe, air enters the upper passage, then traverses the trachea. This area is the narrowest cross-section of the entire airway. The trachea branches into the right and left mainstem bronchi, or bronchial tubes, behind the ribcage. One bronchi enters each lung. The bronchi then divide into two to three more branches, called bronchioles. The bronchioles lead to air sacs called alveolar sacs or alveoli. Their total surface area is estimated to be 70 square meters.

Oxygen is extracted from the air we breathe into the lungs and supplied to millions of alveoli, which pass oxygen molecules into the capillaries. Oxygen then combines with hemoglobin in the red blood cells and is carried to the rest of the body.

Exhaling diffuses carbon dioxide molecules from the capillaries into the alveoli and expels them from the body through the bronchi, trachea, and upper air passage.

Three diseases affect the bronchial tube system: asthma, bronchitis, and emphysema. Asthma is characterized by attacks of breathing difficulty. Bronchitis is an inflammation of the bronchial tubes. Toxins can trigger both asthma and bronchitis, which are reversible in their early stages. The toxins in cigarette smoke can cause both chronic bronchitis and emphysema. Emphysema destroys lung elasticity by damaging the walls separating the alveoli from one another, creating tiny craters. Other alveoli become permanently enlarged. Emphysema is irreversible.

■■ HOW TOXINS ENTER THE LUNGS

The lungs have the greatest exposure of any organ to the environment. The air we breathe contains microorganisms, chemicals, dust, and pollution. Small solid particles and liquid aerosols can easily enter the lungs and be deposited in three ways: impaction, sedimentation, and diffusion. Gases are absorbed directly through the cells lining the respiratory tract.

■ IMPACTION

In impaction, large particles continue in straight paths through the airway passages. Most larger particles land on the surface of the nose and throat area (nasopharynx) or at the branching of the bronchi. These particles become embedded in mucus or trapped by nasal hairs and are eliminated by sneezing, swallowing, or blowing the nose. The nasopharynx removes 95 percent of particles 5 microns or larger.

■ SEDIMENTATION

Medium-sized particles, 1 micron (the size of a cell) to 5 microns in diameter, are deposited in the lungs by sedimentation. Most of these land in the mucus layer of the bronchioles, and are eventually either moved up in the mucus and exhaled, or swallowed. If the particles do reach the alveoli, they can become trapped permanently and may damage the lungs.

■ DIFFUSION

The smallest aerosol particles, less than 0.1 micron in diameter, are deposited in the lungs by diffusion. Many of these particles are exhaled immediately, but those that become trapped can eventually cause lung disease, known as pneumoconiosis. Two types of pneumoconiosis are asbestosis, caused by asbestos fibers, and silicosis, caused by silica dust.

∎ ABSORPTION

Gases are absorbed differently in the respiratory tract, depending on their solubility and flow rate, and the duration of exposure. Most absorption of gases takes place in the upper air passages. Some gases dissolve in the fluid that lines the epithelium (the cell layer lining the respiratory tract).

The nose absorbs gases more readily when air flow is increased, which may account for increased absorption by physically active people. The gas may also alter the lining fluid, so that the rate of absorption is increased.

∎∎ PROTECTIVE DEVICES

The lungs protect themselves against environmental pollutants with filters, epithelial barriers, enzyme systems, and immune responses. Filters include mucus and cilia.

Mucus is produced by glands located beneath the epithelium. Certain cells contain cilia, which are hairlike projections that beat in a synchronized fashion at about a thousand times per minute. Together, mucus traps particles and cilia help to move them out of the lungs. A person can then sneeze and cough out the irritants. However, cilia cannot transport particles if there is insufficient mucus. Influenza virus can paralyze the cilia, leading to secondary bacterial infections. Some people have a condition known as immotile cilia syndrome, which means

their cilia do not move, and they are prone to sinus and respiratory tract infections.

Epithelial barriers consist of special cells in the epithelium. Alveolar macrophages, a type of white cell, ingest particles, and kill bacteria and viruses, which they then present to lymphocytes. The lymphocytes, another type of white cell, destroy them. Alveolar macrophages also contain aryl hydrocarbon hydroxylase, a type of enzyme that detoxifies chemicals.

In addition, an enzyme system helps to protect the lungs. When particles are inhaled, inflammatory enzymes, known as proteases, are released. These proteases can damage the lung cells or the connective tissue in the lungs. Specific proteins known as antiproteases protect the alveoli by combining with proteases to inactivate them. Cigarette smoke destroys the balance between proteases and antiproteases, increasing the activity of the proteases. The most common antiprotease is alpha-1-anti-trypsin. People with a deficiency of this antiprotease are more prone to emphysema.

∎∎ DETOXIFICATION

The lungs contain enzymes from the mixed-function oxidase family, enabling them to metabolize drugs and xenobiotics to more water-soluble chemicals, which can then be excreted by the kidneys.

The lungs also have antioxidant enzymes to counteract free radicals, including superoxide dismutase, glutathione enzymes, and catalase. In addition, alveolar lining fluid, containing transferrin, ceruloplasmin, and glutathione, protects the lungs from oxidant stress. Vitamin E, an antioxidant found in cell membranes, protects the lungs against toxic lipid peroxides produced by the cell membranes of the lungs when attacked by organisms. In patients who smoke cigarettes, the fluid lining the alveloi can be deficient in vitamin E.

Finally, the lungs have immune responses to protect them against inhaled organisms. Lymphocytes in the lungs produce immunoglobulins (antibodies), while other immunoglobulins cross from the blood into the lungs. Immunoglobulins IgA, IgG, and IgE have all been found in the respiratory tract. IgA neutralizes many viruses, and it seems to prevent antigen absorption across the lung cells. T-lymphocytes (white blood cells that help fight infection) help protect the lungs against microbes and tumor cells. T-lymphocytes also release lymphokines, which are molecules that activate and stimulate macrophages (white blood cells that ingest foreign material).

The Gastrointestinal Tract

The gastrointestinal (GI) tract includes the mouth, pharynx, esophagus, stomach, small intestine, large intestine, and rectum. The other portion of the gastrointestinal system is made up of glandular organs that secrete substances into the gastrointestinal tract. These glands include the salivary glands, liver, gallbladder, and pancreas. The function of the gastrointestinal system is to process the food we eat into a form that the circulatory system can distribute to the cells of the body.

The GI tract is a tube that runs through the body from the mouth to the anus. In adults, this tube is approximately 15 feet long. The contents of the lumen, which is the interior of this tube, are technically outside the body. For example, millions of bacteria populate the large intestine. Most of them are beneficial, but if these bacteria should leave the intestine and enter the body, they are harmful and can even be lethal.

Food is taken into the mouth where it is mixed with saliva, which moistens and lubricates the food particles so they may be swallowed easily. The saliva contains an enzyme called amylase that aids in digesting carbohydrates.

The pharynx and esophagus serve as a pathway to deliver the food from the mouth to the stomach. The movement of these two parts of the gastrointestinal tract controls the process of swallowing.

The stomach mixes the food with hydrochloric acid, pepsin, gastrin, and mucus. The pepsin processes protein, and gastrin stimulates the release of hydrochloric acid. These materials break the food down into even smaller particles, and the resulting mixture is known as chyme. In addition to breaking down the particles of food, the hydrochloric acid also kills almost all the bacteria that enter the body with the food. Some do survive and subsequently begin to live and multiply in the large intestine. The stomach also stores food while it is being partially digested. It then delivers fluid and partially digested food to the small intestine in amounts that allow for maximum digestion and absorption.

The last stages of digestion and absorption take place in the small intestine, which is the longest portion of the digestive tract.

GI Tract

The gastrointestinal tract is an important route for the absorption of toxins. In our lifetime the GI tract processes over 25 tons of food, representing the largest load of antigens and xeno- biotics confronting us. The mucosal surface of the stomach and intes- tines is 200 times that of the body surface area, making it very susceptible to toxic exposures.

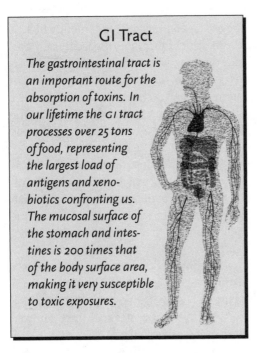

Enzymes from the pancreas break down chyme into monosaccharides, fatty acids, and amino acids. These substances then cross the layer of epithelial cells that line the intestinal wall and enter the blood and lymph, the watery fluid in the lymph vessels.

A small volume of water, minerals, and undigested material passes into the large in- testine. This material is temporarily stored and acted upon by the intestinal bacteria. The large intestine concentrates the mate- rial by removing water. The concentrated material is then eliminated from the body through defecation when the rectum be- comes distended. The eliminated material is called feces and consists of a small amount of food that was not digested or absorbed, toxins, cast-off cells, and bacteria, which contribute to the bulk of the feces.

❙❙ HOW TOXINS ENTER THE GI TRACT

Toxins arrive in the stomach after being in- gested in food or water, or being breathed in through the nose or mouth and swallowed. The absorption of toxins in the stomach de- pends on the amount ingested, as well as the degree of lipid or water solubility, degree of ionization, molecular size, and pH of the toxin. Digestive enzymes, hydrochloric acid, and bile acids also affect the absorption and metabolism of toxins.

The intestines are exposed to bacteria; viruses; yeasts and parasites; food and plant ingredients; and toxins in food, water, and the environment. Foreign chemicals may also be absorbed into the body from the small and large intestines. To be absorbed, chemicals must be made soluble before they come into contact with the intestinal mu- cosa. Unabsorbed chemicals reach their highest concentration in the colon (large in- testine).

Chemicals are usually absorbed slowly from the GI tract, but the amount absorbed depends on how rapidly the chemicals move through it. The faster a chemical passes through, the less is absorbed. The degree of intestinal absorption is also affected by gas- tric emptying time, intestinal motility, the size and condition of the surface area of the small intestine, blood flow to the intestine, diet, genetic factors, and age.

❙❙ PROTECTIVE DEVICES

The GI tract has various defense mecha- nisms against bacteria, viruses, yeasts, para- sites, and chemical toxins. It is protected by enzymes, mucus, normal intestinal bacte-

46

ria, intestinal secretions, and the innermost layer of epithelial cells.

In the intestines, the first barrier to the absorption of chemicals is the unstirred water layer. This layer of immobile fluid coats the intestinal mucosa (mucous membrane). It has a mucus layer and an acid microlayer that is rich in protons (particles with a positive charge). It acts as a barrier to the chemical penetration of the mucosa. Nonpolar, lipid-soluble chemicals diffuse through the unstirred water layer more slowly than they would penetrate a cell membrane. Pesticides, dyes, and food additives are examples of nonpolar chemicals.

The second barrier is gastrointestinal mucus, which protects the intestinal mucosa from physical and chemical injury, and acts as a lubricant. Cells in the esophagus, stomach, small intestine, and large intestine all produce mucus. Mucus consists of 95 percent water, with the remainder made up of salts, proteins, nucleic acids, and mucins. Mucins, composed of carbohydrates, lipids, and proteins, give mucus its viscous, gel-like texture. Mucus is sticky and can trap large molecules, such as metallic chemicals. It can also trap parasites and bacteria, and can bind viruses, helping to eliminate them in the feces.

The third barrier to absorption of chemicals is the small intestine's acid microclimate layer, consisting mostly of protons. This layer has a 5.9 pH, which is acidic compared to the 7.3 pH of the lumen of the small intestine, which is mildly alkaline. The acid microclimate layer may influence the permeability of weak acids and alkalis, by repelling acids and neutralizing alkalis.

The fourth barrier is the concentration of bacteria in the large intestine or colon. More than 400 species of bacteria reside in the colon. Intestinal bacteria metabolize drugs and other chemicals. However, bacteria may metabolize chemicals in a manner completely opposite to the body's metabolism, restoring a xenobiotic to its original form, allowing it to reenter circulation and again become part of the toxic load.

Another defense mechanism is the rapid shedding of intestinal cells. They are some of the most actively dividing cells in the body, with up to 100 cells per hour formed in the intestines, and billions of cells shed every day. Metals and lipid-soluble chemicals may be excreted from the intestines along with the old cells.

■ DETOXIFICATION

Both Phase I and Phase II detoxification systems are found in the GI tract, which is the second major site of detoxification in the body. Phase I changes the chemicals so that Phase II can add a small molecule (see chapter 5, Phases of Detoxification). The GI tract contains the same biotransformation enzymes as the liver, but metabolism in the GI tract is slower than in the liver. Depending on the composition of the toxin, the GI tract can transform a xenobiotic to either a less toxic chemical or a more toxic chemical.

In the stomach, pepsin and hydrochloric acid can help break down chemicals and toxins. The intestines contain bile acids and various enzymes, such as proteases, lipases, and glucuronidases, which can also break down chemicals and toxins.

The mixed-function amine oxidase sys-

The Liver

The liver is essential to sustain life, with more functions than any other gland. Its many functions include:

- metabolism of fats, proteins, and carbohydrates
- metabolism of hormones, endogenous wastes, and foreign chemicals
- synthesis of blood proteins
- formation of bile and lymph
- production of prothrombin and other blood-clotting factors
- formation of urea and ketones
- assimilation and storage of fat-soluble vitamins
- storage of glycogen, which can be released and converted to glucose for energy
- storage of carbohydrates, vitamins, and minerals
- excretion of bilirubin, a breakdown product of hemoglobin
- phagocytization (ingestion) of microorganisms and other foreign material

tem is most active in the duodenum, the first part of the small intestine. Mature enterocytes, the cells lining the intestine, contain the largest amount of cytochrome P-450 activity. The activity of these Phase I enzymes decreases from the duodenum to the colon.

Many factors affect the ability of the intestines to metabolize xenobiotics. For example, when people go on starvation or semi-starvation diets, the activity of many of the metabolic enzymes decreases. Iron deficiency and selenium deficiency can reduce cytochrome P-450 activity. Cruciferous plants (cabbage, cauliflower, broccoli) increase the activity of the mixed-function amine oxidase system. Chemicals can decrease or increase enzyme activity, depending on the type of chemical. Enzyme activity in a portion of the small intestine called the jejunum has been found to be lower in females than in males. The very young and the very old also seem to have less active detoxification enzymes.

The gut itself can act as an organ of excretion for toxins. Cells lining the intestinal walls can secrete xenobiotics into the intestines. Strong acids and digitalis compounds are secreted from the bloodstream into the intestinal lumen, where they are then excreted in the feces.

The Liver

The liver is a dome-shaped gland that fits under the diaphragm, just under the right ribcage. It is considered a gland because it secretes bile, and it is the largest gland in the body.

The liver is divided into two major regions, the right and left lobes. The right lobe, which has three smaller lobes, is larger than the left, which has two smaller lobes. Each of the five lobes is composed of compartments called liver lobules.

The central vein passes through the center of each lobule and drains away waste products from the liver. The cells of the lob-

48

ule closest to the central vein are known as centrilobular hepatocytes (liver cells). Cytochrome P-450 is most highly concentrated in these cells, and detoxification activity is also highest in this area.

On the other side of the liver, the hepatic artery and portal vein are known as the periportal system. The hepatic artery supplies oxygen to the liver directly from the heart and lungs. The cells of the lobule closest to the hepatic artery have the highest concentration of oxygen in the liver. They also have the highest concentration of nutrients because the liver is the first organ to receive nutrients absorbed by the GI tract, delivered by the portal vein. These cells also have the highest exposure to xenobiotics in the liver, as well as higher concentrations of glutathione and transaminase enzymes. The levels of these enzymes are tested in the standard blood chemistry test for liver function.

∎∎ HOW TOXINS ENTER THE LIVER

The liver is situated to receive a majority of the venous blood from the lower body, the kidneys, the spleen, and the gastrointestinal tract. Approximately 1500 ml of blood, containing many different toxins, flows through the liver every minute.

The liver is the main organ for biotransformation of chemicals. However, it is susceptible to tissue injury from the toxic effects of chemicals, and if it becomes overloaded, can be permanently damaged. Some chemicals are toxic to specific parts of the liver.

∎∎ PROTECTIVE DEVICES

Adequate levels of the conjugation enzymes needed for Phase II are protective for the liver. They help prevent the buildup of toxic substances formed as a result of biotransformation during Phase I of detoxification. The presence of adequate antioxidants to quench free radicals is also protective for the liver.

Even when 80 percent of the cells of the liver are damaged, the liver can continue to function, but with reduced efficiency. It has the ability to restore and replace these damaged cells, and can recover if the sources of the toxins are removed.

∎∎ DETOXIFICATION

The bulk of toxic substances are detoxified in the liver. The liver removes chemicals that have been absorbed into the blood, and excretes them into the bile stored in the gallbladder. Both Phase I and Phase II detoxification processes are active in the cells of the liver, and the liver's cytochrome P-450 system is the body's first-line site for the detoxification of foreign chemicals (see chapter 5, Phases of Detoxification).

Over 300 known chemicals can induce (increase) enzyme system activity in the liver. These chemicals can lead to more enzymes being present and a faster rate of detoxification. They also increase the amount of endoplasmic reticulum (membranes in the cell where detoxification occurs) in the liver.

While some chemicals increase the liver's metabolic action, others inhibit the activity of cytochrome P-450 and other detoxification enzymes. Chemicals can cause inhibition in several ways:
- competition between two or more compounds for the same detoxifying enzymes
- inhibition of enzyme synthesis

- inactivation or destruction of enzymes or the endoplasmic reticulum
- overwhelming of the detoxification enzyme systems
- depletion of necessary cofactors for Phase II

Inhibition of cytochrome P-450 can lead to the buildup of toxins in the body. For example, theophylline is a drug used to control asthma and belongs to the same family as caffeine. It can build up to toxic levels if the patient is given erythromycin simultaneously, which inhibits the cytochrome P-450 enzyme system from breaking down the theophylline. Erythromycin and antifungals such as ketoconazole can also inhibit the breakdown of Seldane, an antihistamine. Because the resulting high levels of Seldane can cause heart rhythm disturbances, it has been taken off the market.

The Kidneys

The principal excretory organs in all vertebrates, the kidneys lie in the back of the abdominal wall, one on each side of the backbone. They are bean-shaped, and on the concave side of each one is an area called the hilus, where the renal (kidney) artery enters and the renal vein exits. The adrenal glands sit on top of the kidneys. The kidneys are also regulatory organs, helping to maintain homeostasis (physiological balance between all body organs).

Each of the kidneys consists of the outer cortex and the inner medulla. The cortex receives 85 percent of the total renal blood flow and is composed of nephrons, which are excretory units. Each kidney has over one million nephrons. Each nephron has three parts:

- the vascular or blood circulation component, composed of interconnected capillaries;
- the glomerulus, the filtering tissues of the kidney; and
- the tubules, small tubes or ducts that reabsorb 98 to 99 percent of the salts and water filtered by the glomerulus, for the body's use. The last tubule, the collecting duct, concentrates the remainder of the fluid as urine.

The nephron's tubular element joins the ureter, which exits from the same side of the kidney as the renal vein and artery. The ureter carries the urine to the bladder, a balloon-shaped storage chamber. As urine enters the bladder, its walls of smooth muscle unfold to the volume needed to contain the urine. When the bladder becomes distended, receptors are stimulated to contract the bladder. The urine then flows under voluntary control through the urethra, and out of the body.

Kidneys filter out cellular waste, metabolic waste (mostly breakdown products of protein metabolism), drugs, and toxins from the blood. In addition to filtering the blood and draining wastes, the kidneys eliminate foreign chemicals from the body, and regulate the body's pH balance, calcium metabolism, electrolyte balance, fluid balance, and extracellular volume (circulating fluid outside the cells). The kidneys produce a hormone that stimulates red blood cell production, helps to regulate blood pressure, and also plays a role in vitamin D metabolism.

■■ HOW TOXINS ENTER THE KIDNEYS

The kidneys have an even higher blood flow than the brain, liver, or heart, and receive 25 percent of the body's total blood volume, causing high exposure to chemicals carried in the blood. They reabsorb and redistribute about 99 percent of the blood volume received, and 0.1 percent of the blood filtered becomes urine.

■■ PROTECTIVE DEVICES

An adequate supply of Phase II enzymes is protective for the kidney, as is the intake of adequate fluids. Kidney stones, which can damage the kidneys, can form when there is too little fluid. Accurate pH control of the urine is also protective, as kidney stones tend to form when urine pH is not optimum.

Kidney disease can be quite advanced before it is detected, as the kidneys can lose 80 percent of their function before symptoms appear.

■■ DETOXIFICATION

The kidneys excrete chemicals that have been prepared by Phase II detoxification in other parts of the body. Phase II converts lipid-soluble nonpolar substances into more polar substances. This makes them less fat-soluble and less likely to be reabsorbed by the kidney tubules. They are then available for excretion in the urine.

Some chemicals (for example, ammonia) are secreted by the tubules and move into fluid in the lumen (interior) of the tubule, where they are then eliminated from the body in the urine. Tubule cells are also capable of catabolizing (breaking down) certain organic compounds, which destroys them even though they are not excreted in the urine.

CHAPTER 7

Minor Routes of
Detoxification and Excretion

IN THE PREVIOUS CHAPTER, we have considered the major detoxification pathways of the body. However, there are other methods that the body uses to cleanse and balance itself. Minor routes of detoxification and excretion include:

• hair
• fingernails and toenails
• sweat
• tears
• breast milk

Hair

Furred animals can excrete a large amount of xenobiotics into their hair, which serves as an excretory tissue for essential, nonessential, and potentially toxic elements. These elements are irreversibly incorporated into growing hair, and the amount is proportional to the level of the element in other body tissues. Because of this, hair can be used to estimate the extent of toxic exposures.

In some instances hair is more revealing than blood, because blood tests reveal the concentrations outside the cell and waste material being discarded, rather than the concentrations being stored in the body. The hair serves as a recorded history of what is stored in the body, and contains 200 times the trace elements that the blood does. Blood is an indicator of recent exposures, while hair is indicative of chronic, long-term exposures. Hair grows at a rate of about one-half inch a month, so that a person whose hair is five inches long has an exposure record of approximately 10 months.

▮▮ HAIR ANALYSIS

Toxins in the body, as well as nutritional status, can be determined by hair analysis. Hair elements analysis is an assay of the mineral composition of the hair, and can show physiological excess, deficiency, or maldistribution of elements in the body. Hair levels of potentially toxic elements such as arsenic, cadmium, mercury, and lead correlate highly with symptoms and pathology. (See chapter 16, Chemicals and Metals, for a discussion of heavy metal toxicity.) For these el-

The Death of Napoleon

Forensic medicine makes use of hair analysis to determine toxic exposures. A very famous case involved Napoleon Bonaparte. Over 140 years after his death, hair analysis performed on locks of his hair indicate that Napoleon died of arsenic poisoning.

It was the emperor's habit to bestow locks of his hair as gifts, and in addition, hair was shaved from his head just after his death. A number of these hair samples were analyzed, showing peaks and valleys of arsenic concentration, consistent with arsenic poisoning over a period of time. At the time of his death, his hair contained 13 times the normal amount of arsenic.

Investigators suspect that the arsenic was systematically given him in the wine provided by his caretakers. Napoleon had his own private stock of wine, and people to whom he gave this wine as a gift became ill with symptoms similar to those he was experiencing.

ements, hair levels are better indicators of body stores than levels in blood and urine. However, because head hair is affected by external elements such as shampoo, hair coloring, and permanents, hair exposures must be investigated and the test results interpreted accordingly. Some hair treatments can cause low readings of toxins present in the body.

Most hair analyses test for the toxic elements of aluminum, antimony, arsenic, beryllium, bismuth, cadmium, lead, mercury, nickel, platinum, silver, thallium, thorium, tin, titanium, and uranium. In addition, they test for essential elements and other elements important in nutrition, including barium, boron, calcium, chromium, cobalt, copper, germanium, iodine, iron, lithium, magnesium, manganese, molybdenum, phosphorus, potassium, rubidium, selenium, sodium, strontium, sulfur, vanadium, zinc, and zirconium.

Drugs and prescribed medications are also excreted in the hair. Although it is still in the developmental stages, hair analysis can be used to determine the ingestion and amount of illicit drugs. Reliable hair testing procedures will show minute traces of cocaine, marijuana, heroin, and LSD.

Fingernails and Toenails

Substances taken into the body, both toxic and nontoxic, are deposited in the cells of the nails and become part of the nail. Fingernails and toenails are formed from heavily cornified epidermal layers. The hardness and flexibility of nails are related to the keratin (a protein in hair and nails) content and its orientation pattern, as well as its water content. The high sulfur content of keratin contributes to their hardness. The pink coloration of nails is caused by the capillary network beneath them that is visible through the cornified cells.

The analysis of nails by several different methods can determine nail content, as well

Chemicals in Sweat

Some people complain that their sweat makes their skin hurt or gives them a rash. This is caused by the chemicals they are excreting in their sweat. The analysis of sweat from patients in detoxification units has shown the presence of xenobiotics to which the person had been exposed. Patients undergoing detoxification in sauna programs report smelling and tasting chemicals to which they have previously been exposed.

Some patients in detoxification programs even complain of ill effects from chemicals in the sweat of other patients with them in the sauna room.

Towels used while in the sauna, as well as towels used for showers following sauna time, will have distinctive odors from the chemicals and must be laundered or disposed of promptly.

as identifying depositions in the nails. Forensic testing sometimes involves testing nails for the presence of poisonous elements, such as arsenic. Sometimes depositions are evident on visual inspection of the nail. In some cases only the fingernails are involved; in others, the toenails are also affected. Toxins that affect the nails include:

- *Antimalarials:* pigmentation ranging from yellows to blacks in both fingernails and toenails
- *Arsenic:* in acute poisoning, transverse white striations of the nails; with single broad bands that contain arsenic; in chronic arsenic poisoning, longitudinal dark bands
- *Chlorpromazine* (a tranquilizer): tan or slate blue to deep blue-black or purple on exposed areas of skin, with nail bed involved in severe cases
- *Doxycycline:* brown discoloration and separation of the nail from the nail bed
- *Fluorine:* longitudinal striations, pitting, and mottled appearance of nails of both fingers and toes

- *Gold:* dark brown discoloration of nails, which become soft and fragile with longitudinal streaks
- *PCBs* (polychlorinated biphenyls): nail deformity and black discoloration of the nail bed
- *Silver:* blue-gray discoloration of fingernails; toenails are usually not involved
- *Tetracycline:* yellow pigmentation of nails
- *Thallium:* longitudinal dark bands in the nails

The deposition of chemicals in the nails can be useful when treating some nail disorders, including fungal infections. For example, one medication, griseofulvin, is deposited in the keratin precursor cells. It binds tightly to new keratin, which then becomes resistant to fungal invasions.

Sweat

Our bodies sweat when we get hot in an effort to maintain normal body temperature. Sweat content is almost identical to that of urine, and includes water, lactic acid, and uric acid. Because of this, the skin, which is a major organ of the body, is sometimes referred to as the third kidney. As much as 30 percent of body wastes can be eliminated through sweat.

Xenobiotics and heavy metals are excreted in the sweat when the body is heated. Raising body temperature causes these chemicals to be released from fat cells into the bloodstream. Blood vessels in the skin dilate to allow more blood to flow to the surface, which activates the sweat glands. The sweat glands pour water onto the skin's surface, and as it evaporates, it releases both heat and toxins from the body. Dilating the blood vessels and increasing blood flow increases the nutrient supply to the skin, as well as allowing toxins deep in the body to be carried to the surface and excreted. In addition, the heat inhibits the replication of pathogenic bacteria and viruses, increases oxygen intake and heart rate, and stimulates blood and lymph flow, all of which assist in cleansing the body.

Tears

Tears are another minor route of excretion for the body. They are formed in the lacrimal gland, located above the eye in a depression of the orbital bone. The tears flow over the eyes and into the inferior lacrimal duct, two small tubes in the corner of the eye. They then spill into the nasolacrimal duct, a tube leading into the nose, causing the nose to run when a person cries. If these ducts are overtaxed, tears run down the cheeks. Tears moisten the eyes, wash away irritants, and protect the eyes from infection.

Dr. William Frey of the Dry Eye and Tear Research Center in Minneapolis believes that the chemicals built up during emotional stress are removed from the body in tears, playing a role in the ability to tolerate stress. He has found that the lacrimal gland concentrates and removes manganese, with the level of manganese in tears 30 times higher than in blood serum. He has also found that emotional tears have a different chemical content than irritant tears. Emotional tears, shed in response to emotional stress, contain 24 percent more protein than irritant tears.

Both emotional and irritant tears contain three chemicals known to be released by the body during stress. These are adrenocorticotropic hormone (ACTH), the most reliable indicator of stress; leucine-enkephalin, an endorphin that probably modulates pain sensation; and prolactin, a hormone that regulates milk production in mammals. Prolactin also promotes tear production, which may explain why women cry more easily than men do. Adult women have serum prolactin levels nearly 60 percent higher than those of men; but before puberty, boys and girls have similar prolactin levels and similar crying frequencies.

Breast Milk

Even breast milk, both for humans and other mammals, is a minor route of detoxification and excretion. Toxic substances are excreted in breast milk, just as they are in the sweat and tears. Human breast milk contains 3 to 5 percent fat, and lipid-soluble chemicals can be excreted in this fat. During lactation, stores of body fat release their stored toxins into the bloodstream, where they make their way into the breast milk. Women who have

Pregnancy and Detoxification

Women planning to become pregnant should prepare for pregnancy, particularly those who intend to nurse their babies. They should avoid toxic exposures and, if possible, undergo detoxification procedures before pregnancy. Detoxification baths, a diet of whole foods unadulterated by additives, nutritional supplements, and regular

exercise are excellent preparation measures. (See also Pregnancy Preperation chart in Part VIII.)

Women who are pregnant should under no circumstances undergo detoxification procedures while pregnant, but try to live and eat as cleanly as they can.

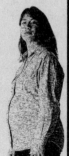

more stored toxins are believed to release more toxins into their breast milk.

Polychlorinated biphenyls (PCBs) and the pesticide DDT have been found in breast milk, as well as toxic metals such as lead. The U.S. Environmental Protection Agency states that the average American breastfed baby ingests nine times the permissible level of dieldrin, a cancer-causing pesticide, and ten times the maximum allowable level of PCBs. PCBs have been found to cause birth defects and cancer in animals.

Cow's milk also contains toxins excreted by the cow. Any chemicals to which a cow is exposed, such as herbicides and pesticides, as well as fertilizers and any chemical treatment of its foods, can be reflected in the milk. Cow's milk containing the same amount of DDT as is frequently found in breast milk would be banned by the Food and Drug Administration. In addition to DDT, cow's milk has been found to be contaminated with pesticides such as dieldrin, heptachlor epoxide (a metabolite of a pesticide), and lindane. Infant formula that is prepared from cow's milk can contain these toxins.

In spite of the possible toxins that can be in breast milk, breastfeeding is still preferable to bottle-feeding. Breast milk contains the nutrients a baby needs in the right proportions, including the amino acids necessary for development of the brain and nervous system. It forms a smaller curd in the baby's stomach and is easier to digest than the cow's milk protein in infant formulas. Breastfed babies are less likely to become ill with diarrhea and gastrointestinal infections. Breastfeeding also decreases the possibility of autoimmune disease, leukemia, sudden infant death syndrome, ear infections, immune system disorders, and respiratory disease. If a breastfed baby does develop a respiratory infection, it is likely to be less severe.

Breastfeeding also offers long-term benefits. It appears to slow the development of celiac disease (a digestive disorder) and to offer protection from Crohn's disease and ulcerative colitis in adulthood. Individuals who were breastfed are less likely to develop insulin-dependent diabetes, lymphoma (malignant tumors of the lymph tissue), and food allergies.

How We Are
Exposed to Toxins

THERE IS NO PLACE in our lives where we do not encounter toxins. This includes our home, workplace or school, leisure, and traveling. In addition, we often encounter toxins when we seek medical treatment. On the surface, these exposure possibilities make living safely sound like an unobtainable, impossible goal. However, the opposite is true. It is being aware of the possibility of toxic exposures that enables us to live cleanly and safely. Unless we are aware of where and what the toxins in our lives might be, we cannot avoid them.

Part III is a very comprehensive section, so that people from all walks of life and in a broad range of situations can learn about their exposures. Detailed information is necessary in order to make this book useful to as many people as possible. It is not an attempt to frighten or overwhelm people, but an effort to help them learn to live safely and to actively pursue a healthy lifestyle. Avoiding toxic exposures helps to keep your toxic burden low, and reduces your need for detoxification procedures.

Because children have different physiology, problems, and needs than adults, they have been given their own chapter. The information will help parents to understand and accommodate their special needs.

CHAPTER 8

Toxins in the Home

THIS CHAPTER WILL HELP you become more aware of the toxin levels in your home. Our homes do not have to be toxic, as many measures can be taken both to prevent and lessen these exposures. Ways to create and maintain a healthy home are discussed in Part VII, Prevention Methods.

We spend at least one-third of our day at home. Our homes can be nontoxic, safe havens but, unless we have taken special precautions, our homes can also be a serious source of toxic exposure. Some homes are more toxic than others. A home is unhealthy if:

- more than one person in the same house has similar symptoms.
- people who spend the most time at home have the most severe symptoms.
- visitors complain of symptoms after they have been in the home.
- symptoms improve or disappear when people leave the home for hours or days.
- symptoms get worse when the house is closed up for the winter.
- symptoms begin after moving into a new

house, after remodeling an old house, or after adding new furnishings.

Common Sources of Home Toxins

▌▌ CHEMICALS AND MINERALS
▌ ASBESTOS
Asbestos may be found in wall and ceiling insulation in homes built before the 1950s. Until the early 1970s it was used for insulating hot-water pipes, steam pipes, furnaces and boilers, and on ceilings and walls. Asbestos was also used in wallboard and spackling compound in houses built before 1977. Resilient floor tiles and older refrigerators, dishwashers, ovens, and toasters may contain asbestos.

Intact asbestos is not a problem unless it starts to crumble or is disturbed. When airborne, asbestos particles can be inhaled or ingested, causing lung cancer or damage to the lungs, and cancer of the gastrointestinal tract.

▌ FORMALDEHYDE
At normal room temperature formaldehyde is a colorless, pungent gas that can irritate

MOST EFFECTIVE DETOXIFICATION METHODS

**Chemical Exposures
in the Home Environment**

- Detox baths or sauna program (chapter **22**)
- Antioxidant nutrients (**23**)
- Fasting or juicing (**24**)
- Exercise (**25**)
- Oxygen therapy (**26**)
- Allergy extracts or hands-on allergy treatment for the specific chemicals (**27**)
- Homeopathic remedies, such as *Sulfuricum acidum* for pollution and *Ignatia* for perfume (**28**)
- Bach Rescue Remedy (**28**)
- Herbal remedies such as elderberry, ginger, milk thistle (**29**)
- Charcoal packs and oral charcoal (**30**)
- Organ cleansing (**31**)

the eyes, nose, and respiratory tract. Formalin, a 37 to 50 percent formaldehyde solution stabilized with methanol, is the major form in which formaldehyde is marketed. It has many industrial uses, particularly in manufacturing. As a result, it is a major indoor pollutant because it is contained in many of the manufactured products found in our homes.

Formaldehyde is found in wooden building materials such as paneling, plywood, chipboard, and particleboard; dry, bare, pressed-wood products made with urea formaldehyde resins; and wet, prepasted wallpaper. Paints, shellacs, waxes, glues, and adhesives are sources of formaldehyde exposures. Formaldehyde is also found in molded plastics, disinfectants, pesticides, newsprint, paper grocery bags, carpets, draperies, and photography darkroom chemicals.

Formaldehyde is even found in personal care products. Cosmetics, nail polish, and nail polish remover are a significant formaldehyde exposure. When wet, fingernail hardeners and nail polishes emit more formaldehyde per unit measure of surface area than particleboard. Unwashed permanent-press fabrics in clothing are also high emitters of formaldehyde. Washing permanent-press fabrics once reduces formaldehyde emissions by over half.

Flooring can represent a serious source of formaldehyde exposure. Manufacturers are now making attempts to reduce the toxicity of carpeting and have either stopped using or significantly reduced the amount of formaldehyde used in the manufacturing process. Researchers from Batelle Memorial Laboratories in Columbus, Ohio, found that urethane-coated wooden floors do not release formaldehyde. However, when wet, the acid-cured resin floor finishes that are frequently used over large areas release up to 1,000 times more formaldehyde than bare formaldehyde-resin wood products such as particleboard and composite woods. The formaldehyde emitted as these floors dry can saturate other surfaces and objects in the room, causing formaldehyde to be released from them long after the floors are dry.

During the 1970s, urea-formaldehyde foam insulation was pumped into walls. Many people subsequently developed burning of the eye, nose, and throat, and skin rashes. Hundreds of families had to leave

Tobacco Smoke

Tobacco smoke is very rich in polonium-210, which gives off radon. Burning only one cigarette can increase the radon decay product levels in a room by 25 percent. Radon decay products can exist at high levels for as long as nine hours after the cigarette is burned. Particulate matter from the smoke can prolong the presence of radon decay products in the air.

their homes. Because of these problems, this insulation is not used in homes today.

Formaldehyde can also cause coughing, runny nose, fatigue, nausea, and nosebleeds. Between 10 and 20 percent of the population is highly sensitive to formaldehyde. Monitors to test formaldehyde levels are available. (See Sources.)

❚ VOLATILE ORGANIC CHEMICALS

Volatile organic chemicals (vocs), alternately called volatile organic compounds, are chemicals that contain carbon and hydrogen. They have a high vapor pressure and are capable of evaporation from a solid or liquid into the air. The indoor level of vocs is two to five times that of the outdoor level. Volatile organic chemicals are found in lacquers, adhesives, waxes, cleaning agents, cosmetics, paint and paint removers, inks, disinfectants, antiseptics, perfumes, mouthwashes, air fresheners, aerosol sprays, permanent-press fabrics, polyesters, synthetic fibers, drapes, pesticides, and plastics.

Tetrachloroethylene, the voc used to dry-clean clothes, has been shown to cause cancer in laboratory animals. Wearing recently dry-cleaned clothes and storing dry-cleaned clothes in closets creates a major exposure to this compound. Tetrachloroethylene can cause headaches, sleepiness, nausea and vomiting, irritation of the eyes, rashes, heart arrhythmias, and numbness.

Paradichlorobenzene is found in many homes, in moth repellent cakes or crystals, toilet disinfectants, and deodorizers. Potential symptoms of overexposure to this voc include eye irritation, swelling around the eyes, profuse rhinitis, anorexia, nausea, vomiting, weight loss, jaundice, and cirrhosis.

VOCs cause eye irritations, headaches, nausea, respiratory symptoms, fatigue, and mood swings. The reproductive system can also be affected, depending on the voc. Low birth weight, birth defects, and sterility are among the reproductive problems caused by vocs. Very little research has been done regarding the effects of chronic low-level exposure to vocs. (See chapter 16, Chemicals and Metals, for information on specific vocs.)

❚ RADON

Radon is an indoor air pollutant that comes from the outdoors. It is a radioactive gas that has no odor, taste, or smell. It can enter houses through cracks in the foundation, through utility service lines as they enter the house, in drinking water, or from building materials with a high radium concentration, such as stones and concrete. (For more information on radon see chapter 14, Water and Air.)

Radon decays to radioactive products that are suspected causes of lung cancer. The

Carbon Monoxide Poisoning

Carbon monoxide is the leading cause of accidental poisoning death in America. According to the Journal of the American Medical Association (JAMA), 1,500 people die annually from accidental carbon monoxide exposure, and an additional 10,000 seek medical attention. The exact number of carbon monoxide incidents is difficult to assess because the symptoms of carbon monoxide poisoning mimic many other common health problems.

U.S. Environmental Protection Agency suggests that a radon level greater than 4 picocuries per liter is unsafe. Kits are available to measure radon levels in a home.

■ CARBON MONOXIDE

Carbon monoxide is generated from the incomplete process of combustion of fuel—natural gas, oil, coal, wood, and kerosene. When combustion takes place in a home, outdoor air should replace the indoor air that is being used in the combustion process. If it cannot, negative pressure builds up and backdrafting occurs as the exhaust gases are drawn back into the house. Backdrafting results when wood stoves, fireplaces, and furnaces burn in houses that are too tightly sealed.

Poorly operating gas stoves, grills, and furnaces produce even more carbon monoxide. However, complete combustion is impossible even in properly adjusted gas furnaces, and there is always some carbon monoxide present in combustion gases.

Kerosene space heaters also produce high amounts of carbon monoxide, even when they are working properly. Carbon monoxide can also enter the house from vent connections in poorly maintained or blocked chimneys. Attached garages in which car engines are run can be another source of carbon monoxide.

Low levels of carbon monoxide poisoning result in symptoms commonly mistaken for common flu and cold symptoms, including shortness of breath on mild exertion, mild headaches, and nausea. Concentrations that might cause headaches in adults (50 parts per million) can kill an infant. Moderate levels of poisoning cause dizziness, mental confusion, severe headaches, nausea, and fainting on mild exertion. At high levels, unconsciousness and death may result.

■ NITROGEN DIOXIDE

Nitrogen dioxide is produced when gas or kerosene stoves burn. The concentration of nitrogen dioxide is two to three times higher in homes with gas cooking stoves than in those with electric ranges. Even the pilot light in gas stoves emits nitrogen dioxide. Tobacco smoking indoors also contributes to nitrogen dioxide levels.

This toxin causes skin, eye, and mucous membrane irritation. It can affect any area of the lung, and can attach to hemoglobin and interfere with its ability to carry oxygen. Nitrogen dioxide also causes impaired defenses against infection, increases airway sensitivity, and oxidizes and injures airway tissues. Children living in homes with gas stoves have higher rates of respiratory infections.

◼◼ HEATING SYSTEMS

All types of home heating systems can be sources of toxins. Gas stoves and furnaces are a common method of heating, and the combustion products and toxic chemicals emitted by these systems are discussed above. All gas appliances, including furnaces, hot water heaters, and gas clothes dryers, should be vented to the outside, and the vent pipe should be as straight as possible. Unvented gas stoves are a fire hazard, in addition to emitting combustion products into the house.

Some people heat with kerosene space heaters. Even a properly adjusted kerosene heater is a fire hazard, and these heaters produce large amounts of carbon monoxide, carbon dioxide, sulfur dioxide, and nitrogen dioxide. Sulfur dioxide can cause bronchospasms. The effects of carbon monoxide and nitrogen dioxide are discussed above. According to Dr. Dean Sheppard of the University of California, San Francisco, School of Medicine, people with asthma should never have a kerosene heater in their homes.

Many people heat with wood, in either fireplaces or wood-burning stoves. Wood contains aliphatic and aromatic hydrocarbons, terpenes, aliphatic and aromatic acids, alcohols, phenols, aldehydes, ketones, esters, ethers, and small amounts of minerals. Burning wood emits ethanol and formaldehyde, as well as the combustion products of its chemicals. These combustion products are estimated to include 17 priority pollutants (chemicals that the Environmental Protection Agency has deemed toxic), 6 that are harmful to the respiratory system, and 4 co-carcinogenic compounds (capable of causing cancer in combination with other toxins). Benzo[a]pyrene is a particulate carcinogen in woodsmoke combustion. In addition, wood ash is radioactive, with many ashes exceeding 100 picocuries per kilogram, the standard for nuclear waste.

Fireplaces produce greater amounts of particulate matter than a closed wood stove, due to their open combustion chambers. All wood-burning stoves made before 1987 and all fireplaces are much more toxic than the new EPA-certified pellet and wood stoves. The new stoves produce 1.5 to 6 grams of particulate matter per hour compared to 40 grams per hour for an old potbellied stove. A stove produces more particulates during the first 20 minutes it burns, until it becomes hotter. Newer stoves with catalytic converters to complete the combustion of flue gases are 70 percent more efficient and reduce soot emission by 84 percent.

A wood stove that is too large for the area being heated will have to be dampered down, creating smoke and decreasing efficiency. When there is the smell of smoke, it means that the stove is not installed properly, the house is too airtight, the wood is not dry, or the stove needs maintenance. It may also mean there is a problem with the chimney.

An improperly burning stove can create creosote buildup from combustible ingredients in the flue gases that were not burned in the fire. Creosote condenses on the inside of stovepipe and chimney walls. Because it is combustible, a buildup of creosote can cause chimney fires.

Pellet stoves are becoming more popular and have the advantage of less ash. However, pellets are more expensive than wood. Most pellets sold now are made of wood, usually pine or a pine and oak combination. In the past, pellets were more toxic because experimental materials were used, including pecan hulls, sunflower seeds, and sometimes trash in addition to binders. These pellets did not work well, contaminated the house, and caused many problems for people, including allergic reactions. Today pellets are made without binders, using sawdust and water. Pellets are formed and then compressed and cured at high temperatures. Pellet stoves emit the same toxins as wood stoves, and their efficiency depends on their construction.

Scrap lumber should never be burned in a fireplace or woodstove because of the chemicals used to treat and preserve the lumber, sometimes including arsenic. Some people burn tightly rolled newspapers, but these release formaldehyde, bleaching agents from the paper, and toxic chemicals from the ink.

■■ RENOVATIONS AND FURNISHINGS

Building a new home or remodeling can involve major toxic exposures unless the building supplies are selected with care. Paneling, plywood, particleboard, and chipboard can be sources of phenolics and formaldehyde. Glues and fillers used with these boards emit volatile organic chemicals (vocs). Joint compound and texturing compounds also contain formaldehyde. (See Formaldehyde, above.)

Paints, stains, varnishes, shellacs, and paint thinners can be problematic because they contain solvents and emit vocs. In addi-

tion, fungicides, pesticides, and mildewcides, which outgas for long periods of time, are added to most paints. Paint removers, both chemical and heat gun removers, are toxic. The chemical removers give off toxic chemicals both from the remover, which contains mineral solvents, and the paint. Heat guns volatilize chemicals in the paint that are then inhaled by people in the house.

Insulation contains fiberglass, which is a particulate hazard, as well as emitting formaldehyde, biocides, and fungicides. Flexible vinyl flooring contains plasticizers that outgas. Grouts and thinset used to install tile contain preservatives that can outgas. Caulking compounds outgas vocs.

Adding new furnishings to our homes can be a source of toxins. Plywood and particleboard that are frequently found in furniture, including sofas, cabinets, tables, and particularly bookcases, outgas formaldehyde, as well as vocs because of the stains and varnishes used.

Many people are sensitive to Scotchgard™ and other spot-preventing chemicals that are frequently applied to upholstered furniture and carpets. Upholstery fabrics may also contain formaldehyde, plasticizers, dye residues, and fungicides. Drapes, bedspreads, and linens must be selected with care to minimize the introduction of more chemicals into the home. Some of these items contain dye residues that can be toxic. Because formaldehyde is used to set dyes and in the manufacture of some fabrics, these items can be significant sources of formaldehyde. Laundering these products before use can significantly lessen exposures.

Toxins in Carpets

While everyone living in a home with a toxic carpet can be affected, crawling babies and toddlers who are in close proximity to the carpet because of their size will absorb a higher level of chemicals. Studies have shown that the amount of lead measured in dust and carpet is an excellent predictor of a toddler's blood level of lead.

◾ CARPETING

Unless they are carefully manufactured and installed, carpets can be a major source of toxins in the home. New carpets can contain more than two dozen chemicals designed to kill bacteria, mold, and insects, as well as to resist stains, bind fibers, and hold colors. Carpeting is often glued down, which can cause problems because the glues are also toxic.

Both when they are new and as they deteriorate, carpets outgas chemicals, including formaldehyde, acetone, benzene, styrene, toluene, and xylene. Even when less toxic carpeting made from natural fibers such as cotton and wool is chosen, it can be a reservoir for chemicals that are tracked in, as well as a haven for mold, household dust, and dust mites. Chemicals tracked in can include pesticides, lead, heavy metals, and polycyclic aromatic hydrocarbons (PAHS), which are aromatic compounds composed of two or more fused benzene rings. (See chapter 16, Chemicals and Metals, for more information on PAHS.)

Having carpets shampooed can increase chemical exposures, particularly while the carpets are wet. Not only can the carpet shampoo or cleaning chemicals cause problems, but the chemicals that outgas from the carpet while it is wet are toxic to some people. With some carpets, formaldehyde emission increases dramatically until the carpet dries. In recent years, manufacturers have made efforts to make carpets less toxic, and there are some safer brands that are now available.

◾◾ HOUSEHOLD SUPPLIES

◾ CLEANING AND LAUNDRY SUPPLIES

Cleaning supplies such as soaps, bathroom cleaners, dishwasher detergents, oven cleaners, drain cleaners, window and glass cleaners, waxes, furniture oils, and metal polishes add to the chemical load found in the home. The cabinets under kitchen and bathroom sinks are frequently "chemical cesspools" because of the cleaning items stored there. Room deodorizers and sprays further add to the chemical load. During their cleaning cycles, fumes from self-cleaning and continuous cleaning ovens increase the chemical load.

Laundry supplies are an important source of chemical exposures in the home. People can be sensitive to any laundry detergent. In addition, laundry detergent frequently contains a scent, which permeates the home as well as remaining on the clothes. Stain and spot removers frequently contain solvents in addition to enzymes and surfactants. These removers can cause irritation of the skin, eyes, and nose.

65

Bleaches are a problem for chlorine-sensitive people and can cause eye and lung irritation, in addition to headache and cerebral symptoms.

Liquid fabric softeners and dryer sheets, both scented and unscented, contain an amazing array of toxic materials that cause health risks from the dryer exhaust, as well as the treated fabrics. These chemicals include:

- carcinogenic chemicals such as benzyl acetate, chloroform, and limonene
- narcotics or chemicals such as alpha-terpineol, benzyl alcohol, camphor, ethyl acetate, linalool, and pentane, which cause central nervous system disorders

■ PERSONAL CARE PRODUCTS

Personal care products and beauty supplies contribute to the chemical levels in a home. Bottles of perfume, cologne, and aftershaves slowly outgas, even from tightly closed bottles. Soaps, shampoos, and deodorants contain numerous chemicals, and frequently contain scents that outgas into the room or cabinet where they are stored.

Most deodorants and antiperspirants contain some type of alcohol. Side effects from using deodorants and antiperspirants can include stinging, burning, itching, cysts, and enlarged sweat and lymph glands.

Makeup constitutes another toxic exposure in the home. Foundations contain oils and pigments, and usually have alcohol, humectants, and preservatives. Rashes or itching on the face, arms, and chest, swollen eyes, and skin swelling and eruptions often result from allergy to foundation. All rouge, whether cake or cream, contains pigments, and may contain perfume, in addition to nu-

Household Hazards

Many items commonly stored inside the house are toxic. Stored paints, paint thinners, shellacs, turpentines, aerosol sprays, charcoal, and lighter fluid all contribute to the level of chemicals in the home.

merous other ingredients. Eye irritation and fungal contamination have been reported from the use of rouge. The powder applied at the end of the makeup process contains pigments, clays, rice or cornstarch, perfume, and many other chemicals, including a type of alcohol. Powders can cause difficulty in breathing for some people.

Lipsticks, even hypoallergenic versions, can cause problems. All lipsticks have various waxes and oils, dyes, pigments, and frequently perfumes. Lipsticks can cause burns, peeling or cracked lips, excessive dryness, rashes, and swollen gums.

Eye shadow contains mineral oils, beeswax, petrolatum, and pigments. Eye irritation is common, and eye shadows are easily contaminated by bacteria. Mascara contains insoluble pigments, carnauba wax, paraffin, perfume, and other ingredients. Tiny fibers of rayon or nylon can make lashes look thicker. Allergic reactions and infections from mascara contaminated by bacteria are common problems.

Hair care products contain many chemicals. At one time castille, coconut, and glycerine soaps were used to wash hair. Shampoos, which are relatively new, are available in different forms. Liquid shampoos contain many chemicals in addition to perfumes. Eye and scalp irritation, hair loss, split hair, shortness of breath, and swelling of the hands, face, and arms can result from shampoo use.

Hair conditioners contain humectants, substances that bring moisture into the hair and reduce brittleness. Cream rinses leave a film on the hair to make it feel soft and look shiny. They may contain lanolin, alcohols, sterols, glyceryl monosterate, spermaceti, glycerine, mineral oil, water, and perfume. Except for individual allergies, these substances are relatively nontoxic.

Hair sprays used by both men and women contain polyvinylpyrrolidone (PVP) dissolved in glycerine with perfume, lanolin, and other chemicals. They can cause headaches, dizziness, hair loss, rash, lung damage, and throat irritation. The popular hair mousses, which are available both as gels and spritzers, contain many different potentially allergenic substances, including alcohols and fragrance. The side effects of these products are much the same as those for hair sprays.

Home permanents contain two solutions, one that curls the hair, and one that neutralizes or stops the acids that curl the hair. Home permanents affect the person receiving the permanent, as well as other members within "smelling distance." These permanents can cause hair damage; swelling of the legs and feet; eye irritation;

rashes of the scalp, neck, forehead, and ears; and swelling of the eyelids.

Hair colorings may be either temporary or permanent. Temporary hair coloring is a rinse that covers the outer layer of the hair only and does not affect the natural color inside the hair shaft. Ear numbness and headaches, in addition to hair turning the wrong color, have been reported with rinses.

Permanent hair coloring products change the color of the hair itself and cannot be shampooed away like the rinses. There are three classes of permanent hair coloring—natural organics, synthetic dyes, and metallics. The natural organics contain henna or chamomile, and rarely cause side effects. The synthetic dyes frequently depend on peroxide to liberate oxygen and activate the dye. These preparations contain the dye itself, the oxidizer, hair conditioners, color modifiers, antioxidants, stabilizers, and other compounds to treat the hair. Women seldom use metallics, which contain copper, because they interfere with permanent waves. However, men frequently use them to darken their hair color, as each use increases the color intensity. Side effects from hair coloring can include scalp irritation, hair breakage, contact dermatitis, hair loss, itching, and swelling of the face.

❚❚ PARTICLES AND INHALANTS
❚ PARTICULATE MATTER
Particulate matter, small enough to be inhaled into the lungs, can be produced by cigarette smoke, gas stoves, wood stoves, fireplaces, kerosene space heaters, and furnaces. Cooking and burning candles and incense can contribute to particulate matter in

Microorganisms in the Home

- Antioxidant nutrients, beneficial bacteria (chapter **23**)
- Healthy high-quality diet (**24**)
- Inhalant and topical oxygen therapy (**26**)
- Allergy extracts or hands-on treatment for specific microorganisms (**27**)
- Homeopathic remedies such as *Gelsemium, Camphora, Cantharis* (**28**)
- Herbal remedies such as alfalfa, black walnut, pau d'arco, garlic, goldenrod (**29**)
- Compresses, packs, and poultices, charcoal therapy (**30**)
- Organ cleansing (**31**)

homes, but tobacco smoke is the highest source of respirable particles indoors. Microorganisms, particularly mold and dust, also contribute to particulate matter. These particles do not simply float through the air, but are stirred up in clouds as people move about, or during vacuuming and dusting.

Particulate matter can cause eye and mucous membrane irritation. At higher levels, it causes lung disease. Particulate matter can also interact with other chemicals to increase the toxicity of both.

■ MOLDS, MICROORGANISMS, DUST, AND PETS

Molds and mildews thrive in wet areas, such as bathrooms, humidifiers, refrigerator drip pans, central air-conditioning systems, the pads of evaporative coolers, heating ducts, ice machines, and any area where there is a water leak. When people breathe, they release moisture into the air, which contributes to mold growth. Moisture is also re-leased from washing machines and dishwashers. Houseplants can contain mold on the plant and in the soil. Watering the plants causes mold spores to be released into the air. Stored magazines and books can be another source of mold.

Two respiratory diseases caused by mold are humidifier fever and hypersensitivity pneumonitis. Mold can also trigger symptoms in people who have asthma, as well as in people who are mold sensitive. Mold symptoms include wet cough, chronic sinusitis, headaches, eustachian tube dysfunction, nasal obstruction, pharyngitis, laryngitis, and a cloudy nasal discharge. Mold can also cause cerebral symptoms, such as depression.

Pollens, dust, and dust mites are common home toxins. These agents can enter on people and pets or can be airborne. Many people have allergic or asthmatic reactions to pollens, dust, and dust mites, as well as to cockroach feces and cockroach parts. Bacteria, viruses, and fungi enter the home in the same way, and these organisms can cause

Household Dust

We are always surrounded by dust, no matter how diligently we clean, and we breathe it continually. An average six-room house accumulates 40 pounds of dust in a year. Dust is formed as materials that make up household articles, furniture, and clothing deteriorate, and as dirt enters from outside. House dust could be considered an occupational hazard for the homemaker.

infection. (For more information on these problems, see chapter 14, Water and Air, and chapter 15, Plants and Organisms.)

Pets increase toxins in the home in several ways. All animals with fur and feathers shed dander—small scales that are the equivalent of human dandruff. This dander is airborne and is allergenic to many people, as is animal saliva. Symptoms of dander sensitivity include itching of the nose; red, watery eyes; itching of the roof of the mouth; and clear nasal discharge.

Many people use flea collars on their dogs and cats in addition to bathing them with flea shampoos and dusting them with flea powder. The collars, powders, and shampoos contain chemicals that are toxic to both humans and animals.

Hamster, gerbil, and guinea pig dander is allergenic, but their bedding (usually cedar chips) is also allergenic to many people because of its terpene content. When animal wastes are excreted in the bedding, the combination can be very toxic. Birds shed feathers to which many people are allergic, and volatile chemicals from their excretions enter the air. In addition, bird feces contain allergens that can cause allergic rhinitis and asthma.

∎∎ WORKSHOPS AND YARDS

Home workshops can add significantly to home exposures. Woodworking shops contribute vocs from paints, stains, varnishes, and shellacs. Sawing and sanding the wood releases terpenes. Mechanical repairs in workshops add solvents, oils, lubricants, and greases to the environment. Many home workshops also add significantly to noise

---

MOST EFFECTIVE DETOXIFICATION METHODS

Pollen, Mold, Dust, Dust Mite, and Animal Dander in the Home

- The nutrients vitamin C, quercetin, and coenzyme Q_{10} (chapter **23**)
- Avoid foods containing mold (**24**)
- Inhalation of oxygen and hydrogen peroxide nose spray (**26**)
- Allergy extracts or hands-on treatment for pollen, mold, dust and dust mite, and animal dander (**27**)
- Homeopathic remedies such as *Dulcamara* for cat allergy and *Blatta orientalis* for allergy to molds and mildew, for dust, mold, and animal dander (**28**)
- Herbal remedies such as eyebright, nettle (**29**)
- Organ cleansing (**31**)

---

pollution when machinery of various types is used, such as power tools, air compressors, and generators. (For further discussion of woodworking, see chapter 10, Toxins from Art and Leisure Activities and Travel.)

The yards around our homes become toxic if lawn chemicals, fertilizers, weed killers, or pesticides are applied to the lawn, trees, or flowerbeds. About 50 percent of American families use yard and garden weed killers. (See Gardening in chapter 10 for more information on toxic exposures.)

Molds grow in soil and are also present on many plants. Massive soil movement from construction, plowing, gardening, and lawn care causes the release of mold spores that can trigger symptoms in a mold-sensitive person. (See chapter 15, Plants and Organisms, for more information.)

CHAPTER 9

Toxins in the Workplace and School

WHEN WE ARE NOT AT HOME, most of us are either at work or at school. The time spent each day at work or school is usually around eight hours. Some people may exceed that time if they are working overtime, or if they return to school for study in the library or other activities.

Exposure to toxins is unfortunately inevitable in the workplace and at school. These toxins come in many forms and the degree to which they affect health can vary widely. Some buildings are more contaminated than others. The identification, evaluation, and control of problem exposures is vital. This chapter will help you become aware of your possible exposures so that you can take steps to eliminate or lessen them. Methods for doing so are discussed in Part VII, Prevention Methods.

Occupational Exposures

The National Institute of Occupational Safety and Health (NIOSH) has developed a list of the ten leading work-related illnesses and injuries. The list includes lung disease, caused by silica dust, asbestos, cotton fibers, and coal dust; occupational cancer; cardiovascular diseases; reproduction and neurotoxic disorders (brain and spinal cord problems); noise-induced hearing loss; skin diseases; and psychological disorders.

Many occupational diseases are caused by exposure to toxic substances. The long-term effects of many of these chemicals are unknown. Scientists have investigated only the acute effects of chemicals; very few chronic studies have been done. At least 80 percent of commercial chemicals have never been tested for toxicity. The synergism (interaction) of chemicals with each other is also not known.

The possibilities of toxic occupational exposures are many and varied, depending on the occupation. It is impossible to create a comprehensive list; however, the following chart contains some of the more common occupations and their associated exposures.

Effects of Occupational Exposures

OCCUPATION	EXPOSURE	EFFECTS
AGRICULTURE		
Agricultural workers and produce handlers	Various plants, including celery, parsnips, citrus fruits	Skin disorders, contact dermatitis, phototoxic skin reactions
	Microorganisms such as bacteria, fungi, protozoa, and viruses	Infectious diseases such as anthrax, rabies, tularemia, hantavirus
	Pesticides, herbicides, fertilizers	Cardiovascular disease; rapid heartbeat, high or low blood pressure, and abnormal heart rhythms; neurological problems
	Sun	Sunburn, skin cancer, heat exhaustion
Mushroom workers	Mold spores	Chronic and acute lung disease; hypersensitivity, pneumonitis with cough, shortness of breath, fever, and acute chills; chronic symptoms of fatigue and weight loss
ANIMALS AND ANIMAL HUSBANDRY		
Veterinarians, hunters, zoo attendants, trappers, animal handlers, ranchers, slaughterhouse employees	Microorganisms such as bacteria, fungi, protozoa, and viruses	Infectious diseases such as anthrax, rabies, tularemia, hantavirus
	Animal dander	Asthma, allergies
AUTOMOTIVE/MECHANICAL		
Mechanics, service station attendants	Solvents, cutting oils, acids, gasoline, detergents	Skin disorders, contact dermatitis, chemical burns, nervous system disorders
	Carbon monoxide	Cardiovascular disease, neurological problems
Tire builders, tire repairers, workers who wear protective rubber clothing	Rubber accelerators	Skin disorders, contact dermatitis

OCCUPATION	EXPOSURE	EFFECTS
CONSTRUCTION		
Building contractors, construction workers, electricians	Formaldehyde, terpenes, solvents, paints, plastics, stains, various glues and adhesives	Skin disorders and rashes; occupational asthma; irritation of ears, nose, and throat; headache; cerebral symptoms; neurological symptoms
	Fiberglass insulation	Skin and lung irritation
Asbestos repair and removal	Asbestos fibers	Lung disease, asbestosis, cancer of lung or GI tract
Construction blasting	Organic nitrates	Cardiovascular disease, angina, heart attack
Lumber industry	Pentachlorphenol (preservative for timber; used as insecticide, herbicide, and defoliant)	Kidney disease
Roofers and road builders	Tars, oils, creosote, liver-toxic solvents	Cerebral symptoms, rashes, liver disease
	Polycyclic aromatic hydro-carbons (PAHS)	Skin rashes, headaches, sweating, vomiting, cancer
Painters	Solvents and propellents	Cardiovascular disease, abnormal heart rhythms or fainting, sudden death
	Liver-toxic solvents	Liver disease
	Organic solvents	Reproductive toxicology, increased risk of congenital malformations in offspring
	Epoxy resins	Skin disorder, contact dermatitis
	Paints, spackling compounds	Neurological problems
HEALTHCARE		
Dentists, dental hygienists	Anesthetic gases	Cerebral symptoms, allergic reactions
	Mercury	Mercury poisoning, renal failure, skin rashes
	X-ray radiation	Skin rashes
	Latex gloves	Anaphylaxis
	Contagious patients	Infectious diseases

OCCUPATION	EXPOSURE	EFFECTS
Healthcare and laboratory workers	Blood, body fluids, soiled linens, contagious patients, puncture wounds	Infectious diseases such as hepatitis, AIDS, tuberculosis, staphylococcal disease
	Latex gloves	Skin rashes, anaphylaxis
	Sulfonamides	Skin disorders, phototoxic skin reactions
	Styrene, alcohols	Headaches, fatigue, poor memory, dizziness
Pharmaceutical workers	Sulfonamides	Skin disorders, phototoxic skin reactions
Anesthesiologists	Liver-toxic chemicals	Liver disease
	Anesthetics	Reproductive toxicology, congenital abnormalities, miscarriage
Radiologists, X-ray technicians	Ionizing radiation	Increased risk of cancer, cataracts
INDUSTRY		
Forklift operators, foundry workers	Carbon monoxide	Cardiovascular disease, neurological problems
Rubber industry	Chlorprene	Reproductive toxicology, abnormal reproduction
	Liver-toxic solvents	Liver disease
	Organic solvents	Reproductive toxicology, congenital abnormalities in offspring
Welders	Welding fumes, carbon dioxide, carbon monoxide, nitrogen dioxide, ozone	Lung irritation and damage, pulmonary edema, metal poisoning, damage and toxicity from free radicals
Welders of cadmium-plated metals	Cadmium	Kidney toxicity, kidney disease
Electronics workers, aircraft assemblers	Epoxy resins	Skin disorders, contact dermatitis
Workers with organic solvents	Liver-toxic solvents	Liver disease
	Organic solvents	Reproductive toxicology, congenital abnormalities in offspring

OCCUPATION	EXPOSURE	EFFECTS
Workers in gas and coke plants, iron and steel foundries	Polycyclic aromatic hydrocarbons (PAHS)	Skin rashes, headaches, sweating, vomiting, cancer
Viscose rayon industries	Carbon disulfide	Cardiovascular disease, accelerated atherosclerosis
Reinforced plastics industry, printing industry	Styrene	Headaches, fatigue, poor memory, dizziness
MANUFACTURING		
Insulation workers, textile manufacturing, manufacture of resins and plastics, particleboard	Formaldehyde	Skin disorders; rashes; occupational asthma; irritation of ears, nose, and throat; headache; cerebral symptoms
Graphite workers, and workers in carbon electrode manufacture	Carbon particles	Lung disease, pneumonoconiosis
Chemical manufacturers	Solvents and propellents (freon)	Cardiovascular disease, abnormal heart rhythms or fainting, sudden death
	Carbon disulfide	Cardiovascular disease, accelerated atherosclerosis
	Carbon tetrachloride	Kidney disease, kidney failure
Manufacture of explosives and pharmaceutical nitrates	Organic nitrates	Cardiovascular disease, angina, heart attack
Electronics workers, aircraft and boat assemblers	Epoxy resins	Skin disorders, contact dermatitis
	Fiberglass	Skin and lung irritation
Manufacture of housing units and camper shells	Styrene	Headaches, fatigue, poor memory, dizziness
Pesticide and solvent manufacturers, and aircraft manufacturers	Liver-toxic solvents	Liver disease
	Organic solvents	Reproductive toxicology, congenital abnormalities in offspring
Battery manufacture and reclamation	Lead, cadmium, sulfuric acid, mercury	Kidney disease, damage to mucous membranes and skin, upper respiratory problems
Manufacturers of electronic tubes, ceramics, and fluorescent light bulbs	Beryllium	Kidney disease and kidney toxicity, lung disease and lung toxicity

OCCUPATION	EXPOSURE	EFFECTS
Paper and textile manufacture	Acrylamide	Peripheral neuropathy
	Formaldehyde	Skin disorders; rashes; occupational asthma; irritation of ears, nose, and throat; headache; cerebral symptoms
Textile workers who work with natural fibers (cotton, flax, hemp, jute)	Inhaled textile fibers	Lung disease, chest tightness, byssinosis (cough)
Electroplating, jewelry manufacture, fluorescent screen manufacturing	Complex salts of platinum	Lung disease, asthma
MILITARY		
Ground forces involved in conflicts	Organic nitrates, noise pollution, chemical and biological exposures, vaccinations, physical and emotional trauma, dust, mold	Cardiovascular disease, angina, headaches, allergic rhinitis, rashes, post-traumatic stress disorder, neurological symptoms
Aircraft personnel	Jet fuel, noise pollution, greases, oils, carbon monoxide	Cardiovascular disease, headaches, allergic reactions, cerebral symptoms, neurological symptoms
Submarine personnel	Carbon monoxide, personal care products of shipmates, oils, greases, munitions	Cardiovascular disease, headaches, allergic reactions, rashes, cerebral symptoms, neurological symptoms
Munitions handlers and workers	Organic nitrates	Cardiovascular disease, angina, heart attack
MINING		
Miners	Carbon monoxide	Cardiovascular disease, neurological problems
	Silicon particles	Silicosis, lung disease
Coal miners	Carbon particles	Lung disease, pneumoconiosis
Uranium miners	Radon gas	Lung cancer
Quarry workers, stone cutters, sandblasters	Silicon particles	Silicosis, lung disease

OCCUPATION	EXPOSURE	EFFECTS
RETAIL		
Grocery clerks	Various plants, including celery, parsnips, citrus fruits	Skin disorders, contact dermatitis, phototoxic skin reactions
	Fumes from cleaning products	Allergic reactions, cerebral symptoms
Retail clerks	Formaldehyde	Skin disorders; rashes; occupational asthma; irritation of ears, nose, and throat; headache; cerebral symptoms
SERVICE		
Beauticians, barbers	Aerosol propellents, formaldehyde, scents, dyes, acetone, alcohols, solvents, halogenated hydrocarbons	Rashes, cerebral symptoms, headaches, allergic reactions, unexplained fatigue
Cosmetics workers	Oil of bergamot, orris root	Skin disorders, allergic reactions
Dry-cleaning workers	Solvents and propellents	Cardiovascular disease, abnormal heart rhythms or fainting, sudden death
Embalmers	Formaldehyde	Skin disorders; rashes; occupational asthma; irritation of ears, nose, and throat; headache; cerebral symptoms
Maids, janitors	Cleaning products, detergents, bleach, deodorants, solvents, various scents, dust, mold	Lung problems, allergic reactions, rashes, headaches, dizziness, cerebral symptoms
Fire fighters	Carbon monoxide	Cardiovascular disease, neurological problems
	Combustion products, solvents	Lung disease, headache
Pesticide applicators	Pesticides, herbicides	Cardiovascular disease, rapid heartbeats, high or low blood pressure, abnormal heart rhythm, neurological problems, wheezing

OCCUPATION	EXPOSURE	EFFECTS
School teachers	Solvents	Cardiovascular disease, abnormal heart rhythms or fainting
	Formaldehyde	Skin disorders; rashes; occupational asthma; irritation of ears, nose, and throat; headaches; cerebral symptoms
	Personal care products of students and other teachers	Headaches, cerebral symptoms, rashes
TRANSPORTATION		
Truck drivers, bus drivers, taxi drivers, delivery van drivers	Carbon monoxide, diesel fuel, gasoline, oils, solvents	Headache, nausea, malaise, fatigue, cerebral symptoms, cardiovascular disease
Railway workers	Tar and creosote	Skin disorders, phototoxic skin reactions
Pilots, flight attendants	Jet fuel, noise pollution, cosmic radiation, personal care products of passengers, carbon monoxide	Sleep dysfunction, respiratory irritation, headaches, cerebral symptoms, allergic reactions, cardiovascular disease, neurological problems

Office Exposures

Indoor air pollution causes more problems than outdoor air pollution. Half the work force now consists of white-collar office workers, who are exposed to more chemicals than in the past.

The leading causes of workplace pollution are faulty ventilation, chemical contamination, biological contamination, and asbestos. In 1981, safety guidelines published by the American Society of Heating, Refrigerating, and Air-conditioning Engineers (ASHRAE) defined acceptable air quality as ambient air that has no known contaminants at harmful concentrations and in

which a majority (80 percent) of the workers have no complaints.

■ VENTILATION

One or more heating, ventilation, and air-conditioning (HVAC) systems are used for most commercial buildings. Fresh outside air enters the building through intake vents. It is then combined with recirculated indoor air and passes in supply ducts through air cleaners and charcoal beds. Air cleaners filter out dust particles, and charcoal beds absorb odors. Air-tempering units regulate the temperature, and then the air is blown into rooms through room vents. Some HVAC

Workplace Toxins

As many as 4 million children and adolescents are legally employed in the United States. The substances to which they are exposed differ somewhat from those of adults. Their usual worksites include food services, automotive services, and retail stores. The most frequent exposures on the job are:

- *cleaning compounds*
- *paints*
- *glues*
- *hydrocarbons*
- *solvents*
- *caustics*
- *bleaches*

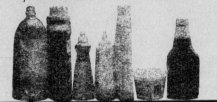

percent more people than they were designed for. These buildings are always described as being "stuffy," and people complain of headaches, fatigue, and eye, nose, and throat irritation. (See Sick-Building Syndrome, below.)

Poor installation or maintenance of the HVAC and local ventilation systems causes workplace pollution problems. Faulty HVAC systems may have water leaks; poor air distribution; and inadequate cooling, heating, and dehumidification. Also, most new buildings do not have windows that open to permit penetration of fresh air.

A common problem arises when the use of the building changes but the ventilation system is not changed to meet new needs. During office reorganization, intake vents may be blocked, which means that the amount of air exhausted is higher than the amount of air brought in, and this causes a vacuum. Contaminated air may then be sucked into the exhaust vents and recirculated. Intake vents are sometimes poorly placed, directly adjacent to exhaust vents, and contaminated air is recirculated back into the building. Intake vents may also be adjacent to sources of chemicals, such as car exhaust fumes containing carbon monoxide and other toxic chemicals.

Ventilation systems are frequently shut down when no one is occupying the building. However, the building itself continues to outgas, as do chemicals from paint, carpeting, and furnishings, and the level of contaminants builds up. If the system has been turned off, it should be restarted and run for several hours before the building is reoccupied.

units may have terminal units (composed of coils) that heat or cool the air.

Air exhaust fans draw the air out of the room and into a parallel system of ducts. Some exhaust air is eliminated through exhaust vents. Recirculated air passes through air filters and enters the building again. Some HVAC units also may humidify or dehumidify the air, depending on the season.

An office building should be ventilated at 15 cubic feet per minute per occupant. As a room is occupied at near maximum levels, ventilation rates should increase. People complain most about office environments that do not have the recommended air exchanges. Floor plans and ventilation systems are designed for a certain number of people, but buildings often contain 30 to 40

Bacteria, fungi, or animal fecal material may contaminate ventilation systems. Molds in air-conditioning systems can cause hypersensitivity pneumonia and humidifier lung. Legionnaire's disease was caused by the growth of a soil bacteria *(Legionella pneumophila)* in air ducts and cooling towers of air-conditioning systems.

▮▮ CHEMICALS

Indoor air pollution is the most serious chemical exposure for office workers. Our energy-efficient, airtight buildings and the increased use of synthetic materials (in carpets, drapes, and particleboard furniture) contribute to this problem. Photocopiers, typewriters, and computer printers have a range of emissions, including vocs. Other major indoor pollutants are identified and discussed in chapters 14, Water and Air, and 16, Chemicals and Metals. Harmful chemicals frequently found in the air in office buildings include:

• *Ammonia:* Commonly used to clean glass and other surfaces, and is also released by blueprint machines. It can burn the nose, throat, and chest and cause wheezing in asthmatics.

• *Benzene:* Found in synthetic fibers, plastics, cigarette smoke, spot removers, and other solvents. Low levels can cause irritation to the liver, kidneys, and gastrointestinal tract (see chapter 16, Chemicals and Metals).

• *Carbon monoxide:* Comes from automobile exhaust that the ventilation system brings into the building, and also present in cigarette smoke. High levels of carbon monoxide cause asphyxiation and death. Low lev-

---

Occupational Exposure to Microorganisms

• Antioxidant nutrients, beneficial bacteria (chapter **23**)

• Healthy high-quality diet (**24**)

• Inhalant and topical oxygen therapy, (**26**)

• Allergy extracts or hands-on treatment for specific microorganisms (**27**)

• Homeopathic remedies such as *Ipecacuanha, Baptisia tinctoria, Engystol* (**28**)

• Herbal remedies such as balm, wormwood, gentian (**29**)

• Compresses, packs, and poultices, charcoal therapy (**30**)

• Organ cleansing (**31**)

---

els cause headaches, dizziness, decreased hearing, personality changes, extra heartbeats, nausea, and vomiting (see chapter 8, Toxins in the Home).

• *Cigarette smoke:* Associated with lung cancer in nonsmokers who are exposed to second-hand smoke, as second-hand smoke contains more chemicals than mainstream smoke (see chapter 14, Water and Air). Fortunately, many buildings are now being designated as nonsmoking.

• *Ethanol:* Found in some duplicating fluids, inhalation can cause dizziness, drowsiness, and headaches. It can also dry out the skin (see chapter 16, Chemicals and Metals).

• *Formaldehyde:* Used in insulation, building materials, resins, textiles, carpets, and furniture, it continues to outgas for years. Exposure symptoms include burning eyes,

Occupational Chemical and Metal Exposures

- Detox baths or sauna program (chapter **22**)
- Antioxidant nutrients, particularly vitamin C (**23**)
- Fasting or juicing (**24**)
- Exercise and massage (**25**)
- Allergy extracts or hands-on allergy treatment for the specific chemicals (**27**)
- Chelation treatment for metal poisoning (**27**)
- Homeopathic remedies such as *Arsenicum album* for pesticide and chemical poisoning, *Alumina* and *Plumbum metallicum* for metal poisoning (**28**)
- Bach Rescue Remedies (**28**)
- Herbal remedies such as apple, garlic, and pectin for lead poisoning (**29**)
- Charcoal packs and oral charcoal (**30**)
- Organ cleansing (**31**)

dizziness, coughing, breathing difficulties, and nausea (see chapter 8, Toxins in the Home). The long-term effects of formaldehyde exposure are unknown.

- *Ozone:* Used as a disinfectant and also produced in offices when oxygen molecules contact high voltages or ultraviolet light. Photocopy machines and laser printers often produce ozone, but grounding them can decrease ozone emissions. Ozone promotes the formation of free radicals in the body, and when inhaled is a respiratory irritant.
- *Particulates:* These are particles small enough to be inhaled into the lungs, such as dust, mold, and particles from tobacco smoke. Cigarette smoke attracts other particulates in the air and allows them to remain airborne for hours, when they might otherwise be removed by the exhaust system (see chapter 14, Water and Air).
- *Radon gas:* Naturally occurring in soil and rocks, radon enters buildings through soil or contaminated groundwater and tap water. Radon has been associated with lung cancer (see chapters 8, Toxins in the Home, and 14, Water and Air).
- *Toluene:* Used in white-out solutions and in some markers and pens, it is a skin and lung irritant and can cause liver damage and neurological disorders (see chapter 16, Chemicals and Metals).
- *Vinyl chloride:* The building block of polyvinyl chloride, which is used in plastic products such as pipes, lighting fixtures, weather-stripping, wall coverings, electrical wires, and synthetic carpeting. Polyvinyl chloride emits vinyl chloride, which is a carcinogen, as it deteriorates and interacts with water (see chapter 16, Chemicals and Metals).

Many chemicals used in offices can irritate or injure the skin, which is the largest organ of the body. Direct chemical irritants, such as solvents, dissolve the skin or extract oils and fat-soluble compounds from the skin. Sensitizing chemicals, which include formaldehyde and duplicating fluids, cause an allergic reaction or sensitize the skin so that even a small quantity can cause a rash. Carbon paper, printer paper, blueprint paper, and carbonless paper forms can also

Sick-Building Syndrome

In "sick buildings," a high percentage of workers complain of nonspecific symptoms of eye, nose, and throat irritation; headaches; fatigue; drowsiness; dizziness; and decreased concentration. Symptoms typically improve over the weekend or vacation time and worsen on return to work. Most cases of sick-building syndrome are in new buildings or buildings remodeled to be more energy-efficient. Studies of these buildings have not shown any chemical levels to be higher than the limits set by the EPA. At first, the symptoms of workers in sick buildings were thought to be caused by hysteria.

In most cases, the exact cause of the sick building is not identified, yet volatile organic chemicals are thought to play a role. Ventilation systems have often been found to be inadequate to meet the needs of the number of people in the buildings or to handle new sources of chemicals, such as copy machines and computers. Pesticides, deodorizers, and scents are sometimes added to ventilation systems for dispersal throughout the building.

Building-related illness refers to those illnesses that have an identified cause. These include hypersensitivity pneumonitis (inflamed lungs caused by an allergy to mold or bird droppings), asthma, Legionnaire's disease (caused by the bacteria Legionella pneumophila), influenza, and carbon monoxide poisoning.

---

cause skin rashes. Toner residue and other chemicals on freshly photocopied material can cause the skin to itch, as well as causing "brain fog."

■■ BUILDING MATERIALS AND FURNISHINGS

- *Asbestos:* Used widely in buildings until the 1970s, it is now found in the air from deteriorating building materials, such as acoustical tile. The U.S. Environmental Protection Agency states that there is no safe level of exposure to asbestos, which causes lung cancer (see chapter 8, Toxins in the Home).

- *Carpeting, drapes, and upholstery:* These office furnishings can be moldy, particularly in very humid climates or where there has been a water leak. They are also "dust catchers," and unless the janitorial staff cleans carefully, can be a significant source of particulates in the air. (See chapter 8, Toxins in the Home, for a detailed discussion of carpeting.)

- *Cubicle dividers:* Many offices are located in large rooms that are divided into individual cubicles with portable dividers, which may be upholstered for noise control. The synthetic fabrics used contain various chemicals, and the dividers can be a source of mold and dust.

- *Fiberglass:* Used for insulation in buildings, fiberglass is a particulate hazard, and when it is inhaled into the lungs it stays there permanently. A lung irritant, it is believed to participate in respiratory tract cancer. It also irritates the skin on contact.

❙❙ ELECTROMAGNETIC FIELDS

Offices usually contain an unnaturally low level of negative air ions. These ions are depleted in offices because the metallic ducts in ventilation systems provide a sink for negative ions. Pollutants such as tobacco smoke also deplete ambient negative ions and increase the ratio of positive to negative ions. When we breathe, excess positive ions attach preferentially to carbon dioxide molecules, speeding up the transfer of carbon dioxide into the bloodstream and acting as a depressant to people.

Computer monitors, or video display terminals (VDTS), contain a transformer that powers the cathode ray tube. It generates enough voltage to impart a positive charge to objects directly in front of it, changing the skin polarity of the person sitting in front of the VDT from negative to positive. This attracts bacteria and viruses to the worker's skin.

We are exposed to a natural electrostatic field when we are outdoors in contact with the negatively charged earth surrounded by the positively charged sky. When we enter a building with a metal frame, this electromagnetic field is shielded by the surrounding metal. This is called the Faraday Cage Effect. Research that was done in Germany in 1967 suggests that the absence of this field can have adverse effects on reaction time and performance.

The modern office also shields out the natural Schumann resonance (natural frequency pulsation of the electromagnetic spectrum) caused by the negative ground plane of the earth and positively charged ionosphere. The Schumann resonance is 7.83 hertz (or 7.83 cycles per second) and coincides with the alpha state of brainwave patterns, which accompany our most alert and creative periods. In an office, the dominant environment is 60 cycles per second, the frequency of the alternating current that flows in the walls, ceiling, and floors. Studies at the University of Chicago have demonstrated that the efficiency of workers may drop to as low as 30 percent of normal when they are in a 60 hertz environment for an extended time.

School Exposures

Toxic exposures at school can affect student behavior and academic performance, as well as health. Children face great environmental health risks because their immune and neurological systems are still developing. They may have a high body burden of air pollutants because they breathe in a relatively large volume of air for their body weight. Most North American schools are polluted and overcrowded. The typical school has about four times the number of occupants as an office building with the same amount of floor space. Except in extremely enlightened school districts with large budgets, little or nothing is done to prevent school pollution.

Both students and teachers are at increased risk of chronic and acute health problems from toxins in the school. Symptoms can include coughing, eye irritation, headaches, asthma attacks, and allergic reactions.

■ SCHOOL BUILDINGS

New schools can be a significant source of volatile organic chemicals and formaldehyde from new furniture, carpet, paint, and building materials. Many parents have noted that their children's performance deteriorated in a new school environment. Remodeling and refurbishing projects can also cause health problems.

Most remodeling projects, such as repainting or recarpeting schools, are done just before school starts or during the school session. The materials are not allowed to properly outgas before students occupy the classrooms. For example, schools usually use enamel paint that has a slick, easy-to-clean surface. Enamel paint takes a minimum of one month to outgas at 100 percent ventilation and at least three months with less than 100 percent ventilation.

Many schools are carpeted in an effort to control and reduce noise. In addition to outgasing chemicals, carpets harbor lead, dust, dust mites, and mold (see chapter 8, Toxins in the Home). Many children are adversely affected by dirty or moldy classroom carpets, as well as from the chemicals released by the carpets.

Some older schools still contain asbestos tiles or asbestos fireproofing. As long as it is intact, the asbestos is not a problem, but when it becomes brittle asbestos becomes dangerous. Renovating can cause asbestos to become airborne (see chapter 8, Toxins in the Home).

Drinking water from water fountains can be exposed to lead in the pipes for long periods during weekends and holidays. This causes a high lead level in the water, particu-

Toxic Schools

School exposures are rarely considered to be a cause of learning and behavioral problems. Many students in remedial programs may have unidentified sensitivities, and behavioral problems are frequently directly related to toxic exposures.

larly in the morning. (See chapter 16, Chemicals and Metals, for further information on lead.)

Most schools have fluorescent lighting. Many students are bothered by these lights, which flicker at a rate of 60 times per second. Several studies have reported that some students demonstrate an increase in hyperactivity when they are exposed to fluorescent lights, and more attentive behavior when fluorescent lights are shut off.

Tar is frequently used when putting on new roofs or patching leaky roofs, and this work is often performed during school hours. Chemically sensitive children can be seriously affected by tar exposure.

When schools become overcrowded, portable classrooms are brought in because they are cheaper than building a new addition. Portable classrooms are typically windowless, and built from inexpensive materials, usually wood products that are high in formaldehyde. These buildings have poor ventilation, worsening indoor air pollution. Many portable classrooms are placed on steel stands instead of a concrete foundation, so that they can be easily moved. This predisposes the space under the portable

Mold, Dust, Dust Mite, and Animal Dander in School

- Vitamin C, quercetin, coenzyme Q_{10} (chapter **23**)
- Inhalation oxygen and hydrogen peroxide nose spray (**26**)
- Allergy extracts or hands-on treatments for mold, dust, dust mite and animal dander (**27**)
- Homeopathic remedies such as *Blatta orientalis, Dulcamara, Silica* (**28**)
- Organ cleansing (**31**)

building to mold and bacterial growth, which can cause illness in both students and teachers.

Many portable classrooms and permanent school buildings are contaminated with mold, particularly in humid climates. HVAC units can become contaminated with mold and spread it throughout the building to carpets, fabrics, and books. If the classroom has had a water leak, there may be mold in the classroom. Mold is one of the most potent and toxic allergens (see chapter 15, Plants and Organisms).

Faulty or inadequate ventilation can contribute to poor air quality in the classroom. Lowered oxygen levels cause drowsiness, fatigue, and poor concentration. Particulate contamination, such as mold, dust, and danders, can be spread through the classroom from dirty air ducts and vents. This can trigger asthma attacks in sensitive children, as well as causing eye and nose irritation.

■■ CLASSROOM EXPOSURES

The major exposure at schools comes from the classroom in which students spend most of their day. Unless a school is particularly informed on possible problems and takes steps to prevent or correct them, these exposures can affect both the learning ability of the children and the health of both the children and teacher.

- *Animals:* Many classrooms have animals, such as guinea pigs, mice or rats, hamsters, and rabbits. Sensitive students can react to animal dander, the bedding material in the cages, or the urine and feces. Many people with allergies to cats also do not tolerate guinea pigs, hamsters, or rabbits (see chapter 8, Toxins in the Home).
- *Classroom chemicals:* Chemicals are used in biology classes (with animals preserved in formaldehyde), chemistry laboratories, or art classrooms. Even if the student is not in the classroom using the chemicals, the fumes can drift into other classrooms and make many students ill. In addition, most schools are treated with pesticides regularly. (See chapter 16, Chemicals and Metals, for information on pesticides and specific chemicals.)
- *Cleaning supplies:* Phenol and formaldehyde are frequently used in bathroom disinfectants in schools. One trip to the bathroom after these supplies have been used can mentally incapacitate a sensitive student for the rest of the day. Their ability to learn can be seriously impaired from the cerebral symptoms caused by these substances.
- *Instructional materials:* Freshly photo-

copied or mimeographed instructional materials are a toxic chemical exposure for many students. Toner and other chemical residues on photocopied materials can cause itching and cerebral symptoms such as brain fog. Mimeographed materials will also have duplicator fluid residues (see Methanol, below.) All paper is a formaldehyde exposure, including the paper in books.

- *Methanol:* Methanol, and sometimes ethanol, are used in duplicating machines, often in poorly ventilated locations. Exposure causes headaches, itchy eyes, and dizziness.
- *Personal care products:* Products used by both students and teachers, including perfumes, after-shave lotions, deodorants, shampoos, hair sprays, and detergent and fabric softener scents in clothes, can cause problems for the sensitive student (see chapter 8, Toxins in the Home).
- *Radon:* Some classrooms contain radon levels above the EPA safety level. Because radon cannot be seen, smelled, or tasted, it is important that classrooms be tested for this gas, which has been linked with lung cancer (see chapter 8, Toxins in the Home, and chapter 14, Water and Air).

■ OUTDOOR ENVIRONMENT

The outdoor environment surrounding schools affects students, particularly elementary students—who usually play outside during recess, sometimes twice a day. This environment also affects secondary students, who sometimes must travel from building to building when they change

Cleaning Mistakes

Even the most well-intentioned cleaning actions can affect the learning ability of children. One teacher, in an attempt to control germs in her classroom, sprayed the desk tops with Lysol. This action dramatically affected a boy in her class, particularly his vision.

He reported that the blackboard looked like a "snowy TV screen" to him, even though he was sitting toward the front of the classroom. In addition, the Lysol gave him cerebral symptoms, causing him to become "spacey" and unable to think clearly. His ability to learn for the entire day was destroyed by this one action.

classes. In addition, elements from the outdoor environment make their way into the classroom.

- *Asphalt:* When a parking lot or adjacent street is resurfaced, asphalt fumes will permeate the classroom. It is a hydrocarbon exposure and chemically sensitive children can develop headaches, cerebral symptoms, and other uncomfortable symptoms.
- *Electromagnetic radiation:* Many schools are located near major transformers and high-tension wires, which are a source of electromagnetic fields (see chapter 18, Radiation, Electromagnetic Fields, and Geopathic Stress).
- *Playground and field chemicals:* Playgrounds are treated on a regular basis with pesticides that may linger for days. High

Chemical Exposures in School

- Detox baths or sauna program (chapter **22**)
- Vitamin C and other antioxidant nutrients (**23**)
- Juicing (**24**)
- Exercise and massage (**25**)
- Allergy extracts or hands-on treatment for the specific chemicals (**27**)
- Homeopathic remedies such as *Arsenicum album, Phosphorus, Plumbum metallicum* (**28**)
- Charcoal packs and oral charcoal (**30**)
- Organ cleansing (**31**)

exposures to pesticides, herbicides, and chemical fertilizers result from playing on grass sprayed with lawn chemicals (see chapter 16, Chemicals and Metals).

- *Traffic:* If schools and playgrounds are near heavily traveled highways, high concentrations of lead from vehicle exhaust may be left in the soil from the days of leaded fuels.

Hydrocarbon levels from exhaust fumes will also be high and can cause headaches, sleepiness, mental confusion, irritation of eyes, nose and throat, nausea, and loss of reasoning ability.

Although the discussion regarding toxins in schools has been primarily in terms of children, adults in the school will be affected by the same toxins. Many teachers and other school workers have suffered symptoms from exposures to these toxins, and their health has sometimes been damaged.

Additionally, students are not always children. Many adults return to school to further their education and receive new training. Toxic exposures at colleges and other post-secondary institutions are similar to those outlined above. In some instances they may be worse, because of the increased numbers of students using science laboratories and taking industrial science and other classes where there are toxic substances and exposures.

Toxins from Art and Leisure Activities and Travel

Toxic exposures occur even during leisure activities and travel. However, many measures can be taken to prevent and lessen these exposures. A discussion of these measures may be found in Part VII, Prevention Methods.

Arts and Crafts

Craft activities often involve exposure to toxins. Toxic art and craft materials enter the body through inhalation and skin contact. Children may put them in their mouths. The Arts Hazard Information Center in New York has documented many cases of symptoms and problems caused from the use of art and craft materials. Examples include a jewelry maker with cadmium poisoning, a batik artist with a chronic cough, and an art teacher who suffered brain damage from solvents and chemicals used in silkscreening.

Paints, dyes, marking pens, oils, glues, waxes, fabrics, plastics, woods, solvents, and adhesives can all contain toxic chemicals. They may also contain fungicides, pesticides, preservatives, and extenders. High doses or chronic exposures to these substances can cause skin rashes, neurological problems, respiratory diseases, lung scarring, birth defects, kidney damage, and impaired physical and mental development.

Many art and craft materials contain toxic metals. Arsenic, cadmium, chromium, cobalt, lead, manganese, titanium, and zinc are used as pigments in paints, dyes, and ceramic glazes. Cadmium may also be in silver solders and fluxes used in making jewelry. Lead is used in making stained glass. Inks may contain cadmium, lead, or chromium. Metals can be inhaled as fumes or dust particles. Acute symptoms of metal exposure can include nausea, headache, diarrhea, and abdominal pain. Chronic exposure can affect vision, hearing, taste, and smell, and cause poor coordination. (See chapter 16, Chemicals and Metals, for information on specific metals.)

Art and craft supplies also contain many volatile organic chemicals (vocs). Airbrush and spray paints are a significant exposure to

Hazardous Hobbies

Hobbies that expose people to toxins include:

- *drawing and sketching*
- *fabric and fiber arts, such as quilting and weaving*
- *gardening*
- *painting*
- *photography*
- *pottery and ceramics*
- *soapstone carving*
- *stained-glass work*
- *woodworking*

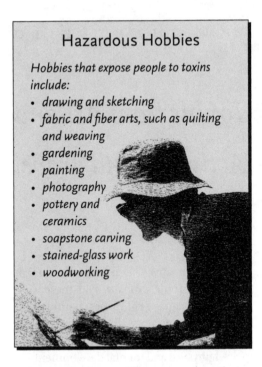

paints and solvents. The user can easily inhale both paint particles and solvent fumes. Toluene, xylene, methylene chloride, petroleum distillate, glycol ethers, alcohols, ketones, and benzene are found in oil- and solvent-based paints, markers, finishes, glues, and coatings, as well as in turpentines and brush cleaners. VOCs can cause eye irritations, headaches, nausea, respiratory symptoms, fatigue, and mood swings. The effects on the reproductive system depend on the voc. Birth defects, low birth weight, and sterility can result from exposures. (See chapter 8, Toxins in the Home, and chapter 16, Chemicals and Metals, for further information.)

A number of arts and crafts involve formaldehyde exposures, including painting, fabric arts, paper crafts, and photography. Formaldehyde is used as a preservative in acrylic paints, fabric finishes, and photographic products, and in the manufacture of all types of paper. In addition, formaldehyde sets dyes, waterproofs fabrics, and makes surfaces smoother, thus making products more appealing to consumers. Even at extremely low levels, formaldehyde can cause asthma, contact dermatitis, nausea, chronic headache, diarrhea, memory lapse, fatigue, drowsiness, eye and respiratory tract irritation, nosebleeds, dry and sore throat, insomnia, and disorientation. (See chapter 8, Toxins in the Home, for further information.)

Many types of art and craft projects involve the use of glue. Glues can be serious toxic exposures, as indicated below.

- *Contact cement:* The solvent type contains neoprene rubber, modified phenolic resin, magnesium oxide, zinc oxide, and a solvent blend of toluene, hexane, and methyl ethyl ketone. Fumes from this glue are toxic, it is poisonous if ingested, and it is a mucous membrane irritant.
- *Epoxy glue:* There are several formulas for epoxy resins that will bond metals, rubber, polyester resins, glass, and ceramics. These glues can cause eye, nose, throat, and skin irritations; lung irritation; skin allergies; and asthma.
- *Glue guns:* Two formulations of glue are used in electric glue guns. One is for a hot gun and it becomes a liquid at a higher temperature than the glue formulated for a "cold" gun. Vapors from these glues are toxic to some individuals and may cause headaches and cerebral symptoms.
- *Krazy Glue™, Miracle Glue™, and Super Glue™:* These cyanoacrylate adhesives do

not usually cause skin rashes, but can seal the skin of the hands and other body parts together. Medical intervention may be necessary if water or acetone do not release the bond. Vapors from these glues are irritating to the eyes, nose, and lungs.

• *Model cement:* These glues may contain nitrocellulose, acetone, cellulose acetate, isopropanol, dibutyl phthalate, hexane, beutyl acetate, tolulol, naphtha, ethanol, and camphor. Inhalation may irritate the lungs. The vapor is irritating to the eyes, mucous membranes, and skin; and continued use can cause liver damage.

• *Rubber cements:* Several formulations are available. They may contain hexane, rubber, and solvents such as toluene, benzene, hexane, ketone, and trichloroethane. They may also contain rosin, ester gum, and antioxidants. Inhalation of large amounts can cause neurological symptoms and damage.

• *Wood glues:* Can contain polyvinyl acetate, dibutyl phthalate, silicone defoamers, methyl cellulose, water, and formaldehyde. They may also contain diethylene glycol dibenzoate. Dibutyl phthalate can cause gastrointestinal upset. The vapor is irritating to the eyes and mucous membranes.

Photograph developers are exposed to many chemicals, including hydroquinone, silver salts, sodium thiosulfate, ammonium thiosulfate, acetic acid, formaldehyde, sodium hydroxide, potassium bromine, sodium carbonate, sodium sulfate, ammonium chloride, boric acid, hydrochloric acid, and sulfuric acid. Sensitive individuals may develop skin rashes, headaches, blurred vision, and cerebral symptoms.

Exposure to Chemicals from Art and Leisure Activities

• Detox baths or sauna program (chapter **22**)
• Vitamin C, other antioxidant nutrients (**23**)
• Fasting or juicing (**24**)
• Exercise and massage (**25**)
• Allergy extracts or hands-on treatment for the specific chemicals (**27**)
• Homeopathic remedies such as *Arsenicum album, Phosphorus* (**28**)
• Herbal remedies such as milk thistle, rosemary (**29**)
• Organ cleansing (**31**)

Exposure to Metals from Art and Leisure Activities

• Detox baths or sauna program (**22**)
• Antioxidant nutrients, cysteine, methionine, or glutathione (**23**)
• Fasting or juicing (**24**)
• Exercise or massage (**25**)
• Allergy extracts or hands-on treatment for the specific metals (**27**)
• Chelation therapy (**27**)
• Homeopathic remedies such as *Alumina, Cadmium metallicum, Hepar sulphuris, Plumbum metallicum* (**28**)
• Herbal remedies such as milk thistle, rosemary (**29**)
• Organ cleansing (**31**)

MOST EFFECTIVE DETOXIFICATION METHODS

Charcoal, pastels, and colored pencils used by artists create a fine dust, which can cause respiratory and eye irritation. Ceramic artists may be affected by the dust produced

Art and Craft Regulations

In 1988, legislation was passed that requires the U.S. Product Safety Commission to regulate the labeling of art and craft materials for health hazards. As of 1990, nontoxic products with an AP or CP seal can be used safely by small children. However, some products that bear the seal, such as metal enamels, ceramic glazes, and clays with talc, are not safe for children to use. In Canada, most consumer products containing toxic materials carry warning labels, but if you use a product frequently it would be wise to obtain a Material Safety Data Sheet from the manufacturer and follow its workplace recommendations.

when cleaning ceramic greenware. The colored glazes used by potters and ceramic artists contain barium carbonate, lead, chromium, uranium, and cadmium. Potters and ceramic artists can also be exposed to asbestos, which is used to insulate kilns. When firing, kilns produce carbon dioxide, sulfur dioxide, formaldehyde, fluorine, and chlorine, as well as lead and cadmium vapors.

Woodworking activities produce sawdust and terpene vapors, which are irritating to many people. Glues, paints, stains, and varnishes used in finishing woodworking projects are also a source of toxins. Headaches, contact dermatitis, respiratory problems, and cerebral symptoms are commonly experienced by sensitive individuals. In addition, the noise from power equipment is a toxic exposure and can cause hearing damage unless ear protection is worn.

Soapstone, used in making jewelry and sculpture, may contain asbestos. When the soapstone is polished, airborne asbestos fibers can be released. Talc, which is finely powdered magnesium silicate, is found in clay. It is also a pigment in paints and varnish. Prolonged inhalation causes lung problems, as it is similar in composition to asbestos. Dry clay contains silica, which can damage the lungs.

Professional artists, art teachers, and art students have the highest exposure to toxins, but they tend to be more careful in the use of their materials than hobbyists. Children and elderly people who use these products less frequently may be more at risk because they are often less informed of the dangers of the chemicals, and their physiology makes them more vulnerable to the effects. Children should use only nontoxic art supplies specifically designed for them. Food-scented art supplies should never be used because they tempt young children to eat them.

Sports Exposures

Although exercise and outdoor activity are usually considered healthful, there are toxic exposures associated with these activities. The following chart shows the exposures connected with some common sports.

Toxic Exposure During Sporting Activities

ACTIVITY	EXPOSURES
Jogging and running	Weather, air pollution, pollens, dust, mold
Working out in gyms, indoor racquetball, tennis, etc.	Indoor air pollution
Cycling	Weather, air pollution, pollens, dust, mold
Hiking and camping	Weather, contaminated water, campfire smoke, sunscreen, insect repellent, chemicals in tent fabric
Boating, water skiing, and fishing	Weather, contaminated water, sunscreen, insect repellent, gasoline fumes, combustion products from engines, oil and oil fumes, materials from engine maintenance, noise pollution
Shooting and hunting	Weather, oils and solvents to clean guns, noise pollution
Snow skiing and snowboarding	Weather, altitude, sunscreen
Racing enthusiasts (drivers and spectators)	Gasoline fumes, carbon monoxide, combustion products from engines, oil and oil fumes, dust, materials from engine maintenance, noise pollution
Sporting events	Noise pollution, weather exposure for outdoor sports; noise pollution, indoor air pollution for indoor sports

Gardening

Many people are avid gardeners in their leisure time, raising flowers or vegetables and fruit. Most gardens require special soil preparation, and gardeners are exposed to mold when they prepare and work with the soil. Many gardeners use pesticides to combat insects in their garden. They may also use chemical fertilizers designed to enhance the growth of their plants, as well as herbicides for weed control.

Although pesticide and fertilizer residues outdoors are broken down by sunlight, flowing water, and soil microbes, yard chemicals can be tracked into homes on shoes, contaminating the home. These chemicals can remain in carpet fibers for years and are a significant pesticide exposure to infants

Exposures While Gardening

- Detox baths for exposure to pesticides, herbicides, fertilizers (chapter **22**)
- Vitamin C, other antioxidant nutrients (**23**)
- Healthy high-quality diet (**24**)
- Massage, other bodywork (**25**)
- Allergy extracts or hands-on treatment for pollens, terpenes, molds (**27**)
- Homeopathic remedies such as *Wyethia* for hayfever, *Allium cepa* for flowers and pollens, *Blatta orientalis* for mold (**28**)
- Herbal remedies such as nettle, milk thistle (**29**)
- Charcoal packs or specific soaks (**30**)
- Organ cleansing (**31**)

crawling on them. A 1995 study in Denver found that children whose yards were treated with pesticides were four times more likely to develop soft tissue cancers than children from households that did not use yard chemicals. (See chapter 16, Chemicals and Metals, for further information.)

Exposure to some plants can cause skin disorders, phototoxic skin reactions, and allergic reactions. Sunburn and heat stroke can also affect gardeners (see chapter 17, Noise, Weather, and Altitude).

Travel

Travel exposes us to toxins while we are on the move, as well as at our lodgings. However, careful planning can minimize these toxins and result in safe and successful traveling.

❚❚ AUTOMOBILE, TRUCK, BUS, AND TRAIN TRAVEL

The majority of North Americans travel frequently in vehicles powered by internal combustion engines. The exhaust from these engines, whether gasoline or diesel, is a toxic exposure. Exhaust from gasoline engines contains paraffins, olefins, sulfur, sulfur dioxide, tars, ammonia, nitrogen dioxide, organic acids, zinc, metallic oxides, and unburned fuel. It also contains fragments of antioxidants, metal deactivators, anti-rust and anti-icing compounds, detergents, and lubricants. Diesel exhaust from diesel vehicles and freight trucks contains nitrogen dioxide, sulfur dioxide, formaldehyde, acrolein, and phenol, in addition to many hydrocarbons. For some, diesel exhaust is more toxic than gasoline exhaust.

Leaks from exhaust and fuel systems often enter older vehicles. Leaks of engine oil, antifreeze, transmission fluid, and power steering and brake fluid can cause additional chemical exposure. When these leaking fluids come in contact with a hot exhaust pipe or manifold, their effects are increased.

The air-conditioning and ventilation system in many vehicles draws in outside, contaminated engine and exhaust air that further adds to the exposure. The ventilation system can also become contaminated by mold, sending spores and mold fragments into the vehicle.

In addition, passengers are exposed to chemicals used by other people in the vehicle. Scented soaps, deodorants, detergents, fabric softeners, perfumes, after-shaves, colognes, hair sprays, and lotions are toxic exposures for sensitive people. In mass-transit vehicles such as buses, trams, and trains, these exposures are sizable. Where smoking is permitted, the confined space increases the severity of the exposure.

Vehicle motion and exposure to exhaust fumes play a role in carsickness. Many people who suffer from carsickness are allergic to the exhaust fumes, which trigger their nausea and headaches. Some people become sleepy when exposed to exhaust fumes. Riders in the front seat are exposed to less fumes than passengers in the back. Several studies have demonstrated that children who suffer from motion sickness are more likely to develop migraine headaches as adults.

❚❚ AIR TRAVEL

❚ AIR QUALITY

Poor air quality in commercial airlines is an increasing problem. Banning smoking on domestic flights has helped, but the problem of inadequate ventilation remains serious. Microorganisms, pollutants, and other materials can build up to dangerous levels. Some of the contaminants found in airplanes include:

- carbon dioxide, from breathing and dry ice
- ozone from the earth's atmosphere
- nitrogen oxides from jet fuel combustion
- volatile organic chemicals (vocs) from fuel and cleaning fluids
- fibers and dust
- bacteria, fungi, and viruses from food and passengers
- tobacco smoke on international flights

Airplane ventilation systems draw out-

MOST EFFECTIVE DETOXIFICATION METHODS

Chemical Exposure While Traveling

- Detox baths (chapter **22**)
- Vitamin C, other antioxidant, nutrients (**23**)
- Allergy extracts or hands-on treatment for the specific chemicals, or for tobacco (**27**)

Mold Exposure While Traveling

- Beneficial bacteria (**23**)
- Allergy extracts or hands-on treatment for mold (**27**)
- The homeopathic remedy *Blatta orientalis* (**28**)

Microorganism Exposure While Traveling

- Vitamin C, other antioxidants, nutrients (**23**)
- Allergy extracts or hands-on treatment for specific microorganisms (**27**)
- Homeopathic remedies such as *Arnica, Gelsemium, Oscillococcinum, Engystol* (**28**)
- Herbal remedies such as echinacea, goldenseal (**29**)

---

door air in through the engines which is mixed with recycled air from the cabin. To save money, airlines use more recycled air and less fresh air. The recycled air passes through a particulate filter, but this does not remove microorganisms.

Criteria for airplane cabin air exchange rates, environmental conditions, and air contaminants have not been established. The Federal Aviation Agency's (FAA) standard for airplane cabin carbon dioxide concentration is twice that allowed for indoor environments.

The American Society of Heating, Refrigeration, and Air-conditioning Engineers (ASHRAE) recommends a ventilation rate of 15 to 20 cubic feet per minute (cfm) per person. Economy-class passengers on a Boeing 747 flight receive less than 7 cfm, while first-class passengers receive 30 to 50 cfm. The ventilation rate for pilots is ten times that of economy class. The recommended maximum carbon dioxide level is 1,000 parts per million (ppm), but without adequate ventilation levels, over 5,000 ppm are not uncommon in airplanes. Related complaints from passengers and flight attendants include sore eyes, scratchy throats, nasal irritation, headaches, cough, shortness of breath, fatigue, and dizziness.

Many flights have ozone levels eight times higher than the recommended amount, causing nose, throat, and lung irritations. Adding filtration systems and using charcoal filters and disposable prefilters to take out volatile organic chemicals and ozone has been suggested by clean air experts.

Low humidity creates serious discomfort for many passengers, causing dry eyes and respiratory and skin irritation. Relative humidity should optimally be between 30 and 65 percent. The U.S. National Academy of Science (NAS) found that the typical relative humidity on planes was 2 to 23 percent. Fresh air brought inside the cabin has less than 1 percent relative humidity. Some moisture is added to the air in cabins as passengers and flight crews breathe and perspire.

On international flights, attendants, passengers, and airline workers are exposed to secondhand smoke. Working as a flight attendant on smoking flights has been said to be like living with a one-pack-per-day smoker. Women who are exposed to passive smoke for three to four hours a day have an increased risk of cervical cancer, in addition to the risk of lung cancer.

▌ MICROORGANISMS

Bacteria, viruses, and fungal spores can be airborne in aircraft cabins, because the particle filters in the ventilation system do not remove particles of this size. Passengers who travel during the winter months are subjected to large quantities of these organisms, increasing their chances of infection. The confined space, recirculated air, delays after boarding, and non-disembarking stops all increase the risk of infection. Documentation of illnesses contracted during a flight is difficult, however, because of incubation time and the dispersion of passengers to many destinations.

Aircraft cabins can be contaminated with these organisms for days, and cabin cleaning procedures do not remove them. The respiratory droplets from coughing, sneezing, and talking accumulate in circulation systems, on bulkhead panels, and on the upholstered seats. These droplets can contain live bacteria and viruses until they dry. Fungal spores enter the air during the motion of takeoff and are inhaled by passengers. Remaining in an unventilated aircraft cabin (such as during takeoff or flight delays when the cabin may not be ventilated) for more than 30 minutes increases the chances of epidemic infection. (See chapter 15, Plants

Flu on Board

Contamination with microorganisms can occur easily on airline flights. On one flight that sat on the ground for three hours in Alaska, 72 percent of passengers developed a strain of flu within three days. One passenger was the source of infection. Flu epidemics frequently spread along major airline travel routes.

and Organisms, for further information on microorganisms.)

■ CHEMICALS

On many international flights, the destination country requires pesticide to be sprayed before passengers are allowed to deplane. Other countries require aerosol spraying of empty cabins every four weeks with a pesticide known as a residual, which leaves long-lasting insect-killing residues in the aircraft cabin and galley. Passengers and flight attendants must then spend long hours on a plane that is thoroughly saturated with pesticide. (See chapter 16, Chemicals and Metals, for further information.)

■ RADIATION

Radiation exposure occurs during airline flights. At typical cruising altitudes of 29,000 to 39,000 feet, the radiation dose is 100 times that at sea level. Pregnant women should not fly frequently because fetuses are more radiation-sensitive than adults. The International Commission on Radiation Protection recommends the maximum permissible dose for air passengers should be no more than 5 millisieverts (500 millirems) a year. An airline passenger making 10 trips a year receives about 3 millisieverts (300 millirems) of exposure. Frequent flyers who log 100,000 miles a year in the air should have their exposure doses monitored regularly. (See chapter 18, Radiation, Electromagnetic Fields, and Geopathic Stress.)

■ ILLNESS AND JET LAG

Airsickness is a problem for some passengers. It is caused both by the motion of the plane and the cabin pressure. For sensitive individuals, exposure to jet fuel and the soaps, perfumes, and fabric softeners on other passengers also plays a role. Other individuals may not feel well while flying because of electromagnetic disturbances. Airplane cabins frequently have a high level of positively charged ions.

Airplane travel can be dangerous for people with heart and respiratory disease. Airplane cabins are pressurized to the equivalent of 7,000 to 8,000 feet in altitude,

Airport Terminals

Airport terminals can be very toxic. Tobacco smoke, cleaning products, personal care products of other travelers, pesticides, jet fuel and exhaust, and mold contribute to the toxicity. Most airports seem to be under perpetual construction, either in the terminal or in the parking facilities. The building materials used can cause problems for many passengers.

which is a problem for individuals with respiratory or heart disease.

Air travel can also disrupt the normal body circadian rhythms, which are based on the 24-hour day. A person traveling across several time zones can become very tired and may develop gastrointestinal symptoms. This is known as jet lag. After a flight from Germany to North America, for example, people need three days to resynchronize their psychomotor performance. It takes eight days to resynchronize if the flight direction is east. Jet lag also causes cerebral symptoms, including disorientation, inability to concentrate, and memory loss. Anxiety, impatience, indecisiveness, and a feeling of vulnerability can also be triggered by jet lag.

▮▮ BOAT TRAVEL

People travel on a wide variety of boats, from the size of row boats to cruise ships. On powered boats, toxic exposure includes oils and reserve fuel tanks, as well as the exhaust from the engines. The contents of the exhaust varies with the engine type. (See Automobile, Truck, Bus, and Train Travel, above.)

On passenger ships, toxic exposures are higher because of the size and complexity of the vessel. In addition to the engine exhaust, cleaning supplies, carpets, drapes, heating and cooling systems, tobacco smoke, and passengers' personal care products can all be toxic exposures.

People suffering from pollen allergies, however, do well on a sea voyage because exposure to pollens is negligible.

The possibility of seasickness is common to all boats, but seasickness is largely caused by the rhythmic action of the water, unlike motion sickness in aircraft or land vehicles.

▮▮ LODGING EXPOSURES

Hotels, motels, cottages, and cabins are often responsible for toxic exposures. Cleaning supplies, room deodorizers, carpets, and drapes may outgas toxic chemicals. All types of lodgings are usually treated with pesticides regularly because guests object to the presence of ants, cockroaches, and other insects in their rooms. In areas where insect populations are high, pesticides may be applied weekly.

If smoking or pets are allowed in the building, the air will include additional chemicals and allergens from the animals. Rooms located close to the swimming pool may smell heavily of chlorine.

The laundry supplies used on the linens, including the laundry soap and fabric softener, can adversely affect sensitive people. Residual fumes from gas dryers can also cause problems. Rooms located close to the laundry room will have higher levels of these chemicals in the air.

Mold can sometimes be a problem in motel and hotel rooms, and is even more of a problem in cabins and cottages. It can result from a leaking roof, shower stall, or even ground contamination. In humid climates, mold control can be very difficult.

Air conditioning and heating systems are sources of mold, bacteria, and dust. Many lodging establishments are lax in cleaning filters and ducts, allowing these substances to build up. Cooling towers for heating, ventilation, and air conditioning systems can harbor bacterial growth unless special precautions are taken. (See chapter 15, Plants and Organisms, for further information.)

The building materials in lodgings can also be sources of toxins. See chapter 8, Toxins in the Home, for a discussion of building materials.

∎∎ FOOD AND WATER

Regardless of your mode of travel and place of lodging, you will be eating food and drinking water. Both food and water can constitute a toxic exposure, especially when your body is not accustomed to the food and water of a new place. If you have food allergies, it will compound the problem.

Food and water are discussed in detail in chapters 13 and 14. Careful planning and prevention methods can assure your good health during a trip.

CHAPTER 11

Toxins from Medical Treatment

As incredible as it may seem, we encounter toxins in almost every type of standard medical treatment. The very treatments that are meant to heal us can be sources of toxic exposures for some individuals. However, proper planning, a healthy lifestyle, and detoxification procedures can minimize the effects of these toxins. Detoxification methods are discussed in Part VI, Ways of Detoxification, and methods of lessening and preventing problems are presented in Part VII, Prevention Methods.

Hospital Exposures

Unfortunately, hospitals, which are supposed to be healing institutions, are some of the most contaminated buildings we can encounter. Because of attempts to maintain sterility and minimize infections, powerful disinfectants are used to clean operating and other hospital rooms, corridors, and restrooms. Sterilizing solutions used on equipment are also quite potent. In addition, standard cleaning supplies, such as soaps, waxes, oils, and strippers, are used through-

out the hospital. Laundry products used on hospital linens contain a high bleach content to kill microorganisms. Regular pesticide applications attempt to keep insect populations at a minimum. All of these chemicals can be toxic, even to patients who are not chemically sensitive.

Hospital furnishings, drapes, and carpets can all be toxic exposures. New items will outgas numerous chemicals, including formaldehyde. Spot-resistant chemicals may be used on drapes, carpets, and upholstery and contribute to outgasing. Older furnishings can be moldy and dusty. In addition, over time, the fabrics absorb fumes from all of the hospital chemicals.

The heating, ventilation, and air-conditioning (HVAC) systems for hospitals are subject to the same problems as HVAC systems in office buildings. The comfort and health of hospital patients depends in part on the efficient functioning of this system. (See chapter 9, Toxins in the Workplace and School, for more information.)

Hospital patients are also exposed to the

personal care products of the staff, their roommates, visitors, and hospital volunteers, adding to their toxic burden. Patients are also exposed to the plants and gifts of other patients. Plants can be a mold exposure, which can increase each time the plant is watered. The scent of plants is caused by terpenes, naturally occurring chemicals within the plant, and many people are sensitive to them. Fortunately, tobacco smoking is forbidden in most hospitals, or allowed only in designated areas.

People entering the hospital for even a brief time are exposed to other patients, some of whom may be very ill, and possibly contagious. Infections acquired in the hospital are called nosocomial infections. Organisms can be carried from patient to patient by the staff, including doctors, nurses, and other hospital workers, largely because people fail to wash their hands between patient visits. Many of the organisms that cause nosocomial infections are resistant to antibiotics and the illnesses they cause are very difficult to treat.

Surgery

Many health problems can be prevented by proper diet, exercise, and early noninvasive treatment. Too many surgeries are the result of ignoring early signs and symptoms of disease, with nothing done to remedy the situation until an operation is the only solution. However, there are circumstances under which surgery is not only necessary, but unavoidable. Broken bones must be set, and more complicated breaks may require surgical procedures. A ruptured appendix must be removed before the person develops

Deficient Diets

Hospital diets may afford different types of problems. If you have food allergies, the dietary staff may not be aware of all of the possible exposures for a given food, and may inadvertently serve it to you. If you have a specialized diet, such as vegetarian, the hospital may not provide adequately balanced meals. Some hospitals serve nutritionally deficient diets, including large amounts of fats, salty food, and low-fiber food. When nutritional needs are not met, patients have more difficulty healing and recovering.

peritonitis. Some congenital defects must be surgically repaired. Intestinal blockages must be opened or removed, and hernias repaired. Detached retinas must be reattached, and cataracts must be removed. People hurt in car accidents, by gunshot wounds, or with other injuries, often need surgical repair.

Regardless of the medical condition and the reason for the surgery, you will encounter toxins both in the operating room and the rest of the hospital. Surgery itself involves exposures to anesthetics, as well as drugs that paralyze and minimize muscle movements. Numerous pharmaceutical drugs are given to lessen the after-effects of the surgery and to speed recovery. All these drugs constitute a major chemical exposure that the liver must detoxify. Chemically sensitive individuals may have difficulty tolerating these substances and this can add to

MOST EFFECTIVE DETOXIFICATION METHODS

Surgery

- Detox baths or sauna (chapter **22**)
- Vitamin C, other antioxidants, nutrients (**23**)
- Healthy high-quality diet (**24**)
- Exercise as tolerated and bodywork (**25**)
- Oxygen therapy (**26**)
- Allergy extracts or hands-on treatments-for all allergens, particularly chemicals (**27**)
- Homeopathic remedies such as *Phosphorus, Pyrogenium, Strontium carbonicum* (**28**)
- Herbal remedies such as milk thistle, echinacea, goldenseal (**29**)
- Charcoal packs or specific soaks (**30**)
- Organ cleansing (**31**)

Radiation Treatment

- Detox baths (**22**)
- NAC and antioxidant nutrients (**23**)
- Healthy high-quality diet (**24**)
- Energy bodywork (**25**)
- Homeopathic remedies such as *Cadmium sulphuratum, Ferrum metallicum, Ipecacuanha* (**28**)
- Herbal remedies such as algin, echinacea, ginseng (**29**)
- Organ cleansing (**31**)

their symptoms, cause complications after surgery, and slow their recovery. Even the latex gloves worn by surgical staff can cause skin rashes or other allergic responses for some patients.

The average hospital patient receives as many as nine prescription drugs during a hospitalization. Painkillers, antibiotics, diuretics, stool softeners, blood pressure medications, and other drugs may be given. Patients may have a reaction to a correctly prescribed drug, or an interaction between two or more drugs. Side effects often add to a patient's symptoms. For more details, see Medications, below.

Radiation Treatment

Radiation is used both for diagnostic and therapeutic procedures. Radiation treatment includes the administration of radioactive substances in the body, as well as X-rays.

Radioactive substances are also used in some diagnostic tests. The radioactive substance is injected into the bloodstream and its progress in the body is followed with monitoring equipment. Radioactive iodine is used in diagnosing thyroid problems, and radioactive thallium is used in special treadmill tests to monitor heart function and the viability of grafts from bypass surgery.

X-rays are used diagnostically to help visualize broken bones and to locate tumors and other pathology. X-rays are a form of ionizing radiation, that selectively damages dividing cells. In dividing cells, the DNA is uncoiled so it can be copied, and in this state is most susceptible to damage. Ionizing radiation can cause mutations in these cells that leads to cancer. For further discussion of ionizing radiation and X-rays, see chapter 18, Radiation, Electromagnetic Fields, and Geopathic Stress.

A very sophisticated diagnostic X-ray technique is the Computerized Axial Tomography Scan (CAT or C.T. scan). This equipment X-rays sequential "slices" to create a very detailed picture of the body. While it is a great diagnostic help, particularly for very deep tumors and other deep pathology, the X-ray exposure is quite high.

Debate continues over whether any dose of radiation is small enough to be safe. For this reason, it is best not to let a health professional X-ray you without good reason. Medical and dental X-rays and fluoroscopic examinations are excellent diagnostic tools when they are needed. Unfortunately, they are greatly overused in both the medical and dental professions. Be certain that your medical or dental care cannot proceed without an X-ray before you agree to one.

The one exception to this may be mammograms. The benefits of early detection of breast cancer may outweigh the dangers of exposure for women at risk for this disease. However, a number of false positives result from mammograms. It is important to be certain that the equipment used delivers low-dose radiation. Ask the technician or radiologist how many millirads of radiation are being delivered to the center of your breast. The amount should be in the range of 1,000 millirads. If it is higher than this, the mammogram should be done using more up-to-date equipment.

X-rays, radioactive cobalt, or radium are used to treat cancer. The radiation is directed at cancerous cells and offshoots so that the tumor is destroyed, but there is minimal damage to normal cells. Normal tissue should survive and recover from the treatment.

Radiation may be used to shrink a tumor before surgery. It may be the only possible

---

Chemotherapy

- Detox baths or sauna (chapter **22**)
- Antioxidant nutrients (**23**)
- Healthy high-quality diet (**24**)
- Exercise or bodywork as tolerated (**25**)
- Oxygen therapy (**26**)
- Homeopathic remedies such as *Arsenicum album, Cadmium sulphuratum, China, Nux vomica* (**28**)
- Herbal remedies such as astragalus, milk thistle, fennel (**29**)
- Charcoal packs, oral charcoal (**30**)
- Organ cleansing, particularly coffee enemas (**31**)

MOST EFFECTIVE DETOXIFICATION METHODS

---

treatment for some types of cancer that do not respond to chemotherapy. The newest equipment available has deeper penetration of tissue, and is better able to pinpoint the tumor with less involvement of surrounding normal tissue. Implants of radioactive substances are sometimes used to destroy tumors or localized skin cancers.

Chemotherapy

The term chemotherapy as it is used today refers to the treatment of malignant disease with cytotoxic drugs. Cytotoxic drugs are general cellular poisons that have a toxic effect on cancer cells and, hopefully, minimal effect on normal cells. Cancer chemotherapy is always a compromise between toxic and therapeutic effects. Chemotherapeutic drugs must reach the tumor and remain there in sufficient concentration long enough to kill the tumor cells. The route of administration must guarantee delivery to

Side Effects of Chemotherapy

Chemotherapeutic drugs often cause unpleasant side effects, which may include severe nausea and vomiting, loss of appetite, diarrhea, constipation, mouth sores, and an altered sense of taste. Some people may lose their hair and have impairment of both sight and hearing.

Neurological problems include seizures; nerve and ear damage; numbness of the hands and feet; and brain dysfunction with slurred speech, confusion, and coma. Liver and kidney damage can occur, and lung scarring is also possible. Blood and platelet counts are frequently lowered, and bone marrow is suppressed.

the appropriate site, and cumulative drug and organ toxicity must be considered.

Excellent results have been obtained from chemotherapy for a few cancers, including Hodgkin's disease, lymphomas, leukemias, and gestational choriocarcinoma. For most forms of cancer, though, the response to chemotherapy alone is poor. It can be a valuable adjunct to radiation therapy in some cases. However, proof of its effectiveness for many cancers is weak, and in some cases nonexistent. Damage to organs and bone marrow can prevent other, less toxic treatments from working.

■ CHEMOTHERAPEUTIC DRUGS

Chemotherapeutic drugs are intended to selectively kill tumor cells. They interfere with the synthesis or function of DNA and poison dividing cells. Unfortunately, nonmalignant cells are frequently killed as well. Classes of chemotherapeutic drugs include alkylating agents, antimetabolites, antibiotics, plant-derived agents, platinum-containing agents, and various antineoplastic agents.

Alkylating agents were the first class of

chemotherapeutic drugs, and were created from mustard gas. They combine with nucleic acids to disrupt cell replication. Although they are the most widely used chemotherapeutic drugs, they frequently fail because cancer cells readily develop a resistance to them. For this reason they are frequently used in combination with other drugs that have a different mechanism of action.

Antimetabolites closely resemble a necessary substance in the body, but when they are taken up by the cell, they disrupt cell function by interfering with metabolic pathways in the synthesis of nucleic acids. Both normal and cancerous cells take them up, however, disrupting the normal metabolic needs of the body.

Anti-tumor antibiotics inhibit DNA synthesis. They are natural products derived from cultures of various species of *Streptomyces* bacteria. However, they are too toxic to use against bacterial infections. They kill microbes and human cells, both normal and cancerous.

Plant-derived cytotoxic drugs include the vinca alkaloids, epipodophyllotoxins, and paclitaxel (Taxol). In their purified form, they are of limited use because of their extreme toxicity. These drugs interfere with DNA and RNA synthesis. Damage or destruction of white blood cells is common with this type of chemotherapeutic agent.

Platinum-containing agents bind to DNA and produce lesions in this genetic material. Tumors vary greatly in their sensitivity to the drugs, and kidney damage is the dose-limiting factor.

Antineoplastic agents consist of chemotherapy drugs that do not fit into any of the other classes. These drugs have varying modes of action, and the mechanism for some is either not known or is poorly understood.

Chemotherapeutic drugs are often given in combination to more effectively combat the resistance of cancer cells, to reduce the size of individual drug doses, and to combine different drug actions. By using drug combination, malignant cells are less resistant to the treatment and normal cells suffer less damage.

Medications

Pharmaceuticals, commonly called drugs or medications, are the main allopathic treatment for most health problems. A drug is any compound that modifies the way the body works, and can be used for prevention, diagnosis, or treatment of a disease. Because of the problem with "recreational drugs" and drug abuse, the word drug now has a negative connotation.

All drugs can become poisonous in high doses, but in low doses some poisons are useful drugs. There are many times when

> **Pharmaceutical Use**
> - Detox baths or sauna (chapter **22**)
> - Vitamin C, other antioxidant nutrients (**23**)
> - Juicing (**24**)
> - Exercise or massage (**25**)
> - Oxygen therapy (**26**)
> - Custom allergy extract or hands-on treatments for specific pharmaceuticals (**27**)
> - Homeopathic remedies such as *Avena sativa, Nitricum acidum, Nux vomica* (**28**)
> - Herbal remedies such as milk thistle (**29**)
> - Organ cleansing (**31**)

MOST EFFECTIVE DETOXIFICATION METHODS

drugs are the indicated therapy and they may be life-saving. The administration of adrenaline for anaphylactic shock and antibiotics for serious infections has allowed many people to recover and continue their lives. Many strokes have been prevented with blood pressure medication. Judicious and skillful prescribing of drugs has a justified place in medicine. However, the practice of treating with drugs is so universal that many people expect always to leave their physician's office with a prescription for some type of medication.

Unfortunately, there have been many adverse drug reactions to prescription drugs. Some reactions are caused by an allergic response. Others are caused by a wrong dosage or from a toxic combination of drugs. Very few studies have been done on drug interaction.

Drugs produce a rapid effect on the body. The magnitude of the effect of a drug de-

Words of Wisdom

The French satirist Voltaire (1694–1778) wrote that "Physicians pour drugs of which they know little, to cure diseases of which they know less, into humans of which they know nothing." While Voltaire was speaking of the physicians of his time, there is still some truth in his words today.

pends on how quickly it reaches high concentration in the bloodstream and target organs. When the blood concentration of a drug rises quickly, its effects are fast, intense, and usually last a short time. Under these circumstances, the effects are usually more toxic than therapeutic.

Most drugs are either extracted from plants or manufactured with synthetic compounds. Modern pharmacologists tend to believe that all the desired medicinal properties of the plant are specific to one chemical in the plant and they consider the other plant compounds as inactive. However, drugs refined from plants are more toxic than the plant source. For example, digitalis is a naturally occurring substance in foxglove from which digoxin is extracted. Digoxin is an extremely pure and potent form of digitalis. The plant extracts do not have the natural safeguards that modify the action of the medicinal portion of the plant. The plant compound is also more dilute and less soluble.

No drug has just one effect. Side effects accompany the medicinal effects of all drugs and must be weighed against the benefits. Drug toxicity is rated by a therapeutic ratio: the ratio of the minimum dose producing toxic side effects to the minimum dose producing desired effects. Most allopathic drugs have a therapeutic ratio of between 10:1 and 20:1. The smaller the number, the smaller the margin of safety. Many drugs have quite small margins of safety. For example, digitalis has a therapeutic ratio of 2:1.

Because of the nature of the drugs commonly prescribed, adverse reactions are inevitable. Drug reactions may include the following symptoms:

- skin rashes
- allergic reaction
- anaphylactic shock
- overgrowth of bacteria or yeast
- organ damage
- dizziness
- headache
- joint pain
- eye damage
- lung disease
- kidney stones
- seizures
- neurological symptoms

Over 60 common medications may cause photosensitivity, a skin reaction similar to sunburn. Prolonged or excessive exposure to direct or artificial sunlight must be avoided while taking these drugs. They include some diuretics, antidepressants, birth control pills, antihistamines, blood pressure medications, diabetes medications, anticancer drugs, sulfa drugs, and topical antiseptic creams.

Many drugs can cause drowsiness or dizziness and may impair a person's ability to drive or operate machinery. Activities may have to be curtailed while taking drugs causing this type of side effect.

Some drugs may cause symptoms of chronic toxicity if taken in excess over long periods of time. This is called a drug-induced disease. Reversing these effects is very difficult and frequently impossible.

Diet can also play a role in the effectiveness of drugs. Calcium- and iron-containing foods and products inactivate tetracycline, causing it to become insoluble and unable to be absorbed by the body. Anti-inflammatory drugs and narcotics must be taken with food or milk to reduce stomach upset. Alcoholic beverages must be avoided with many medications.

Iatrogenic illness is one that is caused by the actions of a physician. Drug reaction, drug interaction, the incorrect dosage, or even the incorrect drug are common causes of iatrogenic illness. The results can be severe, or even fatal.

Sometimes, problems with drugs are caused by the people who take them. Some people take the wrong dose, take borrowed medication, or take double doses because they believe "one of anything never does me any good."

As mentioned earlier, there are times when the use of drugs is indicated and necessary to save a life. However, frequently drugs seem to provide the "easy way out," controlling symptoms with the least amount of effort on the part of the patient. They seem to be a "magic bullet," but are not. Symptoms may be controlled, but the underlying problem is not corrected—and the body will need to detoxify the drugs in addition to coping with the original problem.

For many health problems, less toxic alternatives to pharmaceuticals are available. For example, blood pressure can be improved, if not completely controlled, with a

---

Drug Interactions

In addition to the toxicity of a drug and its possible side effects, drug interactions must be considered. Many people have more than one prescription that they take regularly. These drugs may have been prescribed by more than one physician. Drugs can interact with one another, each influencing the metabolism and absorption of the others. The interaction may make the drugs less effective and less long-acting, or more toxic with intensified action. When drugs are tested, they are tested singly and not in combination with other drugs.

---

specific nutritional program. The oxygenating properties of coenzyme Q_{10} can improve heart disease, while exercise strengthens the cardiovascular system. An herbal tincture of Crataegus can help reduce atherosclerosis. Bodywork can reduce edema and relax tight muscles that are causing pain. Vitamin C can clear some types of headache, and the homeopathic remedy Bryonia will relieve headaches that are worse with motion, including migraines.

Vaccinations

A vaccination is an injection or oral administration of a killed or attenuated (made less infective or virulent) organism or altered bacterial toxins, in order to produce immunity against that organism. The vaccine

Vaccinations

- Detox baths (chapter **22**)
- Vitamins B$_6$ and C, and calcium (**23**)
- Healthy high-quality diet (**24**)
- Allergy extract or hands-on treatment for the vaccination organism (**27**)
- Homeopathic remedies such as *Diptherinum, Ledum, Pulsatilla, Sulphur* (**28**)
- Herbal remedies such as milk thistle (**29**)
- Organ cleansing (**31**)

causes the body to produce antibodies that will protect the person if he or she is exposed to the disease later.

The first vaccinations routinely done were for smallpox. Since that time, vaccinations for measles, mumps, yellow fever, cholera, tetanus, typhoid fever, diphtheria, whooping cough, polio, and influenza have been developed. However, many of these diseases had essentially disappeared by the time the vaccines appeared. Improved sanitation, sewage disposal, water purification, and safe food distribution were instrumental in their decline.

Vaccination has often been presented as the only way to prevent and control some diseases. For example, it was thought that vaccination would eradicate smallpox. However, data from England give a different story. After smallpox vaccination became compulsory in England in 1853, many cases of smallpox caused death among the vacci-

nated. After the law was repealed and vaccinations stopped, the disease all but disappeared and the death rate from smallpox dropped to zero.

The end of the polio epidemic in the United States and Canada was credited to the polio vaccine. However, the epidemic ended in Europe at approximately the same time, and there was no vaccination program for polio in Europe. Cases of polio actually increased in the United States after mass inoculations began in 1955. When a live virus vaccine is used, the virus remains in the throat for one to two weeks and in the feces for approximately two months. The recipients of the vaccine are at risk, and they are potentially contagious as long as the virus is in the feces.

Similar statistics exist for nearly all the vaccines commonly used in North America. The diseases were declining and almost gone when vaccinations began. For example, the measles death rate had decreased by 95 percent before the measles vaccine was introduced in 1967. In 1981, an outbreak of measles occurred in Pecos, New Mexico. Seventy-five percent of those who contracted measles had been fully vaccinated, but the vaccinations did not protect the children. In other epidemics, a high percentage of the victims had also been vaccinated for the disease. For example, 95 percent of the whooping cough victims in a 1999 Los Alamos, New Mexico epidemic had been vaccinated.

In addition to the question of effectiveness, vaccinations may also cause numerous side effects. Fevers, rashes, soreness at the injection site, allergic reactions, and neurological symptoms have all been reported following vaccinations. In some rare instances, brain damage and death have occurred.

Carriers in vaccines are responsible for some of these problems. When a person is vaccinated, the organism or toxin is injected along with carriers for the vaccine material. These carriers include formaldehyde, thimerosal (a type of mercury), aluminum phosphate, monkey kidney cell culture, chick embryo, calf serum, and antibiotics. Some vaccines also contain contaminants from the monkey organs used to prepare the vaccines, including viruses such as SV40 (Simian virus 40). There is ongoing controversy over the role these viruses play in subsequent health problems of the vaccinated person. SV40 has been isolated from the stool of some people who received the oral polio vaccine. Several studies have demonstrated SV40 DNA sequences in some human cancers; other studies refute those findings.

Proponents feel that vaccinations have reduced the incidence of disease to its present low levels and that they are essential for the continued health of our children. Most people have little knowledge of the risks associated with vaccination. Both benefits and risks must be understood in order to make an informed decision.

Dental Work

Although needed regularly for good dental health, dental work can be a toxic exposure. The materials used in the mouth can be toxic, and the dental office itself may present a chemical exposure. With careful investiga-tion, it is possible to find a dentist whose office contains a minimum of chemical odors and contamination. In addition, there are dentists who specialize in helping their patients determine safe and compatible dental materials.

Office supplies, cleaning supplies, room deodorizers, and office furnishings can all be toxic to some people. In addition, such chemicals as formaldehyde, acrylic, phenol, nitrous oxide, and mercury are indigenous to most dental offices. Even low levels of these chemicals can be harmful, but mercury is the most toxic.

The personal care products of the dental staff and other patients can cause problems for some people. Tobacco-sensitive people must check for tobacco odors on the hands of the dentist and/or assistants. Even if faint, the odor can amount to a sizable tobacco exposure during the appointment.

Other toxic exposures from routine dental work can include latex, flavoring and coloring, X-rays, and local anesthetics. Most dentists and their assistants now wear latex rubber gloves to protect themselves from infections. Some dentists also use latex rubber dams in the mouth for various procedures. These constitute a toxic exposure for the latex-sensitive person. (See Latex in chaper 16, Chemicals and Metals, for a detailed discussion.)

Regular prophylaxis, or professional cleaning, to remove plaque and calculus by a dentist or hygienist is important for dental health. However, the polishing material used in the final step of prophylaxis is a paste of pumice, water, flavoring, and coloring.

The flavoring and coloring can be a toxic exposure to some sensitive people.

X-rays can be a toxic exposure, if they are done frequently. However, today's X-ray equipment is relatively safe. (For more information on X-rays and radiation, see Radiation Treatment, earlier in this chapter.)

Local anesthetics are a chemical exposure for all people, but may be a particular problem for chemically sensitive individuals. There are two chemical classes of local anesthetics. If a person is sensitive to an anesthetic in one of the groups, he or she is usually sensitive to all of the anesthetics in that group. Unfortunately, some chemically sensitive people do not tolerate any local anesthetics.

∎∎ DENTAL RESTORATIONS

Restoration materials present the largest toxic exposure in dental work because they become a relatively permanent part of the tooth or jaw. Dental restorations include fillings, crowns, inlays, and bridges.

∎ FILLINGS

The amalgam filling is the most common, but controversial, restoration material used. An amalgam filling contains approximately 50 percent mercury and 20 to 30 percent silver. Zinc, copper, and tin make up the balance. Studies have demonstrated that mercury leaches out of amalgam fillings. In one 1990 study by Vimy and Lorscheider at the University of Calgary Faculty of Medicine in Calgary, Alberta, mercury appeared in the organs and tissues of test animals within 29 days after amalgam fillings were placed in their teeth. High concentrations of the mercury were found in the kidneys and liver of the sheep used in the study.

Mercury is released in minute amounts, particularly when a person is chewing, brushing, or drinking hot liquids. Mercury is also released when an amalgam filling is polished as the final step in prophylaxis. For many people, mercury itself causes problems. For others, it may contribute to toxic overload.

The American Dental Association (ADA), Canadian Dental Association (CDA), and many individual dentists believe that amalgam fillings are safe. The ADA and CDA do admit that mercury leaches out of the fillings, but maintain that the mercury levels are too low to be dangerous. However, any amount of mercury is treated as a hazardous substance. When amalgams are removed, the dentist must dispose of them as hazardous waste. Mercury accumulates in the body, suppressing the immune system and damaging hormones and enzymes. It also damages the brain, thyroid, pituitary, adrenal glands, heart, lungs, and nervous system. (See chapter 16, Chemicals and Metals, for further information.)

When dissimilar metals are in the mouth, such as both gold and amalgam fillings, electric charges build up on the fillings. These charges are a result of the "battery effect" produced between the saliva and the different metals. Continuous exposure to these small currents stresses the endocrine glands and further depresses the immune system.

The usual alternative for amalgam fillings is composite fillings. They bond well with the tooth enamel and can be used for both front and back teeth. The composition of composite fillings varies with the manufacturer, but they are primarily ground glass powder with quartz fillers in a plastic binder. They may also contain methylmethacrylate or aromatic dimethacrylates with additives of urethane, diacrylate, vinyl silane, benzoyl peroxide, and benzophenone ether. Composites are either light or chemically cured, depending on their formulation. The light-cured forms are generally tolerated better by sensitive people.

Temporary fillings contain zinc oxide, eugenol, and trace amounts of alcohol, acetic acid, and silica. These fillings are used while crowns and bridgework are being prepared. The materials in these fillings are toxic to some people.

■ IMPRESSION MATERIALS
If you need a crown, bridge, or dentures, study models have to be made. An impression of your teeth or gums must be taken to prepare the study models. Some impression materials are polysulfide, silicone, or polyether rubber. The rubbers contain several compounds and oils to which people may react. Silicone rubber has less odor than the other rubbers used. The impression materials also contain alginate, flavorings, and colorings, which are harmful for some people.

■ CAST RESTORATIONS
Crowns, inlays, and bridges are all cast restorations. Gold alloy is frequently used to make them. Other metals in the alloy include palladium, silver, and trace amounts of copper, iron, indium, tin, and zinc. Some of these metals cause problems in sensitive

individuals, and nickel should not be a part of the alloy. The cement used to secure cast restorations in the mouth can also be toxic for some people.

■■ DENTURES
In addition to the exposures from impression materials, denture materials themselves can be a toxic exposure. The four basic denture materials include acrylic, vinyl, nylon, and polycarbonamate. Acrylic is the most popular and is used in the construction of both full and partial dentures.

Most acrylic denture materials contain methylmethacrylate, benzoyl peroxide, butyl phthalate, hydroquinone, and ethyl glycol demeth acrylate. Any of these ingredients can be allergenic and cause contact dermatitis and respiratory disease. Headache, arthritis, fatigue, and rashes have also been reported from exposure.

The amount of material used, proximity to soft tissues, and length of time they are worn makes dentures a haven for the yeast *Candida albicans*. At times it is difficult to determine whether problems with dentures are from the denture materials or from a *Candida* infection.

▮▮ ROOT CANALS

Root canal surgery can result in an increase of toxins. Recent studies by Dr. Hal Huggins of Colorado Springs, Colorado, as well as studies done in the 1920s by an American dentist, Dr. Weston Price, provide much evidence for concern. Anaerobic bacteria (bacteria that do not need oxygen to survive) remain in the tubules of the tooth's enamel and produce toxins. A tooth with a single root has over three miles of tubules, which can harbor many toxin-producing bacteria. If these toxins seep out of the tooth and into the body, a variety of symptoms and apparently unrelated health problems can result, including immune system suppression.

In young people and in teeth that have been killed by trauma, the chances of successful root canal surgery are relatively high. Those performed on abscessed or infected teeth have much lower success rates. It is a difficult choice because the only alternative to root canal surgery at present is the extraction of the entire tooth. If it is replaced with an artificial tooth, the materials used for the tooth and its implantation can be toxic for some people.

Cavitations can be another source of dental problems that are sometimes difficult to diagnose. Cavitations are actual holes in the jaw bone, containing necrotic bone, and frequently resulting from an extraction that did not heal properly. Bacteria become trapped and remain in the jaw as a chronic infection. As many as 20 to 30 species of bacteria infect cavitations. Toxins from these bacteria can cause numerous, serious health problems. Cavitations may also occur around root canal teeth. A thin, hard layer of bone over the area frequently prevents the cavitations from being visible on X-ray. EAV (electro acupuncture according to Voll) testing is the best diagnostic tool for cavitations. At present, surgical intervention to remove all the necrotic bone is the only available treatment, although other methods are being researched.

▮▮ BRACES

The braces used to straighten teeth can cause health problems for some people. The bands used on the teeth and the wires attached to them are usually metal, and may contain iron, manganese, nickel, chromium, molybdenum, and titanium, to which some people are sensitive. People may also be sensitive to the glue used to hold the braces on the teeth. Special rubber bands are used to help exert pressure on the teeth in order to move them, causing problems for people with a latex allergy. Even the pressure exerted by the braces can affect some people.

Vision care professionals have reported changes in eyeglass prescriptions after braces have been placed.

The retainers that are worn after braces are removed can also be a problem. They are made from acrylic and wire, which contains the same metals as braces. The acrylic material can cause headache, fatigue, and rashes.

▌▌ FLUORIDE TREATMENTS

Many dentists use fluoride treatments for both children and adults as a decay preventative. This is a controversial treatment. Some authorities feel it has no benefit after age 11, and others feel it benefits people of all ages. Fluoride combines with the tooth's calcium to form calcium fluoride, which is much softer than the normal calcium carbonate.

However, calcium fluoride is less soluble in acid and bacteria are less able to etch the enamel.

A growing number of scientists regard fluoride treatment as the administration of a poison because of the toxicity of fluoride. It has been shown to cause nerve damage and even death in animals that have ingested plants containing fluoride salts. At excessive levels, fluoride causes fluorosis, a condition characterized by bone abnormalities and mottled, soft teeth.

In addition, solutions used for the fluoride treatment contain coloring and flavoring agents to mask the flavor of the fluoride compound. These agents may also be toxic to some sensitive individuals.

CHAPTER 12

Toxins that Affect Children

CHILDREN ARE EXPOSED to toxins in the same ways that adults are exposed—in the home, at school, while traveling, while playing, and during medical treatment. However, the response of children to toxins can be quite different from the response of adults exposed to the same toxins for the same amount of time. In addition to the ways in which children are exposed to toxins, this chapter deals with the special responses of children to toxins.

Exposure Risks for Fetuses, Infants, and Children

An unborn child can be damaged before conception by injury to the sperm and egg, as well as by the mother's exposures during pregnancy. Sperm and ova begin their maturation processes approximately three months before conception. In their book, *The Case for Preconception Care of Men and Women*, Margaret and Arthur Wynn state that there are two periods of heightened vulnerability in developing sperm. The first is 80 to 90 days prior to conception, when ex-

posures of the father to chemicals or radiation can cause increased malformations in offspring as well as an increased risk of cancer. The second is immediately before conception. In the four and a half days surrounding conception, the ovum may be much more vulnerable to damage from toxic chemicals or radiation.

The fetus, newborn, and young child are far more susceptible to chemicals from the environment than are older children and adults. This is because of their larger surface area, rapid cell division, higher metabolic rate and oxygen consumption, and immature host defenses.

The fetus is most susceptible to the effects of chemicals. Developmental abnormalities and cancer that occur after birth can be caused by prenatal exposures. A fetus's detoxification systems are not fully developed and chemicals that can damage the fetus may not be toxic to the mother (for example, thalidomide). Excessive movement and hiccuping in utero are a signal that the fetus is overloaded and reacting to the mother's exposures to foods, chemicals, or biological inhalants.

The timing of the chemical exposure is critical. The first trimester is the time of greatest vulnerability because of the formation and rapid growth of limbs and organs. Unfortunately, many women do not realize they are pregnant during this time and are not careful about exposures.

Babies born to drug- or alcohol-addicted mothers will display growth and mental retardation, irritability and screaming, feeding problems, and failure to thrive. Exposure to second-hand smoke is detrimental both before and during pregnancy, as well as after birth. Prenatal exposure to this smoke increases the risk of miscarriage and several types of placental problems, and causes lower birth weights. There is more sudden infant death syndrome among the children of smokers.

Host defenses, including the immune system, the organs of defense (lungs, skin, and gastrointestinal tract), and the detoxification systems, are immature in fetuses, newborns, and children. Newborns also have immature kidneys, a major organ of detoxification. The immune system is not fully developed at birth, especially the production of immunoglobulins, antibodies that fight infection. Adult levels of IgG (immunoglobulin G) occur by age five to six years. The levels of IgM (immunoglobulin M) reach those of an adult by one year of age. The immune system gradually matures by 10 to 12 years of age.

Children have lower levels of the detoxification enzymes for Phase I and Phase II. Conjugation with glucuronic acid, a Phase II

> ## Bioconcentration in the Fetus
>
> *The mother's activities can seriously affect the fetus. For example, Dr. William Rea of the Environmental Health Center at Dallas, Texas, states that the mother may retain one part per billion of styrofoam if she drinks coffee from a styrofoam cup, whereas her fetus may retain two or three parts per billion. Bioconcentration can occur with many chemicals, increasing the toxic load of the fetus and causing vulnerability to new environmental exposures.*

enzymatic reaction, has been documented to be slower in newborns than in adults. This conjugation capability does not become mature until about three months after birth. The toxins hexachlorophene and PCBS are conjugated with glucuronic acid. Infants cannot detoxify these and other foreign chemicals efficiently until their conjugation capability has matured. (See chapter 5, Phases of Detoxification, for further information.)

▮▮ ABSORPTION OF TOXINS

The absorption of toxins from the respiratory tract is much higher in children than in adults. Children under five have a faster respiratory rate than do adults, breathing in twice as much air—and air pollutants—as an adult per unit of body weight. They tend to do more mouth breathing and bypass the nasal passages, which can filter out some of the particulate matter. Because they are

Methods for Children

- Detox baths or controlled sauna program (chapter **22**)
- Balanced nutrients (**23**)
- Healthy high-quality diet (**24**)
- Exercise or tolerated bodywork (**25**)
- Inhalation oxygen when indicated (**26**)
- Allergy extracts or hands-on treatment for any specific allergies (**27**)
- Homeopathic remedies (**28**)
- Bach Flower Remedies (**28**)
- Herbal remedies (**29**)
- Aromatherapy (**29**)
- Charcoal packs, oral charcoal (**30**)
- Compresses, packs, and poultices (**30**)
- Modified organ cleansing (**31**)

The absorption of chemicals through the gastrointestinal tract is higher in children than in adults. Children often eat food in contaminated areas such as the ground outside and while sitting on the floor. They tend to mouth objects, play in dirt, and spend more time on the floor and ground than do adults. This results in greater exposure to toxic metals such as lead, as well as solvents and pesticides. In addition, they do not always exercise good hygiene, sometimes failing to wash their hands after using the toilet, then putting their dirty hands in their mouths. Children may develop constipation, diarrhea, gas, bloating, and cramps as the result of chemical or dietary overload.

▌▌ METABOLIC RATE

Children have a higher metabolic rate than adults, and their cells divide more rapidly than those of an adult. They are thus more prone to cell mutations and the subsequent risk of cancer, evidenced by the long latency period for many cancers. Conversely, it has been suggested that the rapid growth of children allows improved opportunity for healing of cancers and that children may clear chemicals more easily than the elderly. However, it is known that exposure to many compounds in utero or early life exposure to these compounds, including vinyl chloride, nitrosodimethylamine (an industrial solvent), and ethylene-thiourea (a fungicide), increases cancer risk.

During the last six months of pregnancy and the first two years of life, the brain develops rapidly, causing children to be more at risk from neurotoxins than adults are. This rapid growth time is when the child develops

shorter than adults, they breathe in more dust, soil, and heavy vapors close to the ground.

Children also absorb a greater percentage of toxins from the skin than do adults. Relative to their weight, a child's body surface area is about three times larger than that of an adult. The skin of premature babies is much more permeable than that of adults. Drugs applied to the skin are absorbed two and a half times as much on newborns as on adults. The skin absorption of toxins can be increased by occlusion (prevention of skin breathing by plastic or similar substance) or when the skin is damaged. Diaper use causes skin occlusion, which allows increased absorption of any substance put on the baby's skin, and diaper rashes increase absorption even more. Eczema and dry scaly skin can be triggered by chemicals and food.

The Feingold Diet

The success of the Feingold diet in controlling neurological symptoms clearly demonstrates the effects of food additives on children. In the Feingold diet (developed by the late Dr. Ben Feingold, formerly of Los Angeles Children's Hospital), additives such as food coloring, flavorings, and preservatives are eliminated.

The guidelines for the Feingold diet include eliminating:

• Artificial food dyes and flavors (petroleum-based additives)
• BHA, BHT, TBHQ (petroleum-based preservatives)
• Salicylate-containing foods and non-food products

Symptoms such as bedwetting, asthma, frequent earaches, ADHD, and sleep disorders improved on the Feingold diet.

---

more than 75 percent of adult brain weight or size. Also during this time, nerve sheaths are becoming coated with a protective fatty substance called myelin. This process continues through adolescence. Chemical overload and food sensitivities can affect the brain, causing excessive activity, behavior disturbances, and learning disabilities. Approximately 15 percent of American children have been labeled as learning disabled.

Toxic Exposures

■■ FOOD

Children may be sensitive to many foods, just as adults are. Babies can be sensitized in utero to a food frequently eaten by the mother. Children who are breastfed may receive allergenic food molecules in the breast milk because foods their mothers have eaten cross over into the breast milk. Mothers must restrict their diets to prevent foods to which their child is allergic from being in their milk. Red cheeks and ears shortly after eating are a signal that a baby or small child has consumed a food allergen. Recurrent ear

infections, crying, colic, chronic runny nose, and sleep problems are other symptoms of food allergy in babies and children. The limited diet that some children eat also predisposes them to food allergies, because people who tend to become allergic sensitize to the foods they eat most frequently.

Food dyes appear to cross the blood-brain barrier more readily in children than in adults. Food additives and preservatives can have extreme adverse effects on children, targeting their nervous systems. Artificial sweeteners, such as aspartame, may have more effect on children than on adults. Aspartame can also be a potential problem for the unborn fetus. If the unborn baby has phenylketonuria, a disease in which phenylalanine (one of the building blocks of aspartame) cannot be broken down properly, the baby can be adversely affected by aspartame ingested by the mother. Women who have phenylketonuria and were diet-restricted (consuming very little phenylalanine) as children will invariably have a mentally handicapped baby if they do not limit their

Asthma

Asthma affects more than 4.8 million children in the United States and appears to be increasing. It is the leading cause of absenteeism from school. Between 1980 and 1987, the incidence of asthma among children went up 29 percent and deaths related to asthma increased by 31 percent.

In Canada and in Japan, as many as one out of five children has asthma.

ingestion of phenylalanine during pregnancy.

Children are often more sensitive to food poisoning than adults because they have higher exposure on a body weight basis. Children ingest greater quantities of food proportional to their body size, and they have repetitive eating habits. In January 1993, undercooked hamburger meat was responsible for an *Escherichia coli* infection in the states of Washington, Idaho, California, and Nevada. Children were more seriously affected than the adults, and all the deaths occurred among the children. (For more details, see Bacteria and Viruses in chapter 13, Food.)

❚❚ WATER

Children are affected by toxins in water more than adults are, because they absorb chemicals from the gastrointestinal tract at a higher rate. They also drink two and a half times more water per unit of body weight than adults. Children absorb a greater per-

centage of toxins through their skin when they swim or bathe. Any fat-soluble chemicals in water will be stored in their fat cells, accumulating over time.

Any microorganisms in the water will also affect children. They are more sensitive to intestinal parasites than are adults, because their digestive systems are not mature. Children and adults who work in daycare centers in North America have a high incidence of parasite infection. (See chapter 15, Plants and Organisms, for further information on microorganisms.)

Infants who consume only formula drink one-seventh of their own weight of water per day, equivalent to 2 gallons for a 155-pound man. Breastfed babies do not need to drink extra water, so they avoid ingesting contaminated water.

❚❚ AIR

Because younger children have higher respiratory and metabolic rates, they are very sensitive to the effects of air pollution (see chapter 14, Water and Air). Air pollution is one of the five worst environmental threats to children. They are particularly vulnerable when they are outside because they are three times more active than adults. They inhale more pollutants with their more rapid breathing. Some high-density pollutants, such as automobile exhaust, hover close to the ground, increasing the exposures of children. These toxic pollutants exacerbate asthma. Even children who do not have asthma can experience breathing problems and chest pain.

Asthmatic children may wheeze with exposure to such irritants as perfume, fireplace smoke, and cigarette smoke. Secondhand smoke affects non-asthmatic children as well. Children exposed to cigarette smoke have 50 percent more respiratory infections and a lower rate of increase in lung function as they grow older. Infants with smoking parents are more likely to be hospitalized for bronchitis and pneumonia in their first year of life. Children of smokers have more chronic coughs, ear infections, and behavior problems.

A study reported by Dr. Marvin Boris of New York at the 1985 annual meeting of the American Academy of Environmental Medicine showed that children who live in homes with gas stoves have 15 percent more respiratory problems and ear infections than children who live in homes with electric stoves. (See chapter 8, Toxins in the Home, for further information.)

■■ PLANTS AND ORGANISMS

Because most children spend time playing outdoors, their exposure to plants sometimes exceeds that of adults. Not only will they have skin contact with plants, but young children may taste or even eat plants while outside. Even among older children, their recognition of poisonous plants, such as poison oak or poison ivy, is low.

Children can be quite allergic to pollens, terpenes (naturally occurring chemicals in plants that give them their taste and smell), dust, dust mites, and mold. Playing outside increases their exposure to pollens and terpenes. Unless stringent dust and mold control is exercised in the rooms of sensitive children, they can develop symptoms that keep them from sleeping well. The stuffy nose that can result from these allergies

causes some children to have a horizontal crease across their nose that results from the "allergic salute," an upward swipe by the hand to wipe a drippy nose.

A high mold exposure is received when children play in the dirt, where many molds commonly grow. Playing in the dirt can also expose them to parasites that live in the soil. Children tend to put things in their mouths, including their unwashed hands, which increases exposures.

Bacterial and viral infections often affect children more severely than adults. Children tend to be more susceptible to ear infections, which are rare in adults, and are caused by bacteria and viruses. Often, inflammation caused by food sensitivities lowers resistance and increases the possibility of ear infections. Dr. Talal M. Nsouli of Georgetown University School of Medicine studied children with recurrent middle ear problems in 1994. The study showed that 80 percent of these children had food allergies, and most children were allergic to more than one food. Toddlers with chronic ear infections often have difficulty learning to speak correctly because their hearing is usually impaired, while older children may have difficulty in school for the same reason.

The difference in susceptibility between young children and adults is seen clearly with respiratory syncytial virus (RSV) infections. RSV is a lung infection that can make babies very ill. In adults and many children, it causes only a mild cold. Premature babies and babies with lung disease can develop serious symptoms, including wheezing and difficulty breathing. During a typical RSV season, which occurs from fall to spring,

Sensitive Newborns

Newborns are particularly vulnerable to chemical exposures. Many babies receive massive chemical exposures from their first bedroom, as they breathe in two to three times more air per pound of body weight than do adults. Nurseries for newborn babies are frequently freshly painted or wallpapered and have new carpet installed shortly before the baby is born or while the baby is still young. These materials outgas toxic chemicals for months, as does new nursery furniture. We have seen very sensitive infants who were born after their parents moved into a new mobile home or a new house. Mobile homes seem to be the worst, but any new home can be dangerous for infants.

90,000 babies and children will be hospitalized with RSV in the United States. Of this number, about 2 percent die each year.

(See chapter 15, Plants and Organisms, for further information.)

■ CHEMICALS AND METALS

Because of their larger body surface area relative to their body weight, children are more sensitive to solvents, pesticides, and other chemicals than adults are. In addition, children may inhale more solvent fumes because of their higher respiratory rate. Children should never be in the same area when solvent-containing sprays are used.

Children are very susceptible to the toxic effects of many common cleaning supplies.

For example, some furniture polishes contain mineral spirits, which are very poisonous and toxic to the liver. (See chapter 16, Chemicals and Metals, for further information on specific substances.)

Playing on the floor increases a child's exposure to pesticides used indoors, as they are usually sprayed along baseboards. Pesticide residues may linger on carpets and toys for weeks. Playing outside increases children's exposures to lawn chemicals and fertilizers, as well as pesticides. Rolling around on a lawn that has just been sprayed exposes the skin, eyes, nose, and mouth to toxic chemicals.

Recently, the U.S. National Academy of Science has recommended that changes be made to regulate pesticides used on food products to reflect the "unique characteristics of the diets of infants and children." Their report states that children may be uniquely sensitive to pesticide residues, in part because infants and children consume more calories per body weight and eat a smaller variety of foods than do adults.

The Academy also suggests that the Environmental Protection Agency should make decisions based on health issues rather than on agricultural production. The U.S.-based Environmental Working Group, a nonprofit research organization, reports that much of a person's exposure to pesticides occurs by age five, because children usually eat more fruits and vegetables in relation to their body weight than do adults. The group states that the average child receives up to 35 percent of his or her lifetime dose of some carcinogenic pesticides by the age of five.

Children are also exposed to many chemicals at school. While teachers are also affected by these exposures, children are often more strongly affected because of the differences in their physiology. School exposures are discussed in detail in chapter 9, Toxins in the Workplace and School.

As mentioned earlier in this chapter, prenatal exposure to chemicals can have adverse effects on the fetus. In the mid-1980s, the Michigan Maternal Infant Cohort Study assessed the effects of eating contaminated fish on pregnant women and their newborn infants. Mothers exposed to PCBS through eating the contaminated fish gave birth to babies of lower birth weight and smaller head size, which can be associated with developmental delay.

Developmental effects were still evident five to seven months after the birth of the infants and included depressed responsiveness, impaired visual recognition, and poor short-term memory at seven months of age. At four years of age, problems were still evident in the children, including deficits in weight gain, depressed responsiveness, and reduced performance on the visual recognition-memory test, one of the best validated tests for the assessment of human cognitive function.

Until the 1980s, the chemical compound hexachlorophene was widely used all over the world in antiseptic soaps and baby powders to prevent staph skin infections. It was found to cause neurotoxicity (damage to the brain) and death in premature and full-term infants. Their enhanced susceptibility to hexachlorophene was caused by their undeveloped skin barrier defenses, the large surface area available for absorption, an immature detoxification system, a poorly developed blood-brain barrier, and the application of the powder to inflamed areas such as the buttocks.

Lead poisoning is the most common type of metal poisoning in children. In part, this is because they absorb more lead from the gastrointestinal tract than do adults. It causes severe central nervous system effects in children and is associated with problems of cognitive function. Children may be exposed to lead in air, food, and water.

Before 1995, playing outside could increase children's exposure to lead contained in automobile exhaust. Lead is still in the soil both from past use of leaded gasoline and exterior paint residues. At one time paint contained lead, and many children who ate paint flakes developed lead poisoning. Although lead was banned in housepaint in 1978, some of this paint still exists in older buildings.

Children are particularly susceptible to mercury poisoning. In the 1950s, pregnant women in Minamata Bay, Japan, ate fish contaminated by methyl mercury from factory discharges into the water. The mothers often did not suffer adverse neurological effects, but their children were born with varying degrees of cerebral palsy. Even the mercury content of amalgam fillings may damage the health of children (see Dental Work in chapter 11, Toxins from Medical Treatment).

■■ NOISE, WEATHER, AND ALTITUDE
Noise is a toxin that can damage children's hearing. Some children are born with hear-

ing limitations caused by exposures in utero. Many children's toys emit loud noises above safe levels, and frequent or close play with these toys can damage their hearing. Older children tend to want to listen to music with headphones, which can cause permanent damage at higher volumes. Rock concerts are often injurious to their hearing. Children attending sporting events are adversely affected by the noise levels.

Children are affected by weather and many will react adversely to the influx of positive ions before a storm. Children in damp climates suffer more from mold allergies than children in drier regions. Those with pollen allergies will have more symptoms on windy days.

Children are also more sensitive to temperature extremes than adults because of their large body surface area compared to their body weight. Infants are particularly vulnerable to cold because they are not moving and generating extra body heat as much as older children and adults. In hot weather, children can dehydrate easily because of their larger surface area, and need to drink plenty of fluids. Some children tend not to want to drink water, preferring milk, juices, or soda pop, which do not rehydrate as well as water. Children who are dehydrated cry without tears, and have a dry mouth and decreased urine output.

Some children may be more prone to altitude sickness than adults. Smaller children and infants are more readily affected because of their higher respiratory rates and the lower oxygen levels at higher altitudes.

(See chapter 17, Noise, Weather, and Altitude, for further information.)

■■ RADIATION, ELECTROMAGNETIC FIELDS, AND GEOPATHIC STRESS

Radiation from the sun affects children easily. Infants and children should not be allowed to sunbathe and should be careful with overexposure to the sun. They have less melanin, which protects from the sun. Blistering sunburns in childhood are associated with melanoma (a skin cancer) in adults.

Children are also vulnerable to exposure to electromagnetic energy. For this reason, they should not sleep next to electrical appliances. Even a television set on the other side of the wall from their bed can adversely affect them. At least seven studies conducted in the U.S. since 1979 have demonstrated that there is an increase in childhood cancers among children overexposed to the alternating electrical current used in houses.

(See chapter 18, Radiation, Electromagnetic Fields, and Geopathic Stress, for further information.)

■■ NATURAL BODY FUNCTIONS

Like adults, children are exposed to internal toxins caused by the excess production or imbalance of metabolic body products. Older children who exercise frequently may experience muscle pain from the production of excess lactic acid. Children with a congenital defect in their urea cycle enzymes may develop an excess of ammonia, and children can develop an excess of free radicals by the same mechanisms that occur in adults.

Imbalances in neurotransmitters dramatically affect the behavior of children and their ability to learn. Increased activity, inability to sit still, difficulty concentrating, and an inability to stay focused can be symptoms of a neurotransmitter problem.

(See chapter 20, Toxins Produced in the Body, for further information.)

■■ TOXINS OF THE MIND AND SPIRIT

Unfortunately, children are not spared mind and spirit toxins, but are exposed to them just as adults are. Children can be targets for abuse in the household, including physical, emotional, psychological, and sexual abuse. Children whose parents were abused as children are at higher risk of abuse. Although abuse can occur in very subtle ways, its toxic effects are often deep and long-lasting.

We have seen several children in our office whose parents dislike them intensely. The parents sometimes verbalize this dislike in front of the children. They constantly harass and belittle their children in front of other people. There is no way that these children can feel secure and loved.

Children are subjected to a great deal of stress. Many children today have extremely hectic schedules, with various lessons and sports activities in addition to their schoolwork and programs. Sometimes it is the children who want and revel in these activities, but many times they are the desire of the parent. Activities are viewed by some as a babysitting substitute, while other parents attempt to fulfill their own needs through the activities and accomplishments of the child.

In addition to the stress of extra activities, many children are pressured to excel academically. If children are unable to meet these expectations, parents and sometimes teachers may criticize and belittle them. This pressure often costs the child a healthy sense of self-confidence and self-image when he or she cannot live up to parental expectations. This diminished sense of self-worth may stay with the child for life.

Children are also affected by the stress generated by their parents. Some people have very high-stress jobs and they pass their tension on to their families after work. Many parents have long work schedules, and children have to get up too early and leave home too early in the morning in order to accommodate the schedule of the parent. Children in daycare are often not picked up until dinnertime. Dinner is prepared in a rush and bedtime follows soon after, with almost no chance for parents and children to enjoy each other's company.

Not all relationships in a home are peaceful, and children are quick to pick up on the tension. Many even blame themselves for problems that may be only between their parents. Some children receive little or no nurturing because their parents seldom touch them or make them feel special. Parents may be so turned inward because of their own problems that they do not make time for their children and their needs. They may unintentionally, or unfortunately sometimes intentionally, make a child feel unwanted and in the way.

Children need the security of kind, but firm, discipline. Too many children receive very little discipline and guidance from their parents and grow up unable to recognize boundaries. Others are disciplined too harshly. Their punishment is out of proportion to their "crime." Sadly, love and consideration for others is not a part of some households.

Children learn by example and by emulating their parents. Some children do not have an acceptable role model to copy. Their parents may have poor parenting skills. Their personal lives may be less than exemplary, giving the child a poor example of moral code and behavior.

Although children are often thought of as resilient and expected to bounce back from exposure to toxins of the mind and spirit, many of them are scarred for life. Children from the same household can vary widely in their response to such toxins, as well as in their ability to recover. Adults sometimes assume that children are not adversely affected, and the children do not receive the help they need to detoxify. (See chapter 33, Detoxification for Mind and Spirit, for treatment suggestions.)

PART IV

Sources of External Toxins

EXTERNAL TOXINS are the toxins to which we are exposed in our everyday living. Indoor and outdoor air pollution, xenobiotics (chemicals foreign to the body), toxic metals, and poisons produced by plants or microorganisms are all external toxins. Substances from these sources are found in our air, food, and water. Other external elements, including radiation, electromagnetic fields, altitude, and weather, can also be toxic.

We normally try to minimize our exposures to these toxins. None of us deliberately drinks contaminated water, attempts to find the most polluted air to breathe, or eats spoiled or contaminated food. In our workplaces, if we realize a situation could be harmful to us, we try to avoid it. We do not knowingly pollute our homes so that they become toxic to us. However, many times we are unaware of hazardous situations or are unable to control our exposures. Even if we do not have massive exposures, small exposures over time add to our toxic burden.

In the following chapters, we will help you become more aware of the many exposure possibilities. We do not wish to alarm or frighten you, but to inform you, so that you can conduct your life in the safest, most healthy way possible.

CHAPTER 13

Food

MOST FOODS are healthy for our bodies in their natural, unspoiled state. However, they can become toxic with the growth or addition of contaminants and additives. Food contaminants include microorganisms and the toxins they produce, pesticides, and various other chemicals. Additives are chemicals that can be legally added to food, yet may still be toxic for many people. The hormones and drugs given to livestock become human toxins when we ingest them in our food. For people with food allergies, foods that other people eat without ill effects can be toxic, and even fatal.

Chemical Contamination

Food can be chemically contaminated in a number of ways, including:
- irrigation water used on crops
- pesticides and fertilizers used on crops
- toxic metals from sewer sludge used as fertilizer
- natural and synthetic organic chemicals, and radioactive substances
- the diffusion of small amounts of chemicals through the environment
- large-scale industrial accidents or waste disposal
- food packaging

The Food and Drug Administration (FDA), the Food Safety Inspection Service of the U.S. Department of Agriculture (USDA), and the Environmental Protection Agency (EPA) monitor food contamination in the U.S. In Canada, food contamination issues are monitored by the Health Protection Branch of Health Canada.

The FDA analyzes 234 food items for pesticides, toxic chemicals, industrial chemicals, and radionuclides. However, this amounts to only 1 percent of the food items sold, and current testing methods can detect only half of the pesticides used. Imported foods are analyzed for pesticides banned in the United States. The Global Environment Monitoring System (GEMS) of the United Nations analyzes food contamination from countries around the world.

Exposure to Chemicals in Foods, including Additives, Preservatives, Fertilizers, Pesticides, and Chemicals from Containers

- Saunas and detox baths (chapter **22**)
- Antioxidant nutrients including vitamins A, C, E; coenzyme Q_{10}; proanthocyanidins (**23**)
- High-quality, organic diet (**24**)
- Exercise and massage to mobilize toxins in cells (**25**)
- Oxygen therapy to relieve allergic reactions (**26**)
- Allergy extracts or hands-on treatment for chemicals in foods and food allergies (**27**)
- Homeopathic remedies such as *Zingiber* for contaminated food; *Arsenicum album, Phosphorus* for chemical poisoning (**28**)
- Herbal remedies for liver support such as burdock, milk thistle, rosemary, turmeric
- Charcoal therapy (**30**)
- Organ cleansing (**31**)

∎∎ PESTICIDE RESIDUES

American farmers apply roughly a billion pounds of pesticides to their crops annually. Pesticides, which include insecticides, herbicides, fungicides, and rodenticides, are dangerous because they linger in the environment and remain as residues on food. The FDA, the USDA, and the EPA regulate pesticides in the U.S. In Canada they are regulated by the Ministry of Environment. These agencies are responsible for registering new pesticides. The EPA has estimated that 60

percent of the currently registered herbicides, 90 percent of the fungicides, and 30 percent of the insecticides are potential carcinogens.

Unfortunately, the 612 active pesticides registered before 1984 were not adequately tested. If new evidence is found that a pesticide already in use is more dangerous than previously thought, the EPA initiates a Special Review. This process can take 12 years or more, during which the pesticide can still be used. The re-registration process is very slow, but 66 percent (402 cases) have now been completed. According to the EPA, products continue to be registered, while other products have been voluntarily cancelled, or the pesticide has been deregulated. When re-registration is complete in 2002, the EPA will begin a new program to review every registered pesticide on a 15-year cycle.

The United Nations Food and Agriculture Organization (FAO) and the World Health Organization (WHO) have developed Acceptable Daily Intakes (ADI), which are levels of pesticides that can be ingested over a lifetime without seeming to create a significant risk. The EPA has established a standard known as reference doses (RfDs), which have a safety factor of 100 percent in the calculations. The RfDs and ADIs do not always agree. None of these regulatory agencies have modified their calculations to account for the synergistic or inter-reactive effects of pesticides or chronic health problems. In 1996 the Federal Insecticide, Fungicide and Rodenticide Act (FIFRA) was amended by the Food Quality Protection Act to require that all pesticides meet new safety standards.

Some pesticides have been banned in the United States, the insecticide with DDT the best known. It was banned because it bioaccumulates in the food chain, with animals at the top of the chain the most seriously affected. Predatory birds were found to be most vulnerable, producing thin-shelled, easily broken eggs caused by the DDT they ingested. Although DDT was banned in 1973, all people in the United States have residues of DDT or its metabolite, DDE, in their fat tissue. DDT can still be found in the fatty tissue of such foods as meat, fish, poultry, and in dairy products, because it persists in the soil.

Other pesticide residues are also found in foods. Organophosphates are commonly used insecticides that inhibit acetylcholinesterase in humans and insects. This allows the neurotransmitter acetylcholine to accumulate, causing muscle twitching, cramps, anxiety, restlessness, and mental instability. Organophosphate residues may be found in grains and cereals.

U.S. manufacturers are currently allowed to produce pesticides that are banned, unregistered, or restricted as long as the pesticides are exported. Developing countries then use these pesticides, and up to 70 percent of the foods grown in these countries is imported back into the United States. High demands for produce have increased imports from countries where cleanliness and safety standards for produce are not as rigid. It is becoming increasingly rare that fruits and vegetables purchased in the U.S. have been grown there.

Pesticides represent a unique risk to children. They have higher metabolic rates and generally eat a higher percentage of

Most Contaminated Foods

The Center for Science in the Public Interest in Washington, D.C., has produced a list of the fruits and vegetables that are the most seriously contaminated by pesticides. They were compared by the amount of pesticide in the average serving size, and are ranked in order, with the most contaminated listed first:

- *strawberries*
- *cherries (grown in U.S.)*
- *apples*
- *cantaloupe (grown in Mexico)*
- *apricots*
- *grapes (grown in Chile)*
- *blackberries*
- *pears*
- *raspberries*
- *nectarines*
- *spinach*
- *peaches*

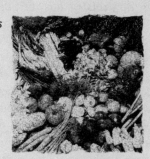

fruits and vegetables in their diet. This can cause them to be affected much more seriously by pesticides. (See chapter 12, Toxins that Affect Children.)

■■ CHEMICAL FERTILIZERS

Fertilizers are used on crops to replace the nutrient balance destroyed by commercial farming methods. Planting the same crop in the same fields year after year produces food

Early Puberty

In Puerto Rico in the spring and summer of 1982, there was an outbreak of early puberty in four- to five-year-old girls. When the children eliminated milk, poultry, and beef from their diet, most of the symptoms disappeared. Estrogens that had been given to animals to fatten them quickly were found to be the culprits.

that may look healthy and appealing, but that is in reality quite nutrient-deficient. This practice removes nutrients from the soil that are vital to the plants' growth. To compensate for the damage to the soil, farmers now rotate crops and apply artificial fertilizers that replace only nitrogen, phosphorous, and potassium. These fertilizers do not replace the lost organic content of the soil.

Consumers are often unaware of the deficiencies due to the attractive appearance of the food. Eating such food will cause people with borderline health or with existing health problems to become vulnerable to more problems because their nutritional needs are not being met.

Many farmers are now using fertilizers obtained from fertilizer manufacturers who have used industrial waste to make their product. While the idea of recycling waste is essentially good, many of these industrial wastes unfortunately contain toxic materials, such as dioxin, lead, and mercury. In investigative articles, the Seattle *Times* documented the nationwide use of arsenic, cadmium, dioxins, lead, radionuclides, and

other hazardous waste in fertilizer. According to the Environmental Working Group of Washington, D.C., between 1990 and 1995, more than 450 fertilizer companies or farms in 38 states received and used shipments of toxic waste totaling more than 270 million pounds. Many states have, as a result of the findings of the Seattle *Times* articles, either passed laws or have regulations pending that would limit toxic waste in fertilizer.

■■ HORMONES AND DRUGS IN LIVESTOCK

Cows, pigs, and poultry are fed hormones and drugs to help them gain weight faster and to mask signs of disease. The majority of North American pigs have pneumonia when they are slaughtered, and many of them are anemic and have ulcers from eating cooked garbage. Cattle often develop pneumonia when they are shipped in unheated trucks. Chickens are crowded indoors in abnormally large flocks without access to the earth or the sun. They are fed processed foods containing hormones and drugs. Even with the use of medications, the USDA estimated in 1992 that 40 percent of poultry is contaminated with *Salmonella*. (See Microorganisms, below.) Turkeys are raised in much the same way as are chickens, and in addition are treated chemically so that frozen turkeys are indistinguishable from fresh turkeys when they are thawed.

Nearly all animals raised as a meat source are given some type of hormone to obtain optimum weight in the shortest time. Pellets containing hormones that promote growth are inserted subcutaneously into the ear of cows, on the rationale that the ears

Pollution and War

During the 1999 bombing of Yugoslavia, bombs struck industrial plants, petrochemical complexes, and electrical transformers in which PCBs were being used as insulating materials. These and other chemicals, estimated to total over 18,000 tons, were released into the environment as a result of the bombing. They could endanger the health of millions of people in Yugoslavia and surrounding countries for years.

A high proportion of the chemicals was discharged into waters that feed into the Danube, a source of drinking water for several countries. These chemicals will also enter the food chain through soil and plant contamination, as people eat the plants, or eat livestock that has ingested contaminated plants.

are not likely to be eaten by humans. The hormones are slowly released into the animal's bloodstream. Since 1988, the European Community has banned imported U.S. meat raised on hormones.

Synthetic bovine growth hormone (BGH) is injected into about 10 percent of U.S. cows to stimulate milk production and to lower milk costs. The National Institutes of Health (NIH) have deemed this hormone to be safe for human consumption. However, opponents maintain that the quality and taste of the milk is adversely affected. They also argue that this synthetic hormone triggers an increased incidence of mastitis, an udder infection that necessitates increased use of antibiotics. The European Union Veterinary Committee, which considers that synthetic bovine growth hormone may be carcinogenic, has banned its sale in Europe.

Livestock ingest more than half of the antibiotics produced in North America each year. Antibiotics are intended to make the animals grow faster and more efficiently by limiting subclinical disease. Most animals

are given antibiotics right up to the time of slaughter, allowing no time for the drugs to clear an animal's system, so that residues will remain in the meat. Cooking does not destroy antibiotics and they may pass into the bodies of humans, causing such symptoms as nausea, diarrhea, and vomiting. Many sensitive individuals react to antibiotic residues in meat.

Because of their tremendous exposure to antibiotics, antibiotic-resistant strains of bacteria develop in the animals which can be passed to humans through the food chain or to humans caring for animals. Antibiotic-resistant bacteria is becoming a serious problem for people in North America. Attempts to regulate antibiotic feed additives in the United States have repeatedly failed, largely because of the lobbying efforts of farm groups and drug companies.

■■ INDUSTRIAL CHEMICALS

There are 210 polychlorinated biphenyls (PCBS) that have had numerous industrial uses, including use as solvents, solvent-carrier heat-transfer fluids, degreasers, dyes in manufacture, moth repellents, germicides, fumigants, insecticides, and chemical intermediates. The EPA banned the use of PCBS in 1977 because of widespread environmental contamination and persistence.

PCBs are still found in freshwater fish from contaminated streams: 20 percent of the fish in the United States is contaminated. Fish is not only consumed directly by people, but also fed to domestic animals. Meat, milk, eggs, and poultry have all been found to be contaminated with PCBS. Animal feeds and food-packaging papers can also be sources of PCBS. These chemicals are fat-soluble and concentrate in fatty tissue, and research has shown that a high percentage of people have PCBS in their fat tissue. PCBs have also been found in human breast milk.

Dr. Russell Jaffe of the Serammune Lab in Reston, Virginia, has reported significant levels of chloroform, carbon tetrachloride, and trichloroethylene in 16 nonorganically grown common foods. Chloroform was originally used as an anesthetic, but was extremely toxic. It is now used as a solvent and cleansing agent, particularly in the rubber industry. Chloroform levels were found to be highest in cheese, butter, potatoes, and tea.

Carbon tetrachloride was once commonly used as a solvent and stain remover. It is now used as a chemical intermediate under strictly controlled conditions. Levels of carbon tetrachloride were highest in butter and olive oil. Trichloroethylene is a solvent used in households, for dry cleaning, and for food extraction, such as the decaffeination of coffee. Butter, beef, and tea contained the highest levels of trichloroethylene.

▌▌ POLYCYCLIC AROMATIC HYDROCARBONS

Polycyclic aromatic hydrocarbons (PAHS) are chemicals that are formed from the incomplete combustion of other hydrocarbons (compounds containing hydrogen and carbon). The hydrogen is consumed, leaving the carbon in a condensed ring, "chicken wire" structure. These compounds are found abundantly in the atmosphere and soil from many sources, including engine exhaust, wood stove smoke, cigarette smoke, and charbroiled foods.

About 100 polycyclic aromatic hydrocarbons have been found in foods. Food that has been in contact with petroleum and coal tar products is contaminated with PAHS. All charbroiled and smoked foods contain PAHS, and seafood may contain PAHS from polluted water. These chemicals are of concern because they can be mutagenic (they change DNA) and carcinogenic.

Epidemiological studies in the United States and Europe have shown an association between consuming foods high in PAHS and gastrointestinal cancer. While some orally ingested PAHS are excreted in the urine and feces, many are absorbed. Absorbed polycyclic aromatic hydrocarbons have been found in the body fat, liver, adrenal glands, and ovaries as long as eight days after their ingestion. (See chapter 16, Chemicals and Metals, for further discussion of PAHS.)

▌▌ TOXIC METALS

Arsenic, cadmium, lead, and mercury have been found in food and all are potentially very toxic. (See chapter 16, Chemicals and

Metals, for further information on these and other metals.)

Arsenic is a natural constituent of soil and is found in many foods. It is also in the water and seafood, particularly shellfish, which contains the largest amount of arsenic. Foods contaminated by pesticides contain arsenic in the form of lead and calcium arsenate. Arsanilic acid is used as a growth additive in cattle and poultry feeds, and may enter the food chain in this way.

Cadmium enters the food chain through root crops and leafy vegetables fertilized with contaminated sludges. Fish, which is contaminated by polluted water, and organ meats concentrate cadmium. Cadmium is stored in the liver and kidneys. It has also been found in breast milk, thereby linking old pollution to new generations.

Food accounts for 55 to 85 percent of a person's lead exposure. Lead solder in cans used to be a major contributor, but its use has been banned since 1991. Some of the lead in food comes from industrial pollution that is released into soil and water and subsequently into the food chain. Bathing and drinking water can constitute a significant lead exposure in North America. Infants and children absorb more lead from food than do adults because the body absorbs lead more efficiently during periods of rapid growth. If the diet is lacking in nutrition, lead absorption also increases. The nutrient-deficient diet that many North American children eat contributes to increased lead absorption.

Fish and other seafood may be contaminated with methylmercury. This most toxic form of mercury is deposited in the brain, and can cause damage to the nervous sys-

---

Mercury in Tuna

The mercury content of the water around the Hawaiian Islands is so high that tuna weighing over 200 pounds cannot be used for food.

---

tem. Emotional disturbances, behavior problems, memory loss, depression, fatigue, lack of concentration, weakness, headache, and gastrointestinal disorders can result.

Microorganisms

Annual statistics regarding food-borne disease in the United States are alarming. The Centers for Disease Control (CDC) in Washington, D.C. estimates that 9,000 Americans die each year from food-borne illnesses, with many more becoming ill from bacterial, chemical, and pesticide residues found in foods of mostly animal origin. No one really knows the true impact of food-borne disease, as it is difficult to recognize. To be officially documented, there must be two or more persons with a similar illness, and a shared food must be implicated as the source of the infecting agent.

There are two main causes of food poisoning: toxins excreted by organisms in the foods, and the transfer of organisms in food to humans, where they then grow.

■■ BACTERIA AND VIRUSES

Bacteria, viruses, and protozoa can all cause food-related illnesses. Most cases of food poisoning can be linked to the presence of harmful bacterias.

The most common cause of food poison-

Baked Potato Scare

A 1994 botulism outbreak in El Paso, Texas was caused by potatoes baked in foil. Potato skins are covered with Clostridium botulinum *spores that can germinate in the anaerobic (low oxygen) conditions allowed by the foil. The potato skin in foil does not get hot enough during baking to destroy the spores, and when the potatoes cool in the absence of air, the spores germinate. Eating the potato soon after cooking, refrigerating foil-wrapped potatoes soon after baking, or baking potatoes without foil prevents the problem.*

ing is *Staphylococcus aureus,* which produces six exotoxins (toxins loosely associated with the bacterial cell). Staphylococcal food poisoning causes nausea, vomiting, diarrhea, gastrointestinal pain, dizziness, and headache. Symptoms appear from 1 to 11 hours after ingestion of the contaminated food and last for 24 to 48 hours.

The foods most frequently contaminated with *Staphylococcus aureus* are meats, cooked ham, milk, and cream-filled bakery goods. Staphylococcal toxins develop in foods at temperatures between 42°F and 130°F. To avoid food poisoning, foods must be refrigerated well within the incubation time (less than four hours). Food that has been frozen, reheated, then refrozen is especially at risk for the growth of staphylococcal bacteria. Boiling kills the bacteria, but will not destroy the heat-stable toxin.

The toxin produced by the bacteria *Clostridium botulinum* is one of the most dangerous to people. It triggers a disease called botulism, which paralyzes the eye, throat, laryngeal, and respiratory muscles. Paralysis of the voluntary muscles, as well as dry mouth, constipation, and urinary retention are other symptoms. Symptoms appear from 12 hours to 10 days after ingestion of the contaminated food. The mortality rate in the past has been as high as 60 to 80 percent, but is now less than 10 percent. Boiling food for 5 minutes or heating at 176°F for 30 minutes will destroy the toxin.

Clostridium botulinum grows in sealed, low-acid food preparations, usually during storage, and causes no change in the color or taste of the food. Home-canned foods, smoked fish, and occasional faulty, commercially canned foods have caused outbreaks of botulism. Infants have developed botulism from eating honey; it is recommended that infants less than one year of age not be fed honey.

Foods may also introduce bacteria into the body, where they then multiply. The most common infections, from *Salmonella,* cause fever, nausea, abdominal cramps, diarrhea that may be bloody, headache, dizziness, and vomiting. This type of food poisoning can be fatal. Symptoms appear 4 to 24 hours after ingestion. *Salmonella* may be found in eggs, poultry, milk and milk products, vegetables, dried coconut, baked goods, and cocoa. Insects, poultry, rodents, and even humans can be carriers, without showing symptoms themselves. *Salmonella* is destroyed by high heat, and thorough cooking of food will help prevent this type of food poisoning.

Bacteria That Infect Food

BACTERIA	SOURCES	SYMPTOMS
Bacillus cereus	Cereals, dried foods, herbs, spices, vegetables, dairy products, meats, meat products	Vomiting, diarrhea, possible fever
Campylobacter jejuni	Raw poultry, meat, raw or inadequately heat-treated milk, water	Fever, abdominal cramps, diarrhea, vomiting
Clostridium botulinum	Smoked fish, canned foods, sealed low-acid foods, honey	Paralysis of eye and respiratory muscles and voluntary muscles, dry mouth, constipation, urine retention
Clostridium perfringens	Meats, poultry, dried foods, spices, herbs, vegetables	Abdominal cramps, diarrhea
Escherichia coli	Undercooked beef, salami, raw milk, unpasteurized apple cider, mayonnaise, cantaloupes, water, vegetables grown in cow manure	Bloody diarrhea, abdominal cramps, vomiting, possible fever
Listeria monocytogenes	Meats, poultry, dairy products, shellfish, vegetables	Focal infections, sepsis, pregnancy infections, encephalitis, cerebritis
Salmonella	Eggs, poultry, dairy products, vegetables, dried coconut, cocoa, baked goods	Fever, nausea, vomiting, abdominal cramps, diarrhea, headache, dizziness
Staphylococcus aureus	Meats, cooked ham, milk, cream-filled baked goods	Nausea, vomiting, diarrhea, gastrointestinal pain, dizziness, headache
Vibrio parahaemolyticus	Fish, shellfish	Abdominal cramps, diarrhea, vomiting
Yersinia enterocolitica	Milk, tofu, pork	Fever, abdominal cramps

E. Coli

In 1993, contaminated beef caused a mass outbreak of an Escherichia coli infection from fast-food hamburgers. Cattle feces at the slaughterhouse had contaminated the beef in the hamburgers, and undercooking allowed the consumption of live organisms. More than 500 people from Washington, Idaho, California, and Nevada developed hemorrhagic colitis with bloody diarrhea, severe abdominal cramps, occasional vomiting, and low-grade or no fever. Four children died from the infection.

Escherichia coli is normally a beneficial bowel bacteria, but pathogenic mutant strains can cause serious illness, even death. These mutant strains are being produced by feeding antibiotics to animals. The bacteria become antibiotic-resistant and very difficult to treat. The U.S. federal meat inspection rules have now been changed to zero tolerance for feces and ingesta (food from the stomach) on meat. The FDA recommends cooking ground beef to 155°F to prevent illness from this strain of *E. coli*. This bacteria can be transmitted from contaminated water, beef, salami, raw milk, unpasteurized apple cider, mayonnaise, cantaloupes, and vegetables grown in cow manure.

Raw sprouts are another frequent source of foodborne illness, with *Salmonella and Escherichia coli* being the most common infecting organisms. Most illnesses have resulted from eating alfalfa and clover sprouts, but all raw sprouts can contain toxic bacteria. The sources of the infecting organisms are thought to be contaminated seeds or contaminated water used to sprout the seeds. These illnesses are usually self-limiting in healthy adults, with diarrhea, nausea, abdominal cramping, and fever lasting for several days. An *E. coli* infection can lead to hemolytic uremic syndrome, with kidney failure or death in children and serious complications in the elderly. *Salmonella* causes serious illness in children, the elderly, and the immunocompromised. Since 1997, there have been 263 cases of salmonellosis from alfalfa/clover sprout mixtures in California, Colorado, Oregon, and Washington. Eight cases of illnesses attributed to *E. coli* from consumption of alfalfa/clover sprouts have occurred in California and Nevada.

■■ PROTOZOA

Shellfish sometimes harbor a paralysis-causing toxin produced by dinoflagellates, a marine protozoan. Mussels, clams, and other shellfish accumulate the protozoa from seawater. The toxin is called paralytic shellfish poison, and it depresses respiration and affects the heart, causing complete cardiac arrest. As little as 4 mg of this toxin can be fatal to a human.

When the population of the protozoa is very high, the surface of the ocean may turn reddish from their color. A "red tide" closure is invoked, prohibiting the harvesting of shellfish from affected areas.

■■ MAD COW DISEASE

The practice of feeding cows animal scraps from slaughterhouses may have led to "mad cow" disease (bovine spongiform enceph-

Danger in a Mug

An unlikely source of organisms in food is the coffee cup. Ceramic mugs harbor bacteria, and plastic mugs with lids are even worse. People usually drink their coffee or tea slowly throughout the day, often leaving a little liquid on the bottom. Sometimes food particles find their way into the coffee. A 1998 University of Arizona study by Drs. Ralph Meer and Charles Gerba showed that these conditions cause a variety of bacteria to multiply in the mugs. These bacteria include Escherichia coli *and other coliform bacteria, indicating poor hygiene. The bacterial count in mugs wiped with communal sponges or dishcloths dramatically increased after cleaning. Washing mugs with soap and water and then drying them is necessary to prevent the bacteria from growing.*

alopathy) in Britain. This protein feed, intended to increase growth rates, was manufactured using material from healthy as well as diseased animals, including brain and nerve tissue. The organism causing the disease is not fully understood and is still being investigated. In some ways the agent is virus-like, and in others it is like a self-replicating protein, referred to as a prion.

To date, approximately 168,000 British cattle have died from this disease. Some humans who ate contaminated beef may have developed Creutzfeldt-Jakob disease (CJD), which is fatal. There is controversy over the possible link of bovine spongiform enceph-

alopathy and CJD. With an incubation period of five to ten years for CJD, it is difficult to assess the relationship between the two diseases. CJD begins with psychiatric symptoms, frequently depression, early in the illness, and is followed by painful sensory symptoms. As the disease progresses, neurological signs appear, including unsteadiness and involuntary movements. Shortly before death, patients become completely immobile and mute.

Nearly all animals in North America raised for human consumption are fattened on rendered products that may contain many disease-causing components in addition to heavy metals, pesticides, plastics, pharmaceuticals, and other chemicals. Minimal inspection is done on the products of the rendering plants, and tests only truth in labeling for the percentage of protein, phosphorous, and calcium.

■■ MYCOTOXINS

Toxins produced by molds are called mycotoxins. The *Aspergillus* genus of mold, including *A. flavus* and *A. niger,* produce several aflatoxins, the best-known mycotoxins. The toxin produced by *A. flavus* is a heat-stable carcinogen commonly found in peanuts. These molds also grow on cereal grains, rice, apples, milk, corn, nuts, and oil seeds. Aflatoxins can cause internal bleeding and are potent liver toxins and carcinogens for most species.

Ergot alkaloids are another type of mycotoxin, produced by *Claviceps purpurea* when it grows on rye. This mycotoxin causes central nervous system disorders called ergotism. When harvesting was delayed during

MOST EFFECTIVE DETOXIFICATION METHODS

**Exposure to Foods
Contaminated by Organisms**

- Saunas or detox baths (chapter **22**)
- Vitamin C, zinc, and other nutrients to support the immune system (**23**)
- Oxygen therapy and oral hydrogen peroxide therapy (**26**)
- Allergy extracts or hands-on treatment for specific organisms (**27**)
- Homeopathic remedies such as Arsenicum album, Ipecacuanha, Lycopodium, Zingiber (**28**)
- Herbal remedies such as angelica, barberry, burdock, chamomile, echinacea, garlic, goldenseal, meadowsweet, and mullein (**29**)
- Charcoal therapy to absorb toxins (**30**)
- Organ cleansing (**31**)

World War II, allowing time for mold to grow, many grains in Siberia were contaminated by *C. purpurea*. People consuming this grain suffered gastrointestinal symptoms, internal hemorrhage, and skin rashes. About 10 percent of the people who ate infected grain died.

■■ FOOD SPOILAGE

Fresh or raw foods normally carry a bacterial population. The type and amount depend on the food, pH, handling, temperature, and time from harvest or slaughter to use. Bacteria destroy cell walls in the food. Enzymes released from cutting and bruising, or from destruction of normal inhibitors, further contribute to deterioration of the food. Nausea, vomiting, diarrhea, and even food poisoning can result from eating spoiled foods.

The spoilage of fresh food is usually obvious, and the consumer can avoid these foods. Dairy products and fish are the most sensitive to spoilage.

Fish is caught, pitchforked, packed in ice for up to 10 days, loaded onto scales, and then onto carts. Fish readily decompose from the action of both enzymes and bacteria. As they age, fish develop a "fishy" odor caused by trimethylamine. When fish spoils, it smells like hydrogen sulfide (or rotten eggs).

Food Additives

At least 2,800 substances are used as food additives, and an average North American consumes about 150 pounds of these substances each year. These additives are added by food processors to thicken and add pliability to foods, to provide leavening, to retard spoilage, to enhance flavor and coloring, and to boost nutritional value (an attempt to replace vitamins lost in processing).

■■ GRAS LIST

In 1958, the Generally Recognized as Safe (GRAS) list was generated by the U.S. Food and Drug Administration from a list of additives in current use. Although the list was circulated to approximately 900 American scientists, just 355 responded, with only 100 making substantive comments. Substances on the GRAS list are those for which no complaints have been filed about an illness related to their ingestion. Once a substance is listed as GRAS, it is not subject to specific regulations, other than for the manufacturer to use appropriate processes.

The Food and Drug Administration

(FDA) did not start to review the scientific literature on GRAS substances until 1969; by 1987 it had reviewed fewer than 500 substances. The Delaney Clause, which is part of the Food Additives Amendment, states that "no additive shall be deemed safe if it is found to induce cancer when ingested by man or animal." However, the FDA ignores potential cancer-causing additives if they are associated with what they consider an insignificant risk to the population eating the food.

In order to save time and money, since 1997 the FDA has allowed manufacturers to notify it of the GRAS status of the additives they are using and to provide some evidence to support it. The current philosophy of the FDA is that allowing the manufacturer to determine what is generally recognized as safe, and making it simpler to obtain FDA approval, will allow the FDA to gain increased awareness of ingredients in the nation's food supply and the cumulative dietary exposure to GRAS substances.

FOOD COLORS

In 1960, the Color Additives Amendment was added to the United States Food, Drug, and Cosmetics Act. Food colors are rigorously tested before the FDA can certify them. Only seven synthetic colors may be legally added to food. Most of these colorings can be allergenic, however, particularly tartrazine (Yellow No. 5). It has been found to cause allergic reactions, especially in people sensitive to aspirin.

High doses of approved synthetic colors cause cancer in animals. In spite of these problems, food manufacturers prefer syn-

Styrofoam Cups

Even temporary food containers can be a source of toxins. Hot coffee and tea will leach chemicals from a Styrofoam cup into the beverage. Phenol-sensitive individuals can react to these chemicals.

thetic dyes to natural dyes because they give more uniform and more intense color.

EXCITOTOXINS

Some food additives are considered to be "excitotoxins" that can play a role in the development of several neurological disorders, including seizures, abnormal nerve development, learning disorders, migraines, neuropsychiatric disorders, as well as neurodegenerative diseases such as ALS, Parkinson's disease, and Alzheimer's disease. Most excitotoxins are amino acids that react with specialized receptors in the brain to destroy certain types of neurons (nerve cells).

Over 75 of these compounds have been identified, including monosodium glutamate (MSG), and aspartame. MSG can be disguised on labels as hydrolyzed vegetable protein, vegetable protein, textured protein, hydrolyzed plant protein, soy protein extract, caseinate, yeast extract, and natural flavoring.

Over 100 million North Americans consume aspartame, and a greater number consume foods containing one or more excitotoxins. Many of these toxins are in almost all

Common Food Additives

ADDITIVE	EFFECTS
Sucrose, corn syrup, dextrose	Cause problems for people with allergies, diabetes, hyperinsulinemia
Sodium chloride (table salt)	Can cause high blood pressure for people who are salt sensitive
Black and white pepper	Allergenic
Caramel	Classified as GRAS, but some people do not tolerate
Carbon dioxide	Can cause shortness of breath, vomiting, high blood pressure, disorientation
Citric acid	Classified as GRAS, but some people do not tolerate
Modified starch	Chemicals used to modify thickening properties can cause sensitivities
Sodium bicarbonate (baking soda)	Classified as GRAS
Yeasts	Allergenic
Yellow mustard	Classified as GRAS, but some people do not tolerate
Calcium sulfate or plaster of Paris (a firming agent)	Ingestion of large amounts can cause intestinal blockage
Calcium phosphate (dough conditioner, firming agent)	Classified as GRAS
Sodium nitrate (in processed meats)	Reacts with other chemicals and foods to create nitrosamines (carcinogens)
Sodium sulfate (in chewing gum base)	Can stimulate gastric mucus production and inactivate pepsin (a digestive enzyme)
Lactic acid (used to acidify foods)	Caustic in concentrated form

**The additives above the double line represent 95%
of the total quantity of food additives used in North America.**

processed foods. Excitotoxins have an effect on the developing brain, and injury from these substances is of particular concern from fetal stage to adolescence. Because the placenta concentrates several of these excitotoxins in the fetus, pregnant women should avoid both aspartame- and MSG-containing products. Many effects of these toxins may not be evident until the child is older and may include immune alterations and loss of the ability to control violence.

■ PRESERVATIVES

Numerous preservatives are added to foods to kill or inhibit the growth of microorganisms and to prevent spoilage by oxidation. Preservatives prevent changes that affect color, flavor, texture, or appearance. All preservatives have the potential to cause problems for sensitive people. About 100 "antispoilant" chemicals are used, including:

• Antioxidants: preservatives for fatty products to prevent off-flavors and off-odors in margarine, lard shortenings, crackers, and potato chips.
• Mold inhibitors: preservatives used in breads, cheeses, syrups, and pie fillings.
• Fungicides: prevent mold and fungus growth on citrus fruits.
• Sequestering agents: prevent physical or chemical changes that affect color, flavor, texture or appearance in soft drinks, and foods such as dairy products.
• General-purpose preservatives: include sulfur dioxide, propylgallate, sugar, salt, and vinegar.

At one time, sulfites were widely used in the United States to keep raw vegetables and fruits in salad bars looking fresh. This practice has been banned because of adverse reactions in asthmatics. In addition, the use of sulfites destroyed some vitamins in foods. However, they are still used on dried fruits and other foods. BHA (butylated hydroxyanisole), which has been linked to cancer, and BHT (butylated hydroxytoluene), which can affect kidney function, are other frequently used preservatives.

Food Packaging Materials

Polyvinyl chloride, which is made from vinyl chloride, a known carcinogen, and acrylonitrile, a suspected carcinogen, are composed of small organic chemicals that are heated into resins at high temperatures. They are found in containers for margarine and cooking oil, food packaging films, bottle closure liners in soft drinks, and the liner in foil-wrapped candies. Acrylonitrile can be trapped in the resin and will diffuse into food during storage. It was also used as a fumigant for foods until 1978. Levels of vinyl chloride are monitored in Britain and have been declining in recent years, but the United States does no monitoring of dietary exposure to vinyl chloride. The amount of acrylonitrile in the average North American diet has not been estimated.

Food containers may be oiled and treated with various chemicals, including pesticides and acrylics, that can then leach into food. Toxic chemicals also migrate into food from plastic storage containers. Phthalates are added to plastics to keep them pliable. Organophosphates similar to organophosphate pesticides are used in large amounts in plastic. Both phthalates and organophosphates leach from the walls of plastic containers, contaminating fluid contents. Water and milk are frequently bottled in plastic containers, and may be contaminated by these substances.

In addition to being contaminated by containers, food is inadvertently contaminated through its packaging by being sold or stored in close proximity to toxic products in supermarkets and shopping malls. The Committee for Universal Security from Santa Cruz, California, has found that foods are absorbing high levels of pollutants by being in the same building with such non-foods as household cleaning supplies, motor oil, shoe polish, detergents, waxes, and furniture polish. Chemicals from dry cleaners can contaminate foods through their packaging as far as a mile from the source, and auto garages, shoe repair shops, electronic stores, and repair shops are among other businesses that can cause serious toxic problems for nearby food stores.

Food Preparation

In some cases, toxins are inadvertently added to foods by their method of preparation. For example, if food is microwaved in soft plastic containers, chemicals from the plastic will migrate into the food. In addition, there is much controversy about the overall safety of microwaving food, which heats the food from the inside out. Some scientists maintain that microwaving changes the structure of food molecules and impairs its quality, whether the food is being cooked or just warmed. They claim that microwaving alters food chemistry and adversely affects people consuming the food, chang-

ing their blood chemistry. Other scientists maintain that while cooking food in a microwave does damage the structure of the food, warming cooked food in a microwave is acceptable.

While frying foods may contribute to the taste and texture of food, it also changes the fat to harmful forms. When oil is allowed to sizzle before adding food, usually at temperatures between 160° and 220°C, both temperature- and light-catalyzed oxidation reactions take place rapidly. Light activates oxygen to form free radicals that start a chain reaction. (See Free Radicals in chapter 20, Toxins Produced in the Body.) Trans-fatty acids, which the body cannot use, are also produced during frying. Oils kept at 215°C for 15 minutes or more consistently produce atherosclerosis in experimental animals. In commercial deep-fat frying vats, the same batch of oil is often kept at a high temperature for days.

Highly refined oils in transparent bottles on supermarket shelves have been degraded by light, have lost most of their nutrient value during refining processes, and are made from the cheapest oils. They are frequently from the most intensely pesticide-sprayed plants, cottonseed oil being one of the worst. These oils are not acceptable for frying. Frying is one of the least healthy methods of food preparation. When frying cannot be avoided, saturated oils (solid fats) are more stable in the presence of light, heat, and air, and will deteriorate less during frying.

Charbroiling or grilling meats and fish over an open flame in which there are fat drippings causes a deposition of polycyclic aromatic hydrocarbons (PAHS) on their surfaces (see above). Significant amounts of PAHS were found on thick T-bone steaks cooked close to the coals for long periods of time. Benzo[a]pyrene is a common PAH in foods, and is found in charcoal-broiled meats, broiled sausage, smoked foods, and roasted coffee. Commonly smoked foods include fish, meat, fowl, and cheeses. Home-smoked or charcoal-broiled foods may contain more PAHS than commercially smoked goods.

Barbecued meats contain several toxins. These meats have been charcoal-grilled with a barbecue sauce spread over their surfaces. In addition to the PAHS deposited during cooking, the sugars in the sauce become charred, which increases their carcinogenic properties. The oil in the barbecue sauce is also changed to a harmful fat. (See Part VII, Prevention, for suggestions on healthy food preparation methods.)

Genetically Modified Foods

Genetically modified (GM) foods are foods that have been genetically engineered to contain a beneficial gene from another species, including other plants, animals, bacteria, and viruses. A gene from another organism is implanted into the plant to provide benefits or improvement, including increased shelf life, decreased need for pesticides, and enhanced nutritional value.

There is much opposition to GM foods in Europe and they are being withdrawn from European supermarkets. In North America at this time, GM foods do not have to be tested for safety and do not have to be labeled. Supermarkets and natural foods re-

Allergens and GM Foods

Not knowing what genes are contained in foods can be very dangerous, particularly for people with allergies. For example, in 1996, genes from Brazil nuts were implanted into soybeans to make them taste nuttier. People who were not allergic to soy, but were allergic to Brazil nuts, reacted violently to the GM soy.

tailers do not know what percentage of their goods contains GM material.

Genetically modified corn and soy have been on the market since 1996. It is estimated that in 1999, 55 percent of the U.S. soybean harvest and 33 percent of the corn crop were GM foods. Other GM crops include potatoes and tomatoes. Genetically modified foods are present in many different foods, including powdered infant formula, pasta, muffin mixes, soft drinks, cooking oils, taco shells, and veggie burgers.

Vyvyan Howard of the University of Liverpool states that the results of GM food testing has shown that the main risk of ingesting GM food is "long-term, low-dose toxicity from subtle changes to the nature of the food chain." Genetic modification can cause unpredictable outcomes. Viral promoters, in the cells of the host plant, which are mechanisms used to switch on the implanted genes, may switch off beneficial genes. Crops would have to be examined on a case-by-case basis, as extrapolation from one to another could be misleading. Standard testing cannot demonstrate the types of problems that are a concern with GM foods.

Reactions to Foods

Food allergies can cause toxic reactions. There are two types of food allergies, both mediated by special antibodies called immunoglobulin G (IgG) and immunoglobulin E (IgE). IgE-mediated food allergies cause life-threatening anaphylaxis (allergic shock), with swelling of the throat, tightness of the chest, and low blood pressure. IgE reactions occur within minutes to several hours after ingesting food.

IgG-mediated food allergies account for about 85 percent of food allergies. A delayed reaction can occur as long as 24 hours after consuming the food. IgG food allergies can cause chronic headaches (often migraine), chronic indigestion, heartburn, fatigue, depression, joint pain, recurrent abdominal pain, canker sores, chronic respiratory symptoms such as wheezing or bronchitis, bedwetting, and bowel symptoms such as diarrhea or constipation.

Many common foods can trigger allergies and contribute to disease. Arthritis is frequently a symptom of food allergy, with wheat, sugar, and the nightshade family (potatoes, tomatoes, eggplant, peppers, pimentos) being the main offenders. Eczema can be triggered by many foods, including wheat and peanuts, but milk should be suspected first. Recurrent ear infections are often caused by an allergic response to food.

Again, milk is a primary culprit. Wheat, egg, soy, and corn cause fluid buildup behind the eardrum, which predisposes children who are allergic to these foods to ear infections.

Eating too much food, or the same food too frequently, can also be toxic and lead to food allergies. Overeating not only leads to obesity and a variety of health problems, it stresses the digestive system, causing it to work overtime and use large amounts of energy. Overeating also tends to wear out the body's enzyme systems, as does eating the same foods repeatedly. This leads to improper food processing by the body, and eventually to food allergies.

Food can have another type of adverse effect on the body. When we eat, a chemical reaction takes place between the blood and the food. Foods contain proteins called lectins, which have agglutinating (clumping) properties that affect red blood cells. The blood group, which is determined by carbohydrates on the red blood cell, in turn determines the compatibility of the food. If we eat a food that is incompatible with our blood group, the lectins begin to agglutinate red blood cells in a target area. There are diets available that take blood groups and these food lectins into consideration. For further information, see Suggested Reading, particularly *Finding the Right Treatment*.

CHAPTER 14

Water and Air

Water

We drink water, cook with it, bathe in it, and inhale it in aerosols or as vapors. Clean drinking water is an absolute necessity for good health and body cleansing.

- Adequate water intake is necessary to flush toxins and waste materials from cells.
- Increased water intake helps detoxify anesthetic agents and medications.
- Adequate fluid levels are necessary for ions in the body to flow and maintain electrical equilibrium.
- Nutrients must be kept in solution, available for cell nourishment and repair.

When it is contaminated, water becomes a toxin. Water can be contaminated with chemicals or microorganisms at the source, in the local water system, and in the home.

In most areas, water is analyzed for dissolved oxygen, fecal coliform bacteria (bacteria from the intestines), suspended sediment, dissolved solids, phosphorus, and for only 60 of 700 chemicals regularly found in our drinking water. It is not monitored for radioactive materials. The level of exposure a person has to these contaminants depends on the fluid intake, absorption rate, and concentrations of chemicals in the water consumed.

▮▮ UNTREATED WATER

Raw untreated water, from groundwater or surface sources, can be contaminated with naturally occurring substances in rocks, such as asbestos, radioactive elements, and metals. Many water sources are also contaminated by various organisms, and toxins produced by human activity.

The area surrounding rivers dramatically affects their quality. Although rivers contain large volumes of moving water, they can be contaminated by landfill runoff, sewage, and agricultural and industrial wastes. Rivers contain biological contaminants from sewage wastes, as well as natural organic pollutants from the land through which they flow.

Toxins Commonly Found in Water

TOXINS	SOURCES
Solvents, pesticides, cleaning preparations, organic chemicals, industrial petrochemicals, salt	Chemical manufacturing, steel mills, sewage treatment plants, mining, hazardous waste disposal sites, chemical dumps
Gasoline	Leaking storage tanks
Asphalt hydrocarbons	Paved areas
Phosphates	Detergents
Nitrates	Runoff from fertilizer and feedlots, sewage treatment systems, seepage from septic systems, natural organic matter
Septic tank degreasers	Leaking septic systems
Fertilizers, pesticides, animal waste	Runoff from lawns, pastures, planted fields, feedlots
Herbicides	Forestry management, highway maintenance
Radioactive elements (radon, radium, uranium)	Natural ores, nuclear power plants, nuclear weapons production sites, hospitals, research laboratories, igneous rocks and sand aquifers, groundwater, surface water
Asbestos	Natural rock formations
Metals	Natural ores, corroded pipes, mineral formations, industrial run-off and waste, mine tailings, galvanizing plants
Inorganic arsenic	Water drainage through mineral formations that contain natural arsenic ores
Inorganic mercury	Discharged into water table and rivers from solid waste treatment plants and water seepage through natural mineral deposits—bacteria then convert it to organic mercury
Sediment containing toxins from source	Silt from fields, construction sites, dam construction, and strip-mined lands, overgrazing, soil erosion, and timber cutting
Pathogens (bacteria, protozoa, viruses, algae, and their toxins)	Sewage, contaminated source water

Lakes are usually fed by streams or other water sources that run into them. They will contain pollution from the area surrounding them, including runoff originating from agricultural wastes, city street pollution, dumps, landfills, and manufacturing and municipal wastes. Lake water may also have a high algae content, as well as being contaminated by exhaust and bilge from boat motors.

Springs can be contaminated by sewage or underground gas and oil wells.

Groundwater, fed by precipitation, is stored naturally in water-bearing rocks called aquifers. The aquifers in which groundwater is stored can be contaminated by underground gasoline tanks, leaking septic systems, poorly located landfills, mine tailings, agricultural runoff, oil field operations, and industrial waste storage tanks. Aquifers near the coast can be contaminated with seawater. It is difficult to trace contamination in an aquifer, and once contamination has occurred it cannot be reversed. Groundwater moves very slowly, and there is no way to dilute the water to decrease the contamination.

◾ ORGANISMS FOUND IN WATER

A variety of organisms are found in rivers, lakes, and groundwater.

Much of the natural water in North America is now contaminated with *Giardia lamblia,* from animal feces. *Giardia* is a microscopic parasite that causes bloating, abdominal cramps, diarrhea, and sometimes vomiting. If not treated, a *Giardia* infection can persist for years.

Cryptosporidium is a parasite found in water contaminated with sewage and animal

---

Exposure to Contaminated Water

- Balanced nutrients (chapter **23**)
- Healthy high-quality diet (**24**)
- Stabilized oxygen or hydrogen peroxide therapy (**26**)
- Allergy extracts or hands-on treatments for chemicals and micro-organisms (**27**)
- Homeopathic remedies such as *Baptisia tinctoria, Zingiber* (**28**)
- Bach Rescue Remedy (**28**)
- Herbal remedies for kidney cleansing (**29**)
- Oral charcoal therapy (**31**)
- Organ cleansing (**31**)

MOST EFFECTIVE DETOXIFICATION METHODS

---

wastes. It makes its way into lakes and rivers and is very resistant to disinfection even by water treatment systems. *Cryptosporidium* causes gastrointestinal illness, with diarrhea, nausea, and stomach cramps. Immunocompromised people will have more severe and persistent symptoms.

In May of 2000, *Escherichia coli* in the drinking water of Walkerton, Ontario caused the worst waterborne outbreak of illness from this organism in North America. At least seven deaths occurred and hundreds of people became ill from ingesting the intestinal bacteria in the water. Other recent deaths are under investigation to see if they are also connected to the outbreak. It is speculated that heavy rains contaminated the town's well with farm manure and a faulty chlorinization system failed to kill the dangerous variety of *E. coli.*

More than one-fifth of Walkerton's resi-

Contaminated Wells

A study done by the EPA in 50 American states between 1988 and 1990 found that 10 percent of community wells and 4 percent of rural wells contained at least one pesticide above the minimum limits of the EPA. Between 1 and 2 percent of the wells tested were contaminated with nitrates (from fertilizer runoff), which can cause methemoglobinemia, a change in red blood cells that prevents them from carrying oxygen. Babies are more sensitive to the effects of methemoglobinemia than are adults. Nitrates are also precursors to nitrosamines, which are known carcinogens.

dents reported nausea, vomiting, and diarrhea. This type of *Escherichia coli* (0157:H7) causes hemorrhagic colitis characterized by the sudden onset of abdominal pain and severe cramps, followed within 24 hours by watery diarrhea that becomes bloody. Most people recover from this infection, but a few individuals develop hemolytic uremic syndrome (HUS), which can lead to kidney failure. There is no known therapy that will stop the progression of HUS. Even with the best and most prompt medical care, HUS has a mortality rate of about 5 percent. Survivors of HUS usually develop serious kidney, neurological, or pancreatic problems that can significantly impair their quality of life.

Other organisms found in water include the bacteria that cause cholera, typhoid, and dysentery and the virus that causes hepatitis, as well as amebas, algae, and fungi. These organisms enter the water supply from human waste from cesspool seepage and runoff containing infected animal urine and feces. Viruses in human waste settle into marine sediments that can become reservoirs. Shellfish, including oysters and clams, bioaccumulate viruses from these reservoirs. (See chapter 15, Plants and Organisms, for further information.)

■■ TAP WATER

Tap water is regulated by the Environmental Protection Agency and is regarded as a utility. Tap water quality depends on the quality of the raw untreated water, the type and number of additives used in the water treatment plant, and contaminants added in transit to the tap.

Groundwater taken from wells is the water source for about half the people in North America. The use of groundwater has increased in the past 30 years, and approximately 75 percent of American cities use groundwater for some or all of their water. In some parts of the country, groundwater is used with little or no treatment. Well water is no longer as safe as it once was because of contamination of deep water tables. In areas of oil shale and coal, well water will contain phenols. It may also contain so many dissolved minerals that it is unfit for drinking.

■ WATER TREATMENTS

When water is not used directly from wells, it is moved from groundwater and surface sources to storage areas for treatment. Some of the substances used to treat water can be toxic themselves.

Fluoride

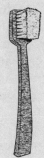

Fluoride is added to drinking water in some areas to prevent tooth decay. In other areas, fluoride occurs naturally in water from dissolved salts in mineral formations. There is controversy over the toxicity of fluoride and whether it can cause other diseases. Opponents to fluoridation claim that long-term exposure to fluorine in drinking water can weaken the immune system and can cause birth defects, genetic damage, cancer, and heart disease. At levels higher than 3 parts per million (PPM), fluoride can cause teeth to turn yellow, brown, or black and the tips to break off. Many water supplies exceed the Environmental Protection Agency's fluoride drinking water standard of 0.7 to 1.2 PPM, and the EPA is considering raising the current standard. (See Dental Work in chapter 11, Toxins from Medical Treatment, for further information on fluoride.)

Copper sulfate, a poison in larger amounts, may be added to control the growth of algae.

Aluminum, in the form of alum, is always added to water to precipitate and remove organic material. Most of the alum precipitates out with the organic material, but even a minute amount of aluminum is very toxic for people with kidney disease.

Since 1908, chlorine has been added to North American water systems as a disinfectant, after it was discovered that it reduced the incidence of infectious diseases in Chicago stockyard cattle. Although chlorination does not kill viruses or protozoa (such as *Giardia lamblia* and *Cryptosporidium*), it is the major method used today to disinfect water in North America. Chlorine-treated water is delivered to 75 percent of North American homes.

Chlorine itself presents a health risk. It can also react with naturally occurring organic materials in the water, such as decaying leaves, to form trihalomethane (THM)

compounds, the most common of which is chloroform. Some trihalomethanes are suspected carcinogens. People who have used chlorinated water all their lives have a higher incidence of bladder and rectal cancer than those who have used unchlorinated water. A California study found that miscarriage rates were higher among women who drank water containing moderate amounts of trihalomethanes. Chlorine has also been implicated in coronary heart disease and atherosclerosis.

Other chemicals, such as ozone, chlorine dioxide, and chloramine may be used instead of chlorine to disinfect the water. Ozonization, the major method of water purification in Europe, is very effective and adds fewer pollutants to the water than other methods. Chlorine dioxide and chloramine are significant pollutants. Chlorine dioxide will remove flavor from water as well as disinfecting it. In excess quantities, it can be highly irritating and corrosive to the skin and mucous membranes of the respiratory tract. Like chlorine, it reacts with organic materials to form trihalomethanes. Chloramine can cause contact dermatitis.

Additional disinfectants may be added to the water to kill microorganisms. Some municipalities also use elaborate filtration systems to remove microorganisms. In spite of all the purification measures used, the Centers for Disease Control in Atlanta, Georgia estimate that every year over a million people in the United States get sick from microorganisms in drinking water, and 900 to 1,000 die as a result.

■ WATER CONTAMINANTS

Corroded pipes between the treatment plant and the consumer can allow lead, copper, asbestos, cadmium, iron, zinc, and nickel to enter the water supply. Lead is one of the most serious toxins found in water. Water in the home can be contaminated with lead from pipes or from lead solder used to join copper pipes. Corrosion of pipes, fittings, and solder adds more lead to the water. Water with an acidic pH leaches more lead from the pipes. Flushing out the tap in the morning for three to five minutes before using the water, and using only cold water for drinking and cooking ensures a lower lead content. Infants and children are more susceptible to the effects of lead. It can affect the formation of blood, the gastrointestinal tract, kidneys, and central nervous system. (See chapter 12, Toxins that Affect Children.)

Copper is widely used in household plumbing materials, and most copper contamination of water occurs from corrosion of these copper pipes by acidic water. It rarely occurs from contamination of the source water. The EPA has set the Maximum Contaminant Level Goal for copper at 1.3 parts per million. Above this level, even for a short time, copper can cause stomach and intestinal distress, liver and kidney damage, and anemia. People with Wilson's disease are particularly sensitive to copper contamination.

Asbestos is no longer used in pipes; however, asbesto fibers released from decaying cement pipes is a potential water contaminant. In areas where the water is acidic, the problem is greater.

Great controversy has existed over plastic pipes and their safety. A variety of toxic volatile chemicals leach into the water from vinyl chloride and polybutylene pipes. In addition, chemicals including pesticides, solvents, and gasoline, can penetrate plastic pipes, as well as iron pipes and most permeable asbestos cement pipe.

The levels of such metals and chemicals as arsenic, cadmium, chromium, fluoride, lead, mercury, nitrate, radium, radon, selenium, trihalomethanes, and uranium are all regulated under the U.S. Safe Drinking Water Act.

The enforcement of current regulations for water is weak. The EPA does not fine all violators of the Safe Drinking Water Act, even though they are required to do so by federal law. Many drinking water suppliers do not notify customers when their water is contaminated. The EPA is under-staffed and under-budgeted to perform enforcement activities. In addition, many states do not fulfill their obligations to ensure water safety.

▮▮ BOTTLED WATER

Bottled water is water that is sealed in a sanitary container and sold for human consumption. It may be sodium-free or contain very low amounts of sodium. About 75 percent of bottled water comes from underground aquifers and springs, and most bottlers use ozone or ultraviolet light, which leave no taste, as disinfecting agents. If the water comes from surface water, the bottling companies are encouraged to use one of three processing methods recommended by the Centers for Disease Control and Prevention: reverse osmosis, one micron absolute filtration, and distillation. (See chapter 35 for a description of these methods and information on the safety of bottled water.)

Federal, state, and trade associations regulate the bottled water industry. The U.S. Food and Drug Administration (FDA) regulates bottled water, which is considered a food product. It randomly inspects water-bottling facilities. States inspect, sample, analyze, and approve sources of water. Only approved sources of water can be used by a bottling plant. The International Bottled Water Association is a trade association that maintains its own set of standards, which are higher than those of the FDA. It performs annual, unannounced plant inspections on its members. Its members distribute 85 percent of the bottled water sold in the United States. All European imports must meet federal and state standards, as well as the standards set by the European Union.

Bottled water is the fastest-growing beverage industry in North America. The International Bottled Water Association estimates that 1 out of 18 people now rely on bottled water as their primary source of drinking water.

Air

Pollution from both indoor and outdoor sources can cause air to become a toxin. Air pollution can cause short-term effects, and long-term or chronic effects, including lung cancer and other respiratory and nonrespiratory symptoms. Acute or short-term effects generally last a few hours to days. Asthma is an example of an acute effect. Chronic effects occur a longer period of time, usually years. Emphysema is a type of chronic effect that can be caused by air pollution.

▮▮ OUTDOOR AIR POLLUTION

Air pollution consists of gases and particulate matter. Carbon monoxide is responsible for half of all air pollution. Other gases include nitrogen oxides, photochemical oxidants, sulfur oxides, and hydrocarbons. Volatile organic chemicals, metals, asbestos, and radionuclides are also found in the air we breathe.

In 1973, the World Health Organization developed a worldwide program to monitor air pollution in order to identify and avoid dangerous levels. The program became part of the United Nation's Global Environmental Monitoring Systems (GEMS). The Environmental Protection Agency has set primary safety standards for various pollutants; however, standards for many toxic chemicals have not been set.

Air quality standards measure six pollutants—total suspended particulates, sulfur dioxide, carbon monoxide, nitrogen dioxide, ozone, and lead. In the United States, the levels of these pollutants, except ozone, have declined over the last 10 years. Many violations of the ozone levels have occurred in the past in large cities, such as Los Angeles.

■ CARBON MONOXIDE

Carbon monoxide is an odorless, colorless gas released when any material burns. Two-thirds of the carbon monoxide in the atmosphere comes from the gasoline burned in vehicles. It enters the bloodstream through the lungs and displaces oxygen from its binding site on the hemoglobin in the red blood cells. Overexposure to carbon monoxide can lead to death from lack of oxygen. (See chapter 8, Toxins in the Home, for further information.)

■ NITROGEN OXIDES

Nitrogen forms several oxides that are emitted from burning coal, oil, and gasoline. During combustion, nitric oxide is produced and then is changed chemically to nitrogen dioxide. Because half the nitrogen dioxide in air comes from transportation sources, concentrations are higher in urban areas than in rural areas. Some nitrogen dioxide is converted to nitric acid, which contributes to acid rain.

Nitrogen oxides can damage the mucous membranes of the eyes, upper respiratory tract, tracheobronchial system, and the alveoli of the lungs. Nitrogen dioxide disrupts some enzyme systems, and is suspected to cause lipid peroxidation, which is the destruction of the lipid cell membranes by free radicals.

■ PHOTOCHEMICAL OXIDANTS

Photochemical oxidants, including ozone, aldehydes, and acrolein, are produced by the action of sunlight on hydrocarbons or volatile organic chemicals and nitrogen oxides in the air. The speed of the reactions increases when temperature and sunlight levels are high.

Ozone can be both a pollutant and a helpful substance, depending on its concentration. It is a major component of smog. Ozone is irritating to the mucous membranes of the eyes and respiratory tract, and has been shown to cause pulmonary edema. (See chapter 26 for a description of the helpful role of ozone.)

Aldehydes are a class of organic compounds that are intermediate between acids and alcohols, and contain less oxygen than an alcohol. Formaldehyde and acetaldehyde are common examples of this class of compound. Most aldehydes are an irritation to the skin and gastrointestinal tract and will attack exposed moist tissue, particularly the eyes and mucous membranes of the upper respiratory tract. The aldehydes of lower molecular weight have low water solubility and can penetrate further into the respiratory tract to affect the lungs.

Acrolein is a special type of aldehyde that is toxic by all routes of contact and ingestion. It is a colorless to yellow liquid at room temperature, has an acrid, choking odor, and is extremely irritating to respiratory tract membranes. Acrolein causes the eyes to water, serving as a warning of its presence. Direct contact to the eye is extremely dangerous, causing corneal damage, swelling of the

Primary Sources of Air Pollution

NATURAL	HUMAN-CAUSED
Smoke from forest fires	Transportation—autos, buses, etc.
Dust from soil	Fuel combustion—factories, refineries, power plants
Ash from volcanoes	Industrial processes
Meteorological phenomena	Waste disposal
Natural gas, including marsh gases	Aerial spraying of farms
Terpenes from plants	Chemical dumps
Ammonia from biological decomposition	Electromagnetic and electrical emissions

eyelid, and a sticky discharge from the eye. It can produce tissue necrosis (death).

■ SULFUR DIOXIDE

Sulfur dioxide is the stable oxide produced when fossil fuels containing sulfur are burned. Coal and oil power plants, pulp and paper mills, and refineries are the main sources. It is a heavy, colorless, pungent gas that can become sulfuric acid when oxidized. Sulfur dioxide is an irritant to the eyes, skin, and respiratory system and can damage the cell walls between alveoli in the lungs. Chronic exposure to sulfur dioxide can cause chronic bronchitis and emphysema.

■ HYDROCARBONS

Hydrocarbons are organic compounds made up of carbon atoms in combination with hydrogen atoms. Because of the ways that carbon atoms can link to each other, very complex arrangements can occur. Some carbon-to-carbon links form aliphatic compounds, which have a chainlike structure. Other carbon-to-carbon links form ringlike structures and are referred to as aromatic compounds.

Petroleum, natural gas, coal, mineral oils, and paraffin wax are examples of hydrocarbons. Many hydrocarbons, both aliphatic and aromatic, are present in polluted air. These compounds come from the emissions of automobiles, trucks, buses, planes, boats, and trains. Industrial processes such as chemical manufacturing also add to the levels of these compounds in the air, as does fuel combustion from factories, refineries, and power plants. Hazardous waste sites and the open burning of refuse further add to hydrocarbon levels in the air.

The composition, properties, and thus the effects of hydrocarbons on people vary widely. Effects can be acute or chronic depending on the circumstances, dose, and length of the exposure. For example, hydro-

MOST EFFECTIVE DETOXIFICATION METHODS

Exposure to Air Pollution

- Detox baths or saunas program (chapter **22**)
- Antioxidant nutrients (**23**)
- Healthy high-quality diet (**24**)
- Oxygen therapy and stabilized oxygen (**26**)
- Allergy extracts or hands-on treatments for chemicals and pollutants (**27**)
- Homeopathic remedies such as *Sulphuricum acidum* (**28**)
- Bach Rescue Remedy (**28**)
- Herbal remedies such as cat's claw, milk thistle, elder (**29**)
- Organ cleansing (**31**)

carbon solvents can damage the skin, liver, blood, central nervous system, and sometimes the lungs and kidneys. Some hydrocarbons are irritants of the skin, lungs, and throat, while others can cause cancer. Symptoms of hydrocarbon exposure include dizziness, lightheadedness, blurred vision, nervousness, sleep problems, nausea and vomiting, disorientation and confusion, irregular heartbeat, unconsciousness, and, in extreme cases, death.

▮ VOLATILE ORGANIC CHEMICALS

Volatile organic chemicals (vocs) generally result from incomplete combustion. They are released from incinerator plants, hazardous waste sites, and through the use of industrial and household solvents. The plastic and semiconductor industries release vocs. Benzene, carbon tetrachloride, chloroform, formaldehyde, methylene chloride, perchloroethylene, trichloroethylene, toluene, and vinyl chloride are all vocs that have been found in the earth's atmosphere. Volatile organic chemicals are a precursor to smog, and many are known or suspected carcinogens.

Common sources of vocs include aerosols, cooking and heating fuel, cleaning compounds, inks, lacquer, paper products, permanent press clothes, textiles, refrigerants, varnishes, and window cleaner. VOCs can cause a variety of symptoms including eye and nose irritation, and central nervous system depression that leads to lethargy, confusion, dizziness, headaches, nausea and unconsciousness. (See chapter 16, Chemicals and Metals, for information on specific chemicals.)

▮ METALS

Arsenic, cadmium, chromium, copper, lead, mercury, and nickel have all been found in air. Arsenic is emitted from coal and oil furnaces. Cadmium, mercury, and nickel come from smelters, while chromium is released from chrome-plating operations. Smoke from refuse incineration contains copper. Lead is released into the air directly, or from contaminated soil and water from residues of leaded gasoline, paint, and lead solder in pipes. (See chapter 16, Chemicals and Metals, for information on specific metals.)

▮ PARTICULATE MATTER

Particulate matter in the air mostly consists of small carbon and dust particles. It can be released from natural sources, such as soil, forest fires, and volcanic eruptions, or from industrial sources, such as fuel combustion, transportation, and solid-waste emissions. Small particles may be inhaled into the lungs, resulting in bronchial irritation and asthma. Toxic gases can be attached to these particles and deposited into the lungs, causing further damage to lung tissue.

■■ INDOOR AIR POLLUTION

In the last few years, it has become evident that indoor air pollution levels for some chemicals may be higher than those outside in most areas. However, the indoor levels of ozone, sulfates, aerosols, sulfur dioxide, and lead are 20 to 80 percent lower than those outdoors. Urban populations spend at least 80 percent of their time indoors, and the most susceptible population groups, such as the elderly and infants, spend even more time indoors.

Indoor air pollutants may come from outdoor air, from materials in the building, or from human activity. Paint, carpets, furniture, plastics, pesticides, cleaning materials, air fresheners, tobacco smoke, and personal and household products are all sources of indoor air pollution. (See chapter 8, Toxins in the Home, and chapter 9, Toxins in the Workplace and School, for additional information on indoor air pollution.)

■ RADON

The gaseous element radon is a common indoor air pollutant that is a member of the natural radioactive uranium series. Radon is found in high concentration in soil and rocks containing uranium, including granite, phosphate, shale, and pitchblende. It creates dangerous radioactive decay products or "daughters," which continue to decay in lung tissue, causing damaging radiation.

Radon enters through cracks in house foundations, joints in concrete slabs, and around gas and water pipes, drains, and

> ## Radon Risk
>
> *In an Environmental Protection Agency survey of 17 states, 25 percent of the homes tested had radon levels above the concentration for which action is recommended. The EPA estimates that 20,000 lung cancer deaths each year may be due to radon exposures, although other studies have not yet been able to prove this link. However, uranium miners who are exposed to high levels of radon have lung cancer rates significantly higher than those of the general population.*

sumps. High radon levels have been found in the United States in Pennsylvania, New England, Colorado, and New Mexico. Canada is the world's largest producer and exporter of uranium. Because of the uranium in the soil and rocks, the Northwest Territories, Saskatchewan, and Ontario have high amounts of radon.

■ CONSTRUCTION AND BUILDING MATERIALS

Since the energy crisis in 1973–74, new buildings are more airtight and more insulation is being added to older buildings. New offices use mechanical ventilation systems rather than relying on open windows. The number of air exchanges in buildings has been reduced to 0.5 per hour. By the 1980s, complaints of health symptoms related to indoor air pollution mushroomed.

Compounding the problems from ventilation deficiencies, many building materials outgas volatile chemicals. Concrete, stone, plywood, particleboard, insulation adhesives, paints, and carpets are all sources of indoor air pollutants. Stone and cinder block may contain radon. Particleboard and plywood outgas formaldehyde from bonding agents. Carpets also outgas formaldehyde, while paints may contain toluene and formaldehyde.

The Environmental Protection Agency recently studied the exposure of people to volatile organic chemicals (vocs) and pesticides. For 11 vocs (including benzene, carbon tetrachloride, chloroform, tetrachloroethylene, styrene, and trichloroethylene) measured both in cities and rural areas, indoor air exposures were higher than outdoor exposures. The pesticide exposures came from indoor sources.

The EPA found that levels of vocs in new buildings were 100 times greater than those found outdoors. Over approximately five months, these levels gradually decreased to two to four times that of outdoor levels.

(See chapter 8, Toxins in the Home, and chapter 9, Toxins in the Workplace and School, for further information on building materials.)

■ INHALANTS

Pollens, dust, dust mites, animal dander, insect parts, and mold are commonly found in indoor air. When they are inhaled, they can cause health problems for many people. (See chapter 8, Toxins in the Home, for a discussion of animal dander.)

Many people are allergic to molds, which are frequent residents of heating, ventilation, and air-conditioning units. Their spores can travel on air currents throughout a building. They grow anywhere there is dampness, particularly in bathrooms, laun-

dry rooms, and kitchens. Mold may be found behind tile and under linoleum. Water leaks are always accompanied by mold growth. (See Molds, Yeasts, and Other Fungi in chapter 15, Plants and Organisms.)

Dust and dust mites can cause allergies, and dust mites trigger asthma in sensitive people. Dust contains minute plant fibers, food remnants, pollen, mold spores, insect fragments, animal danders, fabric fibers, soot, paper and paint fragments, and other microscopic fragments. Symptoms of a dust allergy include sneezing, clear or cloudy nasal discharge, burning of the nasal passages, nasal stuffiness, chronic sinusitis, and cough. Suspect a dust problem if your symptoms are worse:
• indoors, and better outside
• when the furnace is running
• when housecleaning is in progress
• in the morning, improving during the day
• when you first go to bed

Dust mites are microscopic insects that live in dust and feed on dead skin shed by humans. They are harmful only to sensitive people who inhale their airborne feces. They colonize in mattresses, carpets, stuffed toys, and upholstered furniture and thrive in humid climates.

Signs of a dust mite problem include:
• persistently stuffy nose or ears
• repeated sneezing on awakening
• worsening when beds are made
• improvement when outdoors

Some pollen is also present in indoor air. Pollen enters the house through open doors and windows, as well as on clothing, shoes, and pet fur. (See Pollens in chapter 15, Plants and Organisms.)

■ HUMAN ACTIVITIES

Human activities add significantly to indoor air pollution. Carbon monoxide, nitrogen dioxide, nitrogen oxide, carbon dioxide, sulfur dioxide, volatile organic chemicals, and particulates are products of the combustion of natural gas, fuel oil, and in coal heating systems. Gas stoves, hot-water heaters, and dryers also contribute to the problem.

Disinfectants, detergents, cleaning compounds, floor waxes, mothballs, perfumes, room deodorizers, and any scented chemical add to indoor air pollution. Fabric softener dryer sheets contribute to both indoor and outdoor pollution if the dryer is vented to the outside.

Pesticide residues are frequently found in indoor air pollution. Many homes and workplaces are regularly treated with pesticides to kill unwanted insects. While many pesticides are contactants, killing the insects when they crawl over treated areas, most of them are volatile, and their molecules are found in the air of the treated buildings. Depending on their concentrations, these pesticides can cause many problems to people in the buildings. (See chapter 16, Chemicals and Metals, for a detailed discussion of pesticides.)

Photocopiers, correction fluid, refrigerators, blueprint machines, photographic paper, and NCR (carbonless paper) are all potential sources of indoor air pollution. Photocopy machines can emit ozone and volatile organic chemicals.

■ Tobacco Smoke

Tobacco smoke is a major contributor to indoor air pollution. It consists of mainstream smoke (the smoke drawn through the tobacco during active smoking) and sidestream smoke (from burning tobacco). Sidestream smoke contains a higher concentration of gases and particulates than does mainstream smoke. Four thousand different chemicals and particulates have been identified in sidestream smoke, including nicotine, carbon monoxide, ammonia, acetaldehyde, formaldehyde, hydrogen cyanide, nitrogen dioxide, benzo[a]pyrene, phenols, and cadmium.

In a 1975 study published in *Lancet* by Russell and Feyerabend of London, over half of 39 nonsmoking office workers tested had nicotine in their blood plasma during the early afternoon, and almost all had nicotine in their urine, although the urine nicotine levels of smokers were much higher. They concluded that nonsmokers have measurable amounts of nicotine in their body for most of their lives as a result of inhaling sidestream smoke. They further stated that it takes only one or two smokers to contaminate a vehicle or building.

Smoking kills 45,000 people a year in Canada. The U.S. Surgeon General's Office states that cigarettes alone kill 434,000 Americans each year. World War II claimed about the same number of American lives over a four-year period. Cigarette smoking remains the single most preventable cause of cancer death in the United States.

CHAPTER 15

Plants and Organisms

Plants

Plants can be toxic to humans in several ways. The most familiar toxic effect comes from plant pollens when they cause allergic reactions. Aromatic chemicals called terpenes and phenolics, which can also cause allergic symptoms, give plants their characteristic odors and taste. Some plants produce nerve poisons, internal-organ poisons, or skin and eye irritants. In addition, plants accumulate metals or minerals from soil and water, which may be ingested by people.

▌▌ POLLENS

As part of their reproductive cycle, all seed-bearing plants produce pollen. About 100 plant species produce pollen that plays a significant role in allergic reactions and sensitivities. Problem-causing pollen must be abundant, widespread, windborne, light enough to be carried some distance, and contain specific antigens for hypersensitivity.

Trees, grasses, and weeds produce wind-borne pollen that causes allergic symptoms. These plants generally have small, unattractive flowers without nectar or scent. Plants with brightly colored, perfumed flowers are pollinated by insects and birds and their pollen generally does not affect the allergic person.

Pollen allergy symptoms include sneezing; hoarseness; increased mucus production; scratchy throat; hay fever; runny nose; itchy, red, watery eyes; and sinus symptoms of headache, pressure behind the eyeballs, tenderness over the cheekbones, pain in the frontal area, and aching teeth.

Allergic responses to pollens may also include symptoms that are not commonly thought of as pollen related. These include eczema, cold and flulike symptoms, asthma, fatigue, insomnia, depression, cramps and diarrhea, swollen lymph glands, hives, flushing, skipped heartbeats, and panic attacks. During pollen season, some women may experience irregular periods, toxemia during pregnancy, or uterine hemorrhaging, especially if ragweed is pollinating.

PLANT SOURCE	NERVE TOXINS
Spotted hemlock	Coniine
Tobacco	Nicotine
Chrysanthemum	Pyrethrin
Peyote	Pyrrolizidines
Mescal bean	Quinoloizidines
Legumes	Rotenone
Deadly nightshade	Scopolamine and atropine
Western yew tree	Taxol

■■ TERPENES AND PHENOLICS

Terpenes and phenolics, which are present in varying amounts in all plants, have different structures but similar functions in plants. Terpenes are unsaturated hydrocarbons containing an isoprene ring. Phenolics contain a benzene ring, with two or more hydroxyl (OH^-) groups attached to the ring.

Terpenes and phenolics are responsible for the taste and odor of plant and occur in all parts of the plant, including the pollen, but their concentration is highest in the stems, leaves, and flowers. Their function is to attract pollinators, as well as to protect the plant from animal predators. Many of them have an antioxidant function in the plant, protecting it from insect damage and chemical injury. Sensitive people frequently have adverse reactions to pollens, terpenes, and phenolics.

Terpene-sensitive individuals develop their characteristic pollen symptoms long before the specific pollen actually appears. For example, many people in our area of New Mexico complain of juniper symptoms a full month before the juniper trees begin to pollinate. These symptoms coincide with the rise in terpenes.

Terpene-sensitive people will be unable to tolerate the presence of live Christmas trees, cut grass, and many cut flowers. They are usually sensitive to other chemicals, especially those in smoked foods, spicy foods, and scented products. People who are sensitive to phenolics will also be food sensitive. Phenolics occur in both plants and animals, but are more prevalent in plants.

■■ NERVE TOXINS

Some plants produce chemicals that affect the human nervous system, causing a variety of symptoms. These toxins can affect the peripheral nervous system and motor coordination, and may be accompanied by delirium, stupor, and trance states. They may also cause nausea, gastrointestinal disorders, trembling, irregular or abnormally slow heartbeat, impaired respiration, dizziness, speech loss, and fatal paralysis.

Nicotine and pyrethrins both have insecticidal properties, but pyrethrins degrade more quickly and rapidly paralyze insects. Pyrethroids, which are synthetic pyrethrins, have been widely produced in recent years for use as insecticides. They are more toxic to humans than the natural product, and large exposures may cause sensations of burning or prickling of the skin, tremors, and salivation.

Rotenone, found in approximately 70 legumes, also has insecticidal properties but is safe for most mammals, except pigs.

Taxol has been receiving attention re-

PLANT SOURCE	INTERNAL ORGAN TOXINS
Lily-of-the-valley	Convallatoxin
Foxglove	Digitoxin
St. John's wort	Hypericin
Oak	Oxalates
Fescue	Pyrrolizidine alkaloids
Alfalfa	Saponins

cently because of its successful use in cancer chemotherapy for ovarian cancer and metastatic breast cancer.

❚❚ INTERNAL ORGAN TOXINS

The heart, kidney, liver, and stomach are internal organs that can be affected by plant toxins.

Although overdoses cause the heart to stop, convallatoxin and digitoxin in smaller doses strengthen heart beat, which helps eliminate fluids present in congestive heart failure. Digitalis, which is used in treating heart disease, is manufactured from foxglove. The oxalates obstruct the kidney tubules. Saponins cause gastric upset and hypericin and pyrrolizidine alkaloids obstruct veins in the liver. Many of these plant toxins can be processed so that they are beneficial rather than harmful.

❚❚ SKIN AND EYE IRRITANTS

Poison ivy, poison oak, and poison sumac are well-known skin and eye irritants. The toxins in these plants are oily compounds that adhere to the skin. Contact with the foliage of these plants causes a skin rash that may be so severe it is disabling. In sensitive individuals, it may be very difficult to treat and healing can be very slow. People exposed to smoke from the burning plants may require hospitalization to treat lung damage.

Some plants contain photosensitizers—systemic plant poisons that pass unchanged through the liver and collect in the skin capillaries. When the skin is exposed to light, the capillaries leak plasma into surrounding tissues. In severe cases, hair and tissue may be sloughed off. St. John's wort and groundsel are among the plants that can cause this reaction.

Phytophotodermatitis (photosensitization contact dermatitis) can occur after plants containing a chemical used as a defense against fungi and insects are crushed on the skin. When the skin of sensitive people is then exposed to sunlight, a blistering sunburn occurs, followed by a darkened color where the plants touched the skin. Parsnips, dill, celery, parsley, figs, and mus-

Poisonous Plants

Some very common plants, including houseplants, can cause skin rashes in sensitive people. Amaryllis, buttercup, carnation, cyclamen, daffodil, daisy, Ficus benjamina, geranium, holly berry, iris, poinsettia, pyracantha berry, and tulip can all cause a contact rash. If these plants are ingested, nausea, vomiting, diarrhea, and abdominal cramps can result.

tard are some of the plants responsible for this phototoxic reaction.

■ MINERAL ACCUMULATORS

Some plants are toxic because they absorb inorganic materials from soil and water. An example of this type of plant is "locoweed," which accumulates selenium. Animals develop a fatal condition known as the "blind staggers" when they eat enough of the plant to develop selenium poisoning.

Fluorides accumulate in the leaves of plants. This commonly occurs near ore smelters, refineries, and industrial plants that manufacture fertilizers, ceramics, aluminum, glass, and bricks. When animals or humans eat the leaves, symptoms may include headaches, vomiting, diarrhea, fatigue, weakness, excessive thirst, and asthma or bronchitis.

Plants growing on soil treated with nitrate fertilizers under moisture-deficient conditions accumulate nitrates. When humans or animals consume these plants, the nitrate is metabolized to nitrite and enters the bloodstream. The nitrite oxidizes the iron in hemoglobin so that the hemoglobin cannot transport oxygen as efficiently. This condition is called methemoglobinemia. In addition, toxic nitrogen dioxide gas can be generated from these plants when they are stored as silage and undergo fermentation. This exposure can result in "silofiller's disease," a pulmonary edema caused by irritation of the innermost parts of the lungs.

Volcanic activity has given Hawaii and other volcanic islands high levels of mercury in the soil, air, and water. Mercury particularly accumulates in green leafy vegetables,

> **Exposure to Plants**
>
> - Allergy extracts or hands-on treatment for pollens and terpenes (chapter **27**)
> - Homeopathic remedies such as *Sabadilla* and *Wyethia* for hayfever; *Rhus toxicodendron* for poison oak (**28**)
> - Bach Rescue Remedy (**28**)
> - Herbal remedies such as aloe, lobelia, white oak, witch hazel (**29**)
> - Specific compresses, packs, and poultices; specific soaks (**30**)
> - Charcoal poultices (**30**)
> - Organ cleansing (**31**)

MOST EFFECTIVE DETOXIFICATION METHODS

avocados, and papayas. People eating large amounts of these island-grown plants can develop symptoms of mercury poisoning.

Organisms

Organisms such as bacteria, parasites, viruses, molds, yeast, and fungi may be a source of toxins for humans. These organisms live in the soil, water, and air. Under certain conditions, they can cause health problems by generating an infection or by producing toxins. (See also chapter 13, Food, and chapter 14, Water and Air, for a discussion of common organisms found in food and water.) Some insects and arachnids, such as spiders and scorpions, also produce or carry substances that are toxic to people.

■ BACTERIA

Bacteria are single-celled microorganisms that grow in colonies and reproduce by simple division, called binary fission. They may be spheres (cocci), rods (bacilli), curved cells

Common Disease-Causing Bacteria

BACTERIA	DISEASE	TRANSMITTED BY
Clostridium tetani	Tetanus (lockjaw)	Foreign materials in puncture wounds
Clostridium perfringens	Gas gangrene	Soil, foreign material containing C. perfringens spores in muscle injury or wound
Escherichia coli	Traveler's diarrhea	Contaminated food or water
Corynebacterium diphtheriae	Diphtheria	Respiratory tract droplets from person to person or exudate from skin lesions
Shigella dysenteriae	Dysentery	Contaminated food or water, and flies, from person to person
Vibrio cholera	Cholera	Contaminated food or water

(vibrios), or spiral-shaped cells (spirochetes or spirilla). If the bacteria is pathogenic (disease-causing), and if it reaches our bodies in sufficient numbers, a bacterial infection can result.

Bacterial toxins may be divided into two classes: toxins released as the bacteria grow in the human body; and toxins produced in substances that are then ingested. (For more information on ingested bacteria, see chapter 13, Food.)

Bacteria produce several types of toxins. Exotoxins are released from the bacterial cell without destroying the organism. Enterotoxins are exotoxins with an affinity for the cells of the small intestine. Endotoxins are produced within a bacterial cell and are not released unless the bacteria is ruptured. Cy-

totoxins are a specific cell-destroying substance.

Clostridium tetani, a common soil bacteria, enters the body through puncture wounds. The exotoxin that this bacteria synthesizes interferes with the neurotransmitter acetylcholine, causing tetanus or lockjaw, which can be fatal.

Clostridium perfringens causes gas gangrene. The gangrene can develop in traumatic, open lesions, such as bullet wounds or compound fractures, particularly when contaminated with dirt or other foreign materials. The exotoxin passes along the muscle bundles, killing all cells and causing necrotic (dead tissue) areas where the bacteria can grow. The multiplying bacteria produce gas in the tissues that can be heard and felt on palpation. When the bloodstream absorbs the toxin, the resulting systemic illness can be fatal unless treated.

The enterotoxin of the bacillus *Shigella dysenteriae* causes a severe form of dysentery, intestinal hemorrhaging, and gastrointestinal tract paralysis. Enterotoxin-producing *Escherichia coli* is a major cause of traveler's diarrhea. This strain causes less severe illness than other strains. (See chapters 13 and 14 for strains of *E. coli* found in food and water.)

Vibrio cholera produces a potent enterotoxin responsible for cholera. This toxin causes the loss of chloride, potassium, bicarbonate, and water molecules from the cells of the intestinal mucosa, with subsequent diarrhea. The extensive fluid loss, which can be as much as seven liters per day, and electrolyte imbalance can quickly lead to dehydration and death if not treated. Epidemic cholera is spread through water contaminated with this bacteria.

Corynebacterium diphtheriae produces an exotoxin that causes diphtheria and all its systemic effects. This bacteria usually grows on skin tissue and causes the death of cells in the area where it is growing. When the toxin is absorbed into the bloodstream, it causes degenerative lesions in the heart, nervous system, and kidneys. The mortality rate for diphtheria is 0.5 percent if treated on the first day of illness. If it is not treated until the fourth day, the mortality rate goes up to 10 percent.

Most strains of *Pseudomonas aeruginosa* produce an exotoxin that destroys tissues and inhibits protein synthesis. *Pseudomonas* infection is rare in healthy individuals. However, it is an opportunistic pathogen that can be devastating to people with suppressed immune system function.

▌▌ PARASITES

Parasites live on or within other organisms to obtain nourishment and shelter. This relationship may be temporary or permanent, with the parasite depending on the host organism for its entire existence. The parasite receives all the benefit from the association, and the host may or may not be damaged from its presence. Medical parasites include protozoa (one-celled microscopic animals), helminths (worms), and some arthropods (particularly insects).

Some parasites can cause damage through their sheer numbers as they multiply. They obstruct blood vessels, destroy host cells, and compete for nutrients, and their metabolic products cause inflammatory reactions. Only a few parasites release toxins that are harmful to humans; these toxins are described below.

▌ PROTOZOA

Entamoeba histolytica causes amebic dysentery. It produces a cytotoxic enterotoxin that plays a role in tissue invasion. In virulent strains, the destruction and death of tissue cells occurs after contact with this toxin.

A marine species of protozoan organisms belonging to the order of dinoflagellates produces a toxin found in shellfish, commonly known as "red tide." (For more information, see chapter 13, Food.)

▌ HELMINTHS

Helminth comes from the Greek word meaning "worm." The term originally applied only to intestinal worms, but now includes both parasitic and free-living species of worms.

Most helminths produce a toxic substance from secretory glands located near their mouths. These secretions are toxic to humans and are destructive to cells, enabling the worm to digest the host's tissue for food or to migrate through the tissues of the host.

Parasitic worms of medical significance include:
• Annelids – segmented worms that include leeches
• Nematodes – round worms such as hookworms, pinworms, roundworms, and filarial worms
• Flatworms – tapeworms and flukes

▍ PARASITIC INSECTS AND VECTORS

A few insects are considered parasites or act as vectors (intermediate hosts) for human disease.

The louse sucks blood from humans. Their saliva is toxic to humans and causes a red, elevated pimple-like lesion accompanied by severe itching. The louse also acts as a vector for epidemic typhus and trench fever.

Flea bites cause a skin irritation in humans. This irritation may be only a pimple-like lesion or in sensitive individuals can cause a rash. Fleas are also vectors for plague, a bacterial disease of rodents that is transmitted to people by fleas that have bitten infected animals. They may also be mechanical vectors for a number of viral and bacterial diseases.

Bedbug bites produce red itching wheals and blisters. Some individuals may have allergic symptoms, with generalized hives and even asthma.

Certain species of ticks secrete a neurotoxin from their salivary glands, which causes progressive paralysis. Ticks responsible for tick paralysis occur in Australia and North America. The disease has a rapid onset, and although death can occur from respiratory paralysis, most affected people do recover. The paralysis usually reverses quickly after removal of the tick. Most deaths occur from the Australian tick.

The tick that transmits Lyme disease is dependent on deer to reproduce and on mice to become infected. Caused by a spirochete bacteria, *Borrelia burgdorferi*, Lyme disease is not transmitted until the tick has fed for several hours. In addition to the distinctive bull's eye skin lesions at the site of the tick bite, Lyme disease is characterized by fatigue, headache, stiffness, muscle soreness, and swollen lymph glands. Neurological symptoms can develop and persist for weeks to months. Lyme "arthritis," which causes pain and swelling in large joints, may affect the person for years.

Among mosquitoes, only the female mosquito is capable of biting, as the male does not eat during the adult stage. The female's elongated mouthparts are adapted for sucking blood, as she cannot produce fertile eggs without a blood meal. While removing blood, the female mosquito injects saliva into the puncture wound. Antigens in the saliva may cause immediate allergic reactions, as well as delayed skin reactions. A mosquito bite can cause considerable irritation, with redness, itching, and swelling. Mosquitoes are also biological and mechanical vectors for bacterial, helminthic, protozoan, and viral diseases of both humans and animals. Malaria, dengue fever, and yellow fever are spread by mosquitoes.

■ VENOMOUS INSECTS AND ARACHNIDS

Venomous insects cause more fatal poisonings in the United States each year than do all other venomous animals combined. These insects are from the order Hymenoptera and include ants, bees, hornets, wasps, and yellowjackets. They administer water-soluble, nitrogen-containing chemicals through their stinging mechanisms. Fatalities from insect stings are caused by allergic reactions in sensitized individuals, or from toxic overload from multiple stings. These reactions, if severe, can affect the nervous system, cardiovascular system, and respiratory function.

Spiders all produce venom, but most do not produce sufficient quantities to harm humans, although many spider bites cause some irritation. The two most poisonous spiders in North America are the black widow and brown recluse. The black widow spider can be identified by the orange hourglass-shaped spot on its abdomen. Symptoms of black widow spider poisoning include cramps, sweating, dizziness, headache, tremor, nausea, vomiting, pain, and elevated blood pressure. Death occurs rarely, and mainly in children.

The "violin" on the cephalothorax of the brown recluse spider identifies it. This spider usually does not bite unless it is disturbed. The tissue and underlying muscle around the bite of this spider ulcerate and

---

Exposure to Organisms

- Sauna program (chapter **22**)
- Vitamin C and other antioxidant nutrients; beneficial bacteria (**23**)
- Healthy, high-quality foods (**24**)
- Oxygen therapy (**25**)
- Allergy extracts or hands-on treatment for specific organisms (**27**)
- Homeopathic remedies such as *Apis, Camphora, Chenopodium antihelminticum, Pyrogenium* (**28**)
- Herbal remedies such as barberry, black walnut, echinacea, goldenseal, slippery elm bark (**29**)
- Organ cleansing (**31**)

MOST EFFECTIVE DETOXIFICATION METHODS

---

die, leaving a gaping wound. Systemic symptoms, such as anemia, nausea, vomiting, high fever, and convulsions may occur, and in rare instances, death.

Scorpions inject venom into their prey through a stinger at the end of their long tails. The venom causes their stings to be extremely painful. The stings of a few species can be fatal to humans. Scorpions are nocturnal and do not normally sting humans unless bare hands or feet come into contact with them.

■ VIRUSES

Viruses are microorganisms that are not a complete cell. They consist of double-layered shells of protein, lipids, and carbohydrates surrounding either DNA or RNA. They cannot replicate without host cells, and so may be considered a form of parasite. Viruses cause active infections, but can also remain in the body in inactive states for long periods of time, reactivating to again cause acute symptoms and active infections.

Some viruses cause the destruction of cell structures, enabling them to enter the cell. Others create a toxic effect by causing the body to release substances that initiate unpleasant effects. For example, many viruses increase the release of cytokines (substances that help cause the inflammatory response) from the immune cascade, causing the symptoms that are associated with a viral infection, such as muscle aches, fever, and headaches.

■■ MOLDS, YEASTS, AND OTHER FUNGI

Molds, yeasts, and other fungi are plants that lack chlorophyll and reproduce by releasing spores into the air. Many of the organisms in this group also produce harmful toxins.

■ MOLDS

Molds emit mycotoxins, which can cause untoward symptoms and even death in animals and humans. *Fusarium, Trichoderma, Aspergillus,* and *Penicillium* are mold species that produce mycotoxins. However, these toxins are produced only when the molds grow on certain substances. Exposure is usually through ingesting food contaminated by mold. Those mycotoxins that affect humans are described in chapter 13, Food.

Molds are present all year, even when there is snow on the ground. The snow acts as an insulator for molds growing underneath. They are released when the snow melts. The peak spore season is from midsummer through fall, with spores spread by winds and insects, and on the shoes and clothing of people. Molds are found everywhere, both indoors and outdoors, and are particularly abundant in moist areas.

When the numbers of mold spores are high outdoors, they will be high indoors also. Indoor molds become more obvious when buildings are closed and a musty smell signals their presence. Molds are found in the damper parts of homes, including the basement, kitchen, bathroom, atriums, hot tub areas, and utility rooms. Mold spores spread throughout the house by air from these areas.

Flat-roofed houses are particularly mold prone because of water leakage into ceilings and walls. Insulation and wallboard can harbor molds before mold can be detected on the painted surface.

In the southwest United States, some adobe homes are built directly on the soil rather than on a concrete foundation, and the upward seepage of water through the walls encourages mold growth.

In climates with high humidity, mold control can be very difficult. It will grow on the walls and become permanently impregnated into paint and wallpaper. It will also grow on leather products in the house, in addition to wood, books, and many different types of fibers.

Many people are allergic to molds. Common signs of a mold allergy include feeling worse:

• from 5:00 to 9:00 PM
• in damp places indoors and outdoors
• when working in the yard
• from August until frost, even after ragweed season is over

• when eating fermented products or mush-rooms and other fungi

Some symptoms and conditions caused by mold are: nasal symptoms, respiratory complaints, ear infections, rashes, hives, gastrointestinal distress, cerebral symptoms, depression, and allergies.

■ YEAST

Pathogenic yeast, such as *Candida albicans,* produce toxins that can harm humans. *C. albicans* releases over 80 known toxins, many of which are produced to either kill or inhibit competing microorganisms.

Toxic byproducts of candida metabolism include acetaldehyde, ethanol, glycoprotein toxins, polysaccharide protein complexes, tyramine, canditoxin, mannan, and proteinase. Candida toxins weaken the defense system of the body, and the presence of excessive toxins causes the mucous membranes in the gut to leak. Larger protein molecules are absorbed into the bloodstream, stimulating antibody production, and resulting in multiple food and chemical sensitivities.

The most toxic substances produced by *Candida albicans* are acetaldehyde and ethanol. Acetaldehyde, which is chemically related to formaldehyde, disrupts cell membrane function and alters protein synthesis. It is six times more toxic to the brain than ethanol. Ethanol can cause a low-grade intoxication-like state that results in vague neurological symptoms. Because our metabolism cannot convert acetaldehyde or ethanol into useful materials, our body must detoxify them. If the circulating load of these toxins is too great, fatigue, poor memory,

Wild Mushrooms

In the United States, mushroom gathering is not a common activity and mushroom poisoning is rare, with about 350 cases a year, most of them children. In Canada, where mushroom-picking is quite common, there are approximately 150 cases of mushroom poisoning a year. Fatalities have been rare in both countries.

In his book Toxicological Chemistry, *Stanley Manahan reports that in 1988 a liver transplant was performed in the United States on a woman whose liver had been irreversibly damaged from eating wild mushrooms that she and a companion had gathered. They had mistakenly identified the mushrooms as an edible species.*

lightheadedness, inability to concentrate, and depression can result.

■ MUSHROOMS

Mushrooms are fleshy fungi that produce toxins. At one time, the term "toadstool" was supposed to denote a toxic mushroom. There is no scientific basis for this supposition, and care must be exercised in determining which mushrooms are safe for human consumption.

Some mushrooms produce alkaloids that cause central nervous system symptoms, such as narcosis and convulsions, and

Fungus and Infants

Sudden, unexplained lung hemorrhage in infants may be caused by fungal exposure coupled with tobacco or other environmental exposures. The fungi/tobacco combination was a proven cause of hemorrhage in one incident reported by Dr. Will E. Novotny in the March 2000 Archives *of Pediatric and Adolescent Medicine. Other cases have been linked to the fungus* Stachybotrys atra. *Lung hemorrhage in animals has been linked to several fungi. Avoiding the unnecessary exposure of infants to water-damaged and/or mold-laden environments is advised.*

in some cases hallucinations. Muscarine is an alkaloid toxin found in several species of mushrooms. Perspiration, watering eyes, and salivation are symptoms unique to muscarine poisoning. Cramps, diarrhea, headache, and blurred vision may follow.

Psilocybin and psilocin are other alkaloids produced by some mushrooms. Both are hallucinogenic and can produce either a good or a bad "trip," depending on several factors. They can also cause convulsions and narcosis, including stupor and unconsciousness. The length of time the symptoms persist depends on the quantity of mushrooms consumed.

Polypeptides are another class of toxin produced by some mushrooms. These systemic poisons attack the cells of organs, including the heart, liver, and kidneys. Death can result from eating a single cap of a mushroom from the genus *Amanita*. Initial symptoms include violent diarrhea, cramps, and abdominal pain. The victim may also suffer paralysis, delirium, and coma.

▮ OTHER FUNGI

Some fungi can cause diseases in people, and they fall into four classes:

- *Systemic or deep mycosis:* Caused by inhalation of spores and manifesting as respiratory symptoms. If untreated, numerous abscesses or granulomas (modules of inflamed tissue) can form throughout the body. This condition can be fatal.
- *Subcutaneous mycosis:* Caused by direct implantation of spores or filament fragments. Disease begins with a skin abscess or granuloma, which can spread both on the skin or through the lymph system.
- *Cutaneous mycosis:* Fungi can grow in the skin's epidermal layer, hair, and nails. Diseases are chronic and confined to the site of the infection. Some examples of cutaneous mycosis are athlete's foot, ringworm, and fungal infections of the scalp.
- *Superficial mycosis:* Fungi are localized along hair shafts and in hardened, dead epidermal cells.

All of these fungal diseases are caused by microscopic fungi. The more serious types—systemic or deep mycosis and subcutaneous mycosis—require treatment by a physician.

CHAPTER 16

Chemicals and Metals

CHEMICALS INCLUDE both elements and compounds. The 107 elements include such commonly known elements as calcium, chlorine, copper, gold, hydrogen, iodine, iron, magnesium, mercury, nitrogen, oxygen, phosphorus, silver, and sulfur. Some elements can be toxic to humans. For example, approximately 80 elements are classified as metals, and of these the "heavy metals," which include lead, cadmium, and mercury, can be toxic. While metals are chemicals, their properties differ from those of chemical compounds and are thus discussed separately.

Life-giving oxygen, an element that ordinarily possesses two atoms to a molecule, becomes toxic to both plants and animals if there are three atoms to a molecule. This form of oxygen is called ozone and is associated with atmospheric smog pollution. (See chapter 14 for information on ozone as a pollutant.)

Our purpose is not to alarm you, but to inform you so that you can control your chemical exposures. The cleaner your lifestyle, the healthier you will be, and the fewer detoxification procedures you will need to maintain good health.

Chemical Compounds

The substances that we normally call chemicals are usually chemical compounds formed from the elements, which are considered the building blocks of nature. Compounds are composed of two or more elements joined by a chemical bond. The properties of a compound will differ from those of the individual elements forming its structure. There are two types of chemical bonds, each causing the formation of different types of chemical compounds.

Ionic bonds form when electrons are transferred from one atom to another, creating charged particles called ions. The ions are held together in a solid compound by the attracting forces of the oppositely charged ions. Ionic bonds form crystalline compounds, such as table salt (sodium chloride). Some ionic compounds are toxic to humans and animals, including sulfuric acid, barium cyanide, lead acetate, and thallium(I)-carbonate.

Covalent bonds form when electrons are shared between atoms to form a molecule. A water molecule, which consists of two hydrogen atoms joined to one oxygen atom, is a covalent compound.

■ ORGANIC COMPOUNDS

Most carbon-containing compounds, in which the atoms are joined in a covalent bond, are considered organic compounds. The majority of industrial compounds, agricultural compounds, biological materials, and synthetic polymers (very large molecules formed from smaller molecules) are organic compounds. While there are organic compounds that are beneficial to us, many of the compounds that are toxic to us are organic compounds.

Organic compounds are divided into a number of classes. If they contain only hydrogen and carbon, they are called hydrocarbons. There are also oxygen-containing compounds, sulfur-containing compounds, nitrogen-containing compounds, phosphorous-containing compounds, organohalides (compounds containing hydrogen and one of the halogens—chlorine, fluorine, bromine, or iodine), or combinations of these compounds.

A large portion of the chemicals that cause environmental pollution are organic compounds. They are harmful to us because of the damage their chemical makeup causes to our bodies. Subtle differences can cause a large variance in their effect on the body.

■ HARMFUL EFFECTS OF CHEMICALS

Chemicals can interact with different organs and tissues to cause damage. Chemicals can be toxic in many ways, and an individual chemical can be harmful in several different ways. Chemical damage can include:

- dehydration of skin tissue
- burning or death of skin tissue
- damage to eyes and even blinding
- burning of mucous membranes
- lung and respiratory tract damage
- osteosclerosis (abnormal hardening of the bone)
- damage to blood cells and production of blood cells
- glandular malfunction
- liver damage
- kidney damage
- enzyme destruction
- immune system damage
- cancer
- permanent neurological problems
- birth defects
- sterility

Substances that are extremely acid or alkaline are destructive to flesh. Sulfuric acid dehydrates tissue and can cause skin necrosis (death). Ingestion of sulfuric acid can cause severe injury and death. Contact with the eyes can cause loss of vision. Strong alkalis, such as sodium hydroxide, are poisonous and destroy all tissues at the site of exposure. Ingestion of these alkalis results in vomiting, prostration, and collapse. Elemental fluorine is a very strong oxidant that has a strong caustic action on the eyes, skin, and mucous membranes. Chronic absorption can cause mottled enamel of the teeth as well as osteosclerosis and calcification of ligaments. Inhaling fluorine causes lung hemorrhage. Many other chemicals, including allyl alcohol and ozone, damage our lungs if we inhale them.

Other chemicals cause long-term damage that is hidden until overt physical symptoms develop, signaling their presence. Some types of cancer are an example of this type of effect. Some chemicals alter or interfere with our basic body chemistry, causing it to function poorly or to malfunction. For example, if carbon monoxide binds to the hemoglobin in our red blood cells, it can no longer carry oxygen. Fluorine competes with iodine in the body and can cause the thyroid gland to malfunction. Other chemicals destroy the enzymes necessary for our body's biochemical reactions.

Chemicals, particularly environmental chemicals, can also interact and cause effects that are different from those of either chemical alone. If both chemicals have the same physiological action, their effects together may be additive or synergistic (the total effect is greater than the sum of the individual effects). Potentiation occurs when an inactive chemical increases the action of an active chemical. When an active chemical decreases the action of another active chemical, antagonism occurs.

■■ CHEMICAL SENSITIVITIES AND ALLERGIES

Fetuses, children, and elderly people are especially sensitive to chemicals in the environment. Young children have a larger body surface area in relation to their weight, a

---

MOST EFFECTIVE DETOXIFICATION METHODS

Exposure to Chemicals

- Detox baths or sauna programs (chapter **22**)
- Antioxidant nutrients (**23**)
- Healthy high-quality diet (**24**)
- Exercise and bodywork (**25**)
- Oxygen therapy and stabilized oxygen (**26**)
- Allergy extracts or hands-on treatment for specific chemicals (**27**)
- Homeopathic remedies such as *Arsenicum album, Ignatia, Phosphorus* (**28**)
- Bach Rescue Remedy (**28**)
- Herbal remedies such as cat's claw, elder, echinacea, goldenseal, milk thistle (**29**)
- Oral charcoal therapy (**31**)
- Organ cleansing (**31**)

---

higher metabolic rate, an immature host detoxification process, an immature renal system, and an immature immune system. Fetuses and young children are more easily poisoned by lead and pesticides than are adults. (See chapter 12, Toxins that Affect Children, for further information.) Elderly people have impaired host defenses, an increase in fat tissue, a loss of lean body mass, and impaired drug detoxification systems. Females are more susceptible than males to such environmental chemicals as lead, benzene, and alcohol.

Environmental chemical pollution also causes allergic sensitization. For example, people can become sensitized to the chemicals found in polyurethane varnish, foam, and paint. People who live in areas with high levels of pollution have higher IgE levels (an antibody associated with allergy) than people living in areas of low pollution. Asthma is more common in children who live close to roads with high traffic than in children who live further from busy roads.

People develop chemical sensitivity in several different ways:

- An overwhelming exposure to a chemical that causes acute symptoms and may cause chronic symptoms. Subsequent exposures to the same or other chemicals will trigger additional or more severe symptoms.
- Exposure to low levels of a chemical over a long period of time. This results in a cumulative effect and eventually small amounts of a chemical will trigger symptoms.
- Exposure to small amounts of a chemical after a trauma such as childbirth, surgery, immunizations, or severe injury.
- Sensitivity to chemicals sometimes develops after an acute infection (bacterial, viral, fungal, or parasitic).

Chemical Groups and Their Effects

Space limitations will not permit a discussion of all of the classes of chemicals and their effects on the human body. The following section will be limited to some of the more prevalent and toxic chemicals to which we are exposed.

■■ SOLVENTS

Solvents are chemicals used to extract, dissolve, or suspend materials, such as fats and resins, that are not soluble in water. Solvents typically are organic compounds composed of carbon and hydrogen atoms, and repre-

sent a large group of chemicals known as volatile organic chemicals (vocs), which evaporate easily from liquid or solid states. Like all organic compounds, they have irritant properties.

Solvents are lipophilic (fat-soluble) and have an affinity for the central nervous system (cns) because of its high fat content. Solvents dissolved in lipid membranes are relatively protected from enzymatic breakdown and therefore accumulate in the body. CNS symptoms may occur long after an exposure, when the accumulated solvent is released from tissue cells.

Acute organic solvent exposure can cause drowsiness, nausea, headache, dizziness, loss of coordination, rapid heartbeat, psychomotor impairment, loss of consciousness, and eventually death from respiratory failure. In addition, exposure to organic solvents can depress the central nervous system; irritate mucous membranes and tissues; and adversely affect the liver, kidneys, heart, bone marrow, and peripheral nervous system. Exposure to large amounts of solvents can damage the skin, lungs, and eyes. Because solvents are lipophilic, they can also defat the skin by extracting fat from the surface. The chemical structure of the organic solvent and the amount and length of exposure determine its effects.

There is controversy over whether chronic low-level exposure to solvents can be neurotoxic. However, many scientists believe that since exposure at low levels causes symptoms, such as dizziness and slight incoordination, repeated exposure may cause permanent damage, including the death of

Solvent Abuse

Solvents are widely used in inhalant abuse or "huffing"—also known as solvent abuse, volatile substance abuse, glue sniffing, and sniffing. Teenagers, predominantly 14- and 15-year-olds, inhale fumes from a volatile product directly from a container, plastic bag, or saturated rag. An initial euphoria, frequently with hallucinations, is followed by drowsiness and sleep, particularly with repeated inhalations.

This practice leads to central nervous system damage and can result in brain injury and dementia. Loss of cognitive functions, gait disturbance, loss of coordination, lung damage, deafness, and numbness of the hands and feet are only a few of the symptoms that can develop from huffing.

Death can occur from asphyxia, suffocation, aspiration, and sudden sniffing death syndrome. In sudden sniffing death syndrome, the user is startled during inhalation and inhales more deeply. The sudden increase of inhaled chemical produces a surge of epinephrine that can result in a fatal cardiac arrhythmia.

Substances used by huffers include toluene, butane, gasoline (benzene), lighter fluid (butane), model glue (acetone, toluol, ethanol), contact cement (toluene, hexane), permanent-ink felt-tip markers (phenol, toluene, naphtha, xylene), correction fluid (toluene), spray paint (benzene, toluene), paint thinners (acetone, butyl alcohol), and a wide variety of aerosols.

nerve cells (neurons). These cells do not regenerate.

■ ACETONE

Acetone is a clear liquid with a fairly pleasant odor. It is very flammable and explosive and must be kept away from heat and open flames. It is one of 50 top chemicals manufactured in the United States and is widely used as a solvent, in lubricating oils, and in the manufacture of other chemicals. It is also used in glue, airplane "dope," fingernail polish and remover, paints, and lacquer removers.

Acetone can dissolve fats from the skin, resulting in contact dermatitis. Rashes may occur anywhere on the body, but are often seen on the skin of the fingers, from fingernail polish remover. Acetone also causes brittleness, peeling, and splitting of the nails. Inhalation can damage the lungs and high concentrations can irritate the eyes and mucous membranes. If large amounts are inhaled, acetone has a narcotic action and can cause people to feel and act as if they are drunk, and to lose consciousness. Ingestion of acetone causes central nervous system depression and high blood sugar levels. Sometimes acetone poisoning is mistaken for diabetes.

■ BENZENE

Benzene is a common solvent with a pleasant "aromatic" odor. It is the most commercially significant hydrocarbon, and is used as the starting material for the manufacture of numerous products, including phenolic and polyester resins, insecticides, and dyes. Because it is in so many products, benzene is widely distributed in water and air. However, the major exposure to benzene is cigarette smoking. In the past, benzene was commonly used as an inert ingredient in pesticides.

Benzene is an effective replacement for lead in gasoline and an important component of oil-based paints and solvents. It is classified as a hazardous air pollutant, requiring the Environmental Protection Agency to establish exposure standards. In 1978, benzene was banned from use in the manufacture of household goods.

Acute benzene exposure can cause euphoria, excitement, irritability, headache, dizziness, vertigo, nausea, vomiting, skin rash, blisters, irregular heartbeat, loss of consciousness, and coma. Chronic exposure can cause aplastic anemia, in which the bone marrow stops producing red blood cells, or leukemia, (cancer of the bone marrow).

❚ CARBON TETRACHLORIDE
Carbon tetrachloride has an infamous record of human toxicity because of its effect on the liver. In the past, it was used as a dry-cleaning agent, as a degreasing solvent in consumer products, and in home fire extinguishers. Because of its toxic effects, the Federal Drug Administration banned the sale of carbon tetrachloride for all home use in 1970.

Exposure can cause conjunctivitis, headache, dizziness, nausea, vomiting, abdominal cramps, nervousness, narcosis, and coma. When inhaled, carbon tetrachloride affects the central nervous system. When ingested, it affects the liver and gastrointestinal tract. Acute exposure can cause extensive

Ethanol and Pregnancy

When consumed during pregnancy, ethanol is a teratogen that can cause birth defects, including defects of the head and face, and fetal alcohol syndrome. Fetal alcohol syndrome causes central nervous system abnormalities and is also the largest cause of non-genetic mental retardation. It retards physical growth both before and after birth.

kidney and liver damage, in addition to cardiac sensitization, in which the heart becomes more sensitive to any changes in the cardiovascular system.

Fatalities from carbon tetrachloride are caused by kidney failure. Because of its extreme toxicity, carbon tetrachloride is now limited to use as an intermediate compound for chemical manufacturing under controlled conditions.

❚ ETHANOL
Ethanol (grain alcohol) is an organic solvent that depresses the cardiovascular and central nervous systems. It is contained in perfumes and liquor, and used in many types of industry as a solvent. Ethanol is also used as a germicide and in antifreeze, and in recent years has gained fame as a gasoline additive.

Ethanol raises the pain threshold by 35 percent, dilates blood vessels in the skin, increases gastric acid secretion, and may lead to inflammation of the stomach lining or an ulcer. Ethanol weakens all muscles, including the heart muscles, and causes fat deposition throughout the body. It depresses cell production by the bone marrow, leading to a lack of white cells in areas of inflammation. Alcoholics have increased rates of infection. Chronic ingestion causes cirrhosis, a scarring of the liver, which leads to liver failure, and ingesting a large amount in a short period of time can be fatal.

■ ETHYLENE GLYCOL

Ethylene glycol, which is a sweet-tasting solvent, is the major ingredient in antifreeze. It is a humectant and can absorb twice its weight in water. Ethylene glycol is used in chemical synthesis and cosmetics.

Because it has a low vapor pressure, toxic exposures to ethylene glycol are rare. However, inhalation of droplets can be extremely dangerous, and ingestion can be fatal. There have been about 50 human fatalities in the United States from ethylene glycol poisoning. The body metabolizes ethylene glycol to oxalate, a substance that is toxic to the kidneys and may cause renal failure.

Many pets, especially cats, die each year after ingesting leaked or spilled antifreeze, which has an appealing taste to them.

■ FORMALDEHYDE

Formaldehyde is a gas with a pungent, suffocating odor. Because the pure form is unstable, formaldehyde is produced in a 3 to 50 percent aqueous solution known as formalin that is used extensively in industry. The U.S. alone produces 7 to 8 billion pounds annually. Formaldehyde is used in the plastics and resins industries, as well as in cosmetics, disinfectants, mouthwashes, film hardeners, wood preservatives, and biocides. Formaldehyde is also used as a fumigant, as a preservative for tissue and biological specimens, and as an embalming fluid.

Methanol Limp

During Prohibition in the United States, some people desperate for liquor drank methanol as a substitute for grain alcohol (ethanol). The resulting neurological damage caused them to drag one leg when they walked.

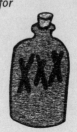

People can become sensitized to formaldehyde by wearing permanent-press fabrics containing melamine-formaldehyde resins. Formaldehyde exposure from off-gassing of building materials, carpets, and new furnishings is a serious health hazard both in homes and in the workplace. (See chapter 8, Toxins in the Home, and chapter 9, Toxins in the Workplace and School, for more information on formaldehyde.)

An irritant, formaldehyde affects the eyes and respiratory tract and causes sensitization of the skin. Formaldehyde is extremely toxic. At concentrations of 0.1 to 5 parts per million it can cause asthma, contact dermatitis, nausea, headache, fatigue, memory lapse, nosebleeds, and disorientation. High exposures can cause serious injury and death.

■ METHANOL

The largest use of methanol (wood alcohol) is in the manufacturing industry for the manufacture of formaldehyde, acetic acid, and other chemicals. It has been added to gasoline in an effort to reduce carbon monoxide emissions. Methanol is added to ethanol to denature it and make it unfit to drink.

Prolonged exposure to methanol fumes, or skin contact, can cause headache, vertigo, nausea, vomiting, abdominal cramps, mild central nervous system depression, sweating, weakness, delirium, and blurred vision. Methanol poisoning can be fatal because it can cause convulsions and cessation of breathing (apnea).

Ingesting just 3 teaspoons of methanol has caused blindness, and 30 teaspoons has caused death. When methanol is metabolized, the metabolite is more toxic than methanol itself.

■ METHYLENE CHLORIDE

Methylene chloride is a colorless liquid with a pungent odor. It is used in varnishes, for degreasing and cleaning fluid, as a solvent in paint and food processing, as an insecticide, as an aerosol propellant, and as a pharmaceutical solvent. It is considered the best liquid paint remover, and some paint strippers are 40 to 50 percent methylene chloride.

Methylene chloride vapor irritates the skin and eyes and causes fatigue, weakness, lightheadedness, and sleepiness. At high concentration it causes a drunkenlike state. The body metabolizes methylene chloride to carbon monoxide, which interferes with oxygen transport in the body. Smokers are doubly affected. Damage to the liver, kidney, and central nervous system can occur.

■ PHENOL

An alcohol attached to a benzene ring, phenol denatures and precipitates proteins. Because it kills bacteria, it is used in many cleaning products. Phenol, which is also called carboxylic acid, is the main ingredient

> ## Phenol
>
> *On a parts per million basis, phenol is as toxic by inhalation as cyanide, and is also extremely toxic by absorption. A man who accidentally spilled phenol on his thighs died within 10 minutes of exposure, although he tried to wash it off with water.*

in Lysol. It is also used in the manufacture of medications of coal tar origin, such as aspirin and sulfa drugs.

Phenol is readily absorbed by the skin, but may also burn the skin on contact. It acts as a local anesthetic, and is a central nervous system depressant. Phenol can cause numbness, nausea, vomiting, cold sweats, headache, irritability, and wheezing. If ingested, it severely burns the membranes of the throat, esophagus, and stomach.

■ POLYCYCLIC AROMATIC HYDROCARBONS

Polycyclic aromatic hydrocarbons (PAHS) are products of tobacco combustion, vehicular exhaust, and industrial combustion. They are lipid-soluble and are absorbed by the skin, lungs, or digestive tract, where they become concentrated in organs with high fat content. The thymus and spleen are particularly affected by the acute effects of PAHS.

When PAHS are metabolized, arene oxides are formed. These are reactive, carcinogenic metabolites that attach to DNA. As early as 1775, it was noted that chimney sweeps and tar workers, both of whom are exposed to PAHS, developed cancer of the scrotum at high rates. Asphalt, coal gas, and coke production workers develop lung cancer at a high rate. PAHs are produced in all these manufacturing processes. (See also chapter 13, Food, for a discussion of PAHs in foods.)

■ STYRENE

Styrene is a liquid at room temperature, with a penetrating odor described by some people as sweet. It is one of the top 20 chemicals manufactured in the U.S. and is used in numerous consumer products, including automobile tires, auto parts, adhesives, bottles, jars, kitchen utensils, boxes, combs, copy paper and toner, cushions, eyeglass lenses, plastic food wrap, photographic film, PVC pipe, and Styrofoam cups and trays.

Styrene is heated to make a variety of plastics, ranging from clear and rigid to multicolored and resistant to impact. One of the problems with using styrene is that it solidifies at relatively low heats. Manufacturers add stabilizers to keep it liquid during shipping. Hydroquinone is frequently used for this purpose, and some researchers question whether people who react to styrene are reacting to the stabilizer rather than the styrene.

Indoor air can be contaminated with small amounts of styrene emitted from a variety of products in the home. There is evidence that styrene migrates from food packaging into the foods. Outdoor air can be contaminated from plants that manufacture styrene, and some rivers have become contaminated with styrene from industrial effluent.

Styrene is absorbed through the skin, respiratory tract, and gastrointestinal tract. Because it is lipophilic, it accumulates in

Tetrachloroethylene

Tetrachloroethylene does not evaporate or break down, and once it contaminates water, its concentration does not decrease over time. It is now classified as a potential human carcinogen.

fatty tissue. Styrene vapor is irritating and damaging to the eyes and mucous membranes. High doses paralyze the respiratory system, first causing dizziness, then loss of consciousness and death. Styrene may be a carcinogen. Some studies report that workers exposed to styrene developed leukemias and lymphomas at a higher rate than the general population; however, other studies do not support this finding.

■ TETRACHLOROETHYLENE

Tetrachloroethylene, also called perchloroethylene (PCE), is a colorless, nonflammable liquid with an ether-like smell. It is used for dry-cleaning and as a degreaser for metals. People who live next door to a dry-cleaning facility receive significant doses of PCE. It is also used in textile processing, as an intermediate in the production of fluorocarbons, and as a solvent. PCE is found in vinyl-coated, asbestos cement pipes, and is sometimes used as an insulating liquid and coolant in electrical transformers.

PCE can be inhaled or absorbed through the skin in limited amounts. It causes eye, nose, throat, and skin irritation; confusion, dizziness, and weakness; respiratory depression; and liver damage. Long-term effects include fatigue, loss of short-term memory, poor muscle coordination, difficulty concentrating, anxiety, nervousness, and irritability.

■ TOLUENE

Toluene is a highly volatile chemical with a structure similar to benzene, but it is less volatile, less flammable, and less toxic. It is now being added to gasoline to improve octane ratings, and it is an ingredient in model glue, markers, and typewriter correction fluid. Toluene is a solvent for paints, inks, resins, and adhesives. It is widely used in the manufacturing of many products, including detergents, dyes, linoleum, perfumes, pharmaceuticals, saccharin, and TNT. Toluene is also contained in cigarette smoke.

Toluene affects the skin, irritating it and causing numbness. It also dries out the skin by defatting the surface layer. Toluene depresses the central nervous system, causing fatigue, weakness, confusion, nausea, headache, and dizziness at high exposure levels. Long-term toluene exposure can cause liver disorders, nerve damage, and irregular heart rate, and has caused death. Ethanol raises blood levels of toluene by blocking its metabolism.

■ TRICHLOROETHYLENE

Trichloroethylene (TCE), which has an odor similar to chloroform, decomposes to form phosgene, a highly toxic gas, and hydrogen chloride, a corrosive gas. It is used in metal degreasers, spot removers, rug cleaners, typewriter correction fluid, and disinfectants. TCE is also used in solvent extraction in many industries and in the manufacture of organic chemicals. It is a common inert ingredient in fungicides and insecticides. In the past it was used as a dry-cleaning agent, general anesthetic, and fumigant. Because of its toxicity, these uses have been discontinued.

TCE depresses the central nervous system and causes headaches, dizziness, and sleepiness. It irritates the eyes, nose, and respiratory tract, and causes liver and kidney damage. At high doses it causes cardiac arrest. With chronic exposure, TCE causes fatigue, memory loss, transient euphoria, and depression. It may be a carcinogen.

■ VINYL CHLORIDE

Vinyl chloride is a flammable, colorless, volatile gas with a sweet odor. It is the raw material for manufacturing polyvinylchloride plastic, which is the polymer in PVC pipe, car and garden hoses, containers for margarine and oils, and plastic food wrap. It is also used as a refrigerant and in the synthesis of organic compounds. In 1974, its use was banned in aerosol cans for hair spray and deodorants.

Vinyl chloride is found in small amounts in alcoholic beverages, butter, vinegar, edible oils, and mineral water. Plastic packaging and PVC pipes are believed to be the source of this contamination. Inhalation of contaminated air around vinyl chloride manufacturing plants and industrial sites where it is used constitute the most significant exposures.

Vinyl chloride irritates the skin and acts as a central nervous system depressant. It will dissolve most fats. It was originally thought that chronic exposure to vinyl chloride caused only bone loss in the fingers, decreased circulation, and skin changes. However, in 1973, companies producing vinyl chloride began to report deaths of workers from angiosarcoma of the liver, a fatal cancer. Further investigation showed vinyl chloride exposure also causes cancer of the lungs and nervous system.

∎ XYLENE

Xylene is heavily used in the chemical industry to manufacture many other chemicals, including solvents, plastics, pesticides, and pharmaceuticals. It may be used alone as a solvent and is also found in household products such as air fresheners, degreasing cleaners, glues, lacquers, marking pens, nail polish, paints, and paint remover.

Because it is released into the air during industrial processing, xylene is a common outdoor air pollutant in industrialized areas. It is one of the most toxic of the aromatic hydrocarbons, which include benzene and toluene.

High concentrations of xylene vapor in the air irritate the eyes, nose, and throat, causing coughing, hoarseness, and fluid in the lungs. Continued inhalation causes symptoms of drunkenness, poor balance, central nervous system depression or agitation, tremors, restlessness, and unconsciousness. Skin exposure to xylene causes redness and blisters, and continued exposure can result in kidney damage. Most fatal poisonings are from inhalation of xylene vapor, with death occurring from respiratory or cardiac arrest.

∎∎ PESTICIDES

Rachel Carson's landmark book *Silent Spring* (1962) changed the way North Americans viewed the use of pesticides. This book led to the increased scientific study of pesticides and to improved government requirements for testing pesticides. Carson is often cred-

Pesticide Use

Since 1960, pesticide use has doubled in the U.S. Herbicide use has increased dramatically, while insecticide use has decreased, with herbicides representing 61 percent of pesticide use and insecticides representing 21 percent. Instead of using mechanical methods of controlling plants, people have turned to chemical methods. U.S. agriculture uses over 900 million pounds of pesticides annually, producing food that is eaten worldwide. In 1998, 35 percent of U.S. food samples contained pesticide residue. In Canada, more than 100 million pounds of pesticides are used annually on crops, lawns, and gardens.

Despite this increased use of chemicals, the quantity of food production has not proportionately increased. One-third of the food crop is still lost to pests, demonstrating that pesticides are of limited effectiveness.

ited with starting the environmental movement.

Pesticides are chemicals used to control weeds, insects, rodents, and other organisms that people consider to be pests. They include rodenticides, insecticides, ascaricides (worm-killers), herbicides, and fungicides. Some chemicals currently used as pesticides were originally developed as nerve gases by Germany before World War II. The three main categories of pesticides are carbamates, organophosphates, and organochlorines. Pesticides are very toxic to humans and can cause numerous health problems.

The agriculture industry uses 90 percent of the pesticides in the U.S. However, pesticides also are used in paints, carpets, mattresses, paper, dentures, shampoos, hair wigs, disposable diapers, and contact lenses. Pesticides are even used in swimming pools to control algae. Many North American families use insecticidal flea collars, sprays, dusts, shampoos, or dips for their pets. Pesticide residues from these products can find their way into the family's carpeting, clothing, bedding, and even food.

Every North American is exposed to pesticides daily. Each year, they cause approximately 80,000 to 90,000 field workers to become ill and 80 to 100 to die. Pesticide residues are found in our food, drinking water, air, clothing, and household furnishings. Exposure to pesticides occurs in most schools, offices, apartment buildings, churches, and factories. The spraying of golf courses, agricultural lands, parks, and neighborhood gardens provides yet another source of pesticide exposure. Cities often have widespread spraying programs.

A single pesticide exposure may not cause problems for most people, but combined exposures do. Many pesticides are broad spectrum and can damage plants, birds, and humans. Pesticides may interact synergistically with each other, tripling or quadrupling the effect of each pesticide.

The concept and use of pesticides is not new. Approximately 2,000 years ago, the Chinese used dried chrysanthemum flowers, which contain pyrethrums, to kill insects. The Romans used salt brine and ashes to sterilize the soil. Tobacco plant extracts (nicotine) have been used for several hundred years to kill insects. Sulfur, copper, mercury, and arsenic were used in the early 1900s as insecticides.

Pesticides contain several different types of ingredients. The active ingredients are those with lethal/toxic action against target pests. The remaining ingredients are considered to be inert, and they are not tested for their effects. Inert ingredients include solvents, propellants, surfactants, emulsifiers, wetting agents, carriers, or diluents. While they have no pesticide action, these ingredients are not inactive. For humans, they may be the most toxic part of a pesticide product.

Companies may use the same active ingredient but different inert ingredients, which are considered trade secrets. The United States Federal Insecticide, Fungicide, and Rodenticide Act (FIFRA) does not require the inert ingredients to be listed. The Environmental Protection Agency (EPA) has categorized inert ingredients into four lists. There are eight ingredients in List 1, which contains the most dangerous compounds. Formaldehyde and malachite green are being phased out, which will leave six compounds on List 1. Lists 2 and 3 are made up of slightly less toxic compounds than those in List 1. Many of these compounds are no longer used in pesticides. The EPA is completing evaluation of these compounds and some are expected to be reclassified or deleted from the list. List 4 is subdivided into two parts. List 4A contains GRAS (generally recognized as safe) substances, and there is sufficient data to substantiate List 4B substances as safe to use in pesticide products.

Gulf War Chemicals

Several research teams have demonstrated that there was a potent synergistic effect between the chemicals to which the Gulf War soldiers were exposed in 1991. They were exposed to chlorpyrifos (Dursban, an organophosphate), they used DEET (an insect repellant), and they took pyridostigmine bromide (an anti-nerve gas agent) *orally when the risk of chemical attack was high. Studies, including those by Mohamed Abou-Donia of Duke University in Durham, North Carolina, and Tom Kurt of the University of Texas Southwestern Medical School in Dallas, Texas, showed that simultaneous exposure to all three agents dramatically increased their neurotoxicity.*

When an inert ingredient reaches List 4B, no further regulatory action is anticipated.

Synergists, added to the active ingredient to increase its effects, decrease the target pest's ability to detoxify the primary pesticide, frequently making the pesticide more toxic to humans. Synergism has also been noted between two chemicals in a pesticide, each of which may be of low or medium toxicity separately, but in combination show increased toxicity.

Pesticides have two types of action: contact and systemic. Contact pesticides act directly on the targeted pest, killing very rapidly. Systemic pesticides are applied to the soil or the leaves of a plant and may be ingested when people eat the fruits, nuts, or seeds. Systemic herbicides affect normal plant metabolism, inhibiting the plant's growth.

■ ORGANOPHOSPHATE PESTICIDES

Organophosphate pesticides were originally developed as chemical warfare agents and range in toxicity from that of table salt to that of nerve gas. They do not persist for years in the environment, as DDT does, but they are highly toxic to humans and other mammals.

Organophosphates have poisoned more people than any other group of pesticides and are readily absorbed through the skin, lungs, and gastrointestinal tract. Exposure is mainly through use and application as insecticides, in crop-surface sprays, aerosols, baits, and fumigants. Organophosphates include parathion, dichlorvos, diazinon, phosmet, and malathion.

Organophosphate pesticides bind to and inactivate acetylcholinesterase (AchE) within nerves. Acetylcholine, a neurotransmitter, is released from one nerve cell and binds to another nerve cell, causing an electrical charge in the second nerve cell, "exciting" it. Acetylcholinesterase breaks down the acetylcholine so that the nerve cell is no longer excited. If AchE is inhibited, acetylcholine can continue to excite the nerve cell, leading to muscle twitching, rigid paralysis, or even death.

Most organophosphate pesticides must be metabolically converted in the liver to become biochemically active. Once activated, organophosphates are rapidly metabolized and excreted. Because of this rapid excretion, they are difficult to detect in the blood

48 hours after exposure, and laboratory tests to determine their presence must be done before this time.

Organophosphate pesticides have severe acute effects:

• When they are absorbed through the skin, they can affect the neuromuscular junction, causing excess sweating, muscular twitching, extreme weakness, and paralysis.

• If organophosphates are inhaled, they affect the respiratory muscles, causing difficulty breathing and a feeling of chest tightness. The smooth muscle in the lung goes into spasms, triggering an asthma attack.

• On ingestion of organophosphates, the muscles of the GI tract and bladder go into spasm, resulting in nausea and vomiting. In some cases the pupils of the eyes constrict.

Central nervous system symptoms can develop from absorption, inhalation, or ingestion, including tremor, confusion, slurred speech, poor balance, and poor coordination. With large exposures, convulsions and death may result.

In chronic exposures, organophosphate pesticides easily cross the blood-brain barrier and enter the central nervous system, causing pathological changes. Neuropathy (damage to nerves) develops, affecting the central and peripheral nervous systems, and may appear up to 85 hours after the original poisoning. Peripheral nerves that control movement and sensation can be affected, but the most common changes include paralysis of the lower legs, wasted muscles, and loss of strength.

Exposure to organophosphates can also cause acute psychosis, loss of memory, schizophrenia, or severe depression. These symptoms can occur up to two months after an acute exposure. The psychiatric effects last at least six months and up to one year, although schizophrenia has persisted longer in some patients.

Many scientists say organophospates do not accumulate in the body, but Dr. William Rea of the Environmental Health Center in Dallas, Texas, has done lab tests that show accumulation. Organophosphate pesticides may also block the body's detoxification mechanism, making related pesticides more toxic.

Dr. Mark Cullen, Head of Occupational Medicine at Yale University, has noted that multiple chemical sensitivities (a syndrome of acquired intolerance to common environmental chemicals, with symptoms involving multiple organ systems) often follows a toxic exposure, and in particular after organophosphate poisoning.

■ CARBAMATE PESTICIDES

Carbamate pesticides are similar to organophosphate pesticides, but are more biodegradable and are less toxic with skin exposures. They are among the most widely used pesticides in the world and have insecticidal, herbicidal, and fungicidal activity, depending on the specific compound. Principally used as herbicides or fungicides, carbamates include baygon, sevin, and aldicarb (Temik).

Like organophosphate pesticides, carbamates inactivate acetylcholinesterase by binding to it, but the body is more rapidly able to reactivate it. Acetylcholinesterase levels become normal within two hours of exposure.

Acute symptoms after carbamate pesticide exposure are lightheadedness, nausea and vomiting, increased sweating, increased salivation, blurred vision, weakness, muscle twitching, small contracted pupils, and convulsions. Some carbamates may cause liver or kidney damage. Recovery from carbamate poisoning is relatively quick. While carbamates do not bioconcentrate in mammals, they do accumulate in fish.

In the presence of nitrates, carbamates can be converted to nitrosamines, which are carcinogens. There is little information about the long-term toxicity or cancer-causing ability of carbamate pesticides.

▌ ORGANOCHLORINE PESTICIDES
Organochlorine pesticides are the oldest type of synthetic pesticides used to control insects. They are very stable in the environment and have a high lipid solubility. Organochlorine pesticides are not as acutely toxic as the carbamates or organophosphate pesticides, but they have a greater potential for chronic toxicity.

Organochlorines are well absorbed orally and they accumulate in the fat tissue of animals, where they remain for long periods. Some organochlorines are carcinogenic and all are central nervous system depressants. Acute symptoms include irritability, dizziness, tremors, convulsions, and headaches. Chronic symptoms can manifest as personality changes, tremor, loss of memory, and a specific movement of the eyes called nystagmus.

In 1939, the organochlorine dichlorodiphenyltrichloroethane (DDT) was discov-

ered to have insecticidal properties, and was used widely for two decades. DDT has been one of the safest pesticides used in terms of acute effects on people. It was used directly on humans to kill lice, and has never caused a fatal poisoning. However, DDT was banned in 1972 because of environmental effects through bioaccumulation. (See chapter 13, Food, for further information on DDT.)

Acute DDT exposure can cause numbness of the face, irritability, dizziness, poor balance, tremor, and convulsions. Subacute doses can cause the testicles to become smaller. No adverse clinical effects have been demonstrated for DDT with long-term low dosing. However, during starvation, DDT is released from fat cells and can cause acute symptoms. Women who develop breast cancer tend to have higher residues of DDE, the breakdown product of DDT, in their breasts than do women who are free of the disease.

▌ CHLORINATED CYCLODIENE
   PESTICIDES
Chlorinated cyclodiene pesticides are used on insects and include chlordane, heptachlor, aldrin, dieldrin, endrin, and endosulfan. They are lipid-soluble and may be stored in human and animal fat for long periods of time. Many of these compounds are neuropoisons, and convulsions are often the first sign of toxicity. Other signs of poisoning are headaches, nausea, vomiting, dizziness, and mild chronic jerking of muscles. There may also be long-term loss of memory and personality changes.

Chronic doses of dieldrin, heptachlor, and chlordane have caused liver cancer in mice. Aldrin, dieldrin, and endrin caused

Weed Killers

One of our patients was formerly employed at a refinery where he became sensitized to many different chemicals. Among these chemicals were the chlorophenoxy compounds used by the highway department to kill roadside weeds. He was so sensitive that he would break out into a rash simply from driving down a highway that had recently been sprayed.

birth defects in the offspring of pregnant mice and hamsters. Aldrin and heptachlor caused death in rodent fetuses. Chlordane contains approximately 10 percent heptachlor. Until 1978, chlordane was the primary insecticide used for termites. It was banned because of its long half-life (of 30 years), which leaves areas where it has been used contaminated over many generations.

■ BOTANICAL PESTICIDES

Botanicals, which are insecticidal chemicals extracted from plants, include nicotine, rotenone, pyrethrum extracts, camphor, and turpentine. They are produced naturally by plants to kill or deter plant-eating insects. Botanicals differ in their chemical structure, stability, and specific toxic effects. They are less toxic to people than other types of pesticides, but can cause problems for chemically sensitive people.

Botanicals are extremely effective insecticides but are more expensive than the other classes of pesticides, making them impractical for large-scale agricultural use. Pyrethroids, which are less costly synthetic

pyrethrums, are now available. They are very effective, but are neurotoxic to humans. Side effects include tingling of the skin.

■ MICROBIAL PESTICIDES

Microbial pesticides can contain a bacteria, fungus, or virus as the active ingredient. Non-viable microbials are also used, which consist mainly of endotoxins in killed bacterial preparations. These pesticides are used to infect and destroy target pests by causing a disease in the pest. They are selective and effective in their action and generally present less risk than conventional pesticides. They can be a toxic exposure for people who are immuno-compromised.

Different types of microbial pesticides are available for different types of pests. For example, several different fungi are used, some that control weeds, and some that control cockroaches. The EPA Office of Pesticide Programs has approved 14 fungi as active ingredients in pesticides.

Bacillus thuringiensis (Bt) is perhaps the most commonly used bacteria to control plant diseases. It can control specific insects in cabbage, corn, and potatoes. In addition to many subspecies of *Bacillus thuringiensis*, other *Bacillus* species are employed, including *B. cereus*, *B. popilliae*, *B. lentiborbus*, *B. subtilis*, and *B. sphaericus*. *Agrobacterium radiobacter*, *Burkkholderia cepacia*, several *Pseudomonas* species, and *Streptomyces griseoviridis* are also approved bacterial pesticides.

Seven viruses have been approved as active pesticide ingredients, among them viruses that control the Douglas-fir tussock moth and the gypsy moth. Portions of viruses are also used as microbial pesticides, and have been approved as safe. They are used to protect potato, papaya, watermelon, and squash crops.

■ HERBICIDES

Herbicides are a type of pesticide used to control unwanted plants. They are toxic to plant enzymes and are generally thought to be nontoxic to humans, although people have died from herbicide poisoning.

Chlorophenoxy compounds are used to kill weeds next to highways and broadleaf weeds in farming. Two compounds in this group (2,4-D and 2,4,5,-T) interfere with the growth hormone system in plants. After ingesting plants contaminated with chlorophenoxy compounds, animals have died from ventricular fibrillation and muscle paralysis. Acute toxicity symptoms of both 2,4,5-T and 2,4-D include muscular weakness, depression, paralysis and coma, loss of appetite, loss of weight, and vomiting. At high doses, 2,4,5-T is toxic to the kidney.

The compound 2,4,5,-T contains a trace of dioxin, one of the most potent toxins known. It is teratogenic (causes physical defects in developing embryos) in rats and can cause headaches, dizziness, digestive disorders, generalized aches and pains, and chloracne, a skin eruption resembling acne. Larger amounts of dioxin have been linked to cancer. Dioxin is released into the atmosphere when vegetation treated with 2,4,5-T is burned.

Dinitrophenols are another class of herbicide. Toxic exposures in humans cause nausea, rapid breathing, sweating, rapid heart rate, and coma. Dinitrophenols disable the mitochondria, which are the powerhouses of cells. With chronic exposures,

these compounds can cause fatigue, sweating, thirst, and weight loss.

Because it is a nonselective herbicide, Paraquat, a dinitrophenol, has been used around the world for weed control in agriculture and along roadsides. Paraquat was also used in Vietnam as a weed-killer. It has been used in the United States and Mexico to destroy marijuana crops. This practice was stopped when it was discovered that irreversible lung damage could result from smoking contaminated marijuana.

The liver and kidneys are damaged with high exposure to Paraquat. Even when the exposure does not involve inhalation, Paraquat causes pulmonary fibrosis (thickening and scarring of lung tissue). It can lead to death when ingested.

■■ LATEX

Although it is not a major chemical contaminant as are some industrial chemicals, health problems with latex are an emerging problem in North America. Many people are sensitizing to latex so that when they are exposed to it, they can have very severe symptoms. Latex is natural rubber, the milky fluid from the rubber tree, *Hevea brasiliensis,* and it contains proteins that are allergenic. In addition, it is treated with accelerants and antioxidants to prevent deterioration. This creates several new allergens. The desirable physical properties of natural latex can be reproduced synthetically, but at a considerably increased price.

We have many exposures to latex, including adhesives, baby bottle nipples and pacifiers, balloons, bandages, blood pressure cuffs, catheters, condoms, diaphragms,

Agent Orange

The combination of 2,4,5-T and 2,4-D is called Agent Orange, which was used in Vietnam. The U.S. military sprayed about 11 million gallons of Agent Orange over South Vietnam between 1965 and 1970, to defoliate trees and destroy crops.

Not only did Agent Orange affect the United States troops on the ground in Vietnam, the pesticide has had lasting effects on the Vietnamese people. The Americans were exposed for months, compared to decades for the Vietnamese.

Damage from Agent Orange is caused by an extremely toxic contaminant, dioxin, created during the manufacturing process. It is believed that the chemicals remained on the ground for 12 years after the Vietnam War, with monsoon rains spreading them into uncontaminated areas through streams and rivers. Many health experts believe that dioxin is now in the food chain of southern Vietnam, both in the water and in fish from contaminated streams.

The effects of Agent Orange constitute the most severe problem in Vietnam remaining from the war. The Vietnamese government estimates that half a million people have died or contracted serious illnesses over the years because of Agent Orange. As many as 70,000 are still affected. The Vietnamese veterans have suffered from the same conditions as the American soldiers. In addition, their children are prone to more birth defects of the skin, nervous system, heart, kidney, and oral clefts (cleft palates). Sudden Infant Death Syndrome, difficult or premature births, and infants born without limbs are also far more common among their children. High numbers of malformed fetuses are delivered, or are spontaneously aborted.

American veterans of Vietnam and their children are also still suffering from the effects of Agent Orange. A 1994 committee report from the Institute of Medicine (IOM), a department of the National Academy of Science in Washington, D.C., states that:

- There is sufficient evidence of an association between Agent Orange and soft-tissue sarcoma, non-Hodgkin's lymphoma, Hodgkin's disease, and chloracne.
- There is limited or suggestive evidence of an association in respiratory cancers (lung, larynx, and trachea), prostate cancer, multiple myeloma (bone marrow tumors), acute and subacute peripheral neuropathy, spina bifida, and porphyria cutanea tarda (a skin rash following sun exposure).

At present, available studies are of insufficient quality, consistency, or statistical significance to permit a conclusion for other types of cancer, spontaneous abortion, birth defects other than spina bifida, infant death and stillbirths, childhood cancer in offspring, nervous sytem disorders, abnormal sperm parameters and infertility, and digestive, circulatory, and respiratory system disorders.

This is not a closed issue, however, and the controversial legacy of Agent Orange continues for both American veterans and the citizens of Vietnam.

Latex Allergy

A latex allergy caused one woman to have a very violent reaction to a Band-Aid. When it was placed over a cut on her finger, she began to feel worse, quickly becoming weak and disoriented. She started to shake and fell on the floor, incoherent. When she began having difficulty breathing, her husband put her in the shower, at which point the Band-Aid became wet and fell off.

After a few minutes she began to feel better and stopped the shower. Because she and her husband had not realized the Band-Aid caused the problem, they placed another one over the cut. When she began to have the same symptoms again, they determined the relationship and removed the Band-Aid. She now uses gauze and paper tape instead of adhesive bandages.

finger cots, hot water bottles, latex gloves, dishwashing gloves, erasers, respirators, rubber dams for dental work, rubber stoppers, rubber bands, shoe soles, sports equipment, stethoscope tubing, and tires. Dipped latex products such as balloons, condoms, and gloves are more allergenic than molded latex products. When latex is dried, it is used to manufacture such products as syringe plungers, baby bottle nipples, and vial stoppers.

Workers in the rubber industry who are exposed to high levels of latex for extended periods of time are at high risk for becoming sensitized to latex. Healthcare workers, medical housekeeping staff, and dental workers are also at high risk to develop latex allergies. Most of these workers wear latex gloves, which are frequently powdered. This powder contains latex particles that further contribute to sensitization and symptoms. Because of the life-threatening reactions it can cause during medical procedures, a latex allergy is a serious problem both for health-care workers and patients.

The Food and Drug Administration has reported that latex glove use increased by 247 percent between 1991 and 1996. People who wear latex gloves frequently develop a skin rash or itchy, dry skin on their hands.

Symptoms of latex allergy include hives, itching, runny nose, red eyes, edema, flushing, wheezing, lightheadedness, tachycardia, and anaphylaxis (allergic shock). Inhalation of latex-laced powder particles, such as those in latex gloves, can trigger asthma or anaphylaxis in a latex-sensitive person.

A latex allergy worsens with repeated exposure, and can be debilitating. Latex is so widespread that it can be difficult to avoid. Latex-allergic people who continue to be exposed to latex products can seriously damage their health. Systemic symptoms will become progressively worse and the danger of anaphylaxis increases with continued exposure.

Genetics apparently determines the potential for an individual to develop a latex

MOST EFFECTIVE DETOXIFICATION METHODS

Metal Exposure or Poisoning

- Detox baths or sauna programs (chapter **22**)
- Sulfur-containing nutrients (**23**)
- Healthy high-quality diet (**24**)
- Exercise and bodywork (**25**)
- Oxygen therapy (**26**)
- Allergy extracts or hands-on treatment for specific metals (**27**)
- Chelation therapy (**27**)
- Homeopathic remedies such as *Alumina, Cadmium metallicum, Hepar sulphuris, Plumbum metallicum* (**28**)
- Herbal remedies such as apple, garlic, pectin (**29**)
- Organ cleansing (**31**)

allergy. In addition, people who have had surgery, particularly on the nervous system, spine, or genitourinary tract, are more likely to develop latex allergy. Latex allergies cross-react with certain foods, including avocados, bananas, chestnuts, kiwi, papaya, and pineapple. People who are allergic to latex may develop symptoms from eating these foods.

Metals

Approximately 80 elements are classified as metals. The physical properties of metals include high reflectivity, electrical and thermal conductivity, and strength. In a water solution, metals can give up a negative particle, or electron, to form a positively charged ion, a cation. It is this property that determines the biological activity and toxicological characteristics of each metal. Metals are frequently used in the workplace, and some cause serious contamination of our environment.

Dr. Henry Schroeder, one of the world's authorities on trace elements, felt 20 years ago that chronic toxic metal exposure could be a more dangerous and insidious problem to human health than are organic substances such as pesticides. This section will discuss the most commonly encountered toxic metals.

Although metals are categorized as heavy, trace, essential, nonessential, or toxic, there is much overlapping between these categories. Heavy metals have a specific gravity greater than 4 or 5.

Trace metals, found in minute quantities in the body, are also essential metals, and are necessary for proper functioning of the body. However, essential metals can be toxic, depending on the amount. For example, copper, iron, and cobalt are all needed by the body, but can be toxic in high amounts. Nonessential metals are not necessary for proper metabolism of the body, and they may also be toxic.

Metals can be inhaled as fumes or dust particulates, and particles less than 1 micron may be absorbed from the lung's alveoli into the bloodstream. Metals can also be ingested in food or water. The gastrointestinal tract may absorb metals if they are sufficiently soluble. A person's age, nutritional status, the amount of food in the intestines, and the intake of metals competing for absorption in the body (for example, zinc and cadmium) affect the absorption rate of metals. More metals are absorbed when less food is present. The chemical form (an element or a compound) of the metal in the body also determines how much metal will be absorbed.

Most metals are excreted through the kidneys, but some are reabsorbed by the kidney tubules. Many metals are bound to plasma proteins and amino acids. Reabsorption is determined by the pH of the urine, the type of protein or amino acid to which the metal is attached, and whether other metals are competing for the same tubular reabsorption site. The gastrointestinal tract also excretes metals. Lead, cadmium, and mercury are absorbed from the blood into the intestines. Metals that are attached to the cells lining the GI tract are excreted when these cells are shed. Metals are also deposited in the hair and are a reliable indication of the body burden of that metal.

Metals can be acutely or chronically toxic. Chronic toxicity is much more difficult to diagnose. In chronic toxicity, a person is exposed to small doses over a long period of time. Symptoms may not develop for months to years. Acute toxicity symptoms may be different from those of chronic toxicity. For example, acute inorganic mercury toxicity may cause nausea, headache, diarrhea, and abdominal pain, while chronic inorganic mercury toxicity causes difficulty in swallowing; abnormal vision, hearing, taste, and smell; and poor coordination in the arms and legs.

Metals inhibit the activity of many enzymes and they can bind to vitamins. Toxic metals may displace essential metals. They tend to accumulate in target organs, and when the level exceeds the threshold level for that organ, symptoms result. Many of the organs affected are those that are normally involved in the detoxification procedures to

Aluminum

Aluminum is the third most abundant element on earth and the most abundant metal. At one time aluminum was very difficult to extract from ore and was considered a very valuable metal. Napoleon's state dinnerware was made from aluminum. When an easy and inexpensive extraction process was discovered in 1886, it became a common and readily available metal.

eliminate the metal from the body, including the kidney, the gastrointestinal tract, and the liver. Metals are often toxic to the organs that cannot detoxify them.

■ ALUMINUM

Aluminum exposures in industry are from metal dust, welding fumes, aluminum-soluble compounds, aluminum alkyls, and aluminum pyro powder. Coal-fired power plants, metal smelters, cement manufacturing plants, and waste incinerators are all sources of aluminum contamination. Aluminum forms clumps or flocs with organic material, and it is often used in water-treatment plants in the form of alum to remove organic material.

Aluminum is found in soft-drink cans, most antacids, other medications, paints, table salt, white flour, animal and plant food, fireworks, and deodorants.

Many people use aluminum foil when cooking. Aluminum is used as a leavening agent in cake mixes, dough, and baking powders. Processed, sliced cheese products of-

Aluminum in Over-the-Counter Drugs

Some antacids contain from 35 to over 200 milligrams of aluminum per dose, and a person taking antacids could ingest as much as 5,000 milligrams of aluminum a day. Patients with kidney disease can develop aluminum poisoning from taking aluminum antacids and must take aluminum-free preparations.

Buffered aspirin contains aluminum. Antidiarrheal medications, hemorrhoid medications, vaginal douches, and lipstick may all contain aluminum.

ten contain aluminum. Teas may contain aluminum, and acidic foods in aluminum containers can leach out the metal. Acidic and alkaline foods can leach aluminum from aluminum cooking pots.

Aluminum increases in concentration as it moves up the food chain. Livestock accumulates aluminum, which is then ingested by people. People ingest on average between 5 and 100 milligrams of aluminum daily from all sources.

Drinking water can also be contaminated with aluminum. Acid rain can leach aluminum from soil, rocks, and sediments in lake bottoms. In northeastern North America, the amount of aluminum in surface water has increased tenfold in the past 80 years. In many Scandinavian lakes, there have been massive fish die-offs because of high aluminum concentrations.

Aluminum also enters the body through inhalation, absorption through the skin, and by gastrointestinal tract absorption. It is excreted in the urine and bile.

Aluminum dust and aluminum pyro powders can be toxic to the lungs. Aluminum oxide exposure has caused pulmonary fibrosis (thickening and scarring of lung tissue) and emphysema. Aluminum builds up in the body as a person ages. Chronic, long-term exposure can cause weak bones, anemia, and abnormalities in calcium, magnesium, and phosphorous metabolism.

Aluminum also interferes with the normal metabolism of nerve cells. Laboratory animals exposed to aluminum may develop neurofibrillary tangles (degenerated nerve cells) as are found in Alzheimer's disease, a loss of memory progressing to dementia. Patients with Alzheimer's may have normal aluminum levels in the brain, blood, and cerebrospinal fluid, but the neurofibrillary tangles will have abnormally high concentrations. However, aluminum has not been proven to cause Alzheimer's disease.

■ CADMIUM

A major source of cadmium exposure is dust from automobile tire erosion. It is also produced from burning waste. Cadmium is found in industrial effluents, plastics, fertilizers, auto exhaust, the coating on nails, rechargeable batteries, solder, coffee, soft or acidic water, and tobacco smoke.

Cadmium is poorly absorbed from the gastrointestinal tract, but inhaled cadmium is absorbed readily. Once absorbed, cadmium is bound to a protein known as metallothionein, which is found in the major organs and protects the body against cadmium's toxic effects. Cadmium accumulates primarily in the kidneys and secondarily in the liver. The half-life of cadmium is 20 years, which means that after 20 years, 50 percent of the original amount of cadmium remains in the body. When cadmium reaches a threshold level, damage to the kidney tubules can occur. Some cadmium is excreted in both the urine and feces, but the mechanism is not understood.

Structurally similar to zinc, cadmium causes damage by displacing or replacing zinc (an essential trace metal) in over 200 enzymes. Cadmium is absorbed more easily when a person has a zinc deficiency.

Cadmium is toxic to the lungs. Acute exposure to cadmium dust or fumes can cause death, while chronic exposure can cause emphysema. Other symptoms of chronic cadmium exposure include liver damage, anemia, high blood pressure, weak bones, bone pain, and shrinking of the testicles.

▮▮ LEAD

All humans now have lead accumulations in their bodies. We are exposed to lead from the soil, air, and water. Lead occurs in two forms: inorganic lead and alkyl lead (formerly used in gasoline). Inorganic lead is used in battery manufacturing and reclamation, radiator repair, the printing industry, firing ranges, copper smelting, paint and pigment manufacturing, the plastics industry, and the rubber industry.

Until 1977 when it became regulated, lead was used in paint for pigmentation and

Lead

Lead poisoning is thought to have occurred since Roman times when wine goblets made of lead were in common use. Because lead has a low melting point, it was one of the first metals smelted. Lead has been used extensively and investigated more thoroughly than any other metal.

to reduce weathering. Leaded paint in older buildings can peel, flake, and chip off, then be ingested by children. Children may also mouth objects contaminated with lead from dust and soil. Soil as far away as 10 feet from a building can be contaminated with lead paint.

Water from leaded pipes, soldered plumbing, and water-cooling systems are additional sources of lead. Lead levels are higher in the morning when the water has been in contact with the lead plumbing all night, so it is important to let water run for a few minutes before using it.

The gastrointestinal tract and the lungs absorb lead. The absorption of lead from the lungs depends on the particle size. Absorption from the GI tract depends on the amount of calcium, iron, fat, and protein in the diet. Infants and children absorb more lead than do adults. When lead is absorbed, the blood transports it to the organs of the body where it is transferred into the bones. Bones and teeth store 90 percent of the lead in the body. The rest is found in the kidneys and liver. Lead storage in the bones may pro-

Metallic Mercury Poisoning

In 1999, 16-year-old twin boys were admitted to a Texas hospital with generalized weakness, intermittent headache, erythema (redness) on both legs, feet, and hands, and intense itching of the legs and feet. Their behavior was occasionally uncooperative. A urine heavy metal screen showed a mercury level of 289 microliters (the normal level is less than 10). The boys had found an old blood pressure manometer, had removed the mercury, and had been playing with it frequently after school for a period of several weeks.

They underwent chelation therapy to remove the mercury and gradually returned to their previous level of health. The Centers for Disease Control have reported many cases of mercury poisoning from contact with metallic mercury or its vapors during the 1980s and 1990s.

tect other organs from lead poisoning, but provides a source for remobilization when the body is under physiologic stress, such as during pregnancy, lactation, or chronic disease.

Blood levels give an indication of recent lead exposure, but do not indicate the total body burden of lead. Hair analysis of lead levels is a more accurate indicator. (See chapter 7 for a discussion of hair analysis.) Lead is excreted by the GI tract, urine, and the shedding of skin and hair. Infants excrete more through the GI tract than do adults.

Lead poisoning causes fatigue, lethargy, insomnia, anemia, hypertension, depression, irritability, headaches, tremor, and memory loss. It also causes subtle behavioral effects. Acute exposure can lead to renal failure, severe GI symptoms, and acute brain symptoms such as coma. GI tract symptoms include abdominal pain and constipation. Chronic exposure to lead can result in intellectual impairment.

In addition, lead affects the central nervous system, peripheral nervous system, GI tract, and kidneys. It causes motor peripheral neuropathy (damage to nerves that control movement). It has caused decreased fertility, spontaneous abortion, stillbirth, and increased infant mortality. Males with toxic levels of lead have decreased sperm counts and a loss of sex drive.

Children are more sensitive to the effects of lead than are adults. Chronic lead levels have been studied by examining shed baby teeth. Dr. Herbert Needleman at the University of Pittsburgh found that children with higher lead levels had lower IQ levels and more learning disabilities. When retested five years later, those children had attended more special education classes.

A person can develop lead poisoning from small doses over a long period of time. The lead level considered toxic has been lowered from 158 micrograms per deciliter (mcg/dl) in 1930 to 10 mcg/dl in 1990. People with blood lead levels above 25 mcg/dl require treatment.

■■ MERCURY

Mercury occurs in three forms: metallic or elemental, inorganic, and organic. Each form has different toxicological characteristics.

■ METALLIC OR ELEMENTAL MERCURY

Metallic mercury is soluble in organic solvents but not in water. It is used in thermometers, electric switching devices, gauges, vacuum pumps, pressure-sensing devices, and in amalgams (silver fillings) used in dentistry.

Mercury is the only metal in liquid state at room temperature and it vaporizes readily. When mercury vapor is inhaled, some is changed to inorganic mercury and some stays in the metallic or elemental form, which is more lipid-soluble. This form of mercury crosses the blood-brain barrier, where it accumulates in the brain. Mercury can damage brain cells, particularly sensation and motor nerve cells. Metallic mercury can also accumulate in the kidneys and adversely affects kidney function.

Exposure to metallic mercury can cause lung damage, with inflammation of the alveoli, bronchioles, and the bronchi. Inhaling mercury fumes may cause fever, chills, shortness of breath, and a metallic taste in the mouth. This is known as metal fume fever and can also occur with the inhalation of other metals. Children younger than 30 months of age have died from pulmonary complications after inhaling mercury vapors.

Metallic mercury is poorly absorbed from the gastrointestinal tract, so there is no

Mad Hatters

Nineteenth-century hatters used mercury to cure beaver hides. Because of their exposure to metallic mercury, they developed neuropsychiatric symptoms and thus the term "mad as a hatter" developed.

danger for children who swallow mercury if a thermometer is broken in the mouth. As much as 204 grams of elemental mercury have been ingested without systemic toxicity. Handling mercury is very dangerous, however, as it is readily absorbed through the skin.

After a mercury-containing dental filling is placed, low levels of mercury release for several years (see chapter 11, Toxins from Medical Treatment). Chronic metallic mercury toxicity causes tremor, gingivitis (inflammation of the gums), and erethism (an abnormal state of excitement), which contributes to insomnia, shyness, memory loss, emotional lability, nervousness, and anorexia.

■ INORGANIC MERCURY

A portion of metallic mercury changes to inorganic mercury in the body. Inorganic mercury is also a constituent of dry cells (batteries) and is used as a detonator for explosives. The most famous form of inorganic mercury is a salt called mercurous chloride, commonly known as calomel. Calomel was used for centuries as a primary medication. Physicians prescribed it orally to treat most major illnesses.

Approximately 10 percent of an oral dose of inorganic mercury is absorbed by the GI tract. Inorganic mercury salts damage the mucous membranes of the mouth, throat, esophagus, and stomach. They also cause gastroenteritis with abdominal pain, vomiting, and bloody diarrhea. Mercury salts tend to accumulate in and damage the kidney, with decreased or no urination occurring in about half of cases. The organs of elimination of inorganic mercury are the GI tract and the kidney, although the mechanism is not understood well.

Although inorganic mercury crosses the blood-brain barrier poorly, chronic toxicity causes behavioral changes, such as tremor, emotional instability, insomnia, depression, and irritability.

■ ORGANIC MERCURY

Microorganisms can convert metallic mercury and inorganic mercury into organic mercury. Organic mercury compounds are lipid-soluble and volatile, and can be absorbed through the lungs. They are also absorbed through the skin.

The most significant compound is methyl mercury, which crosses the placenta and can accumulate in the fetus. Organic mercury also crosses into breast milk in toxic amounts. Over 90 percent of methyl mercury is absorbed from the GI tract because of its lipid solubility. Methyl mercury moves to all body cells, but concentrates in the liver, kidneys, blood, brain, hair, and skin. Hair levels correlate with blood levels, and are a good indicator of exposure.

With chronic exposure, methyl mercury toxicity develops gradually. Methyl mercury inhibits the synthesis of acetylcholine, the major neurotransmitter in the body, causing difficulty with concentration, loss of short- and long-term memory, depression, constriction of visual fields, poor coordination and an abnormal gait, numbness of the hands and feet, deafness, slurred speech, tremors of the hands, weakness, paralysis, decreased sense of smell and taste, and fatigue. The prognosis for improvement is poor, because the body is able to excrete only about 1 percent of its organic mercury burden per day.

Organic mercury was used in the past to treat syphilis and as a diuretic. Today it is used as an antiseptic and a preservative. Mercurochrome is an organic mercury antiseptic which, when applied to large burns, has caused death in children. Organic mercury is also used as a fungicide, in embalming preparations, and in insecticide manufacturing. Until 1990, interior latex paint contained organic mercury as an antimildew agent.

Most organic mercury exposure comes from the diet and it can be concentrated in the food chain. Many people have been poisoned by eating grain treated with an organic mercury fungicide and intended for plant seed only, not for human consumption.

In 1953 through 1960 in Minimata Bay, Japan, 25 infants were born with severe intellectual impairment caused by their mothers consuming fish contaminated with organic mercury from a factory discharge.

Noise, Weather, and Altitude

Noise

Excessive noise, which may be described as unwanted sound, is considered a toxic pollutant. Leading noise sources are road traffic, aircraft, railroads, construction, industry, noise in buildings, and consumer products. Toxic noise levels are found in both urban and rural environments and can affect general health and well-being in the same manner as chronic stress. The effects of noise are determined by its duration, level, and frequency. Long-lasting, high-level, and continuous sounds are the most damaging to hearing. Intermittent sounds allow the ear to regenerate during the intervening quiet periods, but they are often more annoying because of their unpredictability.

Sound consists of an air pressure wave. Any object that vibrates causes waves of compressed and expanded air that induce vibration in the human ear which is interpreted by the brain. The ear consists of three parts—the external ear, the middle ear, and the inner ear. The external ear collects sound waves that travel to the middle ear. The middle ear contains the eardrum with three tiny bones (the hammer, anvil, and stapes) that transmit their vibration to the oval window, which opens into the inner ear. The inner ear contains a spiral tube called the cochlea, that holds fluid and hair and nerve cells, which transmit messages along the auditory nerve to the brain.

Sound pressure or volume varies over a range of more than 1 million units. A logarithmic scale, known as the decibel (dB) scale, is used to classify sound pressure. The human ear responds logarithmically, not linearly, and the perception of volume doubles when sound pressure increases by 10 dB. According to the Environmental Protection Agency, almost half of the U.S. population is frequently exposed to noise levels greater than 55 dB. In the 20th century, noise levels increased by 2 dB in each decade.

Noise at 70 decibels can wake a sleeping person. In the 80 dB range, noise can damage hearing over time. Over 80 dB, noise can

Noise

- Treatment for any allergies to reduce ear inflammation (chapter **27**)
- Hands-on treatment for ear problems (**27**)
- Homeopathic remedies such as *Arnica, Asarum europaeum, Borax, Calendula, Silicea terra* (**28**)
- Packs for ear pain (**30**)

cause ringing in the ears, a feeling of pressure, and muffling of sound. Continued exposure can cause permanent hearing loss. The normal pain threshold for noise is 110 dB, and permanent deafness is caused at 135 dB. Sounds of 140 dB can instantly destroy hearing.

Over 20 million people in North America are exposed to environmental noise that can damage hearing. With exposure to excessive noise, people develop auditory fatigue, which may cause a temporary loss of hearing. Their hearing may recover after several hours away from the noise, but repeated exposure can cause permanent hearing loss.

In addition to causing hearing loss, noise can interfere with speech; interrupt communication; and interfere with sleep, leisure, and other activities. The EPA has recommended noise levels to protect health, calculating these levels with an adequate safety margin. It has chosen 45 dB indoors and 55 dB outdoors (averaged over a 24-hour period) as the maximum levels that will not affect public health.

■ EFFECTS OF NOISE

Excessive noise can damage the inner ear, killing the hair cells and replacing them with scar tissue. This is known as sensineuronal or perceptive hearing loss. Sensineuronal hearing loss is irreversible, and it cannot be corrected. This type of hearing loss is usually job-related.

Conductive hearing loss may develop when the eardrum or middle ear is damaged. This type of hearing loss is usually not occupationally induced. A hearing aid that amplifies sound can help a person with a conductive hearing loss. In some cases, this type of hearing loss is reversible.

In 1999 an international team of scientists in Portugal reported evidence of a new

SOUND	DECIBEL LEVEL
Whisper	25
Conversation	60
Vacuum cleaner	70–85
Hair dryer	80
Electric razor	85
Crowded school bus	85
Gas lawnmower	95
Motorcycle	110
Rock concert	110–130
Jet liner (taking off 200 feet away)	120

occupational disorder they call vibroacoustic disease (VAD). They state that diseases caused by noise and vibration are a major occupational problem throughout the world. VAD is caused by loud, low, rumbling noise or vibration and can result in cardiovascular thickening and blood flow impairment, leading to stroke and heart attack; respiratory disorders, including lung cancer in nonsmokers; epilepsy and balance disturbances; digestive and gastrointestinal dysfunction; psychiatric disturbances; and genetic mutations. Suicide is the most serious psychiatric consequence of VAD. People with VAD are very noise intolerant and may have emotional outbursts when exposed to noises that are uncomfortable to them.

Civilian and military air crews and aircraft technicians are very prone to VAD. The noise generated by constantly running machinery, mass transit stations, commercial parking lots, and hand-held vibrating instruments and machinery are a few of the other types of exposure that can cause VAD. This 20-year study also established that workers wearing hearing protection are at greater risk of developing VAD. The protection does prevent damage to their hearing, but it neutralizes the ears' natural protective functions while the rest of the body remains fully exposed to the effects of the noise.

The body reacts to loud noise as it does to other types of stress. Apart from the ear itself, the heart receives most of the stress, with heart rate and blood pressure increasing. Noise causes the body to produce adrenocorticotropic hormone (ACTH), which can cause stomach ulcers if produced frequently in excess. It can also cause changes

Noise and Emotion

Emotions also affected by noise. People may become distressed or even angry as noise levels go up, and experience a significant degradation in quality of life. The Federal Aviation Administration (FAA) has adopted a 65-dB day-night average sound level as the point above which noise normally becomes unacceptable. However, studies have shown that annoyance may be generated for levels well below 65dB. Fear of possible danger, noise sensitivity, and belief that noise is preventable all affect the way people react to noise.

in breathing patterns, muscle tension, mobility of the GI tract, dilation of the pupils, and secretion of saliva and gastric secretions.

The immune system is affected by excessive noise as well. Levels of eosinophils and other white blood cells and gamma globulin (a plasma protein that fights disease) become very low. Fatigue, headaches, anxiety, and stress are common symptoms of toxic noise levels.

■■ INDUSTRIAL NOISE

The maximum allowed daily average industrial noise is 90 dB for eight hours a day. The U.S. Occupational Safety and Health Administration (OSHA) requires that for every 5 dB above 90, noise exposure must be decreased by half. However, the Environmental Protection Agency (EPA) has requested that the eight-hour noise limit should be 75

Too Loud

As pleasurable as music is, too much of it can damage hearing. At rock concerts, the level of the music may be as high as 130 dB. Symphony concerts may reach 105 dB. Even personal stereo headsets may reach 115 dB if the volume control is at maximum setting. At some school or community dances, loudspeakers produce noise levels of 115 to 120 dB. Music from group exercise classes is frequently at 105 to 110 dB and may exceed 120 dB.

dB. In some cases, OSHA has allowed the substitution of protective hearing devices in lieu of engineering noise control.

■■ RECREATIONAL NOISE

Federal laws protect workers, but no laws control the amount of noise people receive when they leave the workplace. Studies have shown that people who work in noisy environments tend to also pursue noisy leisure activities, and recreational noise often exceeds industrial noise. For many people, hearing loss is more likely at play than at work.

In his 1991 review of noise exposure from leisure activities, W.W. Clark reports in the *Journal of the Acoustical Society of America* that the noise level encountered in recreational hunting and target shooting can exceed federal standards for the workplace. This is one of the most serious sources of recreational noise, with peak sound pressure levels at the ear ranging from about 144 dB up to more than 170 dB. Snowmobiles, motorcycles, and powerboats also produce noise in the range that damages hearing. The noise level in stadiums at sporting events can match that of a rock concert.

■■ NOISE IN THE HOME

The home may be besieged with noise from many sources. Power tools, chain saws, power lawnmowers, and snow blowers can exceed federal standards of 45 dB indoors and 55 dB outdoors. The blender, TV, alarm clock, garbage disposal unit, trash compactor, vacuum cleaner, washer, dryer, dishwasher, coffee bean grinder, blow dryer, electric razor, and stereo all add to the noise level in the home. Individual appliances may produce a safe noise level, but when operated simultaneously, the combined volume can be damaging.

Some children's toys that squeak emit noise as loud as a car horn, up to 108 dB at a distance of 4 inches. Toy cap guns and firecrackers can exceed 140 dB. Many battery-operated toys also pose a risk. If an adult holds a child's toy to his or her ear and cannot tolerate the sound for more than 30 seconds, the toy can be injurious to hearing. Children frequently hold toys close to their own ears, or those of other children. Each exposure to a noise louder than 85 dB, even for an extremely short time, can damage a child's hearing.

■■ HEARING PROBLEMS

One in ten North Americans has some type of hearing impairment. While many of these people are elderly, with 33 percent reporting hearing problems, at least 7 million children and adolescents are affected. In one study done in the early 1980s by Dr. David Lipscomb at the University of Tennessee, college freshmen had hearing losses typical of the elderly. The Swedish Navy has had problems finding sailors who could hear well enough to operate listening devices. There has also been a sharp increase of people in their 40s and 50s who complain that they cannot hear well.

Even newborns can suffer from hearing loss, and about 1 out of 1,000 newborn infants in North America is born deaf. Many more are born with hearing impairment. In infants requiring intensive care at birth, 1 out of every 40 suffers permanent hearing loss.

Studies now show that the fetus can also be harmed by noise. Loud noises, such as rock concerts or those encountered near airfields, may harm hearing and brain development in the unborn child. Edwin W. Rubel from the University of Washington states, "What I feel comfortable saying is that anything that hurts the unprotected ear is not going to be very good for the fetus."

Weather

Weather is considered a toxin because it can profoundly affect the human body. The effects of weather on health have been known for centuries. Hippocrates, who lived around 400 B.C., stated that a physician should proceed as follows: "First he ought to consider what effect each season of the year can produce, for the seasons are not alike but differ widely both in themselves and at their changes. Through these considerations, and

Famous Weather Barometers

Some well-known people have been weather-sensitive. In the 19th century, German poet von Goethe carried a barometer to help him determine what each day's weather might have in store for him. His contemporary, French philosopher Maine de Biran, felt that his sensitive system suffered with every atmospheric change, no matter how slight. Nietzsche, a German philosopher (1844–1900), suffered from weather-induced headaches and was apparently a "living barometer" made irritable by the weather. Winston Churchill and Gertrude Stein both planned their schedules carefully to miss the French mistral winds, which made them tense and irritable.

by learning the weather beforehand, the doctor will have available full knowledge to help him in each specific case." Paracelsus (1493–1541) stated that "He who knows the origins of the winds, of thunder, and of the weather, also knows where diseases come from."

Biometeorology, a new multidisciplinary science, studies the effects of atmospheric phenomena on all life. Biometeorologists consider temperature, humidity, hours of sunshine, precipitation, wind speed, and geomagnetic activity. They also look at the rate of these changes over time. According to Dr.

James Rottom of the Florida International University in North Miami, about 20 percent of the population are weather-sensitive. Other scientists feel that as much as 33 percent of the population are weather-sensitive, which may explain why people can wake up one day feeling happy and the next day depressed, even though nothing has changed in their lives.

Dr. Michael Persinger of the Neuroscience Laboratory in Sudbury, Ontario, states that weather is basically a function of the sun, controlled by the connection between solar sunspot activity and the earth's electromagnetic field. Sunspot activity increases solar wind, which is a stream of hydrogen ions from the sun that cause magnetic storms in the earth's atmosphere. These storms decrease the strength of the earth's electromagnetic fields, affecting short-term weather and long-term climate conditions. Some heart attacks has been related to solar activity and the fluctuation of the earth's magnetic field.

■■ SEASONS

A chronic depression called Seasonal Affective Disorder Syndrome (SADS) occurs in winter when the days are short and gray. People who are affected develop symptoms within the same 60-day period each year. In addition to depression, these people crave carbohydrates and feel better when they eat them; sleep more, but always feel tired; have little or no interest in sex; gain weight; feel overwhelmed by everything; have problems concentrating; may avoid family and friends; and have frequent infections and muscle aches.

Hibernation Response

A milder form of SADS, called Hibernation Response, causes people to feel overweight and depressed in the autumn and winter. It occurs worldwide and is postulated by Peter Whybrow and Rober Bahr in their book, The Hibernation Response, *to be an expression of human adaptation to the rhythmic nature of the earth. Dr. Whybrow states that normal people have a markedly seasonal pattern to their activity.*

More than 36 million North Americans suffer from this problem, and no one knows precisely what causes SADS. Women seem more prone to this disorder than men, and it seems to run in families. Most physicians and researchers agree that the syndrome is related to the changes in light that accompany the seasons. SADS begins when the days become shorter and grayer.

Some researchers believe that the syndrome is related to a hormone called melatonin that is secreted by the pineal gland. This sleep-inducing hormone is produced in the dark, so that the body produces more melatonin during the winter.

Since the mid-1800s, a reverse pattern of SADS has been recognized. These people experience summer depression and winter mania. This may be a relatively common problem, as a peak period of depression and suicide occurs in late spring and summer. This phenomenon may be caused by a dysfunction of energy regulation.

■■ STORMS AND WIND

Storms affect many people adversely, causing symptoms each time a storm front moves through. Electromagnetic discharges from lightning travel more rapidly and much farther than the storm. These discharges, called atmospherics or sferics, fill the air with positive ions and cause static on car radios as far as 150 miles away. Experiments in Israel and Europe have shown that this positively charged air results in slower reaction times, more road and industrial accidents, depression, and increased surgical complications.

In contrast, the negative ions that are produced by sunlight shining through clean air, by waterfalls and heavy rain, and by running water or showers cause feelings of calm and well-being. When people are exposed to negative ions, blood pressure is lowered and productivity is higher.

Studies from Australia indicate that thunderstorms stir up grass particles that trigger severe attacks in asthmatics. In 1987 and 1989, thunderstorm activity caused an increase of asthma outbreaks in Melbourne. The 1989 storm lasted for 16 hours and resulted in a tenfold increase of asthma patients in local hospitals. A similar rise in asthma patients was reported in 1994 in Britain following a 12-hour thunderstorm. An indication of the storm's serious effects is the fact that 44 percent of these patients had not had asthma previously. According to Dr. Cenk Suphioglu of the University of Melbourne in Australia, the culprit that triggered the asthma was starch granules released from rye grass pollen when the pollen grains ruptured in the rainwater.

Storm Warning

Several patients at our clinic have been weather-sensitive. Some were adversely affected by changes in barometric pressure, while others complained of symptoms from the wind. One woman always called after a storm front came through, sure that she was coming down with a virus. We would explain to her that there was a new front and her symptoms were probably caused by the weather change. She rarely had an actual virus, and her symptoms nearly always cleared up with the next weather change.

"Ill winds" have been described for centuries and are called by many names, among them the mistral winds in France, foehn in Bavaria and Switzerland, sirocco in Italy, sharav in Israel, hamsin in the Middle East, chinook in the Rocky Mountains, and the Santa Ana winds in California. These winds are laden with positive ions, which increase the production of the neurotransmitter serotonin in measurable amounts.

Serotonin normally eases tension, elevates mood, reduces aggression, affects mental function, plays a role in maintaining blood flow and pressure, participates in temperature regulation, and controls appetite. However, in the presence of positive ions serotonin is released as a stress hormone. Excessive serotonin causes agitation, irritability, tension, giddiness, runny or stuffy nose, eye problems, breathing problems, sore throat, edema, migraine headache, insomnia, nausea and vomiting, rapid temperature changes, diarrhea, and a constant urge to urinate. These symptoms can begin 12 hours before the wind actually arrives.

■■ HEAT

Heat is a physical stressor and thus a toxin. Heat exhaustion and heat stroke may result from overexposure to heat caused by hot weather or working around heat sources.

Heat stress impairs physical and mental performances and can affect the heart and cardiovascular system, respiratory system, kidneys, and endocrine system. The cardiovascular system must work harder to keep the body cool, while blood pressure will decrease. Some respiratory problems will increase. The secretion of the thyroid gland will decrease, as will kidney activity, if sweating is profuse.

Heat stress adversely affects mental performance well in advance of deteriorating physical performance. This can affect productivity in the workplace.

Symptoms of a heat stroke include high body temperature of 106°F or higher, lack of sweating, and mental symptoms including confusion, disorientation, delirium, and loss of consciousness. There are three types of heat stroke:

- *Exertion heat stroke:* occurs during vigorous exercise during hot weather
- *Nonexertion heat stroke:* occurs during exposure to high temperatures with no opportunity to cool off
- *Drug heat stroke:* occurs when a medication prevents the body from cooling properly

Poor physical condition, insufficient fluid intake, obesity, recent fever or diarrhea, a re-

---

Heat and Aggression

Several studies point to a relationship between temperature and aggression. In normally temperate areas, the incidence of murder, rape, and assault is higher in the hot, humid months of July and August. Hot weather apparently stimulates the thalamus gland, which controls the human thermoregulatory system. Many of the same hormonal systems involved in heat regulation are also involved in aggression.

---

cent move from a cool to a hot climate, recent sleep problems, medications that prevent heat loss, excess protective clothing, diabetes, cardiovascular disease, and impaired ability to sweat all predispose a person to heat stroke. The most important method of cooling for humans is sweating.

Heat also affects human mortality. Because the bodies of the elderly are not as adaptable, they are particularly affected by sudden temperature change, and their death rate increases by as much as 50 percent during a heat wave. Approximately 2,000 people die in the U.S. each year from heat-related causes.

■■ HUMIDITY

Humidity, the moisture content of the atmosphere, affects people as well. High humidity causes hot weather to feel hotter and cold weather to feel colder. Extreme heat and humidity can cause increased fatigue and discomfort that can lead to impairment of alertness, mental function, and physical capacity.

Heat coupled with humidity causes the heart rate to increase. Humidity interferes with the ability of the body to sweat; if the external temperature is also elevated, the body cannot cool itself, leading to heat exhaustion.

In regions with high humidity, mold growth is high, increasing allergic reactions to mold. (For further discussion on mold, see chapter 15, Plants and Organisms.)

Humidity also affects the skin. With combined high heat and humidity, the eccrine sweat glands can become blocked and accumulating sweat is forced into the surrounding tissues. This causes an inflammatory reaction and a rash called "prickly heat." Warm temperatures and low humidity produce dryness of the skin and symptoms ranging from intense itching to an eczema known as "low-humidity dermatosis." Low humidity and cold temperatures promote dryness and chapping of the skin, which becomes itchy. This is often called "winter itch."

COLD

Although people can adapt to cold over time, cold is also a physical stressor. It constricts blood vessels, which causes numbness of exposed skin, hands, and feet. Prolonged exposure to cold can lead to frostbite, lowered body temperature, and ultimately death. Frostbite occurs when a shell of skin and tissue under the skin freezes. Plasma from underlying blood vessels then escapes and forms skin blisters.

Manual performance is lowered with cold exposure, even if the hands are kept warm. Fine motor skills are more affected by cold than are large motor skills, and extreme cold slows reaction time. Cold also decreases mental performance. About 1,000 people die in the U.S. each year from cold-related causes.

HYPOTHERMIA

Hypothermia is a condition in which the body loses heat faster than it can produce it, and is no longer able to produce enough heat to maintain body functions. Hypothermia is the most common cause of death outdoors. Once a person's body temperature drops below 95°F, the person cannot be rewarmed without assistance. Elderly and ill people can develop hypothermia indoors during cold weather, if their homes are not heated sufficiently.

During outdoor winter activities, wind chill can be an important element in hypothermia. The wind chill factor is a temperature rating based on air temperature as well as wind speeds, because wind produces a cooling effect. Hypothermia occurs frequently in temperatures above freezing, from 35° to 50°F. Becoming wet from rain or sweat and then becoming chilled is a common risk factor. Fatigue, hunger, anemia, and exertion are other risk factors.

The first sign of hypothermia is shivering. The person may be pale, and body temperature will be 94.6°F or lower. Soon the person will develop confusion, difficulty speaking, decreased reaction time, and poor judgment. Because of this, people usually do not recognize the danger of their situation. Respiration and pulse decrease, and the person may become apathetic. In the late

Exposure to Altitude

- Vitamin C and oxygenating nutrients including coenzyme Q_{10} (chapter **23**)

- Breathing exercises and oxygen therapy (**26**)

- Homeopathic remedies: for altitude sickness, *Carbo vegetabilis;* for frostbite, *Agaricus muscarius;* for shortness of breath, *Calcarea carbonica;* for snow blindness, *Kali muriaticum*

stages, the person may be unconscious. Many victims of hypothermia go to sleep and die while asleep.

■ COLD FRONTS

Cold fronts can trigger glaucoma and asthma attacks. Angina pectoris, which is heart pain that may radiate down the left arm, increases during autumn and winter. A study of 1.6 million people with circulatory problems demonstrated that these problems peak in January and February.

Dr. Michel Gauquelin of the Laboratory for Cosmic and Psycho-Physiological Rhythms in Paris has correlated cold fronts with heart attacks. He has found that the incidence of heart attacks is almost double during these fronts. Post-operative complications also coincide with fronts—60 percent occurring with cold fronts, and 30 percent with warm fronts. In Yugoslavia and Czechoslovakia, surgeries are scheduled around the weather forecast because cold fronts increase blood-clotting time.

Altitude

The main effects of high altitude result from the composition of the air and the corresponding physiological response of the body. Because it can adversely affect the body, altitude may be considered a toxin.

A mantle of gases composed of 78 percent nitrogen, 21 percent oxygen, and small amounts of argon, carbon dioxide, neon, helium, and other gases surrounds the earth. This mixture, combined with varying amounts of moisture, low-altitude pollutants, and particulate matter, constitutes the earth's atmosphere. These atmospheric gases are compressible, so that the number of molecules a unit of air contains is greater at sea level than at high altitude. Air pressure, therefore, is higher at sea level, and decreases with altitude. Barometric pressure, which is a measure of atmospheric pressure, depends on the molecular concentration of the air.

■■ HYPOXIA

The oxygen content of the air is lower at high altitudes, and the major concern associated with altitude is hypoxia, a deficiency in the amount of oxygen reaching body tissue. Most authorities consider high altitude as 10,000 feet or above. The first response to high altitude is generally an increased rate of breathing, or hyperventilation, in an attempt to take in more oxygen. This leads to a feeling of breathlessness. This is usually accompanied by tachycardia (rapid heartbeat), which increases cardiac output during the first few days at high altitude. Headache is another common symptom and may range from mild to severe. Very few people can ascend high mountains without suffering a headache, accompanied by some degree of mental confusion. Mild hypoxia may also induce increased urine output, which can result in dehydration.

At high altitudes, many people suffer from fatigue and an overwhelming desire to sleep. These symptoms are usually disproportionate to the amount of physical activity undertaken. Sleep is often disturbed because of breathing difficulties, which usually consist of periods of heavy breathing followed by a period of apnea (not breathing). This may wake the person with feelings of suffocation, and leave him or her unrefreshed.

People who live at low elevations and who ascend to higher altitudes less than 10,000 feet may suffer from these same symptoms. Usually, the symptoms pass in a few days as the person becomes acclimated to the new altitude. Older people may experience worse symptoms than younger ones.

■■ ACCLIMATION TO ALTITUDE

The body uses several mechanisms to acclimate to altitude. Increased alveolar ventilation (transport of gases through the alveoli), increased red blood cell and hemoglobin synthesis, the growth of new tissue capillaries, and a shift in the equilibrium of oxygen bound to hemoglobin can allow the body to supply normal amounts of oxygen to the tissues. The result of this acclimation may be an increase in the viscosity (thickness) of the blood flow because of the increase of red blood cells. This makes it more difficult for the heart to pump the blood.

People who live at over 5,000 feet in alti-

Mountain Sickness

Some people ascending to very high altitudes suffer from extreme hypoxia and are considered to have mountain sickness. In addition to the symptoms of hypoxia, a person with mountain sickness may have loss of appetite, nausea, dehydration, malabsorption, fluid in the lungs, cough, swelling of the brain, lassitude, loss of coordination, reduced urine output, and retinal hemorrhages. Without proper treatment and prompt descent to a lower altitude, these symptoms can lead to death.

tude may have mild hypoxia, depending on their state of health and the efficiency of their acclimation. In our clinical experience, we have found the healing response to be slowed in some individuals who live at an elevation of 7,300 feet. However, a general improvement in health occurred when organic germanium, a supplement that improves oxygen utilization, was supplied.

■■ ENVIRONMENTAL HAZARDS

In addition to the lack of oxygen, high altitudes have other environmental hazards. Cold is one hazard. For every increase of approximately 450 feet in altitude, the temperature drops by 1°C. At higher altitudes, the velocity of the wind increases. The normal insulating layer of warm air around the skin is blown away, and skin temperature drops. This can lead to frostbite or hypothermia (see Cold, above). The low humidity at some high altitudes can also increase heat loss through evaporation. Sensitive areas such as lips can quickly dry and crack if they are not protected.

Exposure to solar radiation also increases with higher altitude. Ultraviolet radiation, a segment of solar radiation, and cosmic radiation, a collection of charged particles of very high kinetic energy that bombard the earth, are stronger at high altitudes. Dark clothing, the lower oxygen content of the mountain air, and reflection from snow all enhance the warming effect of solar radiation. Intense solar radiation, particularly in snowy areas, can very quickly cause serious sunburn on exposed skin.

Snow and ice can also lead to snow blindness, a temporary blindness caused when the eyes are exposed to ultraviolet light reflecting from the white surface. Snow blindness can be accompanied by severe pain. If the affected person rests the eyes and remains indoors, recovery is usually complete. However, prolonged exposure can damage the retina, resulting in some permanent loss of vision.

Radiation, Electromagnetic Fields, and Geopathic Stress

Radiation

Radiation is the emission and propagation of waves or particles, such as light, sound, radiant heat, or particles emitted by radioactive material. The electromagnetic spectrum is composed of radiation energy, listed below from lower to higher energy and from longer to shorter wavelength:
- electrical currents
- television waves
- radio waves
- microwaves
- infrared light
- visible light
- ultraviolet radiation
- X-rays
- gamma rays
- cosmic rays

Radiation can be ionizing, which means it has enough energy to ionize matter (removing one or more electrons from an atom or molecule) as it moves through the substance, or nonionizing, which possesses less energy. Gamma rays, X-rays, and cosmic rays are ionizing radiation, while all other members of the electromagnetic spectrum are nonionizing. Both types of radiation have biological effects.

▮▮ IONIZING RADIATION

Ionizing radiation comes from natural and human-caused sources and includes any radiation that comes from an atomic nucleus. It may consist of energetic charged particles, such as alpha and beta particles; non-particulate radiation such as X-rays; and neutrons, which are particles that have no charge.
- *Beta particles:* High-speed electrons emitted during the decay of many radioactive elements, beta particles can penetrate up to almost an inch of human flesh.
- *Alpha particles:* Consisting of two protons and two neutrons, alpha particles are emitted from the nucleus of heavy elements during their radioactive disintegration. They are also emitted from some human-made sources. They lose their energy quickly when they collide and can be stopped by the first layer of skin. If taken into the body by breathing or swallowing,

however, they can inflict more biological damage than other types of radiation.

- *X-rays:* Generated by specialized equipment, they have great penetrating power and can pass though the human body.
- *Gamma rays:* Very high energy X-rays that originate from an atomic nucleus. The only difference between X-rays and gamma rays is their origin.
- *Cosmic rays:* Streams of ionizing radiation of extraterrestrial origin, consisting of protons, alpha particles and other atomic nuclei, but also some high-energy electrons. They have varying penetrating abilities and are more intense at higher altitudes than at sea level.
- *Neutrons:* Very penetrating particles that come mainly from the fission (splitting) of certain atoms inside a nuclear reactor.

❚ NATURAL RADIATION

Everyone in the world is exposed to low-level sources of natural radiation, called background radiation. Normal levels of background radiation range from 1.0 to 3.5 millisieverts per person per year, but in some areas are much higher, including India, Brazil, Iran, and Sudan.

The natural ionizing radiation to which we are exposed comes from the sun (cosmic radiation) and from natural elements, (isotopes) in the earth's crust that decay. The materials used to build our homes, radon gas, and carbon-14 in the atmosphere add to radiation levels. Even natural radioactive elements found in minute amounts in our bodies, such as potassium-42 and other isotopes, add to our radiation exposure.

Nature is made of building blocks of matter called elements, such as oxygen, calcium, lead, and hydrogen. Elements consist of atoms, which contain protons and neutrons in their nucleus, as well as electrons orbiting the nucleus.

Some elements have several forms of atoms, known as isotopes, with different numbers of neutrons in the nucleus, giving the isotope a slightly different atomic weight. They have the same atomic number, however, because they have the same number of protons. Some isotopes are unstable and radioactive. When unstable isotopes change to another isotope (known as a decay product), they eject particles (alpha, beta, and gamma rays).

Radioactive isotopes decay in a known pattern, changing into other elements as protons are lost from the nucleus. The time that it takes half of the atoms to be lost is known as a half-life. It takes the same half-life time for "half of the half" that remains to decay. Half-lives vary from less than 1 second to 4.5 billion years.

The damage that radioactive isotopes

> ## Natural Radiation
>
> *The average background radiation dose in North America is 3.6 millisieverts per person per year (equivalent to 360 millirems of X-rays). Flying across the country gives an additional radiation exposure of 2.5 millirems each way. Although no adverse health effects have been reported from these high natural levels, it is estimated that 2 to 4 percent of the total cancer deaths in North America are caused by natural radiation.*

can do to the body depends on the half-life, the type and energy of radiation emitted, the state of the isotope (gas, liquid, or solid), and the chemical interaction of the isotope with other substances. Radiation imparts energy to tissues as it passes through the body, damaging individual cells or their genetic material, DNA.

A common exposure for many people is caused by radon. Radon is a radioactive gas that decays to polonium, a dangerous isotope that emits alpha particles. When radon is inhaled, alpha radiation is emitted inside the lungs, and can lead to lung cancer. (See chapter 14, Water and Air, for further information on radon.)

■ HUMAN-CAUSED RADIATION

Human-caused radiation comes from two sources, that generated by specialized equipment and that emitted by natural radioactive substances used by humans. People receive ionizing radiation from many sources, such as diagnostic X-rays, fallout from past nuclear weapons testing and nuclear accidents, television receivers, gas stoves, and therapeutic radiation. Coal-burning power plants release tons of radioactive materials, and sewage sludge adds more. Some of the sewage is used to make bricks and on farmers' fields.

Many common household objects contain radioactive substances. While the radioactive elements in these substances are natural, humans added them to the objects. For example, there is americium in some smoke detectors, radium or tritium in clocks, and polonium in tobacco.

For most people, the largest human-caused source of radiation is medical radia-

---

Radiation and Electromagnetic Exposures

- Soda and salt detox baths (chapter **22**)
- Antioxidant nutrients, including vitamins A, C, E; selenium and zinc, cysteine and glutathione (**23**)
- Homeopathic remedies such as *Cadmium sulphuratum, Radium bromatum, Sol, X-ray* (**28**)
- Magnets, diodes, or tachyon beads (**32**)

MOST EFFECTIVE DETOXIFICATION METHODS

---

tion, which is generated by specialized equipment. Dental X-rays account for an average annual dose of 0.03 millisieverts a year, and medical X-rays account for 0.35 millisieverts a year. The sanitary sewage system of hospitals also contains radioactive materials, from patient excreta as a consequence of nuclear medical techniques.

The gastrointestinal tract, bone marrow, and hair are most affected when a person receives radiation therapy. Chronic radiation exposure causes cancer in people of all ages and leukemia in children. It is now known that radiation can cause cancer at lower doses than was originally thought.

Scientists made use of natural radiation when developing the atomic bomb. Atomic bombs are made of isotopes that split apart when struck by neutrons. When an isotope splits in two, the resulting halves possess less total mass than the original isotope. The lost mass is converted to energy in a process known as fission, and emitted as radiation.

Irradiation

Irradiation can bleach and change the color of the food, as well as destroying vitamins and other nutrients. For example, about 30 percent of the vitamin C in foods is destroyed by irradiation. Milk loses 70 percent of vitamins A, B_1, and B_2 when irradiated. Vitamin K is particularly sensitive to radiation, as is vitamin E, all of the B vitamins, amino acids, lipids, and carbohydrates.

Irradiation can affect the flavor of proteins and change the texture of food. It also destroys natural anti-oxidants and causes an off flavor in fatty foods.

Fission can cause a tremendous explosion, as in an atomic bomb, or can be controlled, as in a nuclear reactor.

Severe effects of radiation were first documented in the victims of the atomic bombs at Hiroshima and Nagasaki at the end of World War II. Acute radiation exposure causes vomiting, malaise, fatigue, sweating, diarrhea, headache, and loss of appetite from between hours and two days after irradiation. Doses above 50 Gy (gray—the measurement of an absorbed dose) cause death from injury to the central nervous system within two days. Doses between approximately 10 and 50 Gy cause damage to the intestinal mucosa, intestinal bleeding, and death between six and nine days. Doses from one to several Gy cause suppression of the bone marrow within 48 hours, which leads to anemia, infection because of low levels of white blood cells, and bleeding from reduced platelet count.

Radiation dermatitis, hair loss, and sterility in both males and females also result from acute radiation exposure. Acute radiation affects the organs of the body that have the most rapid cell turnover—the gastrointestinal tract, bone marrow, and hair. The small intestine is the most radiosensitive organ in the GI tract and determines whether a person can survive a massive dose of whole body radiation.

■ FOOD IRRADIATION

Approximately one-third of the food produced in the United States has to be discarded because of spoilage. Irradiation of food prolongs its shelf life by killing insects, bacteria, fungi, and viruses, and by slowing the ripening process. Fumigants and chemical preservatives become unnecessary. Irradiation does not make the food itself radioactive. Food irradiation is the only method of food preservation that the FDA considers not to be an additive. Radioactive isotopes of cesium and cobalt are used to produce the gamma rays employed in food irradiation.

When food is irradiated, unique radiolytic products (URPs), which are chemical molecules that have never before been characterized, are produced. The health risk from some of these URPs is unknown; however, the Food and Drug Administration (FDA) designates formaldehyde and benzene, which are known carcinogens, as "known radiolytic products." Formic acid and quinones are also radiolytic products. Concentrated formic acid solutions are corrosive to skin and can cause lesions to the mouth and esophageal tissue. Quinones are aromatic compounds similar to benzene, but containing more oxygen. (For further information on benzene, see chapter 16, Chemicals and Metals.) In larger amounts, quinones can cause skin irritation, diarrhea, depression of the central nervous system, coma, and death.

Some microorganisms found in food are relatively resistant to radiation. The bacteria *Clostridium botulinum* is among the most radiation-resistant microorganisms. The enzymes in food that cause spoilage are also very radiation-resistant and require a dose five times that required by microorganisms to be inactivated.

The amount of radiation required to decontaminate most food products can be up to 5 million times as much as is transmitted in a typical chest X-ray. These high doses of radiation create free radicals, which are oxygen molecules that have lost one of their paired electrons. They then rob other molecules of electrons, damaging molecules in a chain reaction. (See chapter 20, Toxins Produced in the Body, for a detailed discussion of free radicals.) Foods containing high quantities of water are more vulnerable to the formation of free radicals.

By 1989, 30 countries had approved 40 irradiated food items for human consumption, in an attempt to deal with the problem of food spoilage in developing countries. In the U.S., the FDA has approved irradiation of wheat, wheat flour, pork, potatoes, spices, and whole fruits and vegetables. Only spices are currently being irradiated in significant amounts in the United States. Present laws do not require labeling of irradiated foods used in a mixture. Only whole food that is ir-

Photosensitivity

People taking some types of medication must limit their time in the sun and wear protective clothing. These common drugs cause photosensitivity, a skin reaction that is similar to sunburn. These drugs include some blood-pressure medications, diuretics, antidepressants, birth control pills, antihistamines, sulfa drugs, and topical antiseptic creams.

radiated and then sold unchanged must be labeled.

◼◼ NONIONIZING RADIATION

Ultraviolet, visible, and infrared light; microwaves and radiowaves; television waves; and extremely low frequency (ELF) electromagnetic fields are all sources of nonionizing radiation. Ultraviolet, visible, and infrared light is classified as the optical portion of this radiation, although we can see only visible light. Microwaves and higher frequency radiowaves can produce heating, which does not occur with lower frequency radiowaves and ELF fields. These thermal effects can produce biological effects that affect human health. Biological effects from other properties of this type of radiation are still controversial.

◼ ULTRAVIOLET LIGHT

Although the main source of ultraviolet (UV) radiation is the sun, lesser amounts come from welding arcs, electric arc lights, and

Light Quality

Good lighting should be adequately bright and free from glare, reflection, and flicker. Inadequate light can cause eyestrain, while glare and flicker cause headaches. Quality of light is particularly important for the elderly, as vision deteriorates with age.

special ultraviolet lights. The amount of ultraviolet light the earth receives varies, depending on the time of day, the time of year, and the presence of clouds, snow, or water. Ozone in the earth's atmosphere absorbs the highest intensity uv radiation. Glass and light clothing also filter or reflect ultraviolet radiation.

Ultraviolet radiation helps to produce vitamin D in the skin, but also tans the skin and can cause sunburn. Chronic uv radiation exposure causes the skin to age more rapidly, increasing wrinkling and loss of skin elasticity. It can also lead to skin cancer. Ultraviolet radiation can cause inflammation of the eye, photochemical injury to the retina, and the formation of cataracts.

Studies performed at the University of Miami in the early 1990s, by Drs. Richard Taylor and Wayne Streileim, indicate that too much sunlight can damage the immune system. The amount of ultraviolet light that will cause a severe sunburn can damage or kill Langerhans cells in the skin. These cells are the first defense of the body against chemical toxins or infectious agents that in-

vade the skin. This amount of ultraviolet light also decreases the number of circulating T-cells (white blood cells) and triggers fever blisters (cold sores) on the lips of people with latent *Herpes simplex* infections. One to three severe sunburns before the age of 20 doubles the chance that a person will develop malignant melanoma, a common cancer in North America.

■ VISIBLE LIGHT

This is the part of the electromagnetic spectrum that our eyes can detect. Light bulbs, flashlights, burning candles, campfires, fireflies, and stars all emit visible light, as do fast-moving particles that collide. We have extended daylight hours by lighting our homes and largely ignore the natural light/dark cycle of the earth. Most of us spend very little time outdoors in the sunlight.

The two main sources of light in homes, schools, and workplaces are incandescent lights and fluorescent lights. Incandescent lights work differently than fluorescent lights, and while they emit a wide range of the color spectrum, they are deficient at the blue end of the spectrum and contain virtually no ultraviolet light. Much of their light output is in yellows and reds, with the maximum energy produced as infrared radiation (heat).

Fluorescent light is produced by a high-voltage discharge, causing fluorescence of a chemical that coats the inside of the light tube. To accomplish this, a transformer raises the household current to several thousand volts. The light produced depends on the type of phosphor (a chemical) inside the fluorescent bulb. They produce a limited range of the color spectrum and are deficient

Sunlight as Therapy

While too much sun can cause adverse effects, the proper amount of sunlight can have healing and cleansing effects on the body. Studies have shown that repeated short exposures to the sun lower cholesterol and triglyceride levels, blood pressure, and blood sugar. Fungal infections of the skin are often cured or go into remission after sunlight therapy. White blood cells and antibody levels increase with ultraviolet light treatment or exposure to sunlight in amounts that do not redden skin, and neutrophils are stimulated to engulf bacteria more rapidly.

Sunlight speeds the elimination of toxic chemicals, including metals and pesticides. It also has a dramatic effect on trace minerals, making them more accessible to the body. Jaundice is reduced in both children and adults by controlled exposure to sunlight. Many skin diseases, including acne and psoriasis, improve with exposure to sun. (See chapter 37, Outdoor Environment, for information on safe sun exposure.)

in the reds and blue-violets, where the sun's emission is the strongest.

Fluorescent lights produce a much higher magnetic field than incandescent bulbs. One foot away from a fluorescent light, there is still a measurable magnetic field, and in some settings a person's head may be only a foot away from the light.

Light can cause three types of injury to the eyes: thermal, photochemical, and structural. Very bright pulsed light, such as lasers, arc lights, and flash lamps, can cause thermal injury in the retina. Wavelengths in the blue range of visible light can cause photochemical injury in the retina. People will complain of eye pain, a "gritty" feeling in their eyes and photophobia (light sensitivity). Structural injury is associated with lasers. Although injury can occur anywhere in the eye from the cornea to the retina, laser injuries usually involve small retinal burns.

◼ **INFRARED LIGHT**

Infrared radiation emanates from all objects with a temperature above absolute zero. For example, heat given off by a stove is infrared radiation. The sun is a major source of infrared radiation, some of which is absorbed by water vapor. Too much heat from the sun can adversely affect both plants and animals, causing heat exhaustion—a state of collapse brought on by depletion of blood volume through sweating. Untreated heat exhaustion results in heat stroke. When the heat source is the sun, this phenomenon is known as sunstroke. (See also Heat in chapter 17, Noise, Weather, and Altitude.)

Both heat exhaustion and heat stroke may result from exposure to sources of heat other than the sun. Work situations involving furnaces, boilers, or heat-producing engines are potential problems unless temperature control and protective measures are

Microwave Ovens

Microwave ovens heat by agitating the water molecules in food, causing them to vibrate and produce heat. The microwaves enter through the top of the oven and are scattered evenly throughout the oven. They can pass through nonmetal containers, but are reflected by metal containers. Metal containers should never be used in microwaves, as they cause arcing that can burn out the microwave generating tube.

used. Some common medications, including Haldol, Prozac, and Reglon, interfere with neurotransmitters in the brain's thermoregulatory (heat-control) centers, and people taking these drugs are very prone to heat strokes.

■ MICROWAVE RADIATION,
   RADIOFREQUENCY, AND
   TELEVISION WAVES

Radiofrequency (RF) or radio waves are in the frequency of 3 kHz (kilohertz, or 10^3 hertz) to 300 MH (megahertz, or 10^6 hertz). (A hertz is a unit of frequency equal to one cycle per second.) Microwave radiation (MW) waves are in the frequency of 300 MH to 300 GH (gigahertz or 10^9 hertz). Television waves fall within the radio spectrum waves, with some stations generating 54 to 88 MH and others 174 to as much as 220 MH.

All warm objects emit microwaves, including the earth. When the earth is warmed by the sun, it emits infrared light, as well as energy in the microwave range, which special satellites can detect. These microwaves

are between infrared and conventional radio waves in length, and are similar to the waves used in microwave ovens. Microwaves are also used in radar, meteorology, distance measuring, and communications links spanning moderate distances such as a cellular telephone system.

Microwave frequencies produce a thermal skin effect, allowing people to realize when their skin is becoming warm. Exposure to microwaves is dangerous and can cause burns, cataracts, damage to the nervous system, and sterility. In the microwave telecommunication business, people who work around focused microwaves are in danger of lens damage to their eyes. The danger of long-term exposure to low-level microwaves is not known, but the United States government limits microwave exposure levels, including those from microwave ovens.

Radio waves are the energy emitted by radio stations for receiving units in your home to capture. Stars and gases in space also emit radio waves. The radio spectrum has frequency bands that include AM radio, shortwave radio, citizens band (CB) radio, and FM radio. All wireless technology has its own frequency band, including garage door openers, alarm systems, cordless phones, radio-controlled airplanes and cars, cell phones, air traffic control radar, global positioning systems, and deep space radio communications.

The primary health concerns of RF energy are thermal. Radio waves can produce general heating of the body, heating deep body organs without the skin effect that warns a person of danger. The nonthermal (nonheat) effects of radio waves have been studied, and the data include nervous, reproductive, endocrine, immune, and sensory system effects, including cataracts, decreased birth-weight, behavioral changes, and changes in blood count. However, results are inconclusive and contradictory, with some studies showing harmful results and others showing no effect. For many of the studies, statistically significant results were not possible.

Although their frequencies are different, MW is usually considered a subset of RF, as they occur in the same general area of the electromagnetic spectrum. Because of this, the effects of RF and MW radiation exposures are usually considered together. The biological effects from these exposures depend on the frequency of the radiation, the waveform, and the orientation. RF-MWs have been reported to be cancer promoters and can affect the endocrine system, the blood-brain barrier, and the lens of the eye, producing cataracts.

Acute high exposure to RF-MW radiation has caused memory loss. No long-term studies have been conducted regarding the effects of low-level exposure although ham radio operators have a higher incidence of leukemia than does the general public, and military personnel with RF-MW exposure have increased rates of cancer, especially of the blood and lymphatic tissues.

Personal radio transmitters that produce RF-MWs include cordless telephones, cellular telephones, radio-controlled toys, and business security systems. The antennas of these devices are only one to two inches away from the head and brain of the user. The brain pro-

Mobile Phones

In 1998 Dr. S. Braune of the University of Neurology Clinic in Freiluug, Germany, published a study in Lancet *on the effects of radio frequency emitted by mobile phones. He found a significant elevation in blood pressure among mobile phone users, which he and his colleagues concluded was a result of constriction the arteries caused by the rf electromagnetic fields. This increase could severely affect people with high blood pressure.*

duces electromagnetic fields of its own, and these devices conflict with the brain fields.

■ TELEVISION SETS AND VIDEO DISPLAY TERMINALS

Television sets radiate an electromagnetic field in all directions while plugged in, not just while turned on. The larger screens usually radiate a stronger field, which extends further out into the room. These electromagnetic fields penetrate wood and other building materials, and the radiation will pass into another room as though there is no dividing wall. In his book *Cross Currents*, Dr. Robert Becker of New York states that children's beds should not be placed in an adjoining room on a wall opposite a TV set.

Color television sets can also, if adjusted improperly internally, produce X-rays.

Video display terminals (VDTS), which include computer monitors, produce two

TV Radiation

In animal studies, done in 1987 by Dr. H. Mikolajczyk from the Institute of Occupational medicine in Lodz, Poland, television sets were placed 12 inches above rats and were turned on for 4 hours a day for 76 days for females and 50 days for males. The radiation from the TV sets decreased growth, affected brain function, and, in the males, reduced the size of testicles.

types of electromagnetic fields—very low frequency and extremely low frequency. The radiation fields from VDTs are highest at the back and sides of the terminal, and drop quickly with distance. Copying machines and laser printers also emit strong electromagnetic fields, which drop off rapidly with distance.

The extremely low frequency fields have been associated with miscarriages, cancer, and immune dysfunction. Very low frequency fields have also been associated with reproductive difficulties. While there have been many studies to determine the exact relationship between VDTs and reproduction, results have varied and the statistical correlation is not sufficient.

■ EXTREMELY LOW FREQUENCY (ELF) ELECTROMAGNETIC FIELDS

Power transmissions of electrical current produce both electrical fields and magnetic fields.

ELF fields are produced by alternating currents flowing along electrical lines or into electric appliances. Direct current does not produce ELF fields. ELF electromagnetic fields are difficult to detect without special instruments. Occasionally the fields can be heard as they produce a humming noise, or smelled when they produce ozone.

Extremely low frequency electromagnetic fields have wavelengths of 0 to 300 hertz in frequency. All electricity in North America has a frequency of 60 cycles per second, or 60 hertz, and power transmission equipment and home electrical lines and appliances operate at this frequency. Most of the rest of the world transmits electricity at 50 hertz.

Exposure to ELF fields occurs with the use of electric blankets, household appliances, computers, laser printers, copiers, and from electrical transmission lines. High-voltage transmission lines have very large ELF fields associated with them. The United States has regulations that set aside 100 yards of right-of-way beneath high-voltage tension lines.

Electrical currents generate magnetic fields, and household appliances have higher magnetic fields than do high-voltage transmission lines. Even so, exposure to magnetic fields from high-voltage transmission lines is usually greater than that from home appliances due to the small amounts of time involved in the use of home appliances. When an appliance is turned off, the magnetic fields disappear. However, the electrical field remains as long as the appliance is plugged in.

Many studies have been done exposing

cells and animals to ELF fields, as well as studies on workers in the electrical industries. The results have not been consistent and many are controversial. Electrical workers and their children appear to have a higher risk of brain tumors. Some studies show a higher incidence of childhood leukemia in children who live near power lines that carry high voltage, but other studies refute this. Power-line exposure has also been associated with an increased incidence of suicide. Again, there are conflicting studies. However, known effects of electrical fields include changes in reaction speed, production of enzymes and hormones, behavior, and circadian rhythm. Known effects of magnetic fields (which are generated by electrical fields) include changes in nerve impulses, behavior, cell metabolism, and growth. Cancer-causing changes have also been documented.

These effects support the hypothesis that ELFS act as a cancer promoter. ELF fields interact with the cell membrane and can affect hormones, calcium exchange, and tissue growth. It is postulated that the ELFS suppress the production of melatonin, a cancer inhibitor, by the pineal gland. There are now many studies being performed worldwide, researching the effects of ELF exposures on the risk of cancer.

The state of a person's health and the intensity of the electromagnetic exposure influence symptoms. Repeated exposure can cause dizziness, confusion, hyperactivity, memory loss, sleep disturbances, mood changes, numbness, convulsions, and stress syndromes. Some people develop frequent infections and/or allergies and sensitivities.

Healing EMFs

Not all electromagnetic fields are harmful. Low frequency electromagnetic fields have been used to treat ulcers that expose the bare bone, as well as necrotic hip joints, delayed bone union, and osteoporotic bones.

The following effects indicate that a person has an electromagnetic imbalance:

- symptoms that worsen before a storm and improve after it begins
- malfunction of electrical equipment when the person is near
- inability to wear a watch that will keep the correct time
- symptoms when near fluorescent lights
- symptoms from telephone use
- symptoms when near transformers or high-powered electric lines
- malfunction of hearing aids

Geopathic Stress

Geopathic stress is an invisible toxin that can affect health. First demonstrated in 1929 by a German scientist and dowser, Gustav Freiherr van Pohl, geopathic stress is a localized geomagnetic disturbance caused by tectonic fissures, dislocations, faults, and underground water courses. It is stronger where underground streams intersect.

Van Pohl found a relationship between geopathic irritation zones under the beds of cancer victims and the onset, progress, and severity of their disease. He felt geopathic stress was probably both the cause and an acceleration factor of their cancer.

Animals, Plants, and Geopathic Stress

Animals and plants may also be affected by geopathic stress. The refusal of cattle to graze particular parts of a field is attributed to geopathic stress, as is the preference of sleeping places favored by dogs and cats. The inability to grow plants of any kind in a given area, no matter what measures are tried, may be caused by geopathic stress.

Areas of harmful radiation from the earth itself cause geopathic stress. There is a vertical magnetic field going from the earth to the sky, and it varies considerably in field strength over very short distances. Other geomagnetic energies have random direction and may be horizontal, vertical, or diagonal. These distorted energies can rise up through buildings and houses and affect the occupants, disrupting the body's ability to maintain homeostasis.

Dr. Scott-Morley of the Institute of Bioenergetic Medicine in Dorset, England, states that ionizing radiation from the earth is another form of geopathic stress and is given off by certain types of rock structures such as granite. As mentioned above, subterranean water flows, especially those that cross, produce measurable increases in magnetic anomalies, in electrical conductivity of the soil and air, and in the strength of the electromagnetic waves.

Since van Pohl's time, the study of geopathology has continued. In 1979, the U.S.

Department of Health released a study titled *Geomagnetism, Cancer, Weather, and Cosmic Radiation* by Victor Arches. This study found that cancer death rates and the depth contours of the last ice age glacier in North America, which distorted the earth's geomagnetic field lines, correspond with areas of geopathic stress. Associations between cancer incidence and horizontal geomagnetic flux (geopathic stress) were demonstrated on a worldwide basis. The study estimated that 40 to 50 percent of all human cancer may result from the effects of geopathic stress. A correlation was also found between geopathic stress and birth defects.

Changes in the geomagnetic field of the earth affect the electromagnetic field of the body and its organs. In 1978, Russian scientist A.P. Dubrov, author of *The Geomagnetic Field and Life,* reported that a short-term variation in the geomagnetic field affects the central nervous system and may trigger or affect cardiovascular function, epilepsy attacks, glaucoma, and eclampsia. His study found that these changes may also increase traffic accidents, increase blood pressure, decrease white blood cell counts, and upset genetic homeostasis (the balance between genetic components of cells).

Many conditions have been attributed to geopathic stress, including immune system compromise, cardiovascular problems, fatigue, and cancer. Symptoms in which geopathic stress may be common factors are chronic body pains, headaches, sudden signs of physical aging, irritability, and restless sleep. Some people feel that geopathic stress also plays a role in infertility and miscarriages, learning difficulties, and behavioral and neurological disabilities in children.

Several scientists have developed methods for detecting geopathic stress. Dr. Ludger Mersmann of Bio-Physics Mersmann, Inc., a German firm with offices in Massachusetts, has developed equipment that is able to identify influences of geopathic zones, locate and measure magnetic anomalies, and detect disturbed zones of electromagnetic origin, both in the home and workplace. Mersmann states that the main factor in geopathic stress is a disturbed magnetic field.

PART V

Sources of Internal Toxins

WHEN THINKING of detoxification, most people, including healthcare professionals, tend to consider only external toxins (exogenous toxins) and their effects on the body and on health. However, internal toxins, (endogenous toxins) can affect the body just as adversely as external toxins.

One type of internal toxin is a substance that was originally an external toxin, but that became an internal toxin when it entered and was stored in the body. Materials used for dental restorations or medical implants that are a permanent part of the body, but that are not tolerated by the person, are another type of internal toxin.

Substances produced by the body that become toxic when the body produces an excess, or when the body cannot detoxify and excrete what is produced also become internal toxins. A special category that is often overlooked is toxins of the mind and spirit, which can negatively affect the whole person.

Just as external toxins must be detoxified, so must internal toxins. Some require different cleansing, balancing, and prevention techniques from those required for external toxins. Sometimes treatment will be needed for the causative external toxin, as well as for the internal toxin. A discussion of detoxification methods follows in Part VI, and methods to prevent bioaccumulation are presented in Part VII.

CHAPTER 19

Toxins Stored in the Body

NEARLY EVERYONE has internal toxins stored in their bodies. However, people who have had numerous exposures and whose detoxification pathways work poorly will have a larger body burden. The presence of internal chemical toxins should be considered for people:

- who continue to experience reactions and symptoms after receiving standard treatment for chemical sensitivity and after cleaning their environment.
- with high exposure to toxic chemicals.
- with higher than average toxic chemical levels in the blood, serum, fat tissue, or sweat.
- who have recurrent infections.
- for whom treatment methods for other health problems are working very slowly and poorly.

These people will not regain their health unless detoxification procedures are employed to reduce and eliminate their total toxic body load.

Symptoms of headache, fatigue, irritability, memory loss, mental confusion, "flulike" symptoms, mucous membrane irritation, skin problems, eye inflammation, and musculoskeletal pains can be caused by both internal and external chemical exposures. It is important to determine which type of exposure is predominant for an individual, and to treat accordingly. A discussion of detoxification methods and protocols follows in Parts VI and VIII. Methods for preventing bioaccumulation are presented in Part VII.

Microorganisms

Microorganisms can be classified as both external and internal toxins. They enter the body from external sources, but once in the body, they can be considered internal toxins. These microorganisms can include bacteria, viruses, molds, yeasts, fungi, and parasites. While many parasites are microscopic in size, others can be quite large and visible to the naked eye.

As the microorganism grows and multi-

MOST EFFECTIVE DETOXIFICATION METHODS

Microorganisms Stored as Internal Toxins

- Saunas (chapter **22**)
- Nutrients including vitamin C, coenzyme Q_{10}, zinc (**23**)
- Juicing for high vitamin C content (**24**)
- Moderate exercise (**25**)
- Oxygen therapy (**26**)
- Allergy extracts for stored organisms (**27**)
- Hands-on allergy treatment for stored organisms (**27**)
- Homeopathic remedies for the specific organisms (**28**)
- Herbal remedies such as echinacea, goldenseal (**29**)
- Compresses, packs, and poultices for infected areas (**30**)
- Organ cleansing (**31**)

plies in the body, metabolic products are released. Both the metabolic products and substances released when the microorganisms die are internal toxins. Many symptoms of illness caused by microorganisms are due to our allergic reactions to metabolic products, in addition to the protein in the body of the organism itself.

Microorganisms are covered in greater detail in chapter 15, Plants and Organisms. Following is a brief description of various microorganisms that can become internal toxins.

- *Bacteria:* Bacteria contain and produce toxins that can damage tissue, nerves, systemic immunity, and the endocrine system. The bacterial organisms themselves are often allergenic, and their presence exacerbates the symptoms of the illnesses they cause.
- *Parasites:* Toxic substances are released by parasites that destroy tissue and allow them to migrate through our bodies. Parasites also cause damage and mechanical blockage from their increasing numbers. The protein in their bodies is often allergenic, and the egg-producing reproductive cycles of some parasites add to their allergenicity. The body's reaction to parasites can help rid it of them, but the inflammatory process is toxic in itself and increases the eosinophil (a type of white blood cell) count.
- *Viruses:* A variety of illnesses can result when viruses take over the cells of our bodies. They cause the body to produce toxic chemicals in response to their presence. In some cases, their presence in the cell alters specialized cell functions, which affects the person's health even though the cell is not destroyed.
- *Yeasts:* Yeasts can cause infection and hypersensitivity reactions in the body. They also produce numerous toxins that our bodies are unable to adequately process, causing both physical and mental symptoms. Because the body cannot convert these toxins into useful products, it must detoxify them.
- *Molds:* Many people are allergic to molds and their spores. Some molds produce mycotoxins that can cause bleeding and are potent liver toxins and carcinogens for most species. Mycotoxins can also cause

bruising, rashes, vertigo, convulsions, swelling of the heart, destruction of brain cells, and death.

• *Fungi:* Both the infestations and infections that fungi cause become internal toxins. Fungi are very potent allergens and may produce or indirectly generate toxic substances in an attempt to convert the substance on which they are growing into nutrients.

The protein in all these organisms is foreign to our bodies and stimulates an allergic reaction during the infection, exacerbating the symptoms of the infection. As long as the organisms, either dead or alive, are in our bodies, this protein adversely affects us. Dead and partially digested organisms that remain in the body after an infection are also an internal toxin. Until the cellular debris from the organisms is eliminated from the body, it continues to be an internal toxin.

Xenobiotics

Xenobiotics are chemicals that are foreign to the body. Xenobiotics that have been ingested, inhaled, or absorbed through the skin and stored in the body become internal toxins. It never occurs to most people that the perfumes and after-shave lotions that they lavishly apply to their skins are going to become part of their internal toxins and toxic load. The same is true for scented deodorants, body soaps, and lotions. Toxins in food and water that have been ingested are stored in the body, as are inhaled gasoline fumes and fumes from cleaning supplies.

Xenobiotics can damage the body at the main site of entry, in the detoxifying organ,

Releasing Internal Toxins

Evidence that inhaled substances become internal toxins was graphically provided when one of our patients receiving intravenous vitamin C began to detoxify. The whole room in which she was receiving her IV smelled like the wood smoke to which she had been exposed the previous winter, at least six months before.

We have also seen patients who smelled of the pesticides to which they were exposed, and the substances they excreted in their sweat and breath made people around them sick.

or randomly. The weakest organ, which may be genetically damaged or previously harmed, will be the first affected. The sources of these external toxins and their various effects on the body are discussed in detail in Part IV.

Polar (charged), water-soluble chemicals that are absorbed are excreted from the body. Nonpolar (uncharged), lipid-soluble chemicals are stored readily in the body, in all the fatty tissues and the brain, which has the highest fat content of any organ in the body. This accumulation of lipid-soluble, or lipophilic, chemicals is a form of toxic bioaccumulation.

Bioaccumulation is dependent on the dose, interval, and duration of the chemical exposure, the half-life (the amount of time it takes for half of the chemical to deteriorate), and the lipophilic properties of the xenobi-

Persistent Contaminants

Studies have repeatedly demonstrated the persistence of chemicals in the body. In Michigan in the 1970s, animal feed was contaminated with polybrominated biphenyls (PBBS), which passed into meat and cow's milk that was consumed by people. All the residents examined were found to have PBBS in their fat tissue. When the same residents were examined five years later, the PBB levels in their bodies were unchanged. Only with formal detoxification programs were these levels decreased. The derivatives of Agent Orange (dioxin and TCDD), a defoliant used in Vietnam in the 1960s, have persisted in people for over 35 years. (See Pesticides in chapter 16, Chemicals and Metals.)

otic. In addition, the age, overall health, and quantity and quality of immune and enzyme detoxification responses of the person affect bioaccumulation. An overload of xenobiotics can tax the detoxification systems, depleting nutrients, increasing susceptibility to illness and organ malfunction, and increasing bioaccumulation.

The presence of more than one xenobiotic in the body can have synergistic or antagonistic effects. If the effect is synergistic, the symptoms will be more severe than those caused by either chemical alone. If the effect is antagonistic, the symptoms will be lessened, with each chemical reducing the effect of the other.

Some chemicals compete in the body for storage and removal processes. If introduced simultaneously, they compete for the same detoxification enzymes and metabolism. This can result in one chemical being circulated or deposited in fat tissues while the other is cleared from the body. The deposition of xenobiotics in the body seems to occur in layers, because some chemicals cannot be removed until others have been detoxified. When multiple chemicals are present, detoxification procedures and subsequent removal of chemicals from the body must be done slowly so that the liver and kidneys are able to handle the increased detoxification load. (See chapter 31, Organ Cleansing for a detailed discussion.)

In addition to causing direct symptoms, xenobiotics can adversely affect the immune system, suppressing the bacteria- and virus-killing capability of several types of white blood cells, allowing recurrent infections. Some chemicals decrease the number of responder plasma cells (white blood cell–like cells that function in immune responses) in lymph nodes, while others inhibit phagocytic activity (the ability of white cells to engulf and destroy organisms). Some chemicals that inhibit the synthesis of protein or nucleic acids (RNA and DNA) also prevent or modify the synthesis of antibodies and enzymes that are important to the immune system. When the toxic chemicals are removed from the body with detoxification procedures, the recurrent infections usually stop.

Over 300 toxins have been identified in human fat tissue. When the body is stressed by heat exposure, exercise, stress, fasting, or illness, fat may be released into the bloodstream, along with its toxic materials. Fat is also mobilized during sleep, which may explain the severe morning symptoms of chemically sensitive people who felt well when they went to bed. Because the body is unable to excrete all of these chemicals, they circulate freely, targeting various organs and body systems. Later they return to be stored in the fat cells and cell membranes from which they will be released again.

Some people are acutely affected by the release of stored xenobiotics. Others seem to be only mildly affected; however, their toxic burden may lead to more serious diseases in the future. Numerous studies have shown a relationship between the presence of foreign chemicals in human tissue and the incidence of cancer. The severity of bioaccumulation, individual sensitivity, diet, environment, and age all influence the body's response to the release of toxins.

■■ DENTAL RESTORATIONS

A special type of stored toxin is the dental restorations that many people have in their mouths. Restorations include fillings, inlays, crowns, and bridges. Dental materials used include metals, acrylics, resins, binders, cements, and many other substances. (See chapter 11, Toxins from Medical Treatment, for a description of these materials and their effects on health.) These materials can be toxic and constitute a stored toxin for sensitive people.

Restoration materials remain in the teeth until a dentist removes them. Substances from restorations and their breakdown products can migrate into the gums, jawbone, and bloodstream, where they will

---

Stored Xenobiotics

- Saunas and detox baths (chapter **22**)
- Antioxidant nutrients including vitamins A, C, E; coenzyme Q_{10}; cysteine; proanthocyanidins (**23**)
- Healthy high-quality diet, juicing (**24**)
- Exercise and massage (**25**)
- Oxygen therapy (**26**)
- Allergy extracts for specific xenobiotics (**27**)
- Hands-on allergy treatment for the specific xenobiotics (**27**)
- Homeopathic remedies such as *Sulfuricum acidum;* remedies for specific metal poisoning (**28**)
- Herbal remedies for liver support such as milk thistle, burdock, rosemary (**29**)
- Castor oil packs over the liver (**30**)
- Charcoal therapy when indicated (**30**)
- Organ cleansing (**31**)

MOST EFFECTIVE DETOXIFICATION METHODS

---

affect other parts of the body. Even after restoration materials are removed, detoxification procedures are necessary to eliminate the materials and their breakdown products.

■■ MEDICAL IMPLANTS

Some medical procedures require that additional materials be used to help repair the body, aid its function, enhance its appearance, or replace a missing part. Medical implants include joint replacements, breast implants, pacemakers, and surgical aids such as screws, plates, staples, and reinforcing material. These implants become a permanent part of the body. If the recipient does not tolerate the implant materials, they be-

MOST EFFECTIVE DETOXIFICATION METHODS

Dental Restorations

- Saunas and detox baths (chapter **22**)
- Nutrients including B vitamins, vitamin C, cysteine, glutathione, methionine, MSM, magnesium, selenium, zinc (**23**)
- Healthy high-quality diet; avoid fish; eat eggs, milk, butter, onion, garlic, leafy green vegetables, beets, brussels sprouts, oranges, grapefruit, peas, kelp (**24**)
- Massage to help mobilize toxins (**25**)
- Oxygen therapy (**26**)
- Allergy extracts or hands-on allergy treatment for restoration substances (**27**)
- Chelation treatment for metals after restorations have been removed (**27**)
- Homeopathic remedies for liver support (**28**)
- Herbal remedies for liver support such as milk thistle, burdock, rosemary (**29**)
- Packs and poultices to draw out toxins (**30**)
- Organ cleansing (**31**)

come stored internal toxins that can adversely affect the person's health.

■ METAL IMPLANTS

Should they become diseased or worn out, many joints can now be replaced with an artificial joint. Improved technology allows nearly every joint of the body to be replaced, including shoulder, elbow, finger, hip, knee, and ankle joints. Even artificial jaws are now possible. An alloy of titanium—a lightweight, very strong metal—is frequently used in these artificial joints. The implant connection to the bone may be made of porous metal held in place by screws and

around which bone will grow. Bone cements, a type of epoxy, are also used to secure the joint parts to the bone.

While artificial joints give many people increased range of motion and relief from pain, some people tolerate these artificial joints poorly. They may not tolerate the material from which the implant is made or the bone cement used to anchor the implant, or both. Titanium is, unfortunately, an allergen for many people. Heat in the joint, discomfort, swelling, and pain are indications that there is a tolerance problem with the artificial joint. Some people develop weather sensitivity and can tell when a new front is moving in by the way the artificial joint is responding. Pain and swelling preceding a new front are common symptoms.

One of our elderly patients had a knee replacement that unfortunately became a stored toxin. She did not tolerate the material used in the replacement joint, and for the remainder of her life her knee felt hot to her and to others. The skin around her knee looked red compared to the rest of her skin, and her health began to decline more rapidly after the surgery.

In some surgical procedures, plates and screws are used. Metal plates protect the brain when skull bones are missing. Metal plates and rods may also be used to reinforce shattered bones. Screws hold bones together as well as securing reinforcing metal to bones. When people do not tolerate the metal in these surgical aids, they become a stored internal toxin.

■ SILICONE IMPLANTS

Silicone is a synthetic polymer (long chain molecule) containing a repeating silicon-oxygen backbone. Depending upon the number of units in the backbone chain and the amount of linking of the chains, fluids, emulsions, compounds, lubricants, resins, elastomers, or rubbers can be produced. At one point, it was thought that silicone was a completely inert substance that could be used anywhere in the body with no negative effects. While some scientists and physicians still maintain that silicone has no bioreactivity, many other healthcare professionals and many laypeople with silicone implants and accompanying health problems dispute this claim. About 5 percent of the American population have some type of medical implant, many of which contain silicone.

Many women have elected to use silicone breast implants to augment the size of their breasts. While some women are pleased with the results, many women have experienced serious problems with these implants.

Most silicone breast implants are a flexible silicone pouch filled with silicone gel. If implants are placed on a piece of paper, they will leave an oily spot on the paper. When placed in the body, the silicone gel slowly bleeds from the implant. These tiny gel droplets are picked up by macrophages, a special type of white blood cell, and lymph nodes can become clogged with these cells. The gel droplets also migrate to many other organs. The silicone gel adheres to the protein molecules in the body and does not degrade nor is it excreted. The silicone-protein complexes may set off subtle changes that can end in disease.

Scar tissue may form around the breast

Medical Implants

MOST EFFECTIVE DETOXIFICATION METHODS

- Saunas or detox baths (chapter **22**)
- Antioxidant nutrients including vitamins A, C, E; coenzyme Q_{10}; pycnogenol; cysteine, glutathione, and methionine (**23**)
- Healthy high-quality diet (**24**)
- Massage to help mobilize toxins in cells (**25**)
- Oxygen therapy (**26**)
- Allergy extracts or hands-on treatments for materials in the implants (**27**)
- Homeopathic remedies specific for the implant materials (**28**)
- Herbal remedies for liver support such as milk thistle, goldenseal, burdock (**29**)
- Charcoal therapy when indicated, castor oil packs over affected area (**30**)
- Organ cleansing (**31**)

implants and can contract, squeezing the implants so that they become painful and feel hard. Some implants remain intact, some rupture, and others develop serious leaks. In addition to the pain disturbing their sleep, women may experience morning stiffness and numbness; constipation; abdominal, joint, and muscle pain; headaches; swollen lymph nodes; fever; rashes; chronic fatigue; dry eyes and mouth; skin lesions; and hair loss. Implants may also cause granulomas, which are chronically inflamed tissue. In addition, silicone may prompt the formation of auto-antibodies that attack the joints, connective tissue, muscles, nerves, and other organs.

Hard silicone implants are used during plastic and reconstructive surgery for the chin, cheeks, and nose. Both hard and soft silicone implants are used for the penis, testicular implants for the scrotum, and ear vent tubes. Artificial heart valves are sometimes made of silicone. One-third of ear vent tubes, and one out of five artificial heart valves cause problems for the recipients. Symptoms may include hives, pain, and swelling.

■ PACEMAKERS

A pacemaker is an electrical device for stimulating rhythmic heartbeat when the electrical conduction system of the heart is not functioning properly. It is implanted in the body, usually under the collarbone.

These battery-powered devices emit impulses that trigger heart contractions at a rate that can be pre-set or controlled by an external switch. Many pacemakers can be programmed externally by the physician and are replaced or serviced only if the battery must be changed. If the person does not tolerate the materials from which the pacemaker is manufactured, which may include silicone, the pacemaker becomes a stored internal toxin.

■ MESHES

At one time hernias were repaired by laboriously sewing the tissue and skin layers together to close off the hernia. There was a high incidence of hernia recurrence with this technique, as well as accompanying pain and tightness.

Reinforcing materials are now used to help repair hernias. Porous polypropylene mesh, which allows skin cells to attach and grow around the material, is used. This mesh becomes a permanent part of the body wall, and hernia reoccurrence is less than one percent using this technique. These reinforcing materials can become a stored internal toxin if the person does not tolerate them. Pain and hives in the repaired area may signal a tolerance problem.

CHAPTER 20

Toxins Produced in the Body

Toxins produced in the body result from the byproducts of normal physiological processes. These substances become toxic if their rate of production is too high, or if they are not detoxified or excreted adequately. They can include any of thousands of substances in and produced by the cells of our bodies. Most biochemical reactions in our bodies produce both energy and waste products. These waste products—bilirubin, lactic acid, ammonia, uric acid, creatinine, and urea—can be toxic if their levels become too high.

Internal toxins can also be irritating or harmful compounds formed in the body in response to imbalanced conditions. The metabolic waste products of our cells, including carbon dioxide; dead and digested bacteria, parasites, and viruses; hydrogen peroxide; and cellular debris can become toxic. Hormone and neurotransmitter sensitivity and imbalance are other internal toxins. In addition, free radicals may be created in the body in response to various conditions, such as anesthesia, injury, and pollu-tion. These free radicals are toxic to tissues (see Free Radicals, below).

The toxins created by our bodies cause numerous symptoms, which can include behavior changes, confusion, low energy, fatigue, headache, irritability, memory loss, musculoskeletal pain, skin problems, weakness of unknown origin, gastrointestinal complaints, sleep disturbances, and dysfunction of the endocrine and immune systems.

Metabolic Waste Products

Cellular metabolism produces waste products that must be processed and eliminated by our bodies. If the body does not or cannot efficiently eliminate these substances, they build up and become toxic to the body. These waste products enter the plasma, which is the liquid portion of the blood. The plasma carries the waste products to the kidneys, which, when they are functioning properly, excrete metabolic waste products into the urine as fast as they are produced, preventing their accumulation in the body.

MOST EFFECTIVE DETOXIFICATION METHODS

Metabolic Waste Products

- Sauna and detox baths (chapter **22**)
- Antioxidant nutrients including vitamins A, C, E; coenzyme Q$_{10}$ (**23**)
- Healthy high-quality diet, low-protein diet (**24**)
- Exercise, acupuncture, massage (**25**)
- Oxygen therapy (**26**)
- Allergy extracts or hands-on allergy treatment for waste products such as uric acid and creatinine (**27**)
- Homeopathic remedies to support the liver and kidneys (**28**)
- Herbal remedies to support the liver and kidneys (**29**)
- Packs and poultices over the liver and kidneys (**30**)
- Organ cleansing (**31**)

■ BILIRUBIN

The straw color of plasma comes from its bilirubin content. Bilirubin is a breakdown product of the protein hemoglobin contained in red blood cells, and is normally excreted in the bile as a bile pigment.

If the common bile duct is blocked so that further secretion of bile is inhibited, bilirubin builds up in the blood and diffuses into tissues. This produces a yellowish coloration of the skin and eyes, known as jaundice. Bilirubin is also responsible for the jaundice symptoms of hepatitis, a liver disease that causes the liver to be unable to secrete bilirubin into the bile.

■ UREA

Plasma also contains urea (NH_2-CO-NH_2), a nitrogenous compound that is the break-down product of food or tissue protein and amino acids. This breakdown of proteins and amino acids yields ammonia, which the liver converts to urea with the aid of enzymes. The urea leaves the liver and is excreted in the urine by the kidneys. If kidney function is impaired, the urea in the blood will rise above normal range; this condition is known as uremia.

Blockage of any steps in the conversion and excretion of urea can prove fatal, because the body has no other pathways to synthesize urea and to dispose of ammonia, which is toxic to the brain. Some genetic diseases cause a partial block of each of the six urea cycle enzymes. This enzyme deficiency occurs in one out of every 2,500 newborn infants, causing intellectual impairment, lethargy, convulsions, stupor, and periodic vomiting. It can be fatal. Ammonia toxicity can also occur in adults with liver damage.

If you have excess levels of ammonia, you should seek help from a healthcare professional. Excesses of ammonia/ammonium can be cleansed from the body by an alpha-ketoglutaric acid supplement. This acid is an amino group receptor, and it becomes glutamic acid (an amino acid needed by the body), after accepting the amino group. Vitamin B$_6$, vitamin C, mineral supplements, and increased water intake also help to decrease ammonia levels.

■ URIC ACID

When nucleic acids such as RNA and DNA break down, uric acid is produced, which is excreted in the urine by the kidneys. Sometimes it combines with sodium to form stones, or calculi. Elevated levels of uric acid are associated with gout, a condition in which too much uric acid is produced and its excretion is impaired. Severe pain results from the deposition of sodium urate (a salt of uric acid) crystals in connective tissues and cartilage. One of the most common sites of deposition is between the big toe and the foot.

Uric acid excretion is impaired in people with uremia, nephritis (an inflammation of the kidneys), or lead poisoning. Uric acid formation is increased by leukemia. It is also produced in high levels by rapid cancer breakdown, such as the treatment of a large tumor with chemotherapy.

■■ CREATININE

Creatinine is the end product of muscle metabolism and is generated at a fairly constant rate. It is derived from muscle creatine, the molecule that transfers phosphate in the energy metabolism cycle of the body.

Creatinine is filtered in the kidney and excreted in the urine. Its rate of clearance is an indicator of kidney efficiency. If it is not excreted, it is metabolized to other compounds that are harmful to the body.

Hormone Imbalances

Hormones are highly potent substances that function as biological regulators. They are produced by the endocrine system, which consists of all the glands that secrete hormones. These chemical messengers are released from the glands into the bloodstream. They are then carried by the blood to target cells elsewhere in the body. Hormone production does not occur at a constant rate but in short bursts, depending on the amount

Growth Hormone

Growth hormone, secreted by the anterior pituitary, is the most important hormone for growth. Its effects take place after birth, and it has no effect on the fetus. Growth hormone stimulates cell division in many target organs, including bone, directly promoting bone lengthening. An excess of growth hormone during childhood causes gigantism, and a deficiency results in dwarfism. In adults, an excess of growth hormone cannot lengthen bones, but causes disfiguring bone thickening and overgrowth of other organs known as acromegaly.

and duration of the stimuli triggering their production.

Hormone levels depend on the amount produced and on the ability of the body to remove the excess. Hormones become an internal toxin if their secretion is too low or too high. They also become a toxin if the liver is unable to detoxify them adequately, causing high levels to remain in the body.

Thyroid imbalances are a common hormone problem. If the thyroid gland does not produce enough of the hormone thyroxine, the hypothyroidism that results causes fatigue, sensitivity to cold, constipation, dry hair and skin, hoarseness, constipation, and elevated blood lipids. If the thyroid gland produces too much thyroxine, the resulting hyperthyroidism can cause weight loss, heart palpitations, loss of muscle mass and strength, heat intolerance, fast heart rate, and exophthalmos (bulging eyes).

Hormone Sensitivity and Imbalance

- Detox baths for general detoxification (chapter **22**)
- Vitamins A and E, essential fatty acids (**23**)
- Healthy high-quality diet, avoidance of food allergens (**24**)
- Mild exercise, acupuncture, and massage (**25**)
- Breathing exercises and oxygen therapy (**26**)
- Allergy extracts or hands-on treatment for hormone sensitivities (**27**)
- Homeopathic remedies such as *Calcarea carbonica, Lycopodium, Magnesia phosphorica, Sepia, Sulfur* (**28**)
- Bach Flower Remedies for emotions triggered by hormone sensitivity (**28**)
- Herbs such as alfalfa, black cohosh, blessed thistle, cramp bark (**29**)
- Aromatherapy essences such as chamomile, lavender, sandalwood (**29**)
- Hot and cold compresses and packs on abdomen (**30**)
- Organ cleansing (**31**)

Estrogen, one of the female sex hormones, controls the development of the female body configuration as well as playing a role in the menstrual cycle. An excess of estrogen created by the inability of the liver to degrade and excrete it plays a role in endometriosis. Excess estrogen also contributes to uterine fibroids as well as causing sore breasts. In males, it causes female characteristics to develop, including breasts and a female pattern of body fat distribution.

Testosterone, the sex hormone that controls the development of secondary sex characteristics in the male, is also related to aggression. An excess of testosterone causes males to be overly aggressive. Testosterone directly controls male sex drive, and a deficiency of testosterone can cause problems with erection and ejaculation. Females normally have low concentrations of testosterone in their bodies. With an excess of testosterone and other androgens (male hormones), women develop virilism, in which the female pattern of fat distribution disappears, the voice lowers, breasts become smaller, the clitoris enlarges, and beard growth and male body-hair distribution occur.

An insulin imbalance is a form of internal toxin. A lack of insulin production causes type I diabetes. This usually develops in childhood, and its incidence is increasing. The hormone insulin regulates sugar metabolism, and its imbalance is a major contributor to obesity. Insulin is released from the pancreas in response to a rise in blood sugar levels and attaches to special receptor sites on the cells. This enables sugar to enter the cells, where it is burned for energy or stored in fat cells or muscle cells for later use.

If a person has too few insulin receptor sites or if the receptor sites are insulin resistant, the insulin cannot enter the cells and remains in the bloodstream. This causes type II diabetes. The elevated insulin levels cause the body to store fat and sugar; prevent the release of the neurotransmitter serotonin, which controls the feeling of fullness; and

Neurotransmitters and Autism

Neurotransmitter insufficiency, imbalance, or sensitivity plays a role in many conditions, including autism. One autistic child has been treated extensively with allergy extracts for a neurotransmitter imbalance and sensitivity. He also takes nutrients to help with neurotransmitter insufficiency.

At his first testing appointment, he had to be restrained to prevent his kicking the technician. He now sits quietly on his mother's lap during testing. Initially, he screamed on his arrival at the office. He now chatters, using mostly nonsense words, and at times sings. A dirty, ragged quilt was his constant companion for months. He is now content with a small piece of it tied around his finger.

His mother reports the following improvements:

- *He is calmer at school and is trying to play with his classmates rather than hitting them.*
- *He shows more control at school, and his temper tantrums are less frequent.*
- *He is less obsessive and is learning not to generalize his anger.*
- *He talks more, trying to use more words, and speaking more clearly, sometimes making three-word sentences.*
- *He is learning to read and learning some math.*
- *He is able to write to a limited extent and his letter formation is improving.*
- *He tolerates noise better and can listen to others.*

prevent the pancreas from releasing glucagon, the hormone that signals the liver to stop producing cholesterol. Elevated cholesterol will result.

In addition to imbalances, sensitivity to hormones causes them to become internal toxins. Sensitivities to increased levels of progesterone, estrone, or LH (leutinizing hormone) appear to play a role in premenstrual syndrome (PMS). Premenstrual syndrome refers to the complex of symptoms that affects over 20 million North American women. Symptoms can occur from mid-cycle up to and during the first few days of menstruation, although the beginning of the period usually relieves them. Symptoms

can include depression, irritability, mood swings, swelling and tenderness of the breasts, abdominal bloating and cramping, acne, fatigue, and weight fluctuation.

Most women suffering from PMS have normal hormone levels, but when they are tested and treated with allergy extracts for sensitivity of hormones, their symptoms are relieved.

Neurotransmitter Imbalances

Neurotransmitters are the chemical messengers responsible for the transmission of nerve impulses across the synapse (space) between nerve cells. They are produced in the nerve cells and released from precursors

MOST EFFECTIVE DETOXIFICATION METHODS

Neurotransmitter Sensitivity and Imbalance

- Detox baths for light detoxification (chapter **22**)
- Nutrients such as vitamin C, coenzyme Q₁₀, amino acids (**23**)
- Healthy high-quality diet; avoid food allergens; ensure adequate protein consumption (**24**)
- Light exercise, acupuncture, and massage (**25**)
- Breathing exercises and oxygen therapy (**26**)
- Allergy extracts or hands-on treatment for neurotransmitter sensitivity and imbalance (**27**)
- Homeopathic remedies such as *Arsenicum album, Lac caninum, Nux vomica, Pulsatilla* (**28**)
- Herbal remedies such as bergamot, chamomile, orange blossom, rose otto, (**29**)
- Organ cleansing (**31**)
- Neuro Emotional Technique (**33**)

into the bloodstream. Precursors include amino acids, lecithin, minerals, and vitamins.

After their release, excess neurotransmitters are transformed by enzymes into ineffective substances, diffused into extracellular spaces away from the receptor site, or transported back into the releasing neuron and reabsorbed. If the removal process is impaired, the excess neurotransmitters become internal toxins.

Inhibition of acetylcholinesterase, the enzyme that degrades acetylcholine, causes an accumulation of this major neurotransmitter, resulting in the overstimulation of nerves. Adverse effects occur in the central nervous system, autonomic nervous system, and at the junctions between nerves and muscles. Convulsions, paralysis, and eventually death can occur if the levels of acetylcholine remain very high.

An excess of the neurotransmitter histamine can cause suicidal depression. People lose contact with reality and they may have compulsive or obsessive thoughts. Sexual function is affected; males experience premature ejaculation and females have repeated or sustained orgasms.

An excess of the hormone epinephrine, which also has neurotransmitter functions, causes a decrease in oxygen consumption, clotting time, metabolic rate, and motility of the gastrointestinal tract. It also increases heart rate, respiration, blood sugar levels, and sweating.

Glycine is the third major inhibitory (calming) neurotransmitter in the body, and it is required for optimal growth. It passes easily through the blood-brain barrier and is uniformly distributed in the brain and throughout tissues. It plays a role in detoxification, alleviating the toxic effects of phenol, benzoic acid, and methionine. It also helps to remove lead from the body. However, elevated levels can cause intellectual impairment.

Serotonin is also a major inhibitory neurotransmitter in the brain. Increased serotonin levels produce changes in sleep patterns and sexual activity. For other symptoms of excess serotinin, see Weather in chapter 17.

Just as an excess of neurotransmitter causes serious problems, insufficient neurotransmitters have a toxic effect on the body. The body cannot function properly with insufficient neurotransmitters, and some people do not make enough of these chemicals.

People with low levels of histamine are fearful of themselves, their neighbors, and the world around them. Males can have an erection, but no ejaculation, and women cannot have an orgasm. Children are usually healthy, but are hyperactive and have an increased threshold for pain.

Low epinephrine levels cause emotional disturbances and the inability to respond to emergencies, hard work, and temperature extremes. Deficiency signs of norepinephrine include poor nerve conduction, dizziness, light-headedness, and fainting (from low blood pressure).

Constant hunger is a symptom of serotonin deficiency. This deficiency has also been implicated in depression, obsessive-compulsive disorder, autism, bulimia, social phobias, PMS, anxiety, panic, migraines, schizophrenia, and extreme violence. Serotonin function is severely depressed in people with Alzheimer's disease.

Supplementation with neurotransmitter precursors, particularly amino acids, is helpful in overcoming insufficient neurotransmitter levels. However, some people cannot utilize their neurotransmitters properly because they are sensitive to them. This sensitivity causes or contributes to many problems, including attention deficit hyperactivity disorder (ADHD), depression, sleep problems, anxiety, and Seasonal Affective Disorder (SAD). Sensitivity to neurotransmit-

---

Acid/Alkaline Imbalance

- Detox baths (chapter **22**)
- Nutrients such as multivitamin; buffered vitamin C for acidosis; ascorbic acid for alkalosis (**23**)
- Diets for correction of acidosis or alkalosis, avoidance of food allergens (**24**)
- Exercise and massage (**25**)
- Breathing exercises (**26**)
- Allergy extracts or hands-on treatments for food allergens, acids, alkalis (**27**)
- Homeopathic remedies such as *Natrum phosphoricum* (**28**)
- Herbal remedies to support the blood and kidneys such as blessed thistle, dandelion, hydrangea, gravel root (**29**)
- Organ cleansing (**30**)

MOST EFFECTIVE DETOXIFICATION METHODS

---

ters can be helped with allergy extracts or hands-on allergy treatemts. (See chapter 27, Allergy Treatment and Chelation, for further information.)

Acid/Alkaline Balance

The body functions through a series of biochemical reactions involving acids and alkalis, which control many body processes. An acid-alkaline balance is essential to the proper function of the body. An imbalance is toxic and causes many adverse symptoms.

Acids are substances that have a sour or sharp taste. Vinegar (acetic acid), the hydrochloric acid in the stomach, and the sulfuric acid in car batteries are examples of common acids.

An alkali or base is a compound that is bitter, slippery, and caustic. Household ammonia (ammonium hydroxide) is an alkali. Sodium hydroxide, sometimes called caustic soda, is a common alkali, as is potassium hydroxide, sometimes called caustic potash. Both compounds are also referred to as lye.

The measure of whether a substance is acidic or alkaline (basic) is expressed as its pH. The pH scale ranges from 0 to 14. The neutral point is 7; all values below 7 are acidic, and those above 7 are alkaline or basic.

Acid-alkali reactions are necessary to the biochemistry of the body, and unless they occur at the proper speed and in proportion, the body can develop an acid/alkali imbalance. Such an imbalance can be considered a toxin, since the body cannot function properly and can be damaged.

The pH of different parts of the body is crucial to proper digestion. For best digestive function:
- The mouth should be alkaline for the salivary enzymes to function.
- The stomach should be acidic for protein processing.
- The small intestine should be alkaline for the pancreatic digestive enzymes to function.
- The large intestine should be slightly acidic to maintain proper bowel flora.

■ RESPIRATORY ACIDOSIS AND ALKALOSIS

Respiratory acidosis occurs when the lungs are unable to expel carbon dioxide as fast as it is produced. The carbonic acid level in the blood rises as a result, and arterial concentrations of carbon dioxide and hydrogen ions will be elevated. This happens when holding your breath, when there is impaired gas exchange from partial bronchial obstruction, or from a drug overdose. The body attempts to compensate by deeper, more rapid breathing.

Respiratory alkalosis occurs when carbon dioxide is eliminated faster than it is produced, as happens during hyperventilation. In respiratory alkalosis, the arterial concentrations of carbon dioxide and hydrogen ions are reduced.

■ METABOLIC ACIDOSIS AND ALKALOSIS

Our blood is slightly alkaline, with normal pH ranges as given below.
- arterial blood: 7.40 to 7.45
- capillary blood: 7.35 to 7.40
- venous blood: 7.30 to 7.35

If the pH of the blood rises over 7.45, metabolic alkalosis occurs. This is less common than acidosis and can be caused by the loss of large quantities of hydrochloric acid from the stomach, as occurs with severe vomiting. Excessive alkali therapy in treating peptic ulcers can also cause this condition. The body reduces its rate of respiration to compensate for metabolic alkalosis.

During alkalosis, more carbonate is deposited in the bones, and can result in bone or heel spurs. A major symptom of alkalosis is overexcitability of the nervous system as manifested by a highly nervous condition, hyperventilation, and even seizures. Other symptoms include sore muscles, chronic indigestion, vomiting, menstrual problems, hard dry stools, and thickening of the skin accompanied by burning and itching sensations.

At a blood pH below 7.30, metabolic acidosis occurs, as in diabetic coma when excessive acids are produced in tissue metabolism. This results from abnormal glucose combustion caused by insulin deficiency. The excessive production of lactic acid during severe exercise or hypoxia (a deficiency of oxygen reaching the tissues) also produces metabolic acidosis, as do fasting and diarrhea when excess bicarbonate is lost.

When the blood becomes too acidic, the respiratory center is stimulated by the brain to expel more carbon dioxide. This lowers the carbonic acid level, allowing the blood pH to return to normal range. The lungs provide a rapid mechanism for normalizing blood pH, and breathing becomes deep and rapid.

If metabolic acidosis continues for several hours, dissolution of bone occurs. There is a loss of carbonate from the bones, but little loss of calcium or phosphate. If the metabolic acidosis persists for several days, part of the bone will be dissolved. Other symptoms of acidosis include kidney, liver, and adrenal disorders; ketosis (an excess of ketone bodies, intermediates in lipid metabolism); obesity; and feelings of stress, anger, and fear.

■■ BUFFER SYSTEMS

The pH of the blood is also maintained by buffer systems. A buffer is a chemical which, when in solution, prevents or reduces changes that would otherwise occur when acid or alkali is added to the solution. Buffers are essential for the pH of a solution or system to stay relatively constant. They allow the pH of the blood to stay within the normal range even though acid metabolites are constantly being formed in the tissues. If the body overproduces buffers in response to acidosis, the body can become alkaline.

The major extracellular buffer of the body is the bicarbonate system. Bicarbonate is produced by the pancreas, and carbon dioxide is converted to bicarbonate in the red blood cells.

Hemoglobin in the red blood cells is the next most powerful buffer in the body. When hemoglobin releases its oxygen, it takes up hydrogen ions produced as a result of metabolism of protein and other organic molecules and through the respiratory system, gastrointestinal tract, and urine. The affinity that hemoglobin has for hydrogen ions prevents their uniting with carbon dioxide to form carbonic acid. This helps to compensate for the difference in carbon dioxide concentration from venous to arterial blood.

The kidneys provide another buffering system. In metabolic acidosis, the urine becomes more acidic than normal. Diabetic ketosis, starvation, or severe diarrhea also cause abnormally acidic urine. The normal pH of the urine ranges from 4.8 to 7.4. Acidic urine ranges from 4.4 to 4.8.

In metabolic alkalosis, the urine is more alkaline. The urine can also be alkaline during urinary infections when the infecting organisms split urea molecules and release ammonia.

The kidneys help maintain a stable concentration of hydrogen ions in the plasma by regulating the bicarbonate concentration, by either excreting it or adding new bicarbonate to the blood. If too much acidic urine is produced and excreted, depleting the kidney of

MOST EFFECTIVE DETOXIFICATION METHODS

Lactic Acid Imbalance

- Sauna and detox baths (chapter **22**)
- Nutrients such as calcium, magnesium, zinc (**23**)
- Fasting or juicing (**24**)
- Massage (**25**)
- Breathing exercises, oxygen therapy (**26**)
- Allergy treatments or hands-on treatment for lactic acid (**27**)
- Homeopathic remedies such as *Lacticum acidum* (**28**)
- Aromatherapy body balancing essences such as bergamot, lemon, rose otto (**29**)
- Hot and cold compresses and packs (**30**)
- Organ cleansing (**31**)

hydrogen ions, renal alkalosis results. This sometimes happens in severe kidney disease. Renal acidosis occurs if too much alkaline urine is produced and excreted. Both these conditions negatively affect the filtering of acids and alkalis in the kidney because its efficiency is dependent on an optimal pH. The urine of most North Americans is acidic because of their high meat intake, since phosphoric acid and sulfuric acid are produced from the breakdown of protein, particularly meat.

▍▍ CONNECTIVE TISSUE

Connective tissue, also known as mesenchymal tissue, is made up of cells designed to support, connect, and anchor the structures of the body. Connective tissue also forms a drainage system that takes up cell waste products and discharges them through the lymph system, or sometimes stores them.

The pH of the connective tissue and its acid/alkaline balance are essential to its proper function. When acids build up, some are flushed from the body in the urine. Other acids are locked into the connective tissues and, even though the body continues to make buffers, they cannot penetrate to neutralize the acids. This causes the connective tissue to remain too acidic, and it cannot experience normal pH fluctuations.

Factors that negatively affect the health of connective tissue include:

- the Standard American Diet of processed grains, fast foods high in fat and sugar, and few fruits and vegetables
- drugs, both prescription and recreational
- toxic chemicals, including food additives and insecticides
- stress, including environmental, emotional, or physical
- microorganisms, including viruses, bacteria, parasites, fungi, and yeast

Most North Americans have primary mesenchymal acidosis. The high consumption of meats, sugars, white flour, heat-treated oils, and antibiotics are major contributors to this condition. This acidosis affects the magnesium and potassium balance of the cells, congests the lymphatic system, and leaches calcium from bones. People with high tissue acidity suffer from fatigue and headaches, and are more sensitive to weather patterns.

Lactic Acid Balance

The body uses the sugar glucose as fuel, breaking it down into adenosine triphosphate (ATP) and pyruvate to manufacture energy for the cells. Under aerobic conditions

Protective Mechanisms to Combat Free Radicals

Enzymes are a major protective mechanism against free radicals. Other factors that affect the body's reaction to free radicals are diet, nutrient status, level of oxygenation, integrity of cell membranes, the amount of inflammation in the body; and the status of the circulatory system, down to the smallest capillary.

Free radicals are destroyed or controlled in the body by several mechanisms. They can be converted to oxygen by oxidation or to water by reduction. In the process of oxidation, electrons are lost, while in reduction, electrons are gained. Antioxidant enzymes participate in both these reactions. Enzymes also catalyze reactions

that force free radicals to combine with each other, neturalizing their free radical effects.

Antioxidants such as vitamins, minerals, and some amino acids combat free radicals by donating electrons. Sometimes they are oxidized in the process, but are regenerated by enzymes and other cofactors. Some antioxidants, such as vitamin E, appear to intercept free radicals at the cell membrane, sparing the membrane and lipids from oxidative change. One molecule of vitamine E can protect 1,000 membrane and lipid molecules. Other antioxidants neutralize free radicals by bonding covalently (sharing electrons) with them.

(in the presence of oxygen), pyruvate enters the cells. If the oxygen supply is not adequate, pyruvate breaks down into lactic acid instead of carbon dioxide and water.

Lactic acid levels rise during strenuous exercise when the blood flow and oxygen do not meet the increased needs of the muscles. People who are running sprints or who have been exercising for prolonged periods of time produce excess lactic acid in their muscles, resulting in an increased lactate level in their blood. (Lactate is the ionized form of lactic acid; the two compounds readily convert to either form.) This can cause muscle soreness.

Ingestion of alcohol, low blood oxygen, and severe anemia can also increase lactate concentrations in the blood. Anesthesia also increases lactate levels, as do some liver dis-

eases and a variety of conditions in which hypoxia (low oxygen) occurs.

Lactic acidosis can occur in both diabetics and nondiabetics and, if the condition is not corrected, can lead to fatal metabolic acidosis (see above).

Free Radicals

Free radicals are atoms, ions, or molecules containing at least one unpaired electron in their outermost rings, or orbitals. This is unusual because most electrons occur in stable pairs. Free radicals pull electrons from surrounding molecules, which in turn pull electrons from still other molecules, creating a chain reaction that forms more and more free radicals. Oxygen is a life-giving molecule and we cannot live without it for more than a few minutes. However, because it

Free Radical Excess

- Saunas and detox baths (chapter **22**)
- Antioxidant nutrients including vitamins A, C, E; cysteine, glutathione, and methionine; coenzyme Q_{10}, organic germanium, proanthocyanidins, alpha-lipoic acid, enzymes SOD and catalase (**23**)
- High-quality, organic foods (**24**)
- Exercise and massage (**25**)
- Breathing exercises and oxygen therapy, including inhalation, hydrogen peroxide, and stabilized oxygen (**26**)
- Allergy extracts or hands-on treatment for allergens, particularly chemicals (**27**)
- Organ cleansing (**31**)

contains unpaired electrons, it sometimes forms part of a free radical molecule. White blood cells use these free radicals in small amounts to combat microbial invaders. Free radicals are also produced in the lining of blood vessel walls, to help regulate the contraction of the smooth muscles and maintain proper blood flow.

Free radicals produced in the body are called endogenous, and our bodies cannot function properly without them. They exist in small numbers in cells and are useful in activating many enzyme reactions and controlling some biochemical reactions. Free radicals are also important in hormone and energy production.

Exogenous free radicals are produced in the body in response to external sources of toxins. Air pollution, toxic metals, pesticides, herbicides, cigarette smoke, ionizing radiation, toxic waste and runoff, and oxides

of nitrogen cause the production of exogenous free radicals. Even overexposure to the sun can lead to free radicals.

Diet can also contribute to the formation of free radicals. The body utilizes oxygen and the nutrients from food to create energy. Oxygen molecules containing unpaired electrons are released in the process. If they are produced in large amounts, they can damage the body. Oxidation occurs more readily during the breakdown of fats than that of proteins and carbohydrates. A diet high in fat, and the cooking of fats at high temperature, particularly frying foods in oil, produces large numbers of free radicals. (See Food Preparation in chapter 13, Food.)

In excess, free radicals, both endogenous and exogenous, constitute an internal toxin and can damage the body. Some disorders are attributed to damage caused by excess endogenous free radical reactions. Free radical damage can be of genetic origin, when the body has inadequate enzyme protection from oxygen radicals. Two disorders are thought to be caused by free radical damage to the DNA repair mechanisms. Xeroderma pigmentosum is the development of photosensitive areas with severe sunburns in infancy, leading to malignant tumors. Ataxia-telangiectasia is a multisystem disorder that affects children's motor ability, skin problems, and recurrent infections.

Free radical damage may result from a combination of genetic and environmental factors, in which the genetic problem is not evident or expressed unless there are sufficient or overwhelming environmental exposures. Chemical sensitivity and some degenerative diseases, such as cancer, can result from free radical damage that seems to be only exogenous in origin.

Excess numbers of endogenous or exogenous free radicals in the body can alter metabolism and membranes as well as other tissues, because the loss of electrons changes the chemical properties of molecules. Free radicals can:

- be attracted to cell membranes where they can bind and alter cell function.
- puncture the cell membrane, allowing bacteria and viruses to enter.
- destroy the protective cell membrane.
- cause the breakdown of fat in cell membranes, affecting cell function.
- cause the death of cells.
- cause the breakdown of DNA and mutations in DNA (which contains a person's genetic code).
- cause errors in protein synthesis, leading to changes in protein structure.
- eventually damage the immune system.
- bind to enzymes, inactivating them.
- lead to fluid retention in cells, which contributes to the aging process.
- upset calcium levels.
- exacerbate chemical sensitivity.

CHAPTER 21

Toxins of Mind and Spirit

IN THE PREVIOUS chapters we have discussed toxins that adversely affect the body, and to some extent the mind, as some toxins cause cerebral symptoms. However, there are toxins that can affect the spirit. In this chapter we will discuss the toxins that can harm the mind as well as the spirit, and the very special problems they can cause. Detoxification methods for the mind and spirit are discussed in chapter 33 and prevention methods may be found in Part VII.

Many people are sick because their spirit or the connection to their spirit has been damaged by a toxin. They may be unaware of this and attribute all of their problems, both physical and emotional, to a physical illness. They may indeed have a physical illness, but the root cause is deeper. Their inner nature has been affected and their spirit needs to be detoxified and healed. Their body will not recover good health unless cleansing and balancing of the spirit take place.

Emotional and psychological traumas are often suppressed and forgotten by the conscious mind. However, the spirit, the subconscious, and the cells remember, and their memory of a trauma can adversely affect the immune, nervous, and endocrine systems and thus the person's health.

The founder of modern medicine, Hippocrates, and the Greek philosopher, Aristotle, recognized the role of emotions in health and disease over 2,000 years ago. Over time, however, awareness and acknowledgment of their interconnectedness were lost. Dr. Blair Justice, author of *Who Gets Sick*, stated in 1987 that "Most of medicine continues to pretend that mind and body are separated and that pathways by which attitudes and moods physically affect our organs and tissues are really imaginary . . . and that simple physical explanations will be found to account for major disorders, as if mind and brain have no physical reality."

Popular books such as *Love, Medicine, and Miracles* by Dr. Bernie Siegel link health and well-being with how the mind pictures the body and how people feel about them-

What is Spirit?

Spirit is difficult to define. Some people view it as an extension of the mind. Others believe that it is the soul, while others call it the psyche. Regardless of how it is defined, spirit is the essence of our being. It is the innate quality that makes us who we are. Spirit should not be considered as separate from mind, or from body, because what affects the spirit will eventually affect the mind and body.

selves and their world. We are rediscovering the connection between mind and body.

Psychoneuroimmunology

Scientists of various disciplines have begun to discover new relationships between chemistry, physics, and human physiology. For example, Ilya Prigogine, winner of the Nobel Prize in 1977, demonstrated similarities between the behavior of the chemical reactions and the neurological organization of the brain.

In the early 1980s, the organized study of how the mind, central nervous system, hormonal system, and immune system interact began to develop. Psychoneuroimmunology was formed from the marriage of immunology, neurology, and psychology. Doctors slowly began to acknowledge that the body did not function as separate organs, but as a complete, interdependent whole.

The brain regulates all body functions, and dysregulation of the central nervous system is now known to be a contributing factor in disease. Mental states, thoughts, and moods can cause changes in brain chemistry and cells. When people lose a sense of control or feel helpless about their lives, chemical changes in the body occur. Emotions are not only experienced in the brain; they are also experienced in the body. Emotions affect the body physically just as physical illness affects the emotions. Researchers at the University of Rochester School of Medicine have found that 70 to 80 percent of patients who became ill had given up hope or felt helpless, and that the giving-up complex preceded the onset of symptoms.

People who view their condition as hopeless and themselves as victims seem to conserve oxygen. They develop a slow heart rate, lower blood pressure, and a decreased amount of hydrochloric acid secretion by the stomach. This is called conservation-withdrawal and was initially described by George L. Engel in the 1968 *Bulletin of the Meninger Clinic.*

Dr. Bernie Siegel, author of *Peace, Love, and Healing*, notes that physical illness may be the only control some people feel they have over life. Some illness seems to result when people feel they have no control. People may sometimes use their illness to manipulate others; they may become more ill than the person they view as having control over them. Dr. Stewart Wolf, author of *Mind, Brain, and Medicine*, states that "disease is a way of life" for some people and is their response to the problems of life.

The immune system responds adversely to stress and is unable to identify the source

Immune System Response

The recent research of Dr. George Solomon, of the University of California School of Medicine in Fresno, and Dr. Robert Ader of the University of Rochester School of Medicine in New York, has shown that there is communication and interaction between the brain and the immune system. In addition, the immune system responds to chemical signals from the central nervous system.

Dr. Ader and his colleagues injected mice that had a type of lupus (an autoim-

mune disease) with an immunosuppressive drug and saccharine. The immunosuppressive drug, cyclophosphamide, relieved the symptoms of lupus. Later they injected the mice with saccharine only. The immune system of the mice associated the saccharine with the drug and survived longer and had slower development of lupus than the control mice. The saccharine signaled the mice to suppress their immune system just as though cyclophosphamide were present.

of the stress whether it be an infection, an allergic reaction, or an emotional trauma. Continued stress depresses the function and efficiency of the immune system. People can develop a flight-or-fight reaction on an acute level, producing high levels of adrenalin (epinephrine), noradrenalin (norepinephrine), and cortisol; elevated blood sugar; and other biochemical changes. If chemicals produced by these changes occur inappropriately or chronically, the body suffers.

Disease can occur when our bodies inappropriately use these mechanisms that are meant to protect us. For example, the fight-or-flight response is electrical and biochemical, preparing the body to fight or to run away. Cortisol and serotonin levels, heart rate, and blood pressure go up. A 1992 study by Dr. Frank W. Putnam of the National Institute of Mental Health in Bethesda, Maryland showed that girls who have been sexually abused have higher than normal levels of cortisol for as long as two years after

the abuse. Parts of their fight-or-flight response were still active. Continued high levels of cortisol can depress immune system function.

Tissue Memory

Emotions and memories of past experiences, both good and bad, are stored in the cells of the body. Every cell has memory of what has happened to it. These memories can include symptoms of illness, physical injury, and emotional trauma. Often, the memories of traumatic events have been submerged or "stuffed" so that the person is not consciously aware of them.

Many things may trigger a release of memory from the cells. Bodywork, scents, sights, sounds, words, emotional episodes, or even the administration of an allergy extract may release a memory or trigger a flashback of an event. A person usually experiences body memories first, sensing the physical pain or discomfort felt during the event. Sights and sounds follow; emotions occur last. This can set up a chain reaction as cells release other stored memories and chemicals.

Some psychologists question the validity of emotional tissue memory, feeling that so-called recovered memories are subconscious efforts to resolve old hurts or illusions induced by mental illness or confusion, encouraged by current popular books and psychotherapists. While this may be true in some cases, many victims have been able to find evidence that confirms the reality of their memories. A relative or friend may know of the traumatic event, or physical evidence is found that corroborates the memory.

Stress

Stress has been widely blamed for making society sick today. More important than the stress however, is our response to it. The same external event is perceived differently by different people, and exposures to the stress will vary. High stress does not correlate with a high risk of illness. In *Who Gets Sick,* Dr. Justice discusses a number of studies on stress. In one, people who have a sense of control were found to keep their "stress chemicals" from reaching damaging levels when they were under pressure.

Researchers studied a group of executives experiencing significant stress as their company was broken into a smaller company. Half the group did not become ill. Those who stayed healthy viewed change differently and considered it an opportunity for growth and new experience. They had a sense of control over their future, and they

> **MOST EFFECTIVE DETOXIFICATION METHODS**
>
> **Stress**
>
> - Nutrients for stress, particularly B vitamins (chapter **23**)
> - Bodywork, particularly massage for relaxation (**25**)
> - Breathing exercises to reduce stress (**26**)
> - Sound therapy for calming (**32**)
> - Counseling to learn coping skills (**33**)
> - Neuro Emotional Technique (**33**)
> - Journaling (**33**)
> - Laugh and hug therapy (**33**)
> - Changing focus (**33**)
> - Attending to spirituality (**33**)

were optimistic. In this study, researchers found that people who had a sense of purpose and who believed in the importance and value of what they were doing had fewer symptoms of headaches, anxiety, and sleeping difficulties.

In other studies, people who coped poorly with stress had decreased immune responses because of the stress. People with depressed immune systems are most prone to negative health effects from anxiety, distress, anger, or depression. Acute stress can lower the number of white cells in the immune system, as well as the levels of interferon, a chemical that prevents viruses from reproducing.

Traumatic Events

Specific events can cause emotional trauma. When people undergo a traumatic event early in life, it significantly affects their character and life direction. While some people are able to cope and even increase their inner strength, many suffer long-term damage.

Examples of events that cause emotional trauma are extreme disappointment, loss of a job, separation or divorce, the death of a loved one, physical accidents, and mugging or rape.

Giving up a baby resulting from an unplanned pregnancy can cause deep emotional trauma that can affect a woman for the rest of her life. We have seen many patients in their forties and fifties whose health was suffering and for whom treatment measures were ineffective because of the emotional toxins they carried.

When they were able to find the child they had given up, feel reassured that the adoptive parents had nurtured the child, and understand they were not "bad" people, these women could heal from their emotional burden. They could then begin to heal their physical problems. Until this toxin of the mind and spirit was cleared, none of them had been able to make any progress in healing their physical bodies.

Many things can cause extreme disappointment regardless of a person's age. People may let someone down, betray a loved one or friend, participate in a questionable activity, or misrepresent themselves. Events such as the failure to obtain a goal, possession, or raise can be an extreme disappointment. The inability to establish a relationship, learn a skill, or successfully conclude a project can also be a disappointment.

The loss of a job for any reason can be a devastating blow to the ego for some people, resulting in the loss of self-confidence. People who are unable to find another job often

Bereavement

In Who Gets Sick, *Dr. Justice reported on several studies of recently widowed people. In 1977, it was found that widows and widowers had depressed immune function after the death of their spouses. The function of lymphocytes (a cell of the immune system) is depressed for at least six months after the death of a loved one. In one study, the death rate of recently bereaved widows was 3 to 12 times that of married women. In another study, the death rate was 40 percent higher in the first six months of bereavement for a group of widowers.*

lose even more self-confidence. A person who had a high-paying job may find it humiliating to take another job that pays less.

Separation or divorce can be stressful even if a person chooses to leave an unhappy relationship. Either event forces people to reexamine themselves, their values, life, and relationships. Divorced and widowed people may be alone and lonely, and the change in lifestyle, both emotional and financial, can be traumatic. Changes in social status and activities often result, and people may find themselves isolated and no longer as welcome in their usual social circles. The trauma is increased even more when people they considered friends desert them.

Physical injuries such as those suffered in a serious fall or skiing accident are traumatic and emotional events. The resulting inability or difficulty to perform day-to-day

Post-Traumatic Stress

In May of 2000 a fire in the forest around Los Alamos, New Mexico claimed over 48,000 acres and left 402 families homeless when their homes burned to the ground. The town of Los Alamos was evacuated, as was the suburb of White Rock. The residents of these towns became refugees in surrounding communities for five days, many not knowing whether their homes had survived the fire.

The people who lost their homes and all their possessions, except those they were able to carry with them when they were evacuated, are suffering from post-traumatic stress syndrome. Their symptoms are continuing, and they are having difficulty sleeping and coping. Many of them cry easily, have no appetite, feel ill when they force themselves to eat, and complain of feeling irritable all the time. Depression and grief are a common state for these people, as are feelings of being overwhelmed.

People who did not lose their homes are also having symptoms, but to a lesser degree. Many weep when they talk of the fire and their grief for their neighbors and for the town. Many of them startle and feel anxious when they hear helicopters and planes overhead. The sound of a fire siren sends feelings of fear and dread through everyone in the community.

activities can leave a person feeling helpless and out of control. Automobile accidents often affect people emotionally as well as physically. Long after their physical injuries have healed, some people feel anxious or fearful when they drive or ride in a car.

Mugging and rape are an ultimate violation of a person's body and spirit, evoking fear, terror, and a feeling of helplessness. Mugging or rape are traumatic events that can cause a person to develop post-traumatic stress disorder.

The experience of an event takes place over a period of time; it does not happen all at once. The process of experiencing an event can be blocked at an early stage and remain stored in the body (commonly the brain and muscles) for years. When a person experiences an overwhelming external threat, he or she can suspend emotional reaction, maintaining the interrupted experience in an unassimilated form as long as necessary. Until the event is fully experienced, however, it continues to exert effects.

Post-Traumatic Stress Syndrome

After people experience a psychologically distressing event that is outside the range of usual human experience, they often develop post-traumatic stress syndrome. Common traumas causing this syndrome include a serious threat to life—whether of self, children, spouse, or friends; the sudden destruction of one's home or community; or seeing

MOST EFFECTIVE DETOXIFICATION METHODS

Abuse

- Nutrients for stress, particularly B vitamins (chapter **23**)
- Homeopathic remedies such as *Aconite, Gelsemium, Medorrhinum, Plantina* (**28**)
- Bach Flower Remedies such as Rescue Remedy, and single remedies such as rock rose, mimulus, sweet chestnut (**28**)
- Aromatherapy essences that include basil, cypress, orange, sandalwood, and ylang ylang for anxiety (**29**)
- Color and gem therapy (**32**)
- Counseling (**33**)
- Neuro Emotional Technique and other hands-on emotional techniques (**33**)
- Journaling (**33**)
- Laugh and hug therapy (**33**)
- Attending to spirituality (**33**)
- Forgiveness (**33**)

another person seriously injured or killed in an accident or from physical violence. Traumas may involve rape, assault, airplane crashes, large fires, or bombing.

In addition to fear, terror, and helplessness, symptoms include re-experiencing the traumatic event, avoidance of stimuli associated with it, and increased adrenaline and other fight-or-flight hormones. The person may have recurrent and intrusive recollections or dreams of the event.

People will avoid reminders of the traumatic event. They may feel detached from others and uninterested in previously enjoyed activities. They have difficulty falling asleep or staying asleep, and show hypervig-

ilance and an exaggerated startle effect. To be considered post-traumatic stress syndrome, these disturbances must last at least one month.

Abuse

Abuse can be emotional, psychological, physical, or sexual. Abusive behavior is intended to control and subjugate another person through the use of fear, humiliation, and verbal or physical assault. Abuse occurs most often during childhood, but it is also inflicted on adults. People who have been abused during childhood often enter abusive relationships when they become adults because such a situation feels familiar to them.

■■ EMOTIONAL AND PSYCHOLOGICAL ABUSE

Emotional abuse includes neglect, verbal abuse, and psychological abuse. It can involve constant negative comments, continual or chronic scapegoating, terrorizing, berating, and rejection. Children can also suffer from lack of parental concern, which is a form of rejection. Emotional abuse is difficult to prove and, particularly in children, may only come to attention through concomitant physical abuse.

Adults and children in emotionally abusive relationships are criticized frequently. Their aggressor may yell, threaten, call them names, and throw temper tantrums. The aggressor will often threaten physical harm. If the victim becomes upset, the aggressor may become more threatening.

Emotional abuse can also be very subtle.

Neglect and indifference are a form of abuse that can harm both children and adults. Aggressors often deny that an incident happened and blame any abusive behavior on some reaction of the victim. Some abusers lead their victims to blame themselves for the problems and inadequacies of the abuser. The abuser presents himself or herself as the injured party and heaps guilt on the abused person until the victim may accept the blame. The victim then attempts to placate the abuser and to make up for the "terrible behavior" that so "injured" the abuser.

Abuse tends to make victims feel inadequate and helpless, and so "brainwashed" that they question the accuracy of their own memories and perspective. Self-confidence is seriously undermined. The victim often feels isolated, and many begin to doubt their grasp on reality.

■ PHYSICAL ABUSE

Physical abuse can range in severity from bruises, to knife and gun wounds, to death. It may occur more often when there is another crisis in the home, such as job loss.

Among children less than five years of age, about 10 percent of emergency visits in the Unided States are to treat injuries caused by abuse. Approximately one-third of the cases involve children less than six months old, while one-third are between six months and three years old and one-third are over three years of age. Premature, special needs infants, and stepchildren have been found to be at increased risk.

Babies can be injured or even killed by

Learned Behavior

People who batter their spouses often also abuse their children. Frequently the abusers are victims of childhood abuse themselves, and their battering is a learned behavior. In many cases, with proper treatment they can learn to control and direct their anger constructively.

shaking. In severe cases, a shaken baby may suffer coma, seizures, blindness, or permanent brain injury. Common injuries to older children include bruises, broken bones, burns, and organ damage. Abdominal injuries are the second most common cause of death in abused children. Depriving a child of food and water also constitutes physical abuse.

Children who are thought to be physically abused need to be removed from the situation immediately. Medical personnel in North America are obligated by law to report the incident to police or to a social agency. When children who have been abused are returned to their parents without intervention, 5 percent of the children are killed and 35 percent are seriously reinjured. In 65 to 75 percent of child abuse cases, the abuser is a relative, neighbor, or acquaintance.

Among adults, the man is the perpetrator in 95 percent of domestic assaults. More than 2 million women are assaulted by their male partners each year in the U.S. Even though the woman is the victim, most people expect her to end the violence, and leaving the home is usually her only option.

■■ SEXUAL ABUSE

It is estimated that one in three women and one in four to seven men have been victims of sexual abuse as children. Sexual exploitation of children is known as pedophilia; within the family it is also called incest.

Adult forms of sexual abuse include date and stranger rape. Date rape occurs when a person is forced to have sex on a date. Adult sexual abuse also includes forced sexual acts within a relationship or marriage, with or without violence or physical threats, and without the partner's willing participation or consent.

The sexual abuse of children can take many forms, from exhibitionism to taking obscene or pornographic photographs, to actual sexual penetration. Sexual abuse has been documented in children from 2 months to 18 years old. Physical trauma is seen in one-third of the children and the earlier the abuse, the more psychologically damaging it is. Authorities on sexual abuse estimate that about half the survivors suffer from some type of memory loss. Some develop multiple personalities. Sexual abuse can lead to depression, anxiety, low self-esteem, self-abusive behavior, social problems, sexual problems, and food, chemical, or sexual addictions.

Children and adults who have been sexually abused may develop sexually transmitted diseases, including AIDS. Girls, some of them very young teenagers, can become pregnant. Women who were sexually abused as children tend to suffer from anxiety, depression, suicidal tendencies, mistrust of men, and destructive behavior such as substance abuse, promiscuity, and out-of-wedlock pregnancy.

Suppressed Memory

The traumatic memories that our bodies submerge and store affect us even when we are not conscious of them. As a teenager, one young woman was date raped, became pregnant, and gave up her baby for adoption. Her parents treated her very badly and the whole incident was so devastating to her that she had no conscious memory of it until she was in her early thirties, was married, and had another baby.

While the returning memory was painful to her, she was able to recall the circumstances and to deal with the memories and emotions. She found her child, who was then a teenager, and came to terms with the past. She was then able to heal physical problems that included fatigue and multiple allergies after she cleansed the emotional toxins.

Crises of Spirituality and Faith

Spirituality is the special quality that relates to a person's inner being or soul and includes the concept of guidance from or a relationship with a higher being. It may also include the ability to connect with a higher energy or a higher power. Spirituality can give people their principles, and moral and ethical codes. It gives depth of character, integrity, honor, courage, and motivation.

Faith is the quality that allows us to believe in something we cannot prove by logic.

Whatever spiritual beliefs we may favor, this aspect of our lives must be nurtured and balanced to achieve full happiness and health. When faith has been shaken or lost, people experience grief and sometimes anger. Because it eventually affects health and can injure the body, the loss of spirituality and faith can be considered a toxin.

Many life experiences can damage our faith and connection to our spiritual nature, including traumatic events and physical, emotional, and sexual abuse. The connection to spirit can be damaged from the mistreatment by others, resulting in feelings of low self-worth. Harsh words of conflict and confrontation can make a person feel that the soul has been seared and scarred. Misfortunes, losses, illnesses, deaths, or wars can cause people to feel that they have been deserted by their god, or higher being. Failures can lead to the loss of hope, courage, the innate joy of living, and faith.

Cumulative Life Experiences

We are at this moment what we have been becoming since the day of our birth. Each of us is unique and special because the experiences and exposures in each of our lives have been different. Our personalities and perspectives have been shaped from the things to which we have been exposed.

Everything that we have encountered in life has left its mark on our personality, mind, and body. If we had a traumatic childhood, a stormy adolescence, or a disappointing marriage, these things are reflected in

MOST EFFECTIVE DETOXIFICATION METHODS

Crisis of Spirituality and Faith

- Guided meditation (chapter **26**)
- Sound therapy with inspirational music (**32**)
- Counseling by spiritual leaders (**33**)
- Neuro Emotional Technique (**33**)
- Journaling (**33**)
- Prayer and meditation (**33**)
- Forgiveness (**33**)

our psyche. If we had no stimulation as a child, few challenges as an adolescent, or are buried in a dead-end job as an adult, these things affect our mental state. If we had numerous illnesses as a child, a poor diet as an adolescent, or food or drug addiction as an adult, these things are reflected in our bodies and general health.

All our negative life experiences, when totaled like the sum in an addition problem, can have the effect of a toxin. This cumulative toxin will be different for each person. In a life that has contained much trauma, the toxic effects may be large and powerful if a person has not been able to continually detoxify the emotional burden. In a life that has been relatively healthy and happy, the toxic effects should be much smaller. However, if a person copes with the few stressful experiences poorly, the toxic effect can still be damaging.

Regardless of the size of the toxin from

our cumulative life experiences, it must be cleansed. By cleansing and balancing each of the areas necessary for good health, the negative effects of our experiences will be removed, one by one.

As is evident from the discussion in this chapter, we are truly complex organisms.

The internal relationships between mind, body, and spirit that make us sick can be used to help us heal. Any toxins of the mind and spirit must be cleansed and balanced, just as for other toxic exposures, in order to achieve full health.

PART VI

Ways of Detoxification

In THIS SECTION, we will discuss contemporary ways of detoxification. Each of the many treatments presented addresses a specific health and detoxification need. People with multiple or severe health challenges may need to use several detoxification methods. Others, with minor problems, may need to use only one or two.

After reading to this point, you may have accurately identified most, if not all of your detoxification needs and problems. It is best to have a healthcare professional help you with your detoxification needs and program. Their expertise in helping diagnose your main problem areas can save you valuable time and effort. They may recognize connections or symptoms that you have overlooked. In addition, if your problems are multiple or severe, it is imperative for your health that you have professional guidance.

This section will help you identify which detoxification methods are best for you and understand how they work and how to use them. Part VIII details programs for basic detoxification, as well as for specific health conditions and exposures.

As you begin to detoxify you may initially feel worse. This is a small price to pay, however, because if you do not detoxify your health will not improve. You must rid your body of its toxic burden in order to heal.

Also consider that you must take care of all aspects of your health—physical, mental, emotional, and spiritual—to enjoy the benefits of full health. By utilizing appropriate detoxification treatments and making necessary lifestyle changes, you can achieve vitality, mental clarity, improved body functioning, and the expectation of a longer, healthier life.

CHAPTER 22

Saunas, Baths, and Hydrotherapy

ONE OF THE MOST basic steps of detoxification is promoting heat in the body to release lipophilic (fat-soluble) toxins from the fat cells of the body. This is known as heat depuration, which means to remove a toxic contaminant or to purify with heat. When heat frees toxins from the fat cells where they are stored, they move to the bloodstream where they are flushed out of the body in perspiration, urine, bile, and other body fluids.

This chapter presents several methods of accomplishing this. Not all methods will be available or appropriate for all people. For some of them medical supervision is essential; others can be done on your own at home. The heavier your total toxic burden is, the more imperative it is to have medical supervision for your detoxification program. Detoxification must take place slowly enough that the detoxification mechanisms of the body can handle the increased load, so that you do not sustain organ damage (see Part II, The Body).

Saunas

The use of a sauna is a major part of most detoxification programs because the "heat stress" of a sauna is very effective in releasing toxins from fat cells. Developed in Finland centuries ago, saunas are now used worldwide and are common in health clubs and gyms.

A sauna is a relatively airtight room with wooden platforms and benches. The air is kept fresh by a special ventilation system that preheats outside air before it enters the sauna. For good ventilation, the air should be exchanged six times an hour.

Saunas may be either dry or wet. For a dry sauna, no moisture is added to the sauna room. Electricity is used to generate infrared heat. Dry saunas stimulate a therapeutic sweat that helps flush out toxins and heavy metals. They also stimulate vasodilation of peripheral blood vessels and increase cardiovascular activity, which helps the body rid itself of more toxins. Saunas speed up all metabolism in the body and inhibit the repli-

Caution for Pregnant Women

Pregnant women should not use saunas. The heat may cause neural tube defects in the fetus during the first trimester of pregnancy. Since many women do not know they are pregnant during this time, women of childbearing age should have a pregnancy test before beginning a sauna program. People with heart disease, multiple sclerosis, adrenal exhaustion, lupus, kidney disease, and anemia should also avoid saunas.

cation of pathogenic organisms, such as bacteria and viruses. The immune response is also strengthened because the number of leukocytes (a type of white blood cell) in the blood is increased.

Steam is used in wet saunas. A steam generator or water poured over heated rocks may be used to provide steam. In steam saunas, the humidity is controlled to maintain 50 to 60 grams of water vapor per kilogram of air. The steam raises the body temperature quickly, and is beneficial for arthritic pain and upper respiratory conditions, and humid heat helps the skin.

In modern saunas, the walls and floor are often made of tile and concrete rather than wood. Cleaning is easier, which is important in saunas that are used exclusively for detoxification regimens. The benches and platforms are best made of poplar wood to keep outgasing of terpenes from the wood at a minimum. In saunas where chemically sensitive people are not using the sauna and outgasing is not a consideration, benches

may be made of cedar, which adds an aroma from its terpenes. (See chapter 15, Plants and Organisms, for a discussion of terpenes.)

Sauna facilities may have cooling-off rooms in addition to shower rooms. Some sauna programs involve a gentle cooling-off, whereas others use cold showers, a dip in the lake (even through a hole in the ice), or a roll in the snow. If there are known health problems, cooling off naturally or with a tepid shower is safer.

▮▮ EARLY SAUNA DETOXIFICATION PROGRAMS

The use of saunas for detoxification has been thoroughly investigated. In the 1960s, scientists from the U.S. Environmental Protection Agency (EPA) began to research the effects of recreational drugs, including alcohol, on the body, as well as researching methods that would help people cleanse the harmful effects of drugs. In 1977, a sauna program called "The Sweat Program" was introduced. The program took months to complete.

People in the program began to report the excretion of substances in their sweat that smelled or tasted like medications, recreational drugs, anesthetics, diet pills, food preservatives, and pesticides. They also reported sensations of old sunburns, past illnesses, and physical and emotional conditions from the past.

By 1979, scientists had developed the "Purification Program." This long-term detoxification program was designed to assist in releasing and flushing accumulated toxins from the tissues as well as rebuilding impaired tissues and cells. It is a precise program of exercise; sauna; adequate fluid intake and replacement; a regimented schedule; specific vitamins, minerals, and oils; and a diet with appropriate, lightly cooked fresh vegetables. The sauna, vitamins, and minerals must be taken at the same time each day and adequate sleep is essential while a person is on the program.

Niacin, or vitamin B_3, was an important cornerstone of the program because it appears to help release toxins from the tissues. Niacin also stimulates the cardiovascular system and causes vasodilation of skin capillaries. This causes the skin to flush, especially in areas of old sunburn. This hot flush, accompanied by prickly, itchy skin, can last up to one hour. It is not an allergic reaction. When people continue to take niacin, the flush disappears at a given dose, then returns with less intensity at a graduated higher dose.

Niacin dosing is very important, and only the short-acting form is used. Most people start with 100 milligrams (mg) a day of niacin, taken in one dose, with food. When there is minimal flushing and other symptoms have disappeared or diminished, the niacin dosage is increased. *Caution:* See the discussion on niacin under Nutritional Therapy in chapter 23.

Because toxins and drugs can cause deficiencies of nutrients, the scientists recommended other nutrients in addition to niacin. Drug and chemical residues persist in the body for a long time, and they continue to deplete nutrients while stored. In addition to niacin, the Purification Program included vitamin B complex; additional vitamin B_I; vitamins A, C, and D; and mineral sup-

> ## Sauna Facilities
>
> *Sauna detoxification programs are very effective for reducing the body burden of chemicals and toxins resulting from industrial accumulation or overwhelming exposures. Even if you are unable to go to a specialized detoxification facility, it is still possible for you to detoxify with the help of a local healthcare practitioner.*
>
> *Many physical therapy and bodywork facilities have saunas, and some health clubs have saunas that are clean enough to use. While detoxification will not be as rapid, over a period of time you will detoxify and heal.*

plementation. Calcium, magnesium, iron, zinc, manganese, copper, potassium, and iodine were to replace those minerals lost by sweating.

This program has been incorporated into many detoxification programs offered today. It represented a breakthrough in treatment, as it demonstrated that toxins can be eliminated rather than stored in the body indefinitely.

■■ CURRENT SAUNA DETOXIFICATION PROGRAMS

In North America today, there are several sauna detoxification facilities, which use a regimen of exercise, sauna, shower, and massage or physical therapy. (See Recommended Sources and Organizations for a listing of detoxification facilities in North America.) These facilities are built of environmentally safe materials and they specialize in treating environmentally ill patients rather than patients detoxifying from recreational drugs. The programs have added to the list of nutritional supplements used, as well as employing other aids to detoxification.

The specific nutrients, vitamins, and minerals that are needed for detoxification are discussed more fully in chapter 5, Phases of Detoxification, and chapter 23, Nutrients. The following are some of the additional substances used to aid the elimination process.

• *Sodium potassium bicarbonate:* Helps eliminate toxins in the urine as well as balancing electrolytes.

• *Chlorella:* A single-celled algae that helps eliminate toxins in the feces by binding to toxic metals. It also aids in removing toxic chemicals, enhances immune function, and has antibacterial and antiviral properties.

• *Psyllium seed:* A bulking agent that helps eliminate toxins by binding them in the feces so they are not absorbed back into the bloodstream.

• *Activated charcoal:* Helps eliminate toxins and xenobiotics in the feces and adsorbs many times its weight in toxins.

Two of the first special sauna detoxification units in North America are located in Texas and South Carolina. Dr. William Rea of Dallas, Texas has treated over 2,000 environmentally sensitive patients since the late 1980s. His detoxification unit was the first environmentally safe unit constructed in the U.S. Dr. Rea has helped to develop many of the current methods used in sauna detoxification programs.

Dr. Allan Lieberman of North Charleston, South Carolina also uses a similar sauna program in his detoxification unit. He reported in 1993 that of 80 environmentally ill or acutely chemically sensitive patients who underwent sauna detoxification at his Center for Environmental Medicine:

• 71 percent reported improvement in chemical sensitivity.

• 21 percent reported no change in chemical sensitivity.

• 8 percent reported that chemical sensitivities became worse.

■■ YOUR SAUNA CLEANSING PROGRAM

When using a sauna in a detoxification program, a healthcare professional should guide you. It is imperative that people with a high toxic burden be supervised as they detoxify. The speed of detoxification must not exceed the capabilities of the body's detoxification mechanisms, or it can cause organ damage.

If possible, use a dry sauna that has been constructed to be environmentally safe, with air cleaners attached to the air circulation units. Commercial saunas at health clubs tend to be too hot, have inadequate levels of oxygen, and may be constructed of materials that will outgas chemicals that chemically sensitive people cannot tolerate. However, sometimes it is better to use a sauna that is not perfect than not to undergo detoxification.

One- or two-person dry saunas construc-

Heat and Wound Caution

Should you develop clammy skin, extreme tiredness, weakness, headache, dizziness, cramps, nausea, or vomiting, get out of the sauna and take a cool shower. These are symptoms of heat exhaustion. Should you suddenly stop sweating and your skin becomes hot and dry, get into a lukewarm shower and gradually decrease the temperature. These are the first symptoms of heat stroke.

Do not use a sauna if you have an open cut. Allow it to heal first, as heat therapy will temporarily increase inflammation in the area and delay healing.

ted of wood are available for home use. Infrared units provide the heat source for these saunas. Poplar is the best choice of wood for sensitive people, as it outgases fewer terpenes. Portable saunas, sometimes called cabinet baths, are also available for home use. They are available in both wet and dry models. These saunas allow the head to remain cool and the user to breathe the cleaner outside air. Take care when selecting a portable sauna because plastic parts can outgas.

Dry saunas are recommended because they increase sweating and so speed detoxification. A complete sauna cleansing program should include exercise, time in a dry sauna, and a cleansing shower followed by a massage or physical therapy. Both the exercise and sauna time should be built up gradually so that stress to the body is minimized. The bodywork breaks down chemical storage, mobilizes toxins, and helps break down toxic chemicals through increased metabolism.

Some people experience increased excretion of toxins if they exfoliate the skin. The skin is in contact with pollution, ultraviolet radiation, and dirt. These substances combine with the oils, salts, and toxins that the skin excretes daily, as well as dead skin cells that are being shed. Exfoliation, which involves gently rubbing off the old layers, is accomplished with the aid of a loofa sponge, sisal mitt, or brushes. Exfoliation helps speed the detoxification process by increasing circulation, opening pores, and invigorating the skin. If you use exfoliation, take a shower before beginning your exercise session.

Begin your detoxification session with 20 minutes of exercise. You may have to gradually build up your exercise time if you have previously been sedentary. Light cardiovascular exercise, such as a stationary bike or walking on a treadmill as tolerated, is helpful as is rebounding (jumping on a trampoline) for 3 to 5 minutes a day. Rebounding stimulates lymph flow, which helps remove toxins. Drink at least two 8-ounce glasses of water during your exercise period.

Go into the sauna when you finish exercising. If you are fairly healthy, and heat tolerant, begin your sauna time with 10 minutes. If you are heat intolerant or have multiple chemical sensitivities or a chronic illness, begin with 5 minutes and increase by

Detox Schedule

Some people detoxify in cycles, and detoxification sauna or bath programs may have to be repeated. Sometimes months may pass between episodes.

5 minutes daily. The maximum sauna time should be 30 to 45 minutes to allow for ample sweating and the accompanying release of toxins. The temperature should be kept between 140° and 150°F for environmentally ill people and people with a heavy load of toxins.

While sweating in the sauna, be sure to replace the fluids lost, with a minimum of 8 ounces of water for every 15 minutes you are in the sauna. Continue to drink extra water afterward, as it will help your kidneys flush toxins.

A cleansing shower after your sauna washes off the toxins excreted in the sauna and prevents them from being reabsorbed. Be sure to wash your hair also. It is important to pay attention to body odor during a detoxification program. Toxins that are excreted in the sweat can cause other people in the sauna or exercise room to react. Immediately remove and launder towels used in the sauna or after the shower in hot water; they will be impregnated with excreted toxins.

After the shower, have massage or another type of bodywork to relax the muscles and increase blood circulation, which aids in cleansing. Manual lymph drainage or deep tissue massage particularly helps to mobilize toxins. (See chapter 25, Exercise and Bodywork, for further information.) After completing a sauna program session, allow a period of rest. The body needs a quiet time to adjust and rebalance.

Nutritional supplements aid in sauna cleansing, particularly antioxidants. Oils taken orally help to bind toxins as the liver and bile remove them from the body. The help of a healthcare practitioner is invaluable in helping to determine the proper balance of supplements. However, if a healthcare practitioner is not available to help you, take the following supplements each day:

- *Niacin:* begin with 100 mg a day and increase by 100 mg each day, building up to at least 1,000 mg. Use only the short-acting form of niacin.
- *Vitamin B complex:* 2 capsules, each containing 50 mg of most of the B vitamins
- *Vitamin B_1:* 250 to 500 mg over the amount in the vitamin B complex
- *Vitamin A:* 5,000 IU
- *Vitamin C:* take at least 1,000 mg, increasing gradually to bowel tolerance
- *Vitamin D:* 400 IU
- *Vitamin E:* 400 IU
- *Multimineral supplement:* 1 to 2 capsules
- *Calcium:* 1,000 mg
- *Magnesium:* 500 to 1,000 mg

See also the nutrients listed in chapter 5 for the phases of detoxification, in addition to those listed under Current Sauna Detoxification Programs, above. Take the dose recommended on the product you purchase.

If you are able to have a healthcare professional supervise your detoxification program and your schedule will allow it, sauna daily for 6 to 8 weeks. You will then need to follow a maintenance program of a sauna once or twice a week in order to prevent new bioaccumulation of toxins. If you have no professional supervision for your detoxification program, sauna no more than three times a week.

Some people experience skin reactions during their detoxification program. These may vary from burning and itching to eczema, small abscesses, and urticaria (hives). They may also suffer headaches, fatigue, mental confusion, nausea, insomnia, irritable bowel, and anxiety and panic attacks caused by released xenobiotics (foreign chemicals). Many people report symptoms like those experienced with the original exposure to the xenobiotic. These detoxification reactions can usually be treated successfully with buffered vitamin C. (See chapter 23, Nutrients, for specific directions.) While uncomfortable, these reactions are an indication that you are making progress.

Detoxification Baths

Most people who do not have access to a sauna have a bathtub and can take detoxification baths—sometimes called the "poor man's sauna." Baths are especially useful for people with a toxic bioaccumulation of xenobiotics. The hot water increases blood flow and capillary action near the surface of the skin, causing faster release of toxins. The heat also increases sweating and opens pores, allowing toxin-containing perspiration to be excreted more readily. Although using filtered water or safe well water is preferable for these baths, city water, even if it contains chlorine, is still effective and helpful.

Approach these baths with caution and common sense. It is preferable to have a

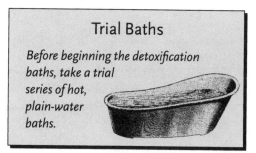

Trial Baths

Before beginning the detoxification baths, take a trial series of hot, plain-water baths.

healthcare professional supervise your detoxification program. If your chemical load is high, baths can make you feel very ill. Have someone in the house with you when you take your detoxification bath in case you develop symptoms and require assistance. Should you experience dizziness, headache, exhaustion, fatigue, nausea, or weakness, stop your bath.

Clean your bathtub with tolerated cleaning products. It should be spotlessly clean for a detoxification bath; you are trying to rid your body of toxins, not absorb more.

Follow these general instructions for both the plain-water baths and the detox baths:

• Wash your body thoroughly with tolerated soap in the shower before you take your bath and scrub with a loofa sponge, sisal mitt, skin brush, or rough washcloth to remove excess body oils, dead skin, and any accumulated toxins. Rinse thoroughly.

• Fill the tub with water as hot as you can tolerate without burning your skin. Cover the tub's overflow valve so the water level will be high enough to immerse your body up to your neck.

• Begin with a 5-minute soak in hot water. *Do not exceed 5 minutes for your first bath.* Gradually increase the time by 5-minute incre-

Take It Slowly

Should you experience immediate intolerable symptoms, drain the bath. Sit in the tub until you feel you can safely stand and get out. If you attempt to get out of the tub while you feel weak, you might fall.

ments until you can soak for 30 minutes without experiencing symptoms. You may feel deceptively well while soaking, but it is extremely important that you do not overstay your time limit. Symptoms sometimes do not occur until the next day.

- Gently massage your muscles with a skin brush while soaking to increase circulation to the skin.
- After soaking, take a cleansing shower. Scrub thoroughly with tolerated soap and rinse well in order to remove any toxins deposited on your skin during the bath. Be sure to also wash your hair. Your body will reabsorb any unremoved toxins. If you continue to perspire, or begin perspiring again, repeat the shower.
- Take your tolerated dose of vitamin C before and after each bath (see chapter 23, Nutrients). This will help your body remove the toxins released into your bloodstream. If you are taking antioxidant nutritional supplements, take them before your bath.
- Drink an 8-ounce glass of water before, during, and after your bath.

Take detox baths three times a week until your general health has improved. Then, use the baths once or twice a week to prevent the accumulation of toxins. If you have unusual chemical exposures, increase the frequency and duration of your baths. This should be done only under the supervision of a health-care professional.

▮▮ TYPES OF DETOXIFICATION BATHS

When you can take a plain hot-water bath for 30 minutes with no symptoms, you may begin detoxification baths. Various substances may be added to the bath to aid in detoxification. Follow the general bath instructions above, adding one of the substances listed below to the bath water. Except for Epsom salts, you may need to rotate the other substances, as their effectiveness may subside quickly if some time is not allowed between their use.

▮ EPSOM SALTS

Epsom salts help eliminate toxins by activating fluid movement in the tissues and increasing perspiration. The salts work as a counter-irritant on the skin to increase blood supply, and also change the pH of the skin surface. In addition, the sulfur component of Epsom salts aids in detoxifying. Sulfur springs have always been recognized for their medicinal and cleansing properties.

Begin with 1/4 cup of Epsom salts. Gradually increase the amount with each bath until you are using 4 cups per tub. Should you experience symptoms at any level, stay at that level until you can soak for 30 minutes with no symptoms.

▮ APPLE CIDER VINEGAR

Vinegar also works as a counter-irritant, increasing blood supply to the skin and changing the skin's pH. Begin with 1/4 cup of apple cider. Gradually increase the amount to 1 cup per tub. Be certain you use only apple cider vinegar, as white vinegar is a chemical product.

■ CLOROX

Use the Clorox brand of liquid bleach only, adding 2 tablespoons to a full bath. Chlorine-sensitive people cannot use Clorox. The oxidizing properties of Clorox aid with detoxification.

■ HYDROGEN PEROXIDE

Use up to 8 ounces of food-grade 35% hydrogen peroxide in a bathtub half-full of warm water. (Hot water causes the hydrogen peroxide to deteriorate too rapidly.) Be aware that this bath taken at bedtime may cause you difficulty getting to sleep. The increase of oxygen at cellular levels can increase the sense of alertness.

■ BAKING SODA

Baking soda, or sodium bicarbonate, creates an alkalinizing bath to restore acid/alkaline balance through osmosis. Use 8 ounces of baking soda to a full bath. These baths are particularly good for cleansing and drying weeping, open sores, and relieving skin irritation and itching. (See Medicated Soaks in chapter 30, Topical Detoxification, for further information.)

■ SODA AND SEA SALT

Soda baths with sea salt are effective for detoxifying X-ray and radiation exposure. Use equal amounts of baking soda and non-iodized sea salt, building up to 1 pound of each.

■ CLAY

Clay is most frequently used in compresses or packs. However, the drawing and alkalizing action of clay baths is also helpful in

Detoxification Showers

Some people are not able to participate in a sauna program, nor do they have a bathtub in which to detoxify. While it is a little more difficult to do and takes longer, people can detoxify by sitting in a very hot shower. You will have to purchase some type of bath stool if your shower stall does not have a bench.

Follow the general directions for hot water baths. In the shower you will not, of course, be able to add any compounds that aid in detoxification. However, you can rid your body of toxins by using a hot water shower to make yourself sweat. Be certain to take a cooler shower and wash your hair afterward to remove toxins.

detoxification baths. Use 1/2 cup of clay to a full bath. Several types of clay are available from health food stores, all appropriate for bathing.

■ GINGER ROOT

Ginger's heating property causes sweating and improves circulation. It also stimulates and draws toxins to the skin surface. Cut a thumb-size piece of ginger root into small pieces, place in a pot of water on the stove, and bring to a boil. Turn off the heat and let steep for 30 minutes. Strain and pour the liquid into a full bath.

■ BURDOCK ROOT

Burdock root baths help the body to excrete uric acid. They also aid in cleansing boils

Preparation for Heat Detoxification

When doing detoxification in a sauna or with baths or showers, it is important to prepare your body ahead of time. Eat a clean diet, with organic foods if they are available to you. Foods high in sulfur, such as garlic, onions, beans, broccoli, cabbage, and eggs, will aid Phase II detoxification in the liver. Fruit and vegetable juicing will also help support your detoxification. (See chapter 24 for further information on diet and juicing.)

Eat very lightly at least one hour prior to having a sauna or bath, to prevent your becoming nauseated. Never sauna or bathe on an empty stomach. Wait at least one hour after a sauna or bath before eating, as digestion will be sluggish following the treatment.

It's important to drink plenty of water to help flush toxins even on days you are not using the sauna or bath. Drink at least eight 8-ounce glasses of pure, tolerated water a day.

Be sure to get adequate rest and sleep during your detoxification program. Mental imagery, relaxation, and breathing exercises will also help your detoxification. (See chapter 26 for breathing exercises.)

and clearing rashes. Simmer a level handful of burdock root in 2 quarts of water for 30 minutes. Strain and pour the liquid into a full bath. Herbal shops and health food stores carry burdock.

▮ OATSTRAW

Oatstraw baths improve skin metabolism, which helps the body to detoxify more quickly. Simmer a heaping handful of oatstraw in 2 quarts of water for 25 minutes. Strain and pour the liquid into a full bath. Oatstraw is available at health food stores and herbal shops.

▮ HERBAL TEA

A number of herbal teas may be used in detoxification baths to aid in eliminating chemicals: catnip, yarrow, peppermint, boneset, blessed thistle, pleurisy root, chamomile, blue vervain, and horsetail. Most of these teas are diaphoretic and promote sweating. Use 1 cup of brewed tea per tub of hot, clean water. Use only *one* of these teas per bath. Sensitive individuals may not tolerate the use of some of these herbs.

Hydrotherapy

Hydrotherapy is the use of water, steam, or ice, and hot and cold temperatures to maintain or restore health. Although the therapeutic use of water dates back to at least the beginning of civilization, Priessnitz, a Silesian peasant and healer, founded hydrotherapy as a science in the early 1800s. He used sprays (strong jets of water directed to a given area), cold purges, sweat baths, wet compresses, and other treatments that are still given today. Many hydrotherapy techniques help with detoxification.

Hydrotherapy makes use of the body's response to heat and cold, utilizing hot water, cold water, or contrast therapy that alternates between the two. The duration and temperature of hydrotherapy application must be adjusted to the individual.

The primary reaction of the body to heat is relaxation, and its secondary reaction is depression, sedation, and atony (lack of muscle tone). The secondary heat effect causes a rapid pulse, decreased perspiration, mental tiredness, drowsiness, and muscular weakness. Heat stimulates the immune system and causes the white blood cells to migrate from the blood vessels into the tissues, cleaning up toxins, including bacteria and viruses, and eliminating waste. It soothes and relaxes the body, and through reflex action affects every organ and system of the body.

The primary reaction of the body to cold is stimulation, and its secondary reaction is invigorating, restorative, and tonic (improves muscle tone). This secondary cold effect causes smooth, soft skin, a sensation of warmth, slowed pulse, easy respirations, warmth of skin, and perspiration. Cold reduces inflammation by vasoconstriction, also reducing inflammatory agents by making the blood vessels less permeable. It tones muscle weakness, and long cold treatments will reduce fever.

Contrast therapy (the alternating of heat and cold) stimulates the adrenals and endocrine system. It reduces congestion, alleviates inflammation, and activates organ function. Contrast therapy is particularly good for improving circulation in the digestive organs and pelvis, and the detoxification capacity of the liver. Hot footbaths with ice on the back of the neck can help to relieve a tension headache.

Hydrotherapy increases the circulation

Hydrotherapy Cautions

Many hydrotherapy techniques can be safely done at home, keeping in mind a few cautions. The young and the old have poor heat regulation, and cannot tolerate severe temperature extremes. Prolonged illness, fatigue, or anemia also reduces a person's tolerance of temperature extremes. Pressure, friction, hot drinks, and exercise can enhance reactions, but the prolonged application of heat or cold can cause tissue damage and block the natural reaction.

of the blood and lymph, cleans the skin, and removes impurities. It can be used to relieve pain, lower fever, decrease cramps, induce sleep, soothe the nervous system, act as a stimulant, increase physical and mental tone, and serve as a local anesthetic. It will also increase urine production and cause bowel evacuation, both of which aid in detoxification.

Hydrotherapy methods should be selected with care, and when possible with the help of a healthcare practitioner, particularly for people with severe problems.

■■ TYPES OF HYDROTHERAPY

Hydrotherapy can include steam baths, saunas, full body immersion, baths, neutral baths, compresses, packs, wet sheet packs, sprays, showers, and colonic irrigation (see Colon in chapter 31, Organ Cleansing). Some of these treatments can be done at home, while others require the help of a trained practitioner. Naturopaths are quite skilled in the use of hydrotherapy.

■ BATHS AND SHOWERS

Baths, including sitz, full-immersion, local, and sweating baths are used. Except for the sweating bath, these baths may be hot, cold, or alternating hot and cold. The sweating bath and hot shower facilitate detoxification and were described earlier in this chapter.

Sweat baths, vapor baths, and steam inhalations clear mucous membrane congestion. Cold baths and showers can reduce inflammation, tone muscles, and reduce fatigue. Alternating hot and cold showers increase circulation and stimulate organ function. They should always begin with hot water and end with cold.

Sometimes neutral baths are used. These are full-immersion baths, with the water temperature from 92°F to 98°F. They are soothing to the nervous system and are effective for treating mental and emotional disturbances, as well as insomnia. According to Dr. Leon Chaitow of London, England, two hours in a neutral bath reduces excessive fluid retention. They also help promote detoxification from drugs and alcohol abuse by helping the body rid itself of toxin-laden fluids.

■ COMPRESSES AND PACKS

Compresses and packs may be hot, cold, or alternating hot and cold. Compresses are usually applied with pressure. Both compresses and packs help to stimulate the immune system and increase the white blood cell count. They are frequently used to treat infections and bruises.

Hot compresses can be applied for 30 minutes or more and changed when they cool off. Cold compresses are usually applied as a cold cloth wrung from ice water. They are refreshed as they warm up. They force blood away from an area when they follow a heat treatment given to stimulate blood flow. (See chapter 30, Topical Detoxification, for further information on compresses.)

Ice packs are a very cold application using ice or gel packs. They help to reduce swelling, inflammation, pain, and congestion. They should be applied to the affected part for 20 minutes out of every hour for the first 24 hours.

Hot packs warm a local area to relieve muscle spasms and pain, and encourage blood flow. Towels soaked in hot water from the tap can be used. The temperature should be around 120°F.

If the temperature of either hot or cold packs is uncomfortable, layers of dry toweling can be used between the pack and the skin.

Full-body wet sheet packs are used cold, but blankets are placed on top to make the patient sweat. The patient stays in the wet sheet until profuse sweating has occurred. This may require several hours, and will occur more rapidly if the patient has exercised or had a hot shower or bath beforehand. Sweating aids cleansing through the skin and is useful in detoxifying environmental toxins, alcohol, and drugs. A warm shower following the sweating period will remove any toxins that are excreted. This technique is best used under the direction of a qualified practitioner.

■ SPRAYS

Sprays are strong jets of water directed at a local or general area; showers are a type of spray. Sprays may be hot, cold, or alternating hot and cold.

Cold sprays to the breastbone or upper legs stimulate the kidneys. Cold sprays or alternating hot and cold sprays on the abdomen stimulate the liver, which will speed detoxification.

CHAPTER 23

Nutrients

VITAMINS AND MINERALS, obtained from the diet or nutritional supplements, are required in the chemical reactions of the detoxification process. Detoxification of xenobiotics (foreign chemicals) requires large amounts of energy, and this energy and the required nutrients usually come from the food we eat. However, if our diets do not contain sufficient nutrients, the concentration of Phase I and Phase II enzymes, amino acids, and peptides is decreased. With lowered enzyme concentrations, the metabolism of xenobiotics decreases. (The nutrients necessary for Phase I and Phase II detoxification are outlined in chapter 5, Phases of Detoxification.)

The body detoxifies naturally every day, and ideally, a wholesome, balanced diet of quality food would supply the needed nutrients. However, many people have such a poor-quality diet or such a restricted diet that their body does not have access to the vitamins and minerals required by the detoxification pathways. Many people eat processed foods in which vitamins and minerals are ei-

ther removed or destroyed during the processing procedures. Some manufacturers attempt to add them back, and while this can help, their levels, balance, and quality are never what they were in the original food.

Even a superior diet may not supply the necessary vitamins and minerals. Many of the foods we purchase at the supermarket are of poor quality. Crops are often raised on soil deficient in nutrients, picked green and artificially ripened, transported long distances, and stored for varying lengths of time. Their vitamin and mineral content can be quite low. Without nutrient supplementation to compensate for the deficits, detoxification will not take place at an adequate level.

In addition, vitamins and minerals are destroyed in the body by drugs, sugar, alcohol, tobacco, and other chemicals such as pollutants and food additives. Not only does this lead to an overall deterioration of health and increased susceptibility to disease, but the nutrients needed for detoxification are not available. If a person has a heavy toxic burden, the nutrient levels needed for detoxification may be high.

In this chapter, we will discuss nutritional supplements that are important in the detoxification process. Some of the nutrients can be found in sufficient amounts in the foods we eat, and others are present in such small amounts that only supplementation will supply them in adequate amounts. In addition to taking quality supplements, it is important to take them properly. (See the end of this chapter for instructions.)

Antioxidants

Antioxidants protect cells against free radicals that can damage tissues and combat free radicals released by damaged tissue. They protect against oxidation damage (the removal of an electron), neutralizing free radicals by binding to their free electrons. They are sometimes called free radical scavengers or free radical quenchers, and include any molecules that neutralize free radicals. (See chapter 20, Toxins Produced in the Body, for a detailed discussion of free radicals.) Antioxidants can also help combat the effects of chemotherapy and radiation therapy.

Antioxidants are very important in the detoxification process, and belong to two classes. The first class consists of essential nutrients obtained from the diet or supplementation:
• vitamin A
• beta-carotene
• vitamin C
• vitamin E
• manganese
• selenium
• zinc

• cysteine or N-acetyl cysteine
• glutathione
• methionine
• alpha-lipoic acid
• bioflavonoids
• coenzyme Q_{10}
• proanthocyanidins
• quercetin

The second class of antioxidants consists of enzymes normally found in the body. These include superoxide dismutase, catalase, glutathione peroxidase, and glutathione S-transferase. Their manufacture in the body depends on the availability of nutrients. Only superoxide dismutase and catalase are available as a supplement. They will be discussed in the section on enzymes later in this chapter.

The discussion of nutrients that follows is limited to a description of nutritional supplements that can help detoxification. They are organized by nutrient type for your easy reference, including vitamins, minerals, amino acids, essential fatty acids, other detoxification nutrients, enzymes, and beneficial bacteria.

Vitamins

■■ VITAMIN A
We can obtain vitamin A through the diet from eggs, milk fat, green and yellow fruits

Vitamin A and Pregnancy

Because vitamin A and its derivatives (such as accutane) can cause fetal defor-mities, pregnant women or women who might be pregnant should take no more than 8,000 IU of vitamin A per day.

and vegetables, fish liver oils, and organ meats, especially liver. Excess vitamin A is stored in the liver and also concentrates in the eyes. Gastrointestinal disease, liver disease, or infections limit the body's ability to use vitamin A.

A reduction of vitamin A levels is detri-mental to the epithelial cells of the skin, glands, and mucous membranes, the lining of hollow organs, and the lining of the respi-ratory, alimentary, and genitourinary tracts. Vitamin A deficiency, often accompanied by protein deficiency, causes night blindness, and itching and burning eyes. Children with vitamin A deficiency are prone to colds and respiratory symptoms, and to diseases such as measles.

Vitamin A deficiency is hard to diagnose, even from blood levels. Malabsorption, para-sites, liver diseases, infectious diseases, pro-longed fever, and renal disease all predis-pose people to vitamin A deficiency. About 40 percent of people in the United States are vitamin A deficient. In a Canadian study reported at the Symposium on Metabolic Functions of Vitamin A at the Massachusetts Institution of Technology in 1969 an au-topsy of 100 subjects from 5 major Canadian cities showed that more than 10 percent had no stores of vitamin A in their livers.

However, excessive intake of vitamin A can also cause symptoms because it is stored in the body. Bone or joint pain, fatigue, in-somnia, hair loss, dryness and fissuring of the lips, poor appetite, weight loss, and an enlarged liver can be caused by an excess of vitamin A.

❚ AID TO DETOXIFICATION

Vitamin A:

• aids in repair and growth of all body tis-sues.

• strengthens the cell wall in mucous mem-branes, the first site of penetration by anti-gens, viruses, bacteria, fungi, chemicals, and air pollutants.

• is an antioxidant that protects the lipid part of the cell membrane, where damage may harm receptor sites for hormones and neu-rotransmitters.

• combats all free radicals, including those released by damaged tissue after surgery and radiation therapy.

• protects against pollution, radioactivity, and cancer formation.

• supports liver detoxification.

❚ DOSE

Vitamin A can be taken in doses of 5,000 to 25,000 International Units (IU) a day. Do not take large doses of vitamin A (more than 50,000 IU a day) for longer than two months. High intake of vitamin A should be closely monitored by a knowledgeable healthcare professional.

❚❚ BETA-CAROTENE

Beta-carotene is found in dark green and or-ange-yellow vegetables such as sweet pota-toes, carrots, cantaloupe, pumpkin, butter-nut and winter squash, broccoli, spinach, and tomatoes. It is also in mangos, papayas, and apricots. Beta-carotene is converted by the liver and intestines into vitamin A.

People with hypothyroidism, diabetes, and liver disorders cannot readily transform beta-carotene into vitamin A. Nitrites from commercial fertilizers also interfere with the conversion, as does alcohol and colestipol, a common cholesterol-lowering drug.

Beta-carotene has different antioxidant properties than vitamin A. It prevents damage to DNA and cell membranes and is also an immune system booster.

■ AID TO DETOXIFICATION
Beta-carotene:
- protects against free radicals.
- is a powerful antioxidant.
- protects against oxidation of low-density lipoproteins (LDL), the "bad" cholesterol.
- protects against heart disease and cancer.
- prevents damage to cellular components, especially DNA and cell membranes.
- helps with detoxification after amalgam removal.

■ DOSE
Beta-carotene can be taken in doses of 25,000 IU from one to three times a day. If the dose is excessive, the skin will become yellow, indicating that the dose should be decreased. This condition is known as carotenemia and is not dangerous.

■■ B VITAMINS

The B vitamins aid in detoxification, but are also essential in maintaining health. B vitamins should always be taken together for balance, but increased amounts of a required B vitamin may be taken for a specific disorder.

■■ THIAMINE (VITAMIN B$_1$)

Cereal grains are good sources of thiamine, but only in the germ and outer coatings. When cereals are refined, the thiamine is lost. Enriched white flour contains 20 percent less thiamine than whole wheat flour. Thiamine is also found in egg yolks, yeast, most nuts, liver, pork, fresh green vegetables, potatoes, and beans. It is destroyed by high temperatures and by baking soda used in foods to control acidity. It is water-soluble, and can be easily lost when the cooking water for grains and vegetables is discarded.

Thiamine is a cofactor (a substance that must be present for another substance to work) in the oxidation process that occurs constantly in each body cell. Thiamine is needed for hydrochloric acid production in the stomach, and it improves the function of the gastrointestinal tract. It is needed for muscle tone of the heart, intestines, and stomach, and for growth. Thiamine assists in blood formation and enhances circulation.

Because nerve tissue is very dependent upon carbohydrate oxidation to function properly, nerve tissue often demonstrates the effects of thiamine deficiency first. Forgetfulness, numbness of the hands and feet, pain and sensitivity, and poor coordination may result. Many other symptoms can also result from a thiamine deficiency, including constipation, fatigue, loss of appetite, and weak and sore muscles.

■ AID TO DETOXIFICATION
Thiamine:
- acts with antioxidants and cysteine to counteract the effects of acetaldehyde and free radicals.

• aids in the absorption and utilization of magnesium.

• protects the body against the effects of alcohol consumption and smoking.

▊ DOSE

Thiamine can be taken in doses of 25 to 50 mg daily. If it is taken for a specific deficiency, doses of 100 to 200 mg are commonly recommended. Thiamine must always be taken with a B-complex vitamin, because all the B vitamins work together.

▊▊ RIBOFLAVIN (VITAMIN B₂)

Riboflavin is found in whole grains, yeast, eggs, cheese, green leafy vegetables, peas, lima beans, liver, and other organ and muscle meats. Fruits contain very little riboflavin. As protein intake increases, the body requires more riboflavin. Riboflavin is sensitive to light and easily destroyed by cooking, antibiotics, alcohol, and oral contraceptives.

Riboflavin is necessary for antibody production, cell respiration, and red blood formation. It is needed for the metabolism of lipids, such as fatty acids, and it helps break down proteins, carbohydrates, and some fats. Riboflavin aids in growth and reproduction, and contributes to healthy nails, hair, and skin.

Deficiency signs include cracks and sores at the corners of the mouth, eye problems, inflammation of the tongue and mouth, and skin lesions. Dizziness, hair loss, insomnia, light sensitivity, and poor digestion have also been attributed to riboflavin deficiency.

▊ AID TO DETOXIFICATION

Riboflavin:

• is converted to two coenzymes that are very active in the liver and are necessary for the formation of oxidizing enzymes that control bodily processes.

• is linked to cytochrome P-450 (as a derivative) as a necessary component (see chapter 5, Phases of Detoxification).

• is needed by some tissues to utilize oxygen.

• helps with detoxification after amalgam removal.

▊ DOSE

Riboflavin can be taken in doses of 25 to 50 mg daily. If larger doses of 100 to 200 mg are taken, a B-complex vitamin that contains approximately 50 mg of each B vitamin should be taken.

▊▊ NIACIN (VITAMIN B₃)

Niacin, niacinamide, and nicotinic acid are all forms of B₃. Niacinamide plays no role in detoxification.

Niacin is found in liver, heart, kidney, beef, rabbit, turkey, chicken, ham, tuna, sunflower seeds, whole wheat grains, broccoli, peas, peanuts, potatoes, tomatoes, and brewer's yeast.

Niacin helps stabilize glucose levels and aids in the production of hydrochloric acid and other substances necessary for digestion. It is needed for enzyme functions in the nervous system; for proper circulation; and for healthy skin, fat metabolism, and the formation of sex hormones.

Niacin decreases fatty acid production. Three to six hours after ingestion, the levels of fatty acids rise in the blood. This mobilizes toxins from the fat and allows them to be excreted.

B vitamin deficiencies, particularly vitamin B₃, cause pellagra, with symptoms including diarrhea, dermatitis, and dementia. In 1915, more than 10,000 people in the U.S. died of pellagra. After ruling out microorganisms as the cause, scientists discovered that pellagra is not an infectious disease but a deficiency disease correctable through diet.

■ AID TO DETOXIFICATION

Niacin:

- is used for electron transfer.
- operates in coenzyme forms to carry hydrogen ions in all cells.
- acts as a coenzyme in the energy cycle of the cell.
- causes vasodilatation (opening up) of capillaries in the skin and can cause histamine release, resulting in the well-known niacin flush. (See niacin discussion in Early Sauna Detoxification Programs in chapter 22.)
- helps control cholesterol levels and is often the first medication recommended for elevated cholesterol levels.
- supports liver detoxification.

■ DOSE

Niacin can be started at a dose of 100 mg daily. It can be increased by 100 mg as tolerated, up to 2,000 to 3,000 mg daily. In detoxification programs, some people are able to take 5,000 mg a day (see chapter 22). Niacin should always be taken with a B-complex vitamin.

■■ PANTOTHENIC ACID
   (VITAMIN B₅)

Pantothenic acid is a B-complex vitamin found in organ meats—heart, liver, kidney, and brain. It is also in soybeans, sunflower seeds, buckwheat, sesame seeds, peas, pea-

---

Niacin Caution

For detoxification, use short-acting niacin. Liver damage can result with the long-acting form. With long-term use, it is important to have regular liver enzyme function tests done.

---

nuts, eggs, and brewer's yeast. Vegetables and fruits contain very little pantothenic acid. Breast milk is rich in pantothenic acid, and bacteria synthesize pantothenic acid in the intestines.

Pantothenic acid is essential for cell metabolism and is used heavily in times of stress. It stimulates the production of adrenal hormones and is essential for adrenal support and prevention of adrenal exhaustion during any type of stress. It also helps the stomach produce hydrochloric acid and aids in the synthesis of cholesterol, fatty acids, and antibodies. Pantothenic acid is an essential element of coenzyme A, which is needed in the utilization of nutrients and production of energy. It is also involved in the production of neurotransmitters and the normal function of the gastrointestinal tract.

Deficiency signs include headache, nausea, fatigue, and tingling in the hands. Deficiencies are believed to be rare but do occur with alcoholism.

■ AID TO DETOXIFICATION

Pantothenic acid:

- helps protect against radiation injury.
- counteracts the side effects and toxicity of antibiotics.
- helps the intestine regain motility after intestinal operations.

Pyridoxine Caution

People have developed numbness in their hands and feet from taking large doses of pyridoxine in the range of 1,200 to 2,000 mg daily.

▌ DOSE

Pantothenic acid can be taken in doses of 25 to 100 mg daily to start, and if recommended can be increased to 1,000 to 1,500 mg. With larger doses, a B-complex vitamin should be taken.

▌▌ PYRIDOXINE (VITAMIN B6)

Pyridoxine is found in all foods, but brewer's yeast, sunflower seeds, whole grains, legumes, liver, lean muscle meats, fish, bananas, and nuts contain the highest amounts. Processing and cooking destroy the pyridoxine in food.

Vitamin B_6 is involved in more bodily processes than any other single nutrient and affects both physical and mental health. When it enters the body, it is converted with the aid of B_2 into the coenzyme pyridoxidal phosphate, the form used by the body. Vitamin B_6 is needed for the proper metabolism and use of protein, fats, carbohydrates, and hormones, such as adrenalin and insulin. It is needed for nervous system function, regulates sodium and potassium balance, and is necessary for DNA and RNA synthesis.

A high-protein diet, antidepressants, and cortisone all increase the need for vitamin B_6. Women need extra pyridoxine while pregnant, on estrogen therapy, taking oral contraceptives, and in the last two weeks of their menstrual cycle. Vitamin B_6 has been used to treat acne and psoriasis, a skin disease. It is also used to treat carpal tunnel syndrome.

A deficiency of B_6 can cause anemia, hearing problems, tremors, irritability, insomnia, nervousness, inability to concentrate, and a skin rash.

▌ AID TO DETOXIFICATION

Vitamin B_6:

• is needed for the metabolism of methionine, a sulfur-containing amino acid.
• helps the transport of amino acids across cell membranes.
• helps the absorption of magnesium and B_{12}.
• supports liver detoxification.

▌ DOSE

Vitamin B_6 can be taken in doses of 25 to 50 mg daily. If higher doses of 100 to 250 mg daily are recommended, a B-complex vitamin should be taken, with approximately 50 mg of each B vitamin.

▌▌ COBALAMIN (VITAMIN B12)

Vitamin B_{12} is found in liver, kidney, beef, clams, oysters, sardines, crab, fish, eggs, and cheeses. Vegans and alcoholics are susceptible to a B_{12} deficiency. People with B_{12} deficiency may show mental apathy, memory loss, paranoia, or even psychosis before clinical anemia develops. Studies have shown that levels of methylmalonic acid and homocysteine may be better indications of B_{12} adequacy in the body than blood B_{12} levels.

Vitamin B_{12} deficiency causes abnormalities in the blood-forming process and nervous system. The red and white blood cell count is decreased and blood cells are enlarged and destroyed rapidly. Nervous system changes include weakness of the arms and legs, decreased sensation, problems with walking and talking (stammering), and jerking of the arms and legs. It can take five years for B_{12} deficiency symptoms to appear.

The stomach secretes a substance known as "intrinsic factor" that binds vitamin B_{12} so that it can be absorbed through the intestinal wall. About 90 percent of patients with pernicious anemia have antibodies against the stomach cells that produce the intrinsic factor. People who are deficient in vitamin B_{12} lack the intrinsic factor and will not be able to absorb oral vitamin B_{12}. For this reason, B_{12} is usually prescribed as an injection. However, a recent study showed that sublingual doses of B_{12} can also be well absorbed.

Although vitamin B_{12} is a water-soluble vitamin, it can be stored by the body. Pregnancy and birth control pills can deplete vitamin B_{12}.

Vitamin B_{12} is necessary for the maintenance of the myelin sheath (fatty covering of the nerve fibers). It plays a role in the formation of DNA and RNA in cells. Vitamin B_{12} contains cobalt and is the only vitamin that contains a mineral. It can increase energy; relieve irritability; and improve memory, concentration, and balance.

■ AID TO DETOXIFICATION
Vitamin B_{12}:
• aids in detoxification of xenobiotics.
• is active in the synthesis of the amino acid methionine.

■ DOSE
Vitamin B_{12} has been used therapeutically in doses of 30 micrograms (mcg) to 5,000 mcg three times a week to once a month. Two injectable forms are available, cyanocobalamin and hydroxycobalamin.

Toxicity, even at large doses, has not been noted. As with other B viamins, a balanced B-complex with 50 mg of each B vitamin should be taken.

■■ FOLIC ACID
Folic acid is a member of the B-complex vitamins. It is also known as folacin and folate. It was first found in green leafy vegetables and was named after foliage. Spinach, liver, kidney, wheat bran, kale, beet greens, turnips, potatoes, broccoli, carrots, cantaloupe, Swiss chard, black-eyed peas, and lima beans are all rich in folic acid.

It is considered "brain food." A folic acid deficiency during pregnancy can cause intellectual impairment in the baby. A folic acid deficiency is also related to mental illness.

Folic acid is involved in protein metabolism and the production of RNA and DNA. Folic acid is also needed for red and white blood cell formation, as well as white blood cell function.

Stress, severe injuries, and surgery can easily deplete folic acid. Birth control pills also cause folic acid deficiency. If folic acid is deficient in a person with anemia, the red blood cells have a shortened life span and are shaped abnormally. People deficient in folate experience weaknesss, fatigue, irritability, and may have memory problems. They may develop graying hair, sore tongue, mouth sores, poor wound healing, mental disease, inflammation of the gastrointestinal tract, and decreased ability to fight infection.

Folic acid deficiency has also been related to developmental delay in children, decreased resistance to infection in infants, and neural tube defects, which affect the formation of the lower end of the spinal cord. The Food and Drug Administration (FDA) has recognized the folic acid and neural tube defect link and allows the fortification of prenatal vitamins with more folic acid (800 mcg), although it still limits the amount of folic acid available in other supplements to 400 mcg. Supplementation must begin *before* conception.

In 1998 the folic acid fortification program of the FDA came into effect. It requires manufacturers to add 0.43 mg to 1.4 mg of folic acid per pound of product to enriched flour, bread, rolls and buns, farina, corn grits, cornmeal, rice, and noodle products. One serving will provide about 10 percent of the daily value for folic acid.

▌ AID TO DETOXIFICATION
Folic acid:
• is needed for the utilization of amino acids.
• plays a role in methylation in Phase II detoxification (see chapter 5, Phases of Detoxification).

▌ DOSE
The usual daily dose for folic acid is 400 mcg. It can be taken in doses of 1 to 5 mg for specific diseases, but a prescription is necessary for the larger doses. Because folic acid given when B_{12} is deficient can cause neurological damage, it is important to take higher doses of folic acid under the supervision of a healthcare professional. Folic acid should always be taken in combination with a balanced B-complex vitamin.

▌▌ VITAMIN C
Vitamin C is a powerful antioxidant that is essential to numerous biochemical reactions and for tissue growth and repair. The largest concentration of vitamin C in the body is in the adrenal glands. Lesser amounts occur in the eyes, white blood cells, pituitary gland, brain, pancreas, liver, cardiac muscle, and blood plasma.

Humans cannot manufacture vitamin C and must obtain it from external sources. Because vitamin C is water-soluble, it is not stored in the body and must be replenished frequently through diet or supplementation. Excess vitamin C is excreted within two to three hours after ingestion.

Vitamin C is contained in asparagus; beet, dandelion, and turnip greens; berries; black currants; broccoli; cantaloupe; citrus fruits; collards; kale; mangos; papayas; pineapple; potatoes; rosehips; spinach; sprouts; sweet peppers; and tomatoes. It is also contained in some herbs. However, it is difficult to obtain enough from the diet, because cooking and exposure to oxygen destroy at least half of the vitamin C in foods.

▌ AID TO DETOXIFICATION
A deficiency in vitamin C decreases the metabolism of xenobiotics by lowering the level of cytochrome P-450 (see chapter 5, Phases of Detoxification).

The diuretic effect of large doses of vitamin C stimulates urine excretion and decreases the amount of fluid in the tissues. This has a cleansing effect on the body. Chemically sensitive people lose more vitamin C from the kidneys than people who have no chemical sensitivities.

Vitamin C:

- combats all free radicals, including those released by damaged tissue after surgery and radiation therapy.
- defends against reactive oxygen free radicals and lipid peroxidation (destruction of fat cells by oxidizing chemicals).
- helps prevent damage from exposure to pollutants.
- detoxifies carbon monoxide and is useful in treatment for carbon monoxide poisoning.
- has a detoxifying action on lead and mercury in the body and protects against mercury toxicity.
- detoxifies sulfur dioxide and carcinogens.
- supports liver detoxification.
- helps detoxify lipophilic (fat-soluble) chemicals stored in the fat cells and cell membranes of the body.
- increases the therapeutic effect of various medications, including antibiotics, so that lower doses can be taken.
- reduces the toxicity of digitalis, sulfa drugs, and aspirin.
- helps detoxify anesthetics and medications.
- cleanses the body from the toxic effects of radiation.
- helps with detoxification after amalgam removal.
- helps prevent and treat cancer.
- helps detoxify carcinogenic nitroso compounds found in the stools of smokers and protects against benzene exposure.
- protects the lung cells against formaldehyde, acrolin, and acetaldehyde from tobacco smoke.

Vitamin C and Allergic Reactions

Buffered vitamin C is particularly effective for clearing allergic reactions. During allergic reactions, 1 gram of vitamin C can be taken every 15 minutes. People with allergies and/or chemical sensitivities often tolerate large amounts, of 20 to 30 or more grams a day.

- helps clear allergic reactions.
- helps clear food poisoning.
- detoxifies bacterial toxins and poisons, such as the botulinum and diphtheria toxins.

■ DOSE

A sensible starting dose of vitamin C is 1 gram (1,000 milligrams) three times daily. Add 1 gram of vitamin C daily, spreading out the doses during the day, until you get diarrhea. Then set your daily dose at 1 gram less than that; this is your bowel tolerance level. When you are under stress, ill, or having allergic reactions, your bowel tolerance will be higher. Bowel-tolerance vitamin C is necessary for adequate detoxification and protection from toxins.

Take the ascorbic acid form of vitamin C with meals and buffered vitamin C between meals. If you take ascorbic acid powder or chewable vitamin C, rinse your mouth afterward to avoid tooth enamel erosion.

Vitamin C can be given intravenously or rectally, as well as orally to help with detoxification. Vitamin C nose drops and eye drops are also very effective for allergy symptoms.

■■ VITAMIN E

Vitamin E is a family of eight related molecules that are divided into two groups—tocopherols and tocotrienols. The alpha tocopherol form is the most potent.

Vitamin E is found in green leafy vegetables, whole grains, milk fat, butter, margarine, vegetable oils, egg yolks, liver, and nuts. When foods are processed, cooked, or stored for long periods of time, significant amounts of vitamin E are lost. Polyunsaturated oils, such as margarine, generate more lipid peroxides (free radicals). Oils produced by high heat, chemicals, and bleaching are prone to peroxidation (oxidation destruction of fatty acids). The use of these oils increases the need for vitamin E from supplements.

Vitamin E is fat-soluble, and has a great affinity for cell membranes, which contain large amounts of unsaturated fatty acids and other fats. It prevents fats from reacting with oxygen to produce free radicals. It is found in large amounts in the brain, pituitary gland, and adrenal glands.

Important in the prevention of cancer and heart disease, vitamin E can also reduce blood pressure, improve circulation, and promote healing. It can relax leg cramps, strengthen capillary walls, maintain healthy nerves, and is essential for tissue repair.

A deficiency of vitamin E increases susceptibility to lung damage caused by ozone. It also may result in damage to red blood cells and destruction of nerves. Menstrual problems and infertility in both men and women can be signs of vitamin E deficiency.

■ AID TO DETOXIFICATION

Vitamin E:

- is the most important antioxidant in the body.
- bonds with oil-based chemicals, ozone, and nitrous oxide.
- enhances detoxification of xenobiotics.
- is a free radical scavenger that improves oxygen transportation by the red blood cells.
- prevents oxidation of ingested fats and lipids in cell membranes and other cell structures.
- joins with lipid molecules to prevent the oxidation of vitamins A and K, and fat-soluble hormones.
- helps increase oxygenation.
- decreases damage to chromosomes and DNA by free radicals, carcinogens, and radiation.
- combats exposure to smog, smoking, sun, or X-rays, which lead to cellular deterioration.
- applied topically helps prevent scars after surgery.
- helps with detoxification after amalgam removal.

■ DOSE

Recommended doses of vitamin E are 400 to 800 IU daily, but up to 1,200 IU can be taken. Always begin vitamin E supplements in small amounts and build up gradually.

Macro and Trace Minerals

Minerals are the elements needed by the body for the formation of blood and bone, proper composition of body fluids, regulation of muscle tone, and maintenance of healthy nerve function. They are necessary for the production of hormones, good digestion, regulation of the heartbeat, and maintenance of water, acid/alkaline balance, and electrolyte balance. They are also essential for the proper utilization of vitamins and other nutrients in our food. Minerals are cofactors that allow the body to function and are vital to almost every function on a cellular level.

The minerals that are required in larger amounts are called macro minerals, and those needed in small quantities are trace minerals. Even though only minute amounts of trace minerals are needed, they are essential to health and body function, including detoxification. All enzyme activities, including detoxification, require minerals. Minerals help draw chemical substances out of the cells and help protect against toxic reactions and heavy metal poisoning.

▌▌ CALCIUM

Calcium is considered a macro mineral and is the most abundant mineral in the human body, with most of it located in the bones and teeth. Dietary calcium is found in milk, cheese, yogurt, sardines, salmon (with bones), green leafy vegetables, tofu, almonds, beans, figs, sunflower seeds, peanuts, raisins, blackstrap molasses, carob, oats, and other foods. It is also found in some herbs in small amounts. Although dairy products are considered to be the only sources of calcium by many people, a variety of vegetables and nuts contain as much or more calcium.

In addition to being necessary for the formation of bones and teeth, calcium is important for the maintenance of a regular heartbeat and transmission of nerve impulses. It is needed for muscle growth and contraction, and prevention of muscle cramps. It can lower cholesterol and help prevent cardiac disease. Calcium activates several enzymes, including lipase, and maintains cell membrane permeability. It is essential in blood clotting and may help lower blood pressure and prevent bone loss associated with osteoporosis.

A deficiency of calcium can lead to brittle nails, eczema, heart palpitations, hypertension, muscle cramps, nervousness, tooth decay, aching joints, cognitive impairment, and hyperactivity. Lack of dietary calcium is also thought to contribute to osteoporosis.

▌ AID TO DETOXIFICATION

Calcium:

- acts as a catalyst for some enzyme synthesis.
- aids in displacement of lead in tissues and protects teeth and bones from lead.
- helps maintain a proper acid/alkaline (pH) balance in tissues.
- regulates movement of nutrients and waste products in and out of cell membranes in its exchange with magnesium, sodium, and potassium.
- absorbs excess stomach acid.
- discourages cell uptake of toxic metals such as lead, cadmium, and mercury.
- supports liver detoxification.

▌ DOSE

The National Academy of Sciences has established new guidelines for calcium that are higher than those previously recommended.

- For ages 19 to 50: 1,000 mg per day.
- For adults over 51: 1,200 mg per day.

Organic Germanium

The oxygenation at the cellular level provided by 150 to 300 mg of organic germanium can clear allergic reactions. Some people may have to repeat this dose in 15 minutes if they do not totally clear. Used daily, organic germanium can also, in many cases, help with chronic pain, such as cancer pain.

Calcium is better absorbed when taken in divided doses throughout the day and before bedtime. Taken at bedtime, it promotes sound sleep.

■■ COPPER

Copper is an essential trace mineral, but can be toxic in excess amounts. Copper is found in meats, seafood, nuts, mushrooms, chocolate, tea, dried yeast, soybeans, and some waters.

In the body, copper is found in the enzyme superoxide dismutase within the cell, and protects against free radical damage to the mitochondria (the energy-producing portion of the cell). Copper is essential to the synthesis of thyroid-stimulating hormone produced by the pituitary gland.

In a study by Dr. Carl Pfeiffer at the Brain Bio Center in Princeton, New Jersey, only premature infants and people who were on intravenous nutrition were found to be copper deficient. Zinc deficiency accentuates copper excess, as zinc and copper are antagonistic. Zinc is lost in food processing and freezing. Copper excess is found in Wilson's disease and may be related to postpartum psychosis, autism, heart attacks, and one type of schizophrenia.

■ AID TO DETOXIFICATION

Copper:

• is necessary in small amounts to form hemoglobin, which carries oxygen in the blood.
• activates the synthesis of several enzymes, including detoxification enzymes.
• helps regulate essential fatty acid metabolism.
• is a cofactor in cysteine-to-cystine production (see Cysteine in Amino Acids, below).

■ DOSE:

Copper is rarely deficient, but when it is needed, 3 mg is the usual daily dose. It must be taken in conjunction with 50 mg of zinc.

■■ ORGANIC GERMANIUM

Germanium appears to be a metal, but has both metallic and non-metallic properties. Inorganic germanium is considered a metalloid and is used in industry as a semiconductor. Germanium is a trace mineral and the form used by the body is chemically bound to an organic compound. Garlic, shiitake mushrooms, onions, and the herbs aloe vera, comfrey, ginseng, and suma contain organic germanium. Inorganic germanium can cause renal toxicity.

Kazuhiko Asai, a Japanese scientist, has prescribed 100 to 300 mg of germanium a day to successfully treat food allergies, candidiasis, chronic viral infections, rheumatoid arthritis, cancer, and AIDS.

■ AID TO DETOXIFICATION

Organic germanium:

• acts as a free-radical scavenger.
• aids in toxic metal detoxification.

- raises the level of glutathione, which is involved in Phase II detoxification (see chapter 5, Phases of Detoxification).
- stimulates energy production.
- increases oxygen utilization at the cell level.
- has been used to treat mercury poisoning.
- has been used to prevent radiation sickness from radiation therapy.
- helps detoxify anesthetics and medications.

∎ DOSE

Germanium can be taken in the 150 mg dose, from one to five capsules daily. A typical maintenance dose is two 150-mg capsules daily. Use only pure organic germanium.

∎∎ IRON

Iron is a trace mineral found in meats, whole-grain cereals, liver and other organ meats, dried fruits, dark green leafy vegetables, legumes, and molasses. Iron cookware is another source of iron. Women and adolescents require twice as much iron as do men. Extra iron is recommended during pregnancy, for female athletes, babies up to one year old, and for people who have lost a significant amount of blood.

Iron combines with protein to make hemoglobin, which gives red blood cells their color and carries oxygen in the blood. Iron stores are recycled when the red blood cells are broken down.

The gene for hematochromatosis, a disease of iron overload, is quite common in the United States population. People with this disease have mild anemia, headache, increasing fatigue, shortness of breath, dizzi-

ness, and weight loss. Iron is deposited in the tissue, including the liver, lungs, pancreas, and heart. People who think they may be suffering from anemia should always be tested to determine whether they have iron deficiency or iron overload.

∎ AID TO DETOXIFICATION

Iron:

- decreases xenobiotic metabolism if deficient.
- is in superoxide dismutase, an antioxidant enzyme.
- is found in cytochrome P-450, needed in Phase I detoxification (see chapter 5, Phases of Detoxification).

∎ DOSE

Iron is recommended in doses of 10 to 18 mg daily for menstruating women, and 10 mg for men. Iron-deficient patients may be recommended to take 50 to 100 mg daily. Most people do not need an iron supplement.

∎∎ MAGNESIUM

A macro mineral, magnesium is found in nuts, whole grains, milk, green vegetables, and seafood. Wheat loses its magnesium in refining. U.S. government studies show that the average American diet supplies only 40 percent of the recommended daily amount of magnesium. Dr. Mildred Seelig, a leading authority on magnesium from North Carolina University Medical Center in Chapel Hill, North Carolina, estimates that 80 percent of the American population has a magnesium deficiency.

Magnesium facilitates the transport of nutrients across the cell membrane. It is needed for producing and transferring energy, contracting muscles, synthesizing

Magnesium and Calcium Treatments

Little known uses for magnesium and calcium include the following:
- *Intravenous magnesium will clear an asthma attack.*
- *One or two capsules of magnesium at bedtime will alleviate constipation.*
- *One capsule each of magnesium and calcium every 4 hours will relieve menstrual cramps.*
- *Liquid magnesium and calcium, given sublingually, will relieve muscle cramps anywhere in the body, as well as the neck tension that can lead to headaches.*

protein, and exciting nerves. As a cofactor, it helps enzymes catalyze many chemical reactions.

Magnesium deficiency depresses thyroid hormone levels and the microsomal lipid concentrations, which decreases xenobiotic metabolism. Magnesium is necessary for over 300 biochemical reactions in the body, so the symptoms of magnesium deficiency can vary widely. They include fatigue, depression, muscle spasms, and irritability. Muscle spasms play a role in migraine headaches, asthma, colitis, coronary artery disease, strokes, uterine hemorrhage, chronic back pain, and hypertension.

Sweating, alcohol ingestion, fast foods, poor intestinal absorption, and diuretics deplete magnesium. Its deficiency is rarely diagnosed. The most accurate test available today is the magnesium-loading test.

Magnesium has been used therapeutically for people with asthma, cardiac arrhythmias, and preeclampsia (a condition of pregnancy associated with high blood pressure, fluid retention, and hyperactive neurological reflexes).

■ AID TO DETOXIFICATION

Magnesium:
- is needed as a cofactor in ammonia detoxification.
- is necessary for the synthesis of glutathione, which is used in Phase II detoxification (see chapter 5, Phases of Detoxification).
- is a mineral activator necessary for many enzymes involved in detoxification.
- is one of the most important minerals in the detoxification of xenobiotics.
- helps with detoxification after amalgam removal.

■ DOSE

Magnesium can be taken in a dose of 800 to 1,200 mg daily. Some people develop diarrhea with higher doses. It is usually taken with calcium in a ratio of two calcium to one magnesium. However, if the deficiency is severe, magnesium can be taken in a one-to-one ratio with calcium.

■■ MANGANESE

Manganese is an essential trace mineral. It is found in avocados, nuts, seeds, dried legumes, spinach, leafy green vegetables, pineapple, blueberries, egg yolks, whole grain cereals, liver, kidney, and muscle meats. Manganese is necessary for bone growth and the formation of cartilage and synovial fluid (the lubricating fluid in joints). It is also necessary for reproduction, lipid metabolism, and the moderation of nervous irritability. It is needed for the synthesis and breakdown of proteins and nucleic acids found in DNA. Manganese is also used by the pancreas to produce insulin.

A deficiency of manganese can cause confusion, convulsions, eye and hearing problems, hypertension, heart problems, memory loss, profuse perspiration, and other symptoms. Deficiencies of manganese are not common, however.

■ AID TO DETOXIFICATION

Manganese:

• is an antioxidant.

• is required in the synthesis of glutathione, which is used in Phase II detoxification (see chapter 5, Phases of Detoxification).

• helps in the production of superoxide dismutase, an antioxidant enzyme.

• helps with detoxification after amalgam removal.

■ DOSE

Manganese can be taken in a single dose of 5 to 20 mg a day.

■■ MOLYBDENUM

Molybdenum is an essential trace mineral found in organic meats, eggs, whole grains, wheat germ, sunflower seeds, buckwheat, leafy vegetables, soybeans, lima beans, and lentils. In areas where molybdenum levels in the soil are low, high rates of cancer occur.

Molybdenum promotes normal cell function and is a component of the metabolic enzyme xanthine oxidase. It is found in the body in the bones, kidneys, and liver. Deficiency can cause impotence in older males and is also associated with mouth and gum disorders.

■ AID TO DETOXIFICATION

Molybdenum:

• opposes toxic accumulation of copper.

• helps in the synthesis and use of sulfur amino acids.

• is a component of enzymes that detoxify sulfites, aldehydes, and aldehyde oxidase.

• is necessary for cells to utilize vitamin C.

• combats chemical sensitivities.

■ DOSE

No recommended daily allowance has been established for molybdenum, but 75 mcg a day is the usual dose. It is usually found in multimineral preparations rather than as a separate nutrient.

■■ SELENIUM

Selenium is one of the most poisonous elements known, but it is an essential trace mineral for animals and humans. It is found in Brazil nuts, broccoli, garlic, brewer's yeast, dairy products, chicken, liver, seafood, and eggs. It is also found in some herbs, and in grains and seeds that are grown in soil containing selenium. When foods are processed, they lose selenium.

Selenium can be toxic to humans in large doses. Too much selenium causes loss of hair, nails, and teeth; skin rashes; arthritis; a metallic taste in the mouth; gastrointestinal disorders; kidney and liver disorders; and paralysis.

A deficiency of selenium can cause exhaustion, growth impairment, infections, high cholesterol, sterility, liver impairment, and pancreatic insufficiency. Cystic fibrosis and hypertension are more common in areas where the selenium content of the soil is low.

Men seem to have a higher need for selenium than women. Breast milk contains six times as much selenium as does cow's milk and twice as much vitamin E. Cancer rates are lower in areas where the selenium content of the soil is high.

■ AID TO DETOXIFICATION
Selenium:
- is found in glutathione peroxidase, which is necessary for the recycling of glutathione.
- is an antioxidant and helps neutralize free radicals.
- protects cell membranes and prevents the breakdown of DNA.
- supports liver detoxification.
- enhances the function of vitamins C and E.
- protects against the toxic effects of organic mercury.
- is needed for the production of coenzyme Q$_{10}$.
- neutralizes the effects of cadmium, a toxic metal.
- helps with detoxification after amalgam removal.

■ DOSE
Selenium can be taken in divided doses of 50 to 200 mcg daily. Up to 400 mcg daily can be taken for a severe deficiency, but should be monitored closely. Do not take more than 400 mcg daily.

■■ ZINC
Zinc is a trace mineral found in meat, liver, fish, oysters, seeds, wheat germ, maple syrup, mushrooms, brewer's yeast, milk, whole grains, nuts, carrots, onions, and other vegetables. Vitamin A is necessary for the utilization of zinc.

Zinc is necessary for gene repair and the growth and development of reproductive organs. It is particularly important for prostate gland function. Zinc is also needed for the proper function of B vitamins and is essential to the synthesis of protein. It can be depleted during chronic infections and inflammatory diseases. Zinc allows acuity of taste and is necessary for bone formation.

■ AID TO DETOXIFICATION
Zinc:
- is an antioxidant.
- helps neutralize free radicals.
- is in alcohol dehydrogenase (a Phase I enzyme that detoxifies aldehydes).
- is found in 90 essential enzymes.
- supports liver detoxification and protects the liver from chemicals.
- reduces lipid peroxidation.
- is a component of superoxide dismutase, an antioxidant enzyme.
- helps with detoxification after amalgam removal.

■ DOSE
Zinc can be taken in a dose of 15 to 50 mg daily. Doses larger than 50 mg daily depress copper levels. Large doses of 150 mg or more suppress the immune system.

Amino Acids

■■ CYSTEINE
Cysteine is a water-soluble amino acid. Like all amino acids, cysteine has an amino (NH$_3$) group and carboxyl group (COOH), but it also has a thiol group, which is sulfur bound to hydrogen. This thiol group is the most important part of the cysteine molecule. Cysteine is a precursor to glutathione, which is used in Phase II detoxification. It is

present in the major protein constituent of the nails, skin, and hair. It aids in the formation of new skin and promotes skin texture and elasticity.

▌ AID TO DETOXIFICATION

Cysteine:

• is one of the most potent antioxidants in the body.
• supports liver detoxification.
• acts as a reducing agent, donating hydrogen atoms to free radicals, neutralizing them.
• protects cell membranes against lipid peroxidation.
• prevents the oxidation of sensitive tissues that leads to aging and cancer.
• helps protect the liver and brain against the effects of alcohol, drugs, and cigarette smoke.
• protects the lung cells against formaldehyde, acrolein, and acetaldehyde from tobacco smoke.
• is used, along with methionine, to treat copper poisoning
• chelates heavy metals.
• detoxifies pesticides, plastics, hydrocarbons, and other chemicals.
• prevents/reduces inflammation of the intestinal lining caused by radiation.
• helps with detoxification after amalgam removal.

▌ DOSE

The recommended dietary allowance of cysteine is 25 mg per pound in adults and 55 mg per pound in children. Dr. Eric Braverman, a noted amino acid researcher from New York, recommends starting with 500 mg of cysteine daily, then building up to 3 to 4 grams daily to treat toxic exposures.

Cysteine Caution

D-cysteine and D-cystine are toxic to humans and should not be used.

People with multiple chemical sensitivities would benefit from cysteine supplementation; however, many of them do not tolerate sulfur-containing amino acids. A molybdenum supplement can increase their tolerance.

■■ N-ACETYL CYSTEINE

N-acetyl cysteine (NAC), a derivative of cysteine, is thought to be an intermediate compound in cysteine metabolism, which is converted back into cysteine in the body. It is not found in food but is synthesized by the body. Like cysteine, NAC boosts glutathione levels, used in Phase II of detoxification. NAC has been studied more extensively than cysteine to determine its usefulness in treating cancer because, unlike cysteine, NAC is patentable.

▌ AID TO DETOXIFICATION

N-acetyl cysteine:

• protects the liver from toxic chemicals.
• has helped to prevent liver and heart toxicity from chemotherapy.
• prevents bleeding and inflammation of the bladder caused by chemotherapy treatment.
• increases survival time if given before cyclophosphamide chemotherapy.
• prevents side effects from radiation treatment, such as hair loss, skin burns, and eye problems.
• decreases the effects of a toxin produced in

the intestine by *Clostridium difficile,* a bacteria related to the overuse of antibiotics.

• is used to prevent liver injury in patients who have overdosed on acetaminophen, phenacetin, and aspirin.

■ DOSE

N-acetyl cysteine comes in capsules that can be taken in doses of 500 mg once or twice daily, but is used in much larger doses, up to 10 grams, for acute poisoning. NAC smells and tastes like rotten eggs. It is nauseating and irritating, causing some people to vomit. Cysteine does not have this smell and is better tolerated.

■■ GLUTATHIONE

All organisms on earth contain glutathione (GSH), a tripeptide made up of the amino acids cysteine, glutamic acid, and glycine. In humans, glutathione is produced in the liver, and the liver, spleen, kidneys, and pancreas contain the largest concentration. The lens and cornea of the eye also contain a large amount. The amount of GSH in the body decreases as people age, and a deficiency can accelerate the aging process.

Glutathione protects the stomach lining against hydrochloric acid. A deficiency also affects the nervous system and can cause symptoms that include tremors, mental disorders, and problems with balance.

■ AID TO DETOXIFICATION

Glutathione is one of the molecules used in Phase II detoxification. The detoxification properties of GSH come from its thiol (sulfur-containing) group of cysteine. The amount of cysteine in the body determines how much GSH is produced. Selenium, magnesium, and zinc are needed for its synthesis and metabolism.

Glutathione helps protect cells against the toxic effects of oxygen and its waste products. Carbon tetrachloride, benzenes, plastics, dyes, and pesticides often form peroxide compounds after Phase I metabolism. These peroxides are then reduced in Phase II metabolism by glutathione peroxidase, an antioxidant enzyme.

Glutathione:

• protects the liver from developing cirrhosis from alcohol.
• protects the liver and lungs from the effects of automobile exhaust.
• protects the lungs against the effects of cigarette smoke.
• helps protect against the toxic effects of radiation treatment.
• prevents ulcers in people taking aspirin and other nonsteroidal drugs.
• prevents breakdown of red blood cells.
• protects against mercury toxicity.
• helps with detoxification after amalgam removal.
• chelates lead and cadmium from the bloodstream.
• detoxifies fungicides, herbicides, carbamate and organophosphate pesticides, nitrates, nitrosamines, flavorings, plastics such as vinyl chloride, arene oxides, steroids, phenolic compounds, and many over-the-counter drugs.

■ DOSE

Glutathione is given in a range of 10 to 90 mg a day, in three divided doses, depending on the severity of illness.

■■ METHIONINE

Methionine is an essential sulfur amino acid that must be supplied in the diet. Methionine is found in sunflower seeds, beans, garlic, egg yolk, wheat germ, milk products, avocados, turkey, pork, beef, fish, and other meats.

L-methionine is a powerful antioxidant and is also needed for the synthesis and transport of lipids. When people are deficient in methionine, triglycerides (a type of lipid containing three fatty acids) build up in the liver and the metabolism of xenobiotics decreases. Methionine is also needed for the synthesis of nucleic acids, collagen, and protein found in all cells.

Methionine protects glutathione levels, because the body can convert methionine to cysteine, a precursor for glutathione. Dr. Eric Braverman from New York uses methionine to treat patients with depression, high copper levels, high cholesterol, chronic pain, allergies, and asthma.

■ AID TO DETOXIFICATION

Methionine:
- aids in detoxifying xenobiotics.
- inactivates free radicals because of its sulfur content and methyl group.
- supports liver detoxification.
- protects cell membranes against lipid peroxidation.
- helps remove heavy metals from the body.
- protects against the toxic effects of radiation treatment.
- helps with detoxification after amalgam removal.

■ DOSE

The recommended dietary allowance of me-

Fatty Acids

There are two types of fatty acids. Saturated fatty acid molecules contain the maximum number of hydrogen atoms and are solid at room temperature. Saturated fats include butter and all other animal fats, coconut oil, and palm kernel oil.

Unsaturated fatty acid molecules are not fully paired with hydrogen, and are liquid at room temperature. Unsaturated fats include corn oil, safflower oil, sunflower oil, soybean oil, peanut oil, cottonseed oil, linseed oil, fish oil, and marine plant oils.

thionine is 25 mg per pound in adults and 55 mg per pound in children. It can be taken in one or two doses a day.

Essential Fatty Acids

Fatty acids, sometimes referred to as vitamin F, are the building blocks of the fats in the human body and in plants. They are structural components of the cell membranes and of the membranes surrounding intracellular structures. Fatty acids also provide a major source of energy for the body and are essential for rebuilding and producing new cells.

Nutrients are considered essential when they have to be supplied to the body because the body cannot synthesize them. Three

Essential Fatty Acids and Menstrual Problems

Because of the hormone fluctuations involved, many problems and symptoms can accompany the menstrual cycle, including premenstrual syndrome, dysmenorrhea (painful periods), and even amenorrhea (absence of periods). The uncomfortable symptoms that can accompany menopause are well known.

A deficiency of essential fatty acids or a problem in fatty acid metabolism can be a causative factor. Supplementation with essential fatty acids, particularly evening primrose oil, can gradually relieve symptoms. Borage oil, flaxseed oil, and black currant oil are also helpful.

Caution: Women with estrogen-related breast cancer should not use evening primrose oil.

unsaturated fatty acids are essential: arachidonic, linolenic, and linoleic. They should make up at least a quarter of the total fats in the diet. Essential fatty acids take part in many biochemical reactions and biological functions.

Essential fatty acids control blood pressure and the formation of plaque in arteries. They stimulate the body's defense against cancer and infections. They increase metabolism, bring oxygen to cells, decrease inflammation, and aid in healing. Premature aging, cardiovascular disease, obesity, and arthritis are associated with a deficiency of essential fatty acids.

Essential fatty acids are necessary for the formation of prostaglandins, hormone-like chemicals that regulate cell activity. Prostaglandins are formed from two types of unsaturated fats, omega-3 and omega-6. The various prostaglandins keep blood platelets from sticking together, reduce the possibility of blood clots, help remove fluid from the body, and dilate blood vessels, improving circulation.

People with an adequate diet produce sufficient prostaglandins from linolenic and linoleic acid. Should there be a block in this metabolism, evening primrose oil, which contains linoleic acid and gammalinolenic acid, and fish oils can bypass the block.

Fish oil is mainly an omega-3 fatty acid, containing EPA (eicosapentaenoic acid) and DHA (docosahexaenoic acid), both of which are omega-3 oils. Fish oil is more beneficial than vegetable omega-3 oils because vegetable omega-3 oils convert to EPA to a much lesser extent. Salmon, mackerel, herring, and sardines provide more omega-3 than other fish. Farm fish raised on soybean meal contain very little omega-3 oil.

Vegetable oils are excellent sources of omega-6 essential fatty acids. Some vegetable oils contain alpha linolenic acid (ALA), an omega-3 oil. The best sources of omega-3 fatty acids are flaxseed (linseed), rapeseed (canola), soybean, and hemp oils. Flaxseed oil is also rich in linoleic acid (omega-6) and contains more linolenic acid (omega-3) than other vegetable oils. Because the conversion of ALA to EPA is quite limited, vegetable oils do not afford the protective effects (such as controlling triglycerides), like that of fish oils. Vegetable oils must always be fresh, as rancid oils can break down to free radicals and carcinogens.

Evening primrose oil contains more gamma-linolenic acid (GLA) than any other food substance. Borage oil and black currant seed oil also contain GLA, but not as much. Evening primrose oil helps prevent PMS, heart disease, hardening of the arteries, and high blood pressure. It reduces pain and inflammation and enhances the release of sex hormones.

■ AID TO DETOXIFICATION

Fish oils and vegetable oils:
- decrease cholesterol and triglycerides.
- speed up transit time of the stool, decreasing the buildup of toxins.

Evening primrose oil:
- helps to relieve PMS, improve eczema, and prevent arthritis.
- helps prevent liver damage caused by alcoholism.
- has been used in the treatment of schizophrenia.

■ DOSE

Doses are given for each type of oil. Select one oil or rotate all three if you are sensitive. *Fish oil:* Take fish oil capsules with a meal, up to four to six a day. Because these omega-3 fatty acids decrease the absorption of vitamin E, also take vitamin E supplements if you are taking fish oil capsules or eating large quantities of fish.

Vegetable oils: Take 1 to 5 Tbsp. of vegetable oil per day. Borage oil, safflower oil, black currant oil, and flaxseed oil are the most helpful.

Evening primrose oil: One to two capsules of evening primrose oil three times a day are recommended. *Caution:* Because it encourages the production of estrogen, women who have estrogen-sensitive breast cancer should avoid or take limited amounts of evening primrose oil.

Other Detoxification Nutrients

Other nutrients are helpful in detoxification but either do not fall into any of the classes discussed or are not used in most formal detoxification programs. Space permits discussion of only a few of these nutrients.

■■ ALOE VERA

Aloe vera has been used for hundreds of years to soothe and heal cuts and burns. This succulent plant has two juices, the yellow sap in the cells beneath the thick green rind, and the gel fillet, which is the water-storage organ. When taken internally, the gel fillet has anti-inflammatory actions, lowers cholesterol and triglycerides, and protects the intestinal tract against ulcers. In commercial aloe vera, the fillet has been processed to contain the least possible amount of aloin from the yellow sap. Aloin is a potent laxative.

Aloe vera has been used internally to successfully treat allergies, anaphylaxis, chronic fatigue syndrome, colds, colic, parasites, staph infections, viral infections, and stasis ulcers. Externally, aloe vera can be used to treat eczema, frostbite, fungal infections, genital herpes, gum infections, shingles, sprains, stings, yeast infections, vaginitis, and warts.

■ AID TO DETOXIFICATION

Aloe vera:

- dilates blood vessels, increasing the oxygen available to cells.
- contains mucopolysaccharides, which form a lining in the colon to prevent toxins from reentering the body; they also help absorb water, electrolytes, and nutrients from the gastrointestinal tract.
- contains acemannan (the active ingredient in the gel fillet), which injects itself into the cell membrane, increasing permeability, so that toxins can leave the cell more easily and nutrients can enter.
- contains proteolytic enzymes, which can break down and digest dead cells.

■ DOSE

Aloe vera can be taken orally in a dose of 2 to 4 Tbsp. of gel daily.

■■ ALPHA-LIPOIC ACID

A vitamin-like substance that the body produces in small amounts naturally, alpha-lipoic acid is sometimes also called thioctic acid. The levels of this substance go down as people age. Alpha-lipoic acid is considered to be the universal antioxidant, because it is soluble in both water and fats. It can help protect both water-soluble and fat-soluble antioxidants, including vitamins C and E, and coenzyme Q_{10}.

Alpha-lipoic acid helps stabilize blood sugar and can treat diabetic neuropathy, a complication of diabetes. It stimulates the uptake of glucose by the cells, helping to combat insulin resistance. It assures proper functioning of two key enzymes that convert food into energy, enhancing energy levels. It also helps prevent food from being deposited as fat.

■ AID TO DETOXIFICATION

Alpha-lipoic acid:

- is an antioxidant.
- helps to neutralize the effects of all free radicals.
- enhances the antioxidant functions of vitamins C and E, and glutathione.
- protects the liver from the effects of alcohol.
- can substitute for vitamins C and E if those vitamins are deficient.

■ DOSE

A daily dose of 100 to 300 mg is the suggested daily dosage. Higher doses may be given in the presence of medical problems such as diabetes, cancer, or AIDS. Vitamin B_1 (thiamine) is a supporting nutrient and should be taken in a B-complex along with alpha-lipoic acid.

■■ BIOFLAVONOIDS

Bioflavonoids (sometimes referred to as vitamin P) are the brightly pigmented substances found in fruit and flowers. They are also found in leaves and stems, and there are over 4,000 of these compounds. High levels of bioflavonoids are found in citrus fruit skin and pulp, apricots, cherries, grapes, green peppers, tomatoes, papaya, and broccoli. Citrus bioflavonoids, such as tangeretin, nobiletin, and sinensetin, have the greatest biological activity. Other bioflavonoids include quercetin, hesperidin, proanthocyanadins and rutin. Quercetin and the proanthocyanidins are two of the most important bioflavonoids and are discussed separately later in this section.

Bioflavonoids support health with their anti-allergenic, anti-cancer, anti-histimine, anti-inflammatory, and anti-viral properties. Bioflavonoids increase capillary wall resistance, improve varicose veins and hemorrhoids, and help prevent blood clots. Bioflavonoids have been used with vitamin C for treating bleeding after childbirth, bleeding gums, heavy periods, hemorrhoids, nosebleeds, and skin diseases.

In addition, bioflavonoids block the "sorbitol" pathway, the accumulation of sorbitol in the lens that is linked to many of the symptoms of diabetes, and they may help protect the lens of the eye from cataracts. They are also capable of improving blood flow in diabetics. Bioflavonoids improve the absorption of vitamin C, and when taken with vitamin C, reduce the symptoms of oral herpes. Alone or with vitamin C, they reinforce collagen and connective tissue, and their anti-oxidant effect prevents LDL cholesterol from building up inside artery walls.

Bioflavonoids could not be classified as a vitamin, because they did not fulfill all of the requirements for a vitamin, and the vitamin P designation was dropped. However, they are frequently called "semi-essential" nutrients because they are as important as essential vitamins and minerals to human health. In the late 1960s, the U.S. Food and Drug Administration declared that bioflavonoids were not a vitamin and had no nutritional value. This is unfortunate because bioflavonoids are very important to the body and this ruling leads people to believe they are unimportant.

■ AID TO DETOXIFICATION
Bioflavonoids:
• are antioxidants.
• can chelate metals.
• protect vitamin C from oxidation.
• decrease capillary fragility. (Cells depend on capillaries to bring nutrients and carry away waste material and toxins.)
• have an antibacterial effect.
• promote circulation and stimulate bile production.

■ DOSE
Although there is no standard recommended dose, most nutritionists suggest taking 100 mg of bioflavonoids for every 500 mg of vitamin C, as they work synergistically.

■■ COENZYME Q10

Coenzyme Q_{10} (CoQ_{10}), also called ubiquinone, is an oil-soluble, vitamin-like substance that plays a critical role in energy production for the body. The function of CoQ_{10} resembles that of vitamin E, and it may be even more powerful as an antioxidant. It stimulates the immune system, increases tissue oxygenation, and aids circulation. The body can produce CoQ_{10}, but it takes high energy to do so, and depletion can occur much faster than the body can resynthesize it. The amount of CoQ_{10} in the body declines with age.

People with diabetes, high blood pressure, periodontal disease, or heart disease have a deficiency of CoQ_{10}, and they improve with oral supplementation. It is a useful treatment for congestive heart failure, angina, and cardiomyopathy, a degenerative disease of the heart muscles. Several studies have shown objective improvement in heart function, decreased incidence of angina attacks, and decreased mortality rate with CoQ_{10} supplementation.

■ AID TO DETOXIFICATION

Coenzyme Q_{10}:

- has antioxidant activity.
- protects cell membranes.
- is a free radical scavenger.
- seems to lower cholesterol and decrease resistance in the blood vessels.
- protects normal tissue against damage caused by chemotherapy agents.
- helps detoxify anesthetics and medications.

■ DOSE

Recommended doses range from 10 mg once daily to 30 mg three times daily. It is best absorbed when taken with oily or fatty foods.

■■ L-CARNITINE

L-carnitine has a chemical structure similar to that of amino acids, and is produced by the liver from the amino acids lysine and methionine. It is also found in organ meats and other meats, and in small amounts in chicken, fish, eggs, and milk. There are negligible amounts in grains and vegetables. It helps convert fat into energy. If there is inadequate L-carnitine, fatty acids can build up within cells and in the blood.

L-carnitine reduces levels of triglyceride and cholesterol in the blood, prevents ketosis (an excess of breakdown products of fat), helps with weight loss, and improves endurance.

A link between some genetic diseases and L-carnitine deficiencies was first discovered in 1972. Muscle diseases, including muscular dystrophy, have been helped with supplementation of L-carnitine. Dr. Ruth McGill of Texas has described an oxidative phosphorylation defect (a defect in the production of energy for the cell) in certain Gulf War veterans and in some patients with multiple chemical sensitivities who have muscular symptoms. This defect has responded to large doses of coenzyme Q_{10} and L-carnitine.

■ AID TO DETOXIFICATION

L-carnitine:

- prevents buildup of plaque on artery walls.
- helps in treating metabolic liver disease.
- enhances the effectiveness of the antioxidants vitamins C and E.
- clears the bloodstream of ammonia.

• reduces the accumulation of lactic acid.

■ DOSE

L-carnitine can be given in divided doses of 1,000 to 3,000 mg a day. For genetic deficiencies, 4,000 mg per day may be recommended.

■■ METHYL-SULFONYL-METHANE

Methyl-sulfonyl-methane (MSM) is a relatively new available supplement and its use is still controversial to some in the healthcare field. MSM is a naturally occurring sulfur compound that is found in the blood and other organs, and has been detected in human urine. MSM is also found in foods, including green vegetables, fruits, grains, meat, fish, and milk, but is lost when food is processed, cooked, or stored.

MSM is a dietary source of sulfur in a form that the body can assimilate. The body uses the sulfur from MSM to create new cells and form connective tissue. It is also required for utilization of the amino acids methionine and cysteine, and for proteins, catalysts, and enzymes that incorporate sulfur into their molecules. Sulfur helps maintain the structure of protein in the body, aids the formation of keratin for nails and hair, aids in the production of immunoglobulin, and catalyzes chemical reactions that change food into energy. Sulfur is an activator of thiamine, vitamin C, biotin, and pantothenic acid. It is also used by the liver in the production of bile and it is a component in insulin production.

■ AID TO DETOXIFICATION

MSM:

• is a free radical scavenger.
• prevents overreaction to medications.

• coats the intestinal tract so parasites cannot attach.
• provides protection against insecticide exposure.
• makes cell walls more permeable, allowing foreign proteins and free radicals to be washed out.
• reduces buildup of lactic acid in the muscles after exercise.

■ DOSE

The recommended dose of MSM is 500 mg twice a day. People with arthritis or a heavy toxic burden may need to take up to 2,000 mg daily.

■■ PROANTHOCYANIDINS

Marketed as pycnogenol or grape pips, proanthocyanidins are a class of nutrients that belong to the flavonoid family. They are found in many plants, but are in the highest concentration in pine bark and grape seeds and skin. Bilberries, cranberries, black currants, green tea, and black tea also contain this flavonoid, as do most fruits and vegetables. However, proanthocyanidins are usually destroyed during normal food handling and cooking.

In addition to their antioxidant properties, proanthocyanidins stabilize collagen and maintain elastin, which are proteins in connective tissue, blood vessels, and muscle. They improve capillary activity, strengthen capillary membranes, and restore flexibility to arterial walls. They bind to collagen fibers (the basic matrix of skin tissue), and help realign these fibers, preventing wrinkling and damage to the skin. Collagen is necessary to maintain healthy bones, cartilage, gums, and eyes.

Proanthocyanidins retard aging, stimulate blood circulation, improve vision, increase flexibility, and reduce bruising. They may reduce the risk of cancer, heart disease, and stroke, and reduce inflammation in arthritis.

❙ AID TO DETOXIFICATION
Proanthocyanidins:

• are a powerful antioxidant and free radical scavenger.
• protect collagen, particularly from free radical damage.
• help protect brain and nerve tissue from oxidation.
• are powerful chelating agents and protect the body from toxic metals.

❙ DOSE
A reasonable supplemental level is 50 to 100 mg per day. For circulatory, capillary, and other health problems, up to 300 mg per day may be recommended.

❙❙ QUERCETIN

Quercetin is a water-soluble plant pigment that is a member of the bioflavonoid family. It is a potent flavonoid found in apples, grapes, broccoli, green peppers, Italian squash, red and yellow onions, tomatoes, cayenne pepper, garlic, black tea, green tea, and red wine.

One of the most powerful anticancer substances discovered to date, quercetin prevents damaging changes in the cells that initiate cancer. It also helps inhibit the spread of cancer cells. In addition, quercetin keeps blood from thickening and forming clots. The pain-promoting inflammatory substances that are produced in the body by rheumatoid arthritis and colitis are blocked by quercetin.

❙ AID TO DETOXIFICATION
Quercetin:

• is an extremely potent antioxidant.
• inhibits the production of free radicals.
• accelerates the production of detoxifying enzymes that rid the body of carcinogenic toxins.
• interferes with an enzyme that neutralizes cortisone, the natural anti-inflammatory produced by the body.
• prevents free radicals from oxidizing low-density lipoproteins (LDL), which are contained in "bad" cholesterol.
• blocks an enzyme that leads to accumulation of sorbitol, which has been linked to nerve, eye, and kidney damage in people with diabetes.
• has a powerful antihistamine action.
• helps protect and potentiate Vitamin C.

❙ DOSE
The usual recommended dose of quercetin is 400 mg two to three times a day. Taking 400 to 500 mg twice daily between meals has a powerful antihistamine and anti-inflammatory effect.

Enzymes

Enzymes participate in virtually every biochemical reaction that takes place in the body. They are catalysts—chemicals that accelerate reactions—and are not used up in the reactions they assist. Enzymes are proteins that contain amino acids. Enzymes enable our bodies to renew old cells, regulate hormones and nerve impulses, metabolize nutrients into building blocks and energy, and remove waste products and toxins. Enzymes are essential to the function of vitamins and minerals and to detoxification processes.

❚❚ METABOLIC ENZYMES

The most common enzymes found in the body are the metabolic enzymes. About 5,000 metabolic enzymes run the body chemistry within cells. All of the organs, tissues, and cells function because of these enzymes, and each tissue has its own specific enzymes. There are many classes of these metabolic enzymes that are important to detoxification. One important detoxification class is the antioxidant enzymes mentioned earlier in this chapter.

Superoxide dismutase (SOD) is an antioxidant enzyme that is the first-line defense against pollution injury. It protects cells by converting the free radical superoxide to oxygen and water. Superoxide dismutase is produced by the body, but it is also found in food sources such as barley grass, broccoli, Brussels sprouts, cabbage, wheatgrass, and most green plants. There are two types of superoxide dismutase, one in which copper and zinc are cofactors and one in which manganese is the cofactor (a substance that must be present for another substance to work). The copper/zinc version protects the cytoplasm (the substance of a cell, exclusive of the nucleus), where free radicals are produced by metabolic activity. The manganese version protects the cells' mitochondria (where energy is produced and the genetic material of the cell is stored).

Catalase, another antioxidant enzyme, breaks down the metabolic waste product hydrogen peroxide, and liberates oxygen to a usable form for the body. Both it and SOD are available in supplement form. SOD must be enteric coated so that it will pass through the stomach acid intact to be absorbed in the small intestine.

Although it is not available as a supplement, glutathione peroxidase is an antioxidant enzyme that is a major defense in the body against peroxides. It requires selenium and converts peroxides to water and oxygen, decreasing lipid peroxidation. Found in red blood cells, glutathione peroxidase protects them from damage, functioning optimally at a pH of 7. It is an antipollutant enzyme that may be induced or suppressed in the chemically sensitive.

The antioxidant enzyme glutathione-S-transferase is a catalyst in reactions in which glutathione participates. It is also a catalyst for binding proteins that serve a storage function for toxic compounds in the liver. Glutathione-S-transferase acts to detoxify toxic intermediates produced by the cytochrome P-450 detoxification process (see chapter 5, Phases of Detoxification) and is a scavenger for alkylating agents such as cancer drugs. This enzyme is not available as a supplement.

❚❚ DIGESTIVE AND FOOD ENZYMES

The body also contains digestive enzymes. These enzymes are secreted in the digestive tract and break down foods so that the vitamins and minerals can be used by the body. These enzymes include protease, amylase, and lipase. Protease is secreted from the

Enzymes from Food

In addition to those it manufactures, the body obtains enzymes from all raw foods. Pineapple and papaya, in particular, contain large amounts of enzymes. Heat destroys enzymes, so the food must be raw for the enzymes to be present and active. For foods to be preserved, enzymes must be destroyed as they will digest the food in which they are contained.

Some hybrid foods are bred to have lower enzyme levels. This will prolong their life in the grocery store, but will have an adverse effect on the people consuming them.

submandibular glands, salivary glands located under the jaw. The parotid glands, salivary glands located near the ear, produce amylase. Lipase is secreted by the sublingual salivary glands located under the tongue. These enzymes are mixed with food as we chew, beginning the digestive process.

Food enzymes include protease, amylase, lipase, and cellulase, and they are not as strong as the digestive enzymes produced in the body. Food enzymes function over a broad pH range (3.0 to 9.0), including the acid environment of the stomach, while pancreatic enzymes (enzymes produced in the pancreas) work only in the alkaline environment of the small intestine. Food enzymes predigest 60 percent of starch, 30 percent of protein, and 10 percent of fat in the stomach. Both digestive and food enzymes work together to cause food to be more completely digested than either can alone.

Protease digests protein and helps acidify the blood. It is found in the saliva, stomach, pancreatic, and intestinal secretions. It also digests organisms, such as the protein coating on certain viruses, toxic debris from dead bacteria, and inflammatory chemicals produced at injury sites.

In addition to the saliva, amylase is found in the pancreatic and intestinal secretions. Different types of amylase break down specific sugars. Amylase digests white blood cells, such as those in an abscess, once the white cells have killed all the bacteria. It can digest viruses, including herpes, and control lymphatic swelling. Amylase also helps control asthma.

Lipase, which is present in fatty foods, is found in the saliva, stomach, and pancreatic secretions. It aids in fat digestion and helps to control fat metabolism. Lipase digests the fat that surrounds viruses and can kill some viruses.

Amylase and lipase can heal hives, contact dermatitis, and psoriasis. They decrease the effects of bee stings and insect bites, and help the lungs clear hardened mucus accumulations.

Cellulase digests soluble fiber found in vegetables and some fruit. It assists in the digestion of raw vegetables, while allowing their fiber to help cleanse the bowel. Chewing releases cellulase from vegetables, allowing access to the food surfaces. Cellulase is not produced in the human body, so must be obtained from food or supplied in an enzyme supplement.

■■ ENZYME SUPPLEMENTS

Enzyme deficiencies are common today. Our foods contain few if any enzymes after cooking, processing, pasteurization, or microwaving. Heating and refining deactivate and destroy enzymes. In addition, each enzyme requires a certain pH to function, and many diets (such as high-protein or high-meat diets) are too acidic for enzymes requiring an alkaline environment.

Environmental toxins and pollutants stress our enzyme systems and affect our detoxification and immune systems, which require enzymes to function. As we grow older, our bodies produce fewer enzymes, reducing digestive absorption, and the body's ability to function efficiently.

Diets containing raw fruits and vegetables are important, but enzyme supplementation is frequently necessary for our bodies to function optimally. Several excellent enzyme supplements are available. They should be stored in a cool place to maintain potency. Refrigeration is not necessary except in extremely hot climates.

■ RECOMMENDED DOSE

Recommended dosages vary from brand to brand, depending on their formulation. The following is a general guide.

- As a dietary supplement, take one to two capsules or tablets with meals three times a day.
- As an anti-inflammatory aid, take four to six capsules or tablets between meals (two hours after a meal or one hour before)

Yogurt

Some beneficial bacteria are found in fermentable dairy products, usually in live culture yogurt. Yogurt has been used in folk medicine as a probiotic source for thousands of years. However, not all yogurt contains live organisms, and there is a wide variation in the strains and their numbers in live culture products. Frozen yogurt contains no live organisms.

three times a day. Your dosage will have to be adjusted according to symptom relief.

Beneficial Bacteria

The gastrointestinal (GI) tract contains a mixture of bacteria, fungi, protozoa, food particles, digestive enzymes, acids, bile, and mucins. The organisms in the GI tract are known as intestinal flora. Beneficial bacteria that are present inhibit pathogenic organisms and prevent them from multiplying and colonizing. They also produce antibiotics and enhance the body's production of antibodies.

Some pathogens of the GI tract are opportunistic organisms. If there is a minor decrease in host resistance, these pathogens colonize the GI tract and resist recolonization by the native bacteria. Pathological intestinal bacteria can produce toxins that can cause hypersensitivity to the bacteria and may initiate autoimmune disease (in which the body attacks its own tissues). This happens when bacteria and tissues in the body share the same antigens (substances that induce an immune reaction). A common example is the antigen shared by heart tissue and the streptococcal bacteria.

A change in intestinal flora can be long-lasting. People treated with antibiotics often have permanent changes in their intestinal flora. Stress also affects intestinal flora. If the pH of the intestines is above 7, abnormal bacterial growth can flourish, interfering with enzyme production that aids food digestion.

Adrenal stress hormones decrease hydrochloric acid production in the stomach, reducing digestive ability and decreasing mucin production in the intestines. Mucin lubricates the surface of the intestines, protecting the underlying mucosa from chemical injury. It also removes bacteria, fungi, viruses, and parasites by binding and trapping them so they can be eliminated in the feces.

An abnormal balance of bacteria in the intestines is known as dysbiosis. It leads to impaired immune defense, damage to the intestinal wall, and the production of acetic acids and hydrogen and methane gases—which can cause bloating, gas, and diarrhea. With intestinal wall trauma, large molecules are able to cross the intestinal barrier and the body produces antibodies to these molecules or develops inflammation because of them. This is known as "leaky gut," and this syndrome has been associated with skin inflammation, arthritis, asthma, bronchitis, and recurrent colds and earaches.

A leaky gut places an increased burden on the liver because of the additional toxins coming in from the intestines. This increases the number of free radicals generated by the detoxification process and can lead to autoimmune diseases or inflammation of the muscles and joints. The large molecules, the antibodies, and the chemicals produced by inflammation must all be filtered by the liver, which is then less able to detoxify foreign chemicals. The overloaded system cannot handle incoming toxins, which accumulate and can damage regulatory enzymes and proteins.

Probiotic literally means "for living," and is a term used for bacteria that are supportive of life. These bacteria have the capacity to prevent or reduce the effects of pathogenic organisms. Probiotics are able to increase in the host while decreasing the number and effects of pathogenic organisms. They promote good digestion, boost immune function, and increase resistance to infection. People who have digestive problems frequently need a probiotic supplement.

■■ LACTOBACILLI

Lactobacilli are one of the five major groups of intestinal bacteria. *Lactobacillus* refers to probiotic bacteria that produce lactic acid. *Lactobacillus acidophilus* or, as it is commonly called, acidophilus, plays an important role in the ecology of the intestines. These bacteria flourish at a pH of around 6.8 and produce an antibiotic that inhibits the growth of disease-causing bacteria such as *Salmonella* and *Staphylococcus*.

Lactobacillus acidophilus produces at least one natural antibiotic, called acidophilin, which helps it fight off harmful bacteria. *Lactobacilli* are effective against 25 different harmful bacteria, including *Salmonella*, *Staphylococcus*, and *Streptococcus*.

Acidophilus can counteract the coated tongue, bad breath, gas, bloating, and diarrhea that are common symptoms of an overgrowth of harmful bacteria. It has also been used to soothe sore throats and reduce cold sores. In addition, acidophilus produces B vitamins, which help fight stress and metabolize food.

Lactobacilli have been used for chronic illnesses in humans and animals. To be successful, a large number of *Lactobacilli* must be used and a utilizable carbohydrate source should be available for the *Lactobacilli* in the intestinal tract. In addition to *Lactobacillus acidophilus*, other probiotic *Lactobacilli* include *L. bifidus, L. brevis, L. bulgaricus, L. casei, L. delbrueckii, L. kefir, L. plantarum, L. salivarius, L. rhamnosus,* and *L. yoghurti*. However, in general, people tolerate a single *Lactobacillus* strain more easily, and *L. acidophilus* or *L. bifidus* are more commonly used.

■ RECOMMENDED DOSE

One-half tsp. of acidophilus powder stirred in water three times a day is recommended (1 tsp. equals 10 to 40 billion organisms, depending on the brand used). Capsules are also available, but large numbers of them may be needed, depending on the organism count per capsule.

■■ BIFIDOBACTERIA

Bifidobacteria make up about 25 percent of the beneficial intestinal bacteria. *Bifidobacteria*, along with *Lactobacillus* species and *Streptococcus faecium*, produce vitamins, enzymes, and antimicrobial substances. An increase in *Bifidobacteria* lowers intestinal pH, blood pressure, and blood levels of cholesterol and triglycerides.

Bacteria Balance

Keeping a balance between beneficial and harmful bacteria in the intestines is important to prevent harmful bacteria from taking over. Poor diet, antibiotics, other medications, alcohol, and tobacco reduce beneficial bacteria. Overeating can also cause an intestinal imbalance.

Bifidobacteria may act to detoxify carcinogens in the intestines. Probiotic *Bifidobacteria* species include *Bifidobacterium bifidum, B. infantis,* and *B. longum*. In one study, the number of *Bifidobacteria* increased by 10 times in a 14-day period when fructo-oligo-saccharide supplements were given. *Lactobacillus* growth also increased, although not as much.

■■ STREPTOCOCCI

Several *Streptococci* species are helpful to the body, rather than causing infections, and are used in probiotic preparations. The major beneficial species is *Streptococcus faecalis*, but *S. faecium, S. lactis,* and *S. thermophilus* are also beneficial and are used in these preparations.

■■ FRUCTO-OLIGO-SACCHARIDES

Fructo-oligo-saccharides (FOS) are discussed here because of their use with probiotics. Fructo-oligo-saccharides are composed of three nondigestible carbohydrates that are approximately half as sweet as sucrose (table sugar). They occur naturally in asparagus, bananas, barley, garlic, Jerusalem artichokes, onions, tomatoes, and wheat, but can be synthesized through the reaction of sucrose with fungal enzymes.

FOS are not digested by carbohydrate enzymes, but pass intact to the colon, where they are used as a growth nutrient by the beneficial bacteria in the intestine, especially the *Bifidobacteria*. Fructo-oligo-saccharides are not used by harmful bacteria such as *Salmonella*, *Escherichia coli*, or *Clostridium perfringens*, and are too large for candida and other yeasts to use.

Fructo-oligo-saccharides decrease intestinal permeability and lower the toxic burden on the liver. They have been useful in treating musculoskeletal diseases.

▐ DOSE

Supplements of *Bifidobacteria* are available in combination with *Lactobacillus acidophilus* and fructo-oligo-saccharides. Supplements of FOS alone or in combination with *Bifidobacteria* and *L. acidophilus* are taken in doses of $1/2$ to 1 level tsp. two to three times a day.

Taking Nutritional Supplements

All vitamins, minerals, and amino acids work together. It is important to take a balance of all the nutrients if you are going to take supplements. It is not generally advisable to take large doses of just one nutrient. An excess of a nutrient can produce the same symptoms as a deficiency. As Dr. Jeffrey Bland of HealthComm in Gig Harbor, Washington says, "Nutrients work in a symphony." It is best to take a good-quality multivitamin that also contains multiminerals, and supplement it with specific nutrients as needed.

▐▐ FORMS

Take nutrients in a form easily assimilated by the body. If a capsule or tablet passes unchanged in the stool, it was not available to the body. Vitamins and minerals that are chelated to amino acids are easily used by the body. Citrates, orotates, aspartates, picolinates, lactates, and gluconates are all easily absorbed.

Specialized liquid nutrients are now available that can be administered rectally. These nutrients are absorbed well, and are particularly helpful for chemically sensitive patients who have difficulty taking and tolerating vitamins orally.

▐▐ ADDITIONAL INGREDIENTS

It is important to take "clean" supplements that do not contain possible allergens, aspartame, and coloring. Look for brands that state that their product is free of common allergens such as wheat, milk, corn, soy, egg, sugar, and yeast. Because supplements are taken daily, they can provide a daily exposure to these common allergens. Avoid products that use aspartame (marketed as Nutra-Sweet and Equal) as the sweetener. These products cause many side effects, including neurological damage. See chapter 13, Food, for additional information on aspartame.

Avoid supplements that have numerous ingredients listed in addition to the nutrients. These ingredients can be potential allergens and are not necessarily active ingredients. Some binders and fillers are necessary to hold tablets together or to extend capsule contents, but there should not be many of these substances. Avoid products that contain artificial colorings and flavor-

Physical Form of Nutrients

FORM	BENEFITS	DRAWBACKS
Powders	More rapidly absorbed and usually contain no binders or fillers; can be encapsulated at home	Taste may be unpleasant
Tablets	Have a long shelf life	Always contain fillers and a binder to hold the tablet together; not absorbed as well as other forms
Capsules	Easier to swallow and absorb than tablets; contain fewer fillers and binders	Capsule portion is usually made from meat sources such as beef or pork; some vegetable capsules are now available
Liquids	Absorbed well; helpful for people who have difficulty with or cannot swallow tablets or capsules	Often contain sugars, flavorings, and colorings
Chewables	Helpful for children	Often contain sugars, flavorings, and colorings
Time-release capsules or tablets	Portions of the vitamin content are released over a period of time	Many people have insufficient stomach acid to dissolve the coating and release the vitamin

ings. In some instances, children's chewable supplements contain artificial sweeteners and flavorings to mask the taste so the child will be willing to chew them. However, some chewable supplements do have natural flavors that are pleasant.

Sensitive people may have to avoid supplements containing herbs. Herbs can be ex-cellent for individuals who tolerate them, however, and they contain small amounts of various vitamins and minerals.

■■ TIMED DOSES

The timing of taking nutrients is important for maximum absorption. Vitamins and minerals are best taken with meals. If they are taken between meals, they can cause an upset stomach and are not absorbed as well. Amino acids should be taken just before meals. Nutritional supplements should be taken in equal amounts spaced throughout the day to avoid taking large amounts at one time and to assure the body of their continued availability.

When enzymes are taken to help digestion, they are taken during or just after a meal. If taken between meals they have an anti-inflammatory action that is useful for bruises, strains, sprains, and arthritic pain.

The timing necessary for taking probiotics varies with the brand. Some are taken on an empty stomach before meals, and others are to be taken with meals. People taking antibiotics always need a probiotic supplement. The antibiotic kills both the "good" and "bad" bacteria, making it necessary to replace the good bacteria. However, the probiotic and antibiotic should not be taken at the same time.

Nutrient Detoxification Programs

Several companies have developed nutritional products that contain all of the vitamins, minerals, and other nutrients necessary to encourage and maximize detoxification. These products provide nutritional support for liver metabolism, detoxification, and intestinal function.

The formulas are vegetarian, low in allergenicity, sodium, and saturated fats, and they contain no cholesterol. They are balanced formulas that provide carbohydrates; easily digested, balanced protein; essential fatty acids; and the vitamins and minerals that both support energy metabolism and correct deficiencies that may result from maldigestion. They also contain full-spectrum antioxidants and a complete complement of B vitamins essential for intestinal and liver energy production. They do not contain enzymes and probiotics. (See Sources for listing of these products.)

These formulas are designed to help support the body's enzymatic processing and elimination of toxic substances. They compensate for nutrient deficits resulting from maldigestion and malabsorption, protect against free radicals associated with detoxification, and help sustain tissue rebuilding. They help detoxify by removing waste, but do not allow the release of fat-stored chemicals. Detoxification methods must be used to cause the release of stored chemicals.

Nutrients for Organ Support

The preceding discussion of nutrients makes obvious to all of us just how important they are to our health, not only for detoxification, but also for the total healthy functioning of our bodies. Each nutrient has specific roles to play in our metabolism, and many of them have effects on our organs.

The chart on the following pages will allow you to determine the nutrients that affect the organs of primary importance in detoxification. as you undertake cleansing and strengthening these organs, be certain you are supplying them with optimal amounts of the needed nutrients. Use nutritional supplements if your diet alone is not sufficient to supply the needed quantities. (See chapter 31 for information on organ cleansing.

Nutrients for Cleansing and Strengthening Organs

ORGAN AFFECTED	NUTRIENT	ACTION
Liver	Vitamin B complex	All B vitamins are essential for normal liver function.
	Vitamin E	Powerful antioxidant, protects liver from damage
	Zinc	Protects liver from chemical damage
	Amino acids	Necessary for liver function
	L-carnitine	Helps prevent accumulation of fat in liver
	Coenzyme Q_{10}	Supplies oxygen to the liver, potent liver protector
	L-cysteine	Detoxifies liver toxins and protects glutathione, prevents accumulation of fat in the liver
	Essential fatty acids	Combat inflammation of the liver, lower serum fats
	Glutathione	Protects the liver
	Lecithin	Protects cells of the liver, aids in preventing fatty liver
	L-lysine	Protects the liver
	L-methionine	Detoxifies liver toxins and protects glutathione, prevents accumulation of fat in the liver
	Phosphatidyl choline	Prevents fatty buildup, important for energy production in the liver
	SOD	Helpful in liver disorders
	Taurine	Antioxidant, protects against free radicals
Colon/ intestines	Vitamin A	Protects and heals the lining of the colon
	Vitamin B complex	Needed for proper muscle tone of the intestines
	Vitamin C	Needed for healing intestines
	Vitamin E	Protects cell membranes that line the colon wall

ORGAN AFFECTED	NUTRIENT	ACTION
Colon (cont.)	Calcium	Aids in preventing colon cancer
	Magnesium	Works with calcium, aids in preventing colon cancer
	Zinc	Aids in repair of intestinal tissue
	Acidophilus	Needed for digestion and manufacture of B vitamins
	Amino acids	Necessary for repair of mucous membranes of the intestine
	Enzymes	Prevent leaky gut and reduce inflammation
	L-glutamine	Major metabolic fuel for intestinal cells, maintains villi (the absorptive surfaces)
	Primrose oil or flaxseed oil	Supplies essential fatty acid, to protect the intestinal lining
Kidneys	Vitamin A	Promotes healing of the urinary tract lining
	Vitamin C	Acidifies urine, which helps prevent stone formation
	Vitamin E	A powerful antioxidant
	Magnesium	Can lower urinary oxalate, a mineral common in kidney stones
	Potassium	Acts as a kidney stimulant
	Zinc	Inhibitor of crystallization, which can lead to stone formation
	L-arginine	Aids kidney disorders
	L-methionine	Reduces kidney stones by destroying free radicals, improves kidney circulation
Lungs	Vitamin A	Needed for repair of lung tissue
	Beta-carotene	Needed for protection and repair of lung tissue
	Vitamin B$_{12}$	Decreases inflammation of lungs
	Vitamin C	Needed to protect lung tissue and fight infection, aids in healing of inflamed tissue

ORGAN AFFECTED	NUTRIENT	ACTION
Lungs (cont.)	Vitamin D	Needed for tissue repair
	Vitamin E	Oxygen carrier, potent antioxidant; deficiency leads to destruction of cell membranes
	Calcium	May increase vital capacity of the lungs, has a dilating effect on bronchial muscles
	Magnesium	Works with calcium
	Selenium	Destroyer of free radicals created from air pollutants
	Amino acids	Important for repair of lung tissue
	Coenzyme Q_{10}	Powerful antioxidant, enhances oxygen in the lungs, improves circulation and breathing
	Enzymes	Keep infections in check by cleansing the lungs, reduce inflammation
	L-cysteine	Aids in repair of lung tissue and reduces inflammation
	L-methionine	Aids in repair of lung tissue and reduces inflammation
	Proantho-cyanidins	Powerful antioxidant and anti-inflammatory
	Quercetin	Antihistaminic effect, stabilizes cells to stop inflammation
	Selenium	Powerful antioxidant
	Zinc	Needed for tissue repair
Skin	Vitamin A	Strengthens skin tissues, needed for healing of skin tissue
	Vitamin B complex	Important for healthy skin tone, improves blood flow to skin surface
	Vitamin C	Necessary for collagen production, strengthens capillaries that feed skin
	Vitamin D	Promotes healing and tissue repair

ORGAN AFFECTED	NUTRIENT	ACTION
Skin (cont.)	Vitamin E	Aids in healing of skin and prevention of scarring, protects against free radicals
	Chromium	Aids in reducing infections of the skin
	Potassium	Deficiency associated with acne
	Selenium	Encourages skin elasticity, powerful antioxidant, protects against ultraviolet damage
	Zinc	Aids in healing of tissues, helps to prevent scarring, necessary for oil-producing glands of the skin
	L-cysteine	Sulfur content needed for healthy skin
	Essential fatty acids	Needed to keep skin smooth and soft, repairs damaged skin cells, dissolves fatty deposits that block pores
	Proantho-cyanidins	Free radical scavengers, strengthen collagen
	SOD	Free radical destroyer, helpful for age spots
Lymph	Vitamin A	Supports tissue, including lymph tissue
	Beta-carotene	Converts to vitamin A, neutralizes free radicals
	Vitamin B complex	Increases efficiency of lymph system, activates many enzymes needed for healing
	Vitamin C	Tissue growth and repair, attacks free radicals in biologic fluids
	Vitamin E	Necessary for tissue repair, works synergistically with vitamin C, prevents cell damage
	Iron	Essential for catalase, an enzyme in white blood cells
	Selenium	Protects immune system, aids in production of antibodies, an antioxidant
	Zinc	Essential for immune system and white blood cells, which circulate in the lymph
	Bioflavonoids	Essential to connective tissue

ORGAN AFFECTED	NUTRIENT	ACTION
Blood	Vitamin B_5	Important in red blood cell production
	Vitamin B_{12}	Essential for red blood cell formation
	Folic acid	Needed for red blood cell formation
	Vitamin C	Important in iron absorption, helps prevent blood clotting
	Vitamin E	Important for red blood cell survival, prolongs life span of red blood cells
	Calcium	Essential in blood thickness
	Copper	Needed in red blood cell production
	Iron	In hemoglobin of red blood cells
	Magnesium	Works with calcium, strengthens heart beat
	Coenzyme Q_{10}	Improves oxygenation

CHAPTER 24

Diet, Fasting, and Juicing

THE "D" IN DIET can remind us that diet is a very important part of detoxification. The two "d's" are intertwined. What we eat can make and keep us healthy, but it can also help us detoxify. The body cannot detoxify xenobiotics (foreign chemicals) if we are constantly adding to our toxic burden with the foods we consume. The body also cannot detoxify if it does not have the proper "fuel" and energy. The detoxification processes in the body require large amounts of energy, and this energy comes from the nutrients in the food we eat. If we eliminate foods that contribute to our toxicity and eat those that help cleanse the body, our health will improve.

In this chapter, diet and its connection to detoxification and the maintenance of health will be discussed. This knowledge will help you to plan a clean diet for your detoxification program and to improve and maintain your health. (For information on healthy ways to prepare foods, see chapter 35, Food and Water, in Part VII, Prevention.)

Diet

Diet directly affects the ability of the body to detoxify.

- High protein intake enhances the removal of xenobiotics, while a protein deficiency lowers glutathione levels and reduces Phase II conjugation by the gluthathione pathway. (See chapter 5, Phases of Detoxification.)

- Low carbohydrate intake decreases the rate of cytochrome P-450 activity in the liver. The best form of carbohydrate for a detoxification program is a complex carbohydrate that is not readily absorbed and does not ferment in the intestines.

- Fatty acids work with carbohydrates to support the energy requirements for detoxification. Fatty acids that do not increase blood fat levels increase liver energy production. The liver can digest, assimilate, and oxidize triglycerides (a compound composed of glycerine and fatty acids) as a source of metabolic energy. Increasing liver energy levels increases detoxification.

Washing Produce

Wash fresh produce in water to which salt, Clorox bleach (this brand only because other brands contain contaminates), Neo-Life Green soap or Nature Clean Fruit and Veggie Wash (see Sources), or diluted 35 percent food-grade hydrogen peroxide (see chapter 26, Breathing and Oxygen) has been added to help kill parasites and microorganisms and remove any pesticides and other unwanted residues.

Use 1 Tbsp. of salt to every 5 cups of water; ½ tsp. of Clorox to a gallon of water; 1 tsp. of NeoLife Green to a quart of water;

1 ounce of Nature Clean to a gallon of water; or 1 ounce of 35 percent hydrogen peroxide to a gallon of water. Allow produce to soak in one of these solutions for 15 to 30 minutes, then rinse well and follow with two 30-minute plain water soaks. With hydrogen peroxide, it is not necessary to leave the food to soak or to rinse it afterward. Dry the produce, and either store or cook it.

Always discard the outer leaves of leafy vegetables, as it is impossible to remove all pesticide and fertilizer residues from them. Peel fruits and vegetables, especially if they are not organic and are waxed.

If you have food allergies, you will need to address this problem, because allergenic substances slow down detoxification processes. In chapter 13, Food, both food allergies and possible toxins in foods were discussed.

▮▮ MAKING HEALTHY FOOD CHOICES

For detoxification and to enjoy optimum health, incorporate the practices shown in the chart on the following page into your daily eating habits. In addition, it is important to eat in a relaxed atmosphere, sitting down, rather than on the go. Never eat when you are upset or right after you have exercised. Be sure to read labels; you will be amazed at what food processors are putting in your food!

It is important to eat a variety of pure, clean, quality foods. Eating the same foods day after day predisposes people to develop allergies to those foods, as well as taxing their enzyme systems.

Unless you have colitis or a digestive problem that prevents you from doing so, eat some raw foods daily to increase your enzyme intake. Chew your food well, including a moderate amount of liquids so that your saliva, which contains the first digestive enzymes, is mixed well with your food.

▮ FRUITS AND VEGETABLES

Fresh fruits and vegetables contain no additives and more nutrition than frozen or canned foods. Frozen foods are purer than canned, although both contain some additives. More vitamins and minerals are retained in fresh and frozen foods than in canned foods.

Natural whole foods are less contami-

Diet Tips for Detoxification and Health

AVOID	CHOOSE
All refined sugar and any food or mixtures that contain refined sugar, including sucrose, dextrose, corn syrup, brown sugar, turbinado, nutritive corn sweetener	Unsweetened foods or foods sweetened with fruit juices, limited amounts of honey, herbal sweetener, stevia
Caffeine in regular coffee and tea, dark and other carbonated drinks, chocolate, cocoa and aspirin compounds	Water, unsweetened fruit juices, some herbal teas, roasted grain coffee substitutes; carob; white willow bark
Soft drinks and fruit-flavored drinks	Unsweetened fruit juices, sparkling water
Alcohol in all forms	Sparkling water with a twist of lemon or lime
High salt intake	Season with herbs and spices; cut salt use in half
Artificial sweeteners, colors, flavors	Natural whole foods, free of any type of additive
Chemical additives and preservatives, including MSG (monosodium glutamate), BHA, BHT, nitrates, nitrites	Only foods that will spoil and eat them before they do; this also avoids micro-organisms and enzyme changes that accompany food spoilage
Processed foods and mixes	Natural whole foods, fresh foods instead of frozen, frozen instead of canned
Refined carbohydrates, such as white flour and white rice	Whole grains, flour ground from whole grains
Fruits and vegetables that have been waxed, sprayed, fumigated, or dyed	Organically grown fruits and vegetables
Saturated fats and artificial fats	Healthy forms of fats and oils such as expeller-pressed, cold-pressed, or unrefined
Fried foods and overconsumption of fat	Low-fat meals; broil, bake, steam, or stirfry food
Processed meats containing fillers, sandwich meats, reconstituted meats	Good-quality meats and poultry free of antibiotics, hormones, and drugs

nated than processed foods and are a good source of fiber. Natural whole foods should be eaten raw when possible, as cooking destroys vitamins, enzymes, and some minerals. Foods high in fiber, such as oat bran and all beans, are effective for lowering cholesterol levels. They also aid digestion, and reduce the risk of some cancers and heart disease.

Whenever possible, eat organically grown fruits and vegetables, which are usually picked ripe and have not lost their nutrients from artificial ripening and prolonged storage. They contain the enzymes necessary for their digestion and none of the harmful chemicals found in pesticides and chemical fertilizers. (See chapter 13, Food, for detailed discussions of pesticides and chemicals in food, as well as genetically modified foods.)

Eat whole vegetables and fruit instead of juices. The whole foods contain natural enzyme activity that helps with digestion and they provide adequate fiber. They also provide healthful snacks containing vitamins that help the body effectively use other nutrients. However, fruit juices are preferable to soft drinks or fruit-flavored drinks. Fruit juices contain more vitamins, less sugar, and contain no chemicals or synthetic ingredients.

■ MEATS, POULTRY, AND FISH

Meat, poultry, and fish provide protein for the growth and repair of body tissue and for the structure of body cells. Good-quality meats and poultry should be free of antibiotics, hormones, and drugs that are given to animals to increase their weight and rate of growth. (For further information, see chap-

ter 13, Food.) They should be from animals fed good-quality grains that are not contaminated with pesticides and other chemicals. Be wary of buying meat from animals that have been given "protein feed," prepared from slaughterhouse scraps. This practice may have led to "mad cow" disease. (For further information, see Microorganisms in chapter 13, Food.)

Fresh fish should have been caught in water uncontaminated by industrial waste. It should have no bruises or signs of drying and should be rinsed before use, as many fish are dipped in a formaldehyde solution to preserve them.

■ CARBOHYDRATES

Refined carbohydrates, such as most white rice and white flour, lack fiber and nutrition, contain chemical residues, and have been bleached. Whole grains and unprocessed products from whole grains contain fiber, vitamins, and minerals needed for enzyme formation and cell repair, and are a rich source of starch, the highest-quality complex carbohydrate.

■ FATS

Saturated fat and overconsumption of fat contributes to obesity, heart disease, hypertension, atherosclerosis, and cancer. If the fat is from an animal source, it may contain a high percentage of environmental toxins and drugs. Frying foods contributes to the overconsumption of fat, destroys the nutritive value of oil, and alters its chemical structure. It oxidizes all types of fats that can then cause damage to tissues, including blood vessels and interstitial tissue.

Low-fat meals counter obesity and high cholesterol levels, and may protect against heart disease and cancer. Healthy forms of fats and oils, such as expeller-pressed, cold-pressed, or unrefined, are a concentrated source of energy. They are also a source of essential fatty acids and provide transport and absorption of fat-soluble vitamins by the body cells.

Artificial fat has been produced in recent years in an attempt to help people lower their fat intake. Marketed as olestra, it has no calories, but may cause abdominal cramping and loose stools. It can inhibit the absorption of vitamins A, D, E, and K, and beta-carotene and other carotinoids. The long-term effects of consuming this substance are unknown.

■ SUGAR

To avoid sugar, you must remember that any word that ends in "ose" is a sugar. Refined sugar disturbs glucose metabolism leading to hypoglycemia, carbohydrate imbalance, and elevated cholesterol, blood pressure, and triglyceride levels. It is addictive, causing craving of sweets, has no nutritive value other than calories, and causes obesity and increased risk of diseases such as diabetes and cancer. Sugar causes tooth decay, creates an added load for the pancreas and adrenal glands, and contributes to yeast overgrowth and bowel dysbiosis.

Hyperactivity, irritability, mood swings, depression, and anxiety can be traced to high sugar intake, and it depletes minerals, B vitamins, and vitamin C. Sugar also interferes with white cell immune function, weakens muscles, and contributes to fatigue.

■ SALT

High salt intake is an acquired taste and can create an imbalance with potassium metab-olism. It is linked to high blood pressure, which can lead to stroke or heart attack if a person is salt-sensitive.

■ FOOD ADDITIVES AND
  TREATMENTS

Artificial sweeteners, colors, and flavors damage cells and can be carcinogenic. They are chemicals and not food, thus are non-nutritional and can cause allergic reactions. Chemical additives and preservatives, including MSG (monosodium glutamate), BHA, BHT, nitrates, and nitrites damage cells and can be carcinogenic. MSG can increase the likelihood of high blood pressure. In addition to affecting liver and kidney function, BHA and BHT are allergenic.

Processed foods and mixes contain chemicals and toxins added as preservatives and stabilizers. They may also contain artificial or imitation flavors that are chemical and non-nutritive, as well as being high in salt and sugar, and low in nutrition. They are likely to contain several common food allergens. Processed foods and mixes frequently contain chemicals that have leached into the food from the packaging material and may be contaminated from processing, packing, and storage.

Fruits and vegetables that have been waxed, sprayed, fumigated, or dyed contain toxic chemicals that may be carcinogenic. Those that are waxed are permanently covered with insoluble waxes and oils that can seal in pesticide residues. Dyes color foods permanently and some dyes can be allergenic and carcinogenic.

■ CAFFEINE

Caffeine has numerous adverse effects on the body, and it is addictive. Caffeine disturbs glucose metabolism and elevates blood sugar levels, contributing to hypoglycemia and diabetes. It disrupts liver and endocrine gland function and exhausts adrenal glands, causing fatigue. Caffeine causes headaches when stopped suddenly and can cause morning headaches that are relieved by a dose of caffeine. It causes nervousness, irritability, loss of sleep, and can cause heart rhythm disturbances and palpitations. It may exacerbate the symptoms of PMS.

In addition to contributing to fibrocystic breast disease, caffeine weakens muscle and interferes with immune function, affecting allergies. It increases the production of stomach acid and can aggravate ulcers. Increased triglycerides, cholesterol, and blood pressure are often seen with caffeine consumption, and it constricts blood vessels and causes cell degeneration.

Consumption of caffeine causes the body to demand extra minerals, particularly potassium, and interferes with mineral absorption. An increased incidence of some cancers, including bladder, pancreatic, and ovarian cancers, is related to caffeine intake.

■ ALCOHOL

Alcohol is addictive, high in calories, low in nutrition, and contains additives. It slows fat metabolism, causing fat buildup in the liver, and increases blood pressure, triglyceride, and cholesterol levels. It has a toxic effect on the liver during its metabolism and predisposes alcohol users to cirrhosis. Alcohol interferes with glucose metabolism and predisposes people to hypoglycemia. It depletes B vitamins and vitamin C and demands extra minerals, especially zinc, magnesium, and manganese.

Alcohol causes fatigue and weakened muscles, can predispose to chronic fatigue and adrenal insufficiency, and lowers immune function. Gastrointestinal problems, including gastritis, abdominal pain, ulcers, deficiency of hydrochloric acid and digestive enzymes, as well as a predisposition to headaches, occur with alcohol consumption. It is notorious for reducing sexual performance and causing impotency. Alcohol also causes degeneration and cell death and has been implicated in malignancies of the mouth.

■ WATER

Drink primarily pure, tolerated water. Juices, sodas, teas, milk, and coffee are not a substitute for water. If you are dehydrated, metabolism slows down and hampers the function of cells and organs. Dehydration also inhibits the removal of toxins and old cells, and healing.

The following formula can be used to calculate the minimum amount of water needed to maintain health. (People undergoing detoxification procedures should drink at least one or two extra glasses of water per day.) Body weight (in pounds) ÷ 2 = ounces of water to be consumed in a day. For example, 120 pounds ÷ 2 = 60 ounces of water or seven and a half to eight, 8-ounce glasses of water per day.

Macrobiotics

A macrobiotic diet is a very helpful detoxification aid for some people. George Ohsawa coined the term macrobiotics in California in the 1920s. Today, there are two main schools of macrobiotics—those of Michio and Aveline Kushi in Boston, and Herman and Cornellia Aihara in northern California.

Macrobiotic Detoxification

On a macrobiotic diet, people will have periodic discharges of old diseased cells and tissue, chemicals, drugs, and mucus that have accumulated in the body and are being eliminated. People often taste and smell chemicals and drugs to which they have been exposed. One woman excreted hair dye that she had absorbed through her scalp.

The macrobiotic program is more than just a diet; it involves a whole lifestyle.

The underlying principle of the macrobiotic diet is called "the order of the universe," and relates to the way in which food can affect our mind and body. There must be a balance between yin, which is female and represents contractiveness, and yang, which is male and represents expansiveness. Any food can be yin or yang, depending on its properties compared to other foods. External conditions, such as season, and a food's size and age, also determine whether it is yin or yang. By eating the proper food, people can achieve an internal balance between yin and yang.

The macrobiotic diet stresses eating foods grown in the same conditions as those in which one lives, and eating as much native food in its natural season as possible. For example, people who live in the northern United States and Canada should not eat oranges, and bananas are not recommended for anyone in Canada or the U.S. Eating nonnative foods may cause imbalances in the body, resulting in colds or flu.

The macrobiotic diet consists of 50 to 60 percent whole grains, 20 to 30 percent locally grown vegetables, 5 to 10 percent beans and sea vegetables, 5 to 10 percent soups, and 5 percent condiments and other foods, including fish occasionally, if desired. The macrobiotic diet is made of whole foods that are eaten raw in small quantities, or boiled, sautéed with oil, or steamed to preserve nutrients. Highly processed foods, sugar, commercial table salt, dairy products, red meat, and poultry are avoided in the macrobiotic diet. The macrobiotic diet is balanced and contains more vitamins, minerals, amino acids, and essential fatty acids than the standard North American diet. On the macrobiotic diet, the body does not have to work at balancing or buffering foods and can spend this energy detoxifying and healing.

Dr. Sherry Rogers, of the Northeast Center for Environmental Medicine in Syracuse, New York, has found that many people with severe chemical toxicity have healed and detoxified on a macrobiotic diet. They were able to correct vitamin and mineral deficiencies and gradually became more chemically tolerant. Sea vegetables (seaweed) contain many minerals that help the body rid itself of toxic metals, such as lead and mercury. A macrobiotic diet promotes slow and gentle healing; it may take a year or more for people on a macrobiotic diet to heal totally.

Macrobiotic diets must be tailored precisely to each person. If you are considering starting a macrobiotic diet, you should see a macrobiotic counselor. There are also many helpful books on macrobiotic ways to prepare and cook foods. The macrobiotic program also includes massage, body scrubs with a hot ginger-soaked towel, deep breathing exercises with yoga and meditation, and exercise. Walking outside in bare feet, wearing cotton clothing, thinking calming thoughts, and doing meridian stretches (see Meridian Bodywork in chapter 25, Exercise and Bodywork) are other parts of the program.

Diet Tips for Specific Health Conditions

Diet is the most important treatment for many health problems. Proper diet can heal people without the aid of pharmaceuticals, which add to the toxic burden. The diets and diet tips below are healing and detoxifying for some of the toxins discussed in chapters 19 and 20.

■■ METABOLIC WASTE PRODUCTS

The waste products from body metabolism become toxins when the body cannot or does not excrete them properly. (For more information on waste products, see chapter 20, Toxins Produced in the Body.)

■ AMMONIA/AMMONIUM EXCESS

A low-protein diet, of 1 gram per kilogram of body weight for adults and 1.5 grams per kilogram of body weight for children, will aid in reducing ammonia excess. Protein is more easily utilized as free-form amino acids. Good protein sources include beans, lentils, millet, peas, soybeans, and whole grains. Animal protein should be avoided or limited, as it puts stress on the kidneys.

■ URIC ACID EXCESS

Gout, the condition that results from the crystallization of the waste product uric acid in the joints, can be helped with diet. Eat raw fruits and vegetables for two weeks when an attack strikes. Cherries and strawberries neutralize uric acid. Eat grains, seeds, and nuts, and drink as much tolerated water as possible.

Avoid purine foods that contribute to uric acid formation, including asparagus, mushrooms, consommé, anchovies, herring, mussels, sardines, meat gravies and broths, and sweetbreads. Do not eat meat, fried foods, roasted nuts, cakes, pies, white flour, or sugar. Avoid alcohol and limit caffeine, dried beans, lentils, fish, eggs, poultry, oatmeal, peas, cauliflower, spinach, and yeast products.

■ CREATININE EXCESS

High levels of creatinine, the end product of muscle metabolism, in urine indicate kidney problems. Diet can reduce stress on the kidney, helping it to heal, and eventually helping to lower these levels. A diet of approximately 75 percent raw foods (especially asparagus, bananas, celery, cucumbers, garlic, papaya, parsley, potatoes, watercress), as well as sprouts, most green vegetables, watermelon, and pumpkin seeds is beneficial. Watermelon should be eaten separately to speed its movement through the system, preventing the formation of toxins. Legumes, seeds, and soybeans contain arginine, an amino acid helpful to the kidney.

Reduce your intake of potassium and phosphates and do not use salt or salt substitutes. Avoid chocolate, cocoa, tea, eggs, fish, meat, beet greens, spinach, rhubarb, and Swiss chard. Reduce or eliminate animal protein. Beans, lentils, millet, peas, soybeans, and whole grains are good sources of protein, and the use of a free-form amino acid supplement can be helpful. Avoid dairy products unless they are soured, such as buttermilk, cottage cheese, or low-fat yogurt.

■■ HORMONES AND NEUROTRANSMITTERS

■ MENOPAUSE AND ESTROGEN

A common imbalance problem occurs as women's estrogen levels decline with age. Changes in diet can provide estrogenic effects so that estrogen hormone replacement therapy is not necessary.

Plant estrogens, called phytoestrogens, isoflavones, or lignans can provide estrogenic effects without increasing the risk of breast cancer. Soy and flaxseed contain larger quantities of plant estrogens than other foods. Three to eight servings of soy and/or flaxseed daily reduce menopausal symptoms, decrease the risk of breast cancer, lower cholesterol levels, and approximate a "bone-protective dose" of pharmaceutical estrogen.

Many recipes utilize soy and flaxseed, including snack bars, trail mix, shakes, cakes, cereals, main dishes, soups, vegetables, pancakes, blintzes, crepes, dips, pâtés, and desserts. Obtaining phytoestrogens from the diet does not mean a sacrifice and can be an adventure in taste.

Other dietary measures help alleviate menopausal symptoms. Because sugar, caffeine, and alcohol can make mood swings worse and trigger hot flashes, eat a diet high in complex carbohydrates and low in fat. Avoid dairy products, as both dairy and meat promote hot flashes and can contribute to loss of bone calcium. Blackstrap molasses, broccoli, dandelion greens, kelp, salmon

> ## Soy Equivalents
>
> *One portion of soy equals:*
> - *1/3 cup soybeans*
> - *1/3 cup dry-roasted soy nuts*
> - *1 cup of soy milk*
> - *¼ cake tofu*
> - *1 soyburger*
> - *¼ cup texturized vegetable protein (TVP)*
> - *2 soy hot dogs*
> - *½ cup soy flour*
>
> *One Tbsp. of flaxseed is approximately equal to a portion of soy.*

with bones, and sardines are sources of natural calcium. Seeds and nuts provide essential fatty acids.

■ HYPERINSULINEMIA

Hyperinsulinemia is an emerging problem that appears to be rampant in North America. Insulin is a hormone that can become a toxin when levels are too high. When we eat, our pancreas releases insulin, which attaches to our cells so that sugar can enter the cells. Insulin levels drop when insulin attaches to the cells and triggers the brain to release a neurotransmitter, serotonin, which signals us that we are full.

Some people either do not have enough insulin receptor sites or their cells are insulin-resistant and the insulin cannot attach. As a result, the circulating insulin levels in their blood are too high, and serotonin is not released, so that the person always feels hungry.

Both insulin and serotonin levels can be controlled with diet. An insulin-control diet also helps control serotonin because of their interaction. An insulin-control diet involves eating more protein than carbohydrates and fats. Most of these diets call for 2 to 5 ounces of protein per meal. The amount of carbohydrates and fats consumed are regulated in order to control insulin release. Several successful insulin-control diets have been formulated, each with a slightly different approach to controlling insulin release. Hyperinsulinemia and these diets are discussed in detail in *Finding the Right Treatment* by Jacqueline Krohn and Frances Taylor.

■■ ACID/ALKALINE BALANCE

Dietary habits can dramatically change tissue acid/alkali balance. Incorporate the following items into your dietary habits to maintain a balanced digestive system.

- Chew food until you can feel the saliva begin to break up the foods.
- Drink minimally with meals and do not use liquid to wash down partially chewed foods.
- Avoid foods with high toxic residues. Unless they are organic, animal and dairy products contain the most toxins. Fruits, vegetables, nuts, seeds, and grains contain the least.
- Eat preservative-free, high-quality foods.
- Eat a variety of foods and rotate them if you have food allergies.
- Eat in moderation. Any food or drink in excess affects the balance of the body.
- Eat only a few foods in one meal. Eating many varieties of food in the same meal taxes the enzymes needed for digestion.
- Eat fruit before noon to avoid fermentation problems.

■ ACID IMBALANCE

The diet presented in the chart on the following page will reduce tissue acidity and can change the tissue acid/alkali balance by as much as 85 percent. However, it is not for everyone. People with hyperinsulinemia may not do well on this diet.

At breakfast, eat only grains. At lunch, eat only grains and steamed vegetables. At dinner, you may eat grains, steamed vegetables, and limited amounts of fish and chicken.

Avoid the following foods while deacidifying the tissues:
- milk and cheese
- red meats, particularly pork; it requires six hours to pass through the stomach and is full of homotoxins, which are very similar to human tissue
- peanuts and peanut butter
- bread and white flour
- sugars, except very limited amounts of honey or pure maple syrup
- tea, coffee, and alcohol
- fried food of any kind
- citrus fruits, except lemon
- raw vegetables, as they further inflame the digestive system.

After the tissue pH has normalized, as determined by checking the blood, urine, and saliva pH, protein foods such as beans and legumes can be added. This is usually possible after 21 days.

■ ALKALINE IMBALANCE

Although it is less common, the body can become too alkaline. Consuming more acid-forming foods helps bring the pH of the body back into the normal range.

Low-level acid-forming and low-level al-

Diet to Reduce Excess Acidity

FOODS	PREPARATION
Steamed vegetables	All vegetables you can tolerate. Do not use aluminum or the microwave to prepare your vegetables. Drink the broth from the steamer seasoned with a little sea salt at 11 AM Sip slowly.
Grains	One to two cups of cooked millet, brown rice, quinoa, or amaranth per day. You may also eat rice crisps or rye crackers containing only rye and water. Avoid oats (acidic), corn in any form (too difficult to digest), and wheat.
Fish	Poached, baked, steamed, or broiled deep-sea fish. Do not eat shellfish.
Chicken	Baked, broiled, or steamed; white meat only, with the skin removed.
Butter	Mix butter with equal parts of a cold-pressed oil.
Lemon	One lemon squeezed into 1 quart of water daily. Sip throughout the day so that you finish the quart before bedtime. Lemon will increase or decrease the body pH, depending on the need.
Water	Pure tolerated water is a must for everyone, regardless of health status. The pH of the water should be between 6.7 and 7 (this can be determined using pH paper).
Limited herbal teas	Consume in the evening in small sips.

kaline-forming foods are almost neutral and have very little effect on changing the pH of the body. Citrus fruits would seem to be acid-forming foods, but in fact their citric acid has an alkalinizing effect on the body.

Alkaline-forming foods are omitted until the pH is normalized. These include avocados, corn, dates, fresh coconut, raisins, most fresh fruits and vegetables, honey, maple syrup, molasses, soy products, and umeboshi plums. Low-level alkaline-forming foods include almonds, Brazil nuts, chestnuts, lima beans, buckwheat, millet, soured dairy products, and blackstrap molasses.

Fasting

Fasting is the deliberate abstention from food, giving the body a rest and freeing the

Diet to Reduce Excess Alkalinity	
FOOD TYPES	SPECIFIC FOODS TO EAT
Acid-forming foods	Asparagus, beans, brussels sprouts, sauerkraut, chickpeas, legumes, lentils, nuts and most seeds, cranberries, prunes, plums, olives, eggs, milk, fish, shellfish, meat, organ meats, poultry, oatmeal, flour and flour-based products, noodles, pasta, cornstarch, cocoa, sugar, all foods with sugar added, catsup, pepper, mustard, alcohol, coffee, tea, soft drinks, vinegar
Low-level acid-forming foods	Butter, cheeses, ice cream, ice milk, dried or sulfured fruit (most), dried coconut, canned or glazed fruit, grains (most), seeds and nuts (most), lamb's quarters (a salad green)

large amounts of energy used by the digestive organs for use elsewhere. It gives the body a chance to reestablish metabolic order and is an extremely rapid method of detoxification. Fasting also helps the body to heal and to resist diseases, infections, and toxins.

Sensible fasting gives the body an opportunity to return to its natural state of homeostasis, or balance. During a fast, toxins are drawn out of the cells and tissues throughout the whole body. Eliminating waste products allows an increase in cellular oxygenation and improves cellular nutrition. The body produces new healthy cells to replace diseased and discarded ones. Conditions that the body could not correct on a normal diet are improved, and the body is cleansed and renewed. Often, however, some type of heat therapy is also necessary, as fasting will not release or remove all of the lipid-soluble toxins in fat tissues. (See chapter 22, Saunas, Baths, and Hydrotherapy, for further information.)

❚❚ BENEFITS OF FASTING

The benefits and healing properties of fasting have been known for centuries. Fasting is mentioned in all ancient medical texts, and Hippocrates prescribed fasting as a means of achieving good health. It has been employed in religious observance both in the past and today. Animals instinctively fast when they are sick or injured. They will ignore available food until their health has improved.

The benefits of fasting are too numerous to list them all; however, the following are the more important benefits. Fasting:
• accelerates the detoxification process.
• cleanses metabolic wastes and toxins.
• cleanses the digestive tract and improves digestion and assimilation.
• increases energy levels.
• rejuvenates the cells and the entire body.
• increases resistance to disease.
• refreshes the mind and spirit.

Many people adopt a schedule of liquids-

Fasting Safety

Most people detoxify adequately by drinking "juices" of fresh fruits and vegetables made in a blender, and herbal teas. These drinks are not true juices because they contain the pulp and fiber from the fruits and vegetables. However, they supply nutrients that support the body while requiring minimal digestion.

Using these substances is safer than a water fast and helps maintain body energy levels. They also stimulate the body to release toxins, produce more thorough detoxification, and allow more rapid recovery.

only one day each week, or liquids-only for a three-day period once each month, for an ongoing healing process rather than postponing action until a health crisis occurs. Although fasting can be done at any time of the year, it is wise to pick a time when you can fit in some extra planning and preparation. While you are fasting, you may feel colder than you normally do, so winter may prove to be an uncomfortable time to fast.

▌▌CONTRAINDICATIONS TO FASTING

Exercising common sense will prevent problems with fasting. Malnourished and undernourished people should not fast, nor should people with an eating disorder, children, pregnant women, and nursing mothers. People with weak hearts or who have had a recent heart attack, and people with lowered immunity should not fast. Before and after surgery is not a good time to fast. Low blood pressure, anemia, bleeding ulcers, some types of cancer, diabetes, epilepsy, liver and kidney disease, tuberculosis, ulcerative colitis, and gout are all contraindications for fasting.

People with many food allergies should exercise caution and fast only under medical supervision. People are always addicted to the foods to which they are allergic. Because of this allergy/addiction phenomenon, these people can go through severe withdrawal symptoms when they first begin a fast.

▌▌TYPES OF FASTING

Short-term fasting lasts from one to three days. More than three days is considered long-term fasting. While true fasting requires that no food or liquid be consumed, this is not advised because the body adapts by lowering the metabolism and eventually consuming its reserves of fat and lean tissue (muscles, connective tissue, and organs).

The toxins concentrated in our fat cells and organs are released rapidly during a true fast. If detoxification is intense, it can temporarily increase sickness. However, for some people this can be immediately helpful. To avoid problems caused by too-rapid detoxification, most people drink water or unsweetened herbal teas during their fast. More liberal fasting includes drinking the juice of fresh fruit and vegetables as well.

Warning: Do not attempt a long-term fast without medical supervision.

Fasting Support

Attitude is also crucial to fasting, both your own and that of those around you. People who do not understand fasting may have a negative attitude and tell you that you are going to starve to death or ruin your health.

Many people, including your own family and friends, may tease you and try to tempt you. Because aromas of food may be hard to resist, it helps to have an agreement that you do not have to cook or be present when meals are prepared or consumed.

◼◼ PREPARING FOR A FAST

Fasting is more likely to be successful if it is entered into gradually by those new to fasting and those whose health is suffering. A good first step is to remove alcohol, caffeine, and sugar from the diet. Ideally, smokers would stop smoking. Avoiding animal food, such as meats, milk, and eggs, also eases the transition. Eating only fruits and vegetables for several days before beginning the actual fast will allow detoxification to begin more slowly. Some people try several short fasts, before beginning a longer and stricter fast.

◼◼ DURING THE FAST

Do not take vitamins and minerals while fasting, as they can interfere with the cleansing process during fasting. They can stress the digestive system and cause nausea on an empty stomach.

If possible, discontinue any medications you are taking. The body has to expend energy to remove them rather than directing the energy to detoxification. If you are taking prescription medication, check with your physician before beginning a fast.

Be certain to get plenty of rest while you are fasting. However, it is important that you incorporate some type of mild exercise to help keep body fluids circulating, even though your energy levels may be less than normal. Blood and lymph must circulate through the tissues in order to remove toxins. Walking is an excellent exercise during a fast. Some people are able to jog, bicycle, or swim during a fast.

◼◼ FASTING MENUS

When you are fasting, drink at least eight glasses of liquid during the day. Should you decide to do a water fast, use only distilled or filtered water. If you fast for more than two or three days, you should use a mixture of:

2 Tbsp. fresh lemon or lime juice

1 Tbsp. raw honey or unprocessed pure maple syrup

8 ounces filtered or distilled tolerated water

$1/8$ tsp. cayenne pepper (optional)

The lemon or lime juice stimulates liver detoxification, and helps rid tissues of toxins. The honey or syrup provides minimal simple carbohydrates for energy. The cayenne pepper aids digestion and improves circulation. This mixture makes the water taste better as well, because the toxins released in the mouth tend to make water taste a little stale after several days of fasting.

Drink this mixture 6 to 10 times a day, and continue to drink at least four 8-ounce glasses of plain water per day in addition.

If you are using "juices" from fresh fruits and vegetables for your fast, dilute them half and half with distilled water to prevent the digestive process from being overloaded. Either of the drinks below may be used as a fasting drink. Use fresh fruits and vegetables if they are available.

❚ BASIC VEGETABLE DRINK

Chop or grate the following vegetables into 2 quarts of boiling water:

    2 large red potatoes (skins included)
    3 stalks celery
    3 medium beets
    4 carrots

If desired, add any of the following vegetables to those listed above: 1 cup shredded cabbage, 1 turnip, 1 onion, or beet tops from 2 beets.

Season moderately with your favorite herbs. Cover and simmer 45 minutes. When slightly cooled, mix in a blender and drink warm. You may need to add additional water. The consistency should be that of a thin gruel rather than a thick soup.

❚ BASIC GREEN DRINK
  IN A FRUIT BASE

To 8 ounces fresh or unsweetened canned pineapple juice in a blender, add any mixture of the following, as desired. Use fresh ingredients rather than dried, and prepare each serving fresh.

    1 celery stalk with leaves
    radish tops from 5 radishes
    carrot tops from 1 carrot
    1/2 ounce comfrey

    1/2 ounce burdock
    1/2 ounce parsley
    1/2 ounce chard
    1/2 ounce plantain
    1/2 ounce dandelion
    1/2 ounce sprouts
    1/2 ounce marshmallow
    1/2 ounce wheatgrass
    1/2 ounce raspberry leaves

Add ice to the blender if you wish. Blend thoroughly and sip.

❚❚ SYMPTOMS DURING FASTING

Fasting does involve a little discomfort. Your stomach will growl and rumble, and maybe even hurt. This simply means that your stomach is empty. These feelings will pass with time, and sometimes drinking water or juice will satisfy your urge to eat.

During your fast your tongue may become coated, and your breath may become quite strong. The more you detoxify, the worse the coating on your tongue and your breath will become. You may brush your teeth and tongue, but do not use a mouthwash. If you have dentures, continue to wear them to prevent gum shrinkage.

You may also experience increased body odor from the toxins being released through your skin. Do not use cosmetics of any kind, deodorants, or perfumes, but take extra showers, using mild soap. Even your urine may become darker and develop a strong smell, but increasing your water intake will help. Because you are not eating solid food, you may not have bowel movements, but do not take a laxative. If you do have a bowel movement, it may be foul smelling and full of mucus, or stringy or rubbery. This is toxic material from your colon that the fast has forced out of your body.

Because you will be undergoing intense detoxification, during which toxins from past exposures are being released into the bloodstream, you may not feel very well during your fast. Vomiting, nausea, aches, pains, fatigue, nasal discharge, diarrhea, and other symptoms are possible. However, if you continue the fast, these will pass. Remember that if you vomit or have diarrhea, you lose fluid and you must drink more to replace it. Should you begin to have symptoms several days after stopping your fast and being symptom-free, this is a signal that your body is continuing to detoxify.

■■ BREAKING A FAST

An important aspect of fasting is the breaking of it. Even with a short fast, it is best to return gradually to solid foods over three to four days. For longer fasts, the return of hunger signals that it is time to break the fast. Continuing a fast past this time exhausts the reserves of the body and it will begin to break down tissue protein to obtain the energy it needs. Although some people may feel some hunger the entire time they fast, the hunger signaling the need for the fast to end will be more intense and urgent.

When breaking your fast, be careful not to overeat. Always eat lightly and chew foods and liquids well. Chewing stimulates the production of saliva and mixes it with the food or liquid. Eat slowly and do not eat too many different foods at any one meal. Many people are continually hungry for a few days

after a long fast, but this feeling will soon normalize. The menu below is helpful for breaking a fast.

■ FAST-BREAKING MENU

1st day: 1 piece of fruit for breakfast
Vegetable salad for lunch

2nd day: 1 piece of fruit for breakfast
Vegetable salad for lunch
Vegetable soup for dinner
Add 1 more fruit during the day

3rd day: Eat larger portions of fruit and salad for breakfast and lunch
Add nuts and soured milk products (such as yogurt)
Baked potato or squash soup for dinner

4th day: Return to a regular diet on a gradual basis. Add protein-rich foods last. Avoid any food allergens and eat moderate amounts of a variety of foods.

Juicing

Juicing is a detoxification method considered by some to be a fast and by others to be a juice diet. It involves refraining from the use of all other nourishment and drinking fruit and vegetable juices rather than water. It detoxifies more effectively than a water fast, and the juices can be more enjoyable to drink than water.

Easily utilized by the body, juices require minimal digestion, and supply nutrients that support the body while stimulating it to release toxins. In addition, juices contain elements that remove toxins and aid cellular rejuvenation better than water alone. Juice fasting is safer than water fasting, and offers

Blender Drinks and Juice Fasts

A blender will not make true juice because it pulverizes rather than removes the fiber. Even if a juicer is not available to you, fruit and vegetable preparations made in a blender will aid detoxification. A fast using blender preparations is not considered a true "juice fast," however, because the blender does not remove the fiber and pulp.

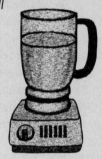

quicker recovery because it supports the body nutritionally during cleansing and maintains energy levels.

Juices are concentrated nutrition. The nutritional part of the plant is separated from the indigestible fiber, and the vitamins and nutrients, including antioxidants, from many fruits or vegetables, are contained within a small volume of liquid. Because juice contains no bulk, it is digested in a short time with no strain on the digestive system. The carbohydrate, protein, and fat in the juice, although in small quantities, supply the body with the energy it needs to carry out daily activities. Even an exercise program can be continued. With a water fast, in contrast, energy levels decrease rapidly without nutrients and the feeling of lethargy makes physical activity difficult. The nutrients in juice supply energy to the detoxification systems and body functions, and pro-

mote cleansing and cellular regeneration.

Juices are prepared from raw fruits and vegetables in a special machine called a juicer. This machine will extract the juice from the fiber. For juices that are high in natural sugar, such as pineapple, apple, grape, and carrot, drinking them without the fiber can cause blood sugar problems for people who are hypoglycemic and hyperinsulinemic.

Vegetable juices are the best rebuilders of cells and fruit juices are the best detoxifiers. You can drink them separately or blended in a mix. For the best results, you must prepare your own juice from fresh, washed organic fruits and vegetables. Commercially prepared juices are not made from quality fruits and vegetables and may contain mold, pesticide residue, and bird and animal droppings. In addition, the enzymes contained in the fresh fruits and vegetables to help you digest them are destroyed in processing.

Not all fruits and vegetables juice well. Bananas and avocados turn into mush and clog a juicer. They can be used in a blender, but result in a thick mixture that will have to be diluted. Apples, apricots, berries, cherries, grapes, mango, melons, papaya, peaches, pears, pineapple, and plums are the best fruits for juicing. Citrus fruits are too acidic for some people, but they may be used sparingly if diluted well.

Many vegetables make good juice, including alfalfa sprouts, asparagus, beets and beet tops, bell peppers, broccoli, brussels sprouts, cabbage, carrots, cauliflower, celery, cucumber, dandelion greens, eggplant, garlic, kale, kohlrabi, lettuce, onions, parsley, parsnips, potatoes, radishes, spinach, Swiss chard, tomatoes, turnips and turnip greens, zucchini, and watercress. Juices made from green vegetables are very high in chlorophyll and are felt by many practitioners to be very healing for blood disorders and the digestive tract.

Juices can be combined to make appealing drinks. However, many fruits and vegetables do not combine palatably. Apples and carrots work well in either fruit or vegetable blends. Very sweet juice mixtures should always be diluted. Vegetable juices can be consumed hot, but some of the nutrients are destroyed.

If you do a juice fast, you should drink between 32 ounces and a maximum of 64 ounces of juice a day, and at least four 8-ounce glasses of water. If the juice has a high sugar content, such as fruit and carrot juices, you may need to limit the amount you drink.

■ GREEN VEGETABLE DRINK

Run the vegetables through your juicer:

2–3 cups of two or three of the following green vegetables: alfalfa sprouts, beet greens, broccoli, chard, kale, parsley, spinach, watercress

3–5 carrots

Most people prefer this blend cold. You may adjust amounts to obtain the quantity of juice that you wish.

Creative Juicing

Juicer combinations are endless and limited only by your creativity. The recipes given here are simply a few suggestions to spark your imagination.

■ HEAVENLY FRUIT BLEND

Put the following fruits through your juicer:

1 bunch unseeded grapes

3 oranges (peeled)

4 lemons (peeled)

Add 1 cup distilled or tolerated water and $1/8$ to $1/4$ cup honey. Increase the amount of water if the juice is too strong.

■ TROPICAL VEGETABLE BLEND

Combine the following in your juicer:

8 small carrots

2 stalks celery

1 cup sliced pineapple

CHAPTER 25

Exercise and Bodywork

Exercise

Exercise? But I can't because:

I'm too tired!

My back/head/feet hurt!

I'm too old to start!

I look bad!

I don't have time!

It won't help!

I don't feel like it!

I get enough exercise at work!

It's too hot/ too cold!

Do any of these excuses sound familiar? We have all used one or more of them to avoid exercise. Some of us may have used all of them—and all on the same day!

Exercise plays an important role in cleansing our bodies. However, we cannot limit exercising to times when we have a problem. It should be a lifelong habit and an enjoyable activity. Lack of exercise allows toxins to build up in our bodies, destroying the balance. Another effect is that calcium leaches from the bones and is excreted in the urine, which can contribute to osteoporosis.

Physical activity stimulates the develop-
ment and maintenance of bone tissue, muscle mass, strength, and endurance. It helps to excrete toxins and restore balance in many body systems. Exercise is a powerful tool for detoxifying the body and improving and maintaining good health.

▮▮ TYPES OF EXERCISE

Many types of exercise can help with detoxification. Pick one that is comfortable for you and that will not be too difficult for you to do or to include in your schedule. For any type of exercise, wear comfortable clothes and shoes that fit and support your body. Shower immediately after exercising so that you do not reabsorb the toxins from your sweat. Wash your clothes as well, to remove toxins; never wear sweat-stained clothes while exercising.

The types of exercise described below do not include every possibility.

▮ AEROBIC EXERCISE

Aerobic exercise is the best type of exercise for your whole body. Brisk walking, running, swimming, cycling, and cross-country skiing are all good forms of aerobic exercise. It should form part of your routine at least three times a week for 10 to 20 minutes at a time. To be aerobic, the exercise must raise your heartbeat to the proper range. However, you should always be able to carry on a conversation while you exercise. If you cannot, you are exercising too hard.

Aerobic exercise will:

• rapidly cleanse chemical toxins from the blood.
• increase oxygen utilization and the function of oxygen-dependent metabolic pathways.
• allow your heart and blood vessels to function more efficiently.
• enhance endocrine function.
• cause a lower resting pulse rate.
• increase your endurance.
• stimulate the production of endorphins, which help to mask pain and bring about a feeling of euphoria.

▌ Walking

Brisk walking is the very best exercise for toning muscles, strengthening bones, and increasing energy. The heart works at a safe "exercising" rate to improve cardiovascular fitness. Walking is a lower impact exercise than running and is easier on the knees and ankles.

A regular walking program will promote cleansing by:

• increasing oxygen uptake.
• improving circulation and muscle tone.
• improving resting and active pulses.
• stimulating elimination.
• making the digestive system healthier.
• promoting weight loss.
• building endurance.

Heart Rate Formula

The formula for determining your proper heart rate is:

Ideal exercise heartbeat rate per minute = 220 minus your age.

This figure multiplied by 0.6 gives the low number for your pulse range. Multiply by 0.85 to get the high number for your pulse range. (For example, if you are 43, your exercise pulse rate should be between 177 × 0.6 and 177 × 0.85, or between 106 and 150.) Any rate between those two numbers is within your target heart rate zone. Moderate aerobic exercise for a longer period of time is more effective than strenuous exercise in short bursts.

• releasing toxins in the sweat and from the lungs.

In addition to its physical benefits, walking aids emotional cleansing. It can reduce anxiety and tension, and even alleviate depression.

If you choose walking for exercise, find a safe place to walk. Pollen-sensitive patients may have difficulty walking in heavily vegetated areas during pollen season. Chemically sensitive patients should find an area away from traffic. If you walk after dark, walk in a well-lit area, both for protection and so you can see obstacles in your path. Wear reflective tape on your shoes and shirt or jacket to make you more visible to motorists.

▌ Running

Running is a popular exercise in North America. Estimates place the number of jog-

Benefits of Exercise

PHYSICAL BENEFITS	MENTAL/EMOTIONAL BENEFITS
• Speeds up removal of toxins and waste materials from the cells	• Improves overall mental health
• Increases blood flow that carries nutrients and oxygen to every cell	• Elevates mood with releases of endorphins
• Increases lymph circulation	• Relieves depression
• Increases levels of high-density lipoprotein (HDL) cholesterol (the "good" cholesterol)	• Increases sense of well-being
	• Improves self-image and self-confidence
• Helps lower blood pressure	• Increased oxygen levels improve mental abilities, learning potential, and cognitive skills
• Helps prevent heart attacks	
• Helps maintain appropriate blood sugar levels	• Improves memory
	• Enhances sense of personal achievement
• Increases body temperature	
• Prevents the formation of gallstones by increasing the solubility of cholesterol in bile	• Improves reaction time
	• Makes the mind more creative and playful
• Restores lung power, endurance, and strength	• Decreases feelings of inertia
• Increases muscle flexibility and strength	• Reduces mental stress
• Improves bone structure and support for the body	• Reduces tension and anxiety
	• Decreases anger and hostility
• Can shorten the duration of an allergic inflammatory cascade	
• Can reverse adult-onset diabetes	
• Aids in weight-reduction programs	

gers at just over 33 million in the United States.

Running:
- increases the elimination of toxins.
- increases oxygenation to cells.
- improves circulation.
- improves lung capacity.
- increases muscle and reduces body fat.
- strengthens legs, muscles, and bones.

If you follow a sensible program, running can be good for you. Even though it is a high-impact exercise, if done properly it usually entails very little risk. You should warm up with gentle stretching exercises before you run to prevent strains and sprains. Warming up causes muscles and tendons to become more flexible and to elongate to accommodate the longer range of motion required for running. Be careful not to overdo the initial stretching to prevent injury.

Watch for warning signs of injury. Pain in the knee, hip, or ankle is a sign that the joint could be injured if it is not rested. Burning pain in muscles while exercising and extended cramping after exercising indicate that the exercise is too strenuous. Take additional nutrients such as magnesium, vitamin C, and coenzyme Q_{10}, wait a few days, then run a shorter distance more slowly. Pain that persists for more than 48 hours should be checked by a physician.

I *Swimming*

Regular long-distance swimming produces the same benefits as running, cycling, or cross-country skiing. You can get into good shape by swimming twice a week for at least 15 minutes each time. The water makes exercise easier, especially for those who are overweight, because the water supports your weight. The water pressure can improve circulation by 25 percent, and painful joints move more easily in water.

Exercise in the pool may be in the form of swimming laps, running, walking, jumping, or using a kickboard. The water acts as a cushion for these activities, absorbing the shock from jumping and providing low-impact exercise. Because water has more resistance than air, walking or running in water makes your leg muscles, heart, and lungs work hard even though your speed will be slower. Water exercise sessions are available at many public pools.

Swimming:
- increases oxygenation to cells.
- improves circulation.
- increases cardiorespiratory endurance.
- improves lung capacity.
- increases muscle strength.
- reduces body fat.

When you use the pool for exercise, there are a few precautions to consider. Either begin your exercise slowly in the water, or do gentle warm-up activities before you get in the water. Wear padded goggles to help protect your eyes. Some swimmers are more comfortable using a nose clip to prevent water from entering the nose. If you are allergic to chlorine, take a chlorine extract before and after swimming (see chapter 27, Allergy Treatment and Chelation), and shower immediately after the swimming session, making sure to shampoo your hair, as well.

I *Cycling*

Bicycle riding is an excellent aerobic exercise and has the added benefit of also being useful for transportation. It is not a weight-

Exercise Injury

Homeopathy offers remedies for injuries and other problems from exercising.
- *Bone pain or injury to the ankle:* Strontium carbonium
- *First-aid remedy, for injury or trauma worse with motion:* Bryonia
- *Muscle soreness after exercise:* Magnesia phosphorica
- *Pain and/or exhaustion after exercise:* Lacticum acidum
- *Pain better with movement, trauma to joints, back pain:* Rhus toxico-dendron
- *Tennis elbow, frozen shoulder, trick knees, or overuse of joints:* Ruta graveolens
- *Tennis elbow, or sore muscles:* Bellis perennis
- *Trauma, sore bruised feeling, or muscle fatigue:* Arnica

Two homeopathic ointments are helpful for exercise injuries:
- *Minor sports injuries, sprains, bruises, and inflammation:* Traumeel®
- *Temporary relief of bruises; minor muscle and joint aches and pains; swelling from minor falls, blows, sprains, and strains; simple headache; sports injury; and overexercising:* Arnica gel®

Aloe vera, an herb, decreases inflammation associated with athletic injuries, such as joint sprains, tendonitis, and blisters.

bearing activity and therefore is less stressful to your joints. Bicycling provides almost as much benefit as walking and jogging. However, since it is not weight bearing, it does not help strengthen bones or prevent osteoporosis.

Cycling:
- increases circulation.
- improves blood transport.
- increases oxygenation to cells.
- increases elimination of toxins.

If you are concerned about air quality in your area, stationary bicycles offer more environmental control than outdoor bicycles. The best stationary bicycles have fan blades in the wheel and handlebars that move. The fan generates the pedaling resistance, and the handlebars exercise your upper body. This type of bicycle offers you the option of exercising your legs or your upper body separately. There are also no pauses in stationary pedaling, as there are when you ride on the street.

▌ Cross-country Skiing

Cross-country skiing is considered to be one of the most complete forms of exercise. Unlike downhill skiing, almost anyone can cross-country ski, as the techniques are quite simple. Because you use both your arms and legs, you receive roughly twice the workout you would walking or running at the same speed. It is good for the heart and lungs, and you avoid the shock and stress to the feet and ankles that are involved in running.

There are exercise machines available that allow the same movements as cross-country skiing, and that can be used indoors all year.

Cross-country skiing:
- improves circulation.
- increases cardiorespiratory endurance.
- oxygenates tissues.
- strengthens muscles.
- increases endurance.
- reduces body fat.
- promotes sweating.

■■ TRADITIONAL CHINESE EXERCISES

Traditional Chinese exercises are commonly used in Asian countries, such as Japan, China, and Korea. They can be an excellent form of exercise, and they emphasize balance, agility, and coordination. While there are several forms of more physically intense exercise, the two that are the most helpful for body balancing and health are Chi Kung and Tai Chi.

■ CHI KUNG (QIGONG)

Chi Kung (pronounced Chee-kung) is a Chinese term applied to exercises that work with the chi, or vital life energy. The common goal of Chi Kung exercises is to stimulate and balance the internal flow of chi along the energy pathways. It is believed that fascia, the most pervasive tissue within the body, is the means by which the chi is distributed along these pathways. The pathways correspond to the well-documented classical acupuncture meridians, which often run parallel to the cardiovascular system.

The unobstructed flow of chi is vital to health. Blockages of chi can cause an overload of the energy system and consequently disease. Sedentary lifestyle, bad posture, toxicity, stress, and many other factors can cause blockages. Chi Kung can help to treat disease and enhance detoxification, but it also teaches people how to remain well.

Chi Kung exercises range from simple, gentle calisthenic-type exercises to very complex exercises where the practitioner manipulates heart rate, brain wave frequency, and other organ functions. It combines movement, deep relaxation, and breathing. When practiced regularly, Chi Kung can aid detoxification, reverse damage from injuries and disease, increase strength and flexibility, promote relaxation and awareness, and instigate and promote healing.

Regular Chi Kung practice can:
- facilitate the free flow of energy throughout the body, promoting blood, lymph, and nerve impulse flow, all of which help detoxification.
- initiate the "relaxation response" that decreases heart rate and blood pressure, dilates the capillaries and optimizes availability of oxygen to the tissues.
- alter the neurochemistry of the body to moderate pain, depression, and the cravings of addiction, as well as increasing immune capability.
- enhance the efficiency of the immune and detoxification systems by increasing the rate and flow of fluid through the lymph system.
- improve resistance to infection and disease by increasing the elimination of toxic metabolic byproducts from the tissues, organs, and glands via the lymph system.
- increase cell metabolism and tissue regeneration through increased oxygen and blood supply to the organs, tissues, and brain.
- coordinate the hemispheres of the brain,

reducing anxiety, promoting deeper sleep, and increasing mental clarity.

• increase mental focus and decrease sympathetic nervous system activity.

• moderate gland and cerebrospinal fluid system of the brain and spinal cord, which mediate pain and mood, and improve and strengthen immune function.

• massage the organs in the abdominal cavity through abdominal breathing, stimulating the stomach and intestines, improving digestion and absorption, and reducing blood congestion in the lower abdomen.

Chi Kung includes a form of meditation, in addition to exercises. Meditation can be done standing, sitting, or lying down. It helps to maintain health and coordinate body, mind, and spirit in a healthy person. In a sick person, meditation mobilizes healing resources. Healing energy is circulated through deep breathing, deep relaxation, intention, and visualization.

■ TAI CHI

Tai Chi is a part of Chinese medicine and philosophy that, in turn, is part of Taoism. Tai Chi was originally designed as a system of self-defense, and intended as exercise that is controlled by the mind. Tai Chi is a series of postures linked with continuous slow, fluid, and graceful movements. Its series of consecutive moves have been described as "meditation in motion" or "swimming in air."

The relaxed style of exercise allows chi to flow to all parts of the body. This flow clears the meridian channels, which connect to the principle organs, improving function. The movements also realign the physical structures of the body, enhancing their function.

Most people view Tai Chi as a mild exercise, but the primary goal of Tai Chi is to achieve health and tranquility while developing the mind through movement. It involves as much time to learn well as other martial arts, such as karate or tae kwon do.

As with Chi Kung, both physical and mental benefits come from practicing Tai Chi. Without changing breathing rhythm or increasing heart activity, Tai Chi:

• increases blood circulation that both nourishes the muscles and helps with detoxification.

• exercises the cardiopulmonary system.

• stimulates glandular activity and the nervous system.

• improves joint movement.

• promotes good posture.

• reduces tension and anxiety.

• enables the mind to function with greater clarity, concentration, and awareness.

Tai Chi has five essential qualities: slowness, lightness, balance, calmness, and clarity. In Tai Chi, the emphasis is on the attention of the mind, combined with the movement and coordination of breath, which guides the physical form.

Should you decide to try Tai Chi, you will be surprised by how easy it is to begin, as well as by the resulting feeling of well-being. In the beginning, it requires no physical strength and is suitable for men and women of all ages and in almost any state of health.

■■ EXERCISE FOR THE ENVIRONMENTALLY ILL

For those who are acutely sick with environmental illness, a limited amount of gentle to moderate exercise will help to alleviate the inflammatory processes of allergic reactions. Too much exercise places an added burden on the adrenal glands, which are already stressed from the allergic state. A five-minute brisk walk or a few minutes on an exercise bicycle can be enough to clear an allergic reaction and provide some detoxification benefits. If you are housebound, you can still achieve aerobic benefits if you walk briskly about a safe room, flail your arms vigorously, or do bicycle exercises.

The advantages of exercise for the sensitive patient are:
- increased oxygen uptake and utilization
- increased blood transport to carry nutrients and oxygen to the cells, and waste products and toxins away from the cells
- increased stimulation of endorphins, for a feeling of well-being

Non-aerobic forms of exercise are also helpful for the environmentally ill person. The stretching forms of yoga, Tai Chi, and Chi Kung all provide gentle exercise that can benefit but not overly stress people with health problems.

Bodywork

Bodywork is a general term describing a group of therapies that are used to correct the structure and improve the function of the human body. These methods all involve the therapeutic use of touch. Touch is a primal need that is as necessary for growth as food, clothing, and shelter. It is the first sense to develop in humans, and may be the last to fade. Infants cannot survive and thrive without touch. Less than 50 years ago, infant mortality was almost 100 percent for infants under one year in United States orphanages.

Touch can be as simple as a hug or a pat on the back, or it can involve massage, acupressure, or therapeutic touch, but it connects us with others, gives us comfort, and helps us to heal. In addition to its direct physical benefits, bodywork can help us to realize that our bodies are living, growing systems that continually change. They are dynamic processes interacting with our physical and emotional environments.

∎∎ BENEFITS OF BODYWORK

To survive and function, every cell must continuously receive nutrients, oxygen, hormones, antibodies, immune modulators, and water. In addition, toxic wastes must be taken away from the cell. Bodywork increases circulation, which facilitates cleansing and the removal of waste material. This cellular cycle of receiving and expelling also involves movement. Through bodywork, lazy muscles are encouraged to work and connective tissue is softened and stretched.

The cleansing action of bodywork:
- improves blood and lymph circulation.
- increases the oxygen supply to cells.
- increases availability of nutrients to cells, muscles, and bones.
- acts as a mechanical cleanser, pushing out wastes.
- promotes elimination of toxic waste.
- relieves congestion and excess fluid in tissues.
- improves liver function, which aids detoxification.
- eliminates waste fluid from muscles.
- balances the nervous system, which affects all body systems.

Bodywork can heal and cleanse on all levels. Touching the body also touches the mind and the emotions. Bodywork gives physical, emotional, and mental benefits. Physical benefits include increased detoxification, a strengthened immune system, improved muscle tone, reduced blood pressure and physical stress, and increased flexibility and movement. Emotional and mental benefits include the reduction of stress and anxiety, improved self-image, and increased ability to concentrate.

❚❚ TYPES OF BODYWORK

All types of bodywork directly affect the nerves, organs, and circulation, and indirectly affect the body as a whole. They have one thing in common—touching the skin, which stimulates the body's natural self-healing abilities. Contact with the skin stimulates specific receptors, resulting in a specific reaction. The exact receptors that are stimulated and the resulting effect depend on the manner of skin contact.

Before beginning bodywork, you and your bodywork practitioner must be aware of your general physical, mental, and emotional condition. Your practitioner also needs to know what medications you are taking or have taken recently. There are many different types of bodywork, varying in vigor and depth. If bodywork is entered into too enthusiastically, it is not uncommon for a person to develop nausea or a headache. Shorter, more frequent sessions may be necessary in order to avoid the effects of too-rapid detoxification. Common sense dictates the appropriate type of therapy. If you are in doubt, be sure to ask questions.

Because of overlapping in techniques, bodywork is difficult to categorize. Only a few of the basic types of bodywork are discussed here. These include:
- soft tissue
- connective tissue–fascia
- meridians
- energy and healing touch

❚ SOFT-TISSUE BODYWORK

There are as many types of soft-tissue bodywork, or massage, as there are nationalities. Soft-tissue massage may range from gentle, nurturing stroking to more vigorous classic Swedish massage. All of the techniques balance the body's energy flow, and help to detoxify and rejuvenate the body.

❚ Swedish Massage

Swedish massage is the most familiar style of soft-tissue bodywork. It involves treatment of the entire external body, except the reproductive organs and body orifices. The person is always draped and may undress to a personally comfortable degree. Oil, powder, or alcohol are often used to help the therapist's hands glide over the skin surface. Swedish massage has a set pattern of stretching the limbs and an active stimulation of skin and soft tissue.

Strokes are rhythmic, follow muscle groups, and always end with stroking toward the heart. The basic strokes include:
- *Effleurage:* gliding across the skin with no attempt to move deep muscles.
- *Petrissage:* gently lifting muscle mass and gently wringing or squeezing it.
- *Friction:* small circular movements that move the tissues under the skin.
- *Tapotement:* gentle tapping that provides contrast and tension release.
- *Vibration:* delicate movement to promote relaxation.

Bodywork Contraindications

Some physical conditions prevent vigorous, stimulating, or deep bodywork. Before beginning bodywork, evaluate your condition and any accompanying problems. If you are under a physician's care, always request an opinion regarding your readiness for bodywork.

As a general rule, do not seek stimulating, vigorous, or deep bodywork if you have a fever, a concussion, an external injury to the skin, a sprain, an incompletely knit broken bone, inflammation, high blood pressure, or circulatory problems. Body-work is not recommended if you are in poor health or extremely weak physical condition, or have an unidentified severe pain.

It also may not be wise to have bodywork when you have recently consumed alcohol or smoked and have either a completely empty or an extremely full stomach. These activities all affect the vascular system. Alcohol is a vasodilator and smoking constricts the blood vessels. When you eat, the blood is diverted from the skin to the digestive system. With an empty stomach, you could become hypoglycemic.

❙ Manual Lymphatic Drainage
Caution: This technique must only be practiced by a completely trained professional.

Developed in the 1930s by Dr. Emil Vodder of Denmark, manual lymphatic drainage (MLD) can be regarded as one of the large-surface massage methods. It moves metabolic waste through the body and accelerates movement of lymphatic fluid. It involves manual techniques that are not used in any other classical form of massage.

In MLD, the skin is always kneaded, never stroked. The technique consists of a combination of round or oval, small or large, and deep or shallow circular movements, all of which knead the skin. The sensitivity and intuition of the practitioner are vital to the length of treatment of a particular body part, the use of pressure, and the speed of movements.

Because the effect of MLD is largely derived from mechanically displacing fluids and any toxic substances they carry, the techniques developed and taught by Vodder must be executed precisely. The amount of pressure used depends on the state of the tissue to be treated; the softer the tissue, the softer the massage. Normally only the skin is moved, as 40 percent of the lymph is within superficial layers.

The basic principles of manual lymphatic drainage are as follows.

• The proximal area (closest to the center of the body) is treated before the distal areas (farther from the center of the body), so that the proximal area is emptied to make room for fluid flowing in from the distal ends.

• The techniques and variations are repeated rhythmically, usually five to seven times, either at the same location in stationary circles or in expanding spirals, following the direction of the muscle fiber.

• As a rule, no reddening of the skin should appear, and MLD should *not* elicit pain.

335

MLD can be used to reduce edema and swelling, move metabolic waste through the body, and promote rapid recovery from illness or disease. Its strength lies in its stimulation of the natural cleansing system of the body, which helps the body rid itself of accumulated toxins.

■ CONNECTIVE TISSUE–FASCIA BODYWORK

In addition to the skeletal system, the other supportive structure in the body is connective tissue, or fascia. It fastens muscles to bones and bones to joints, surrounds every nerve and vessel, holds all internal structures in place, and envelops the body as a whole. Connective tissue has many different shapes and properties. It can be quite diffuse and watery, or it can form a tough, flexible meshwork. Tendons and ligaments have extraordinary tensile strength, superior to steel wire.

Connective tissue has limits on its ability to regenerate and maintain resilient properties. Poor nutrition and sedentary habits weaken all the connective tissues of the body, stiffen them, and can shorten their effectiveness, even in a young adult. Over time, connective tissue may eventually dry and become rigid, restricting the motion of muscles and joints.

Many deep-tissue techniques for manipulating the connective tissue framework have been developed and used with success. Direct pressure and stretching are among the most effective means for increasing energy levels and pliability in all forms of connective tissue. This happens in several ways:

- Warmth from the practitioner's hands contributes some thermal energy.
- Temperature and viscosity far beneath the skin surface are affected by deep manipulation, pressure, motion, and friction.
- Squeezing, stretching, and contorting the connective tissues causes flushing and assists with cleansing.
- Large amounts of toxins and wastes can be moved out of the intercellular fluids and into the bloodstream, where they can be eliminated.

■ Rolfing

One popular connective tissue massage is rolfing, developed by Dr. Ida Rolf, who established the Rolfing Institute in Boulder, Colorado, in 1972. Rolfing addresses the structural properties of connective tissue. Lack of use, misuse, poor postural habits, and chronic strains may cause asymmetries and imbalances. Some connective tissues may thicken and shorten; others weaken and lengthen. Muscle sacs develop excess fiber, and ligaments overextend and cannot support the joints. Sheets of fascia bunch up and become glued to themselves or to their neighbors with hydrogen bonds.

When these various related problems become widespread, a deep-tissue practitioner can rearrange and actually "sculpt" these deformed and glued structures. Rolfers use fingers, knuckles, forearms, elbows, and sometimes even tools to exert pressure or stretching forces on the connective tissue in an effort to energize and reshape it. This pressure and stretching, carefully applied at specific points and in specific directions, softens and lengthens the connective tissues to make them more malleable. The release of thickened and strained areas proceeds systematically, session by session, area by area. The process of rolfing can be somewhat painful if the connective tissue requires extensive reshaping.

The rate of metabolism of the entire body system can be improved with rolfing. A more efficient distribution of weight and a broader range of motion are then possible. Rolfing releases toxins from connective tissue where they are stored when there is insufficient drainage in the body. The rolfing action mobilizes them so that they are accessible to be cleared from the body.

■ MERIDIAN BODYWORK

All living things possess a vital energy. The Chinese call it *chi*, Japanese call it *ki*, East Indians call it *prana*, and Tibetans call it *rlun*. Wilhelm Reich, an Austrian psychoanalyst (1878–1957), called it *orgone*, and today's scientists are calling it bioplasma. It has been described as an electromagnetic energy that influences both the body and the psyche.

Meridians are the pathways along which this vital energy flows. Scientific research has not yet identified a physical phenomenon demonstrating this pathway, but it has been observed that many of the meridian pathways run closely parallel to the pathways of one or more main nerve branches. With slight curves, or brief horizontal jags, meridians move along a vertical plane. The meridians are bilateral, duplicating themselves on each side of the body. Both the vital energy and the circulatory systems of blood and lymph flow through them.

Of the 59 meridians, the 12 organ meridians and two of the extra meridians are most commonly used in treatment. The organ meridians are: lung, large intestine, stomach, spleen, heart, small intestine, urinary bladder, kidney, pericardium (of the cardiovascular system), triple warmer (endocrine system), gallbladder, and liver. The two extra meridians are the governing vessel and the conception vessel. The governing vessel is the confluence of all the yang meridians and it is said to "govern" over them. Stiffness and pain in the spinal column and febrile conditions are associated with obstruction of governing vessel chi. The conception vessel is the confluence of the yin meridians, and symptoms associated with the liver and kidneys result from abnormalities in the chi of this channel.

The organ meridians are named for the organ affected or controlled by the energy flow along that particular meridian. In addition, meridians are classified as either yin, where the energy mainly flows upward, or yang, where the energy mainly flows downward. The terms and concept of yin and yang come from Chinese medicine. Yin is female energy, more passive and receiving; yang is male energy, active, aggressive, and outgoing.

The circulation of energy and nutrients starts at the first organ meridian, the lung, and over a 24-hour period moves through all the meridians. This cycle repeats continuously throughout life. Each meridian has a two-hour interval in which a maximum of vital energy is reached. Each cycle also has a sequential directional flow, moving from a yin meridian to a yang meridian.

If the flow of chi through a meridian is not optimal because the body is toxic, the person will experience symptoms during the two-hour interval when the energy is at its maximum for that meridian. It is a signal

Acupuncture

In addition to its role as an anesthetic for surgery in China, acupuncture has been used successfully for centuries as a preventive form of medicine and to facilitate the body's repair of diseased conditions. In cases of paralysis, acupuncture assists nerves in the affected area to recover their ability to transmit impulses. In organ congestion, stimulation along various points of the meridian allows the organ to receive energy and dispel blockage.

that the organ associated with that particular meridian needs detoxification.

❚ *Acupuncture*

To balance the energy in the body, slim needles are applied to specific points along meridians. By both the placement and the manipulation of the needles (twirling, vibrating, heating, and electric current), the therapist can sedate, stimulate, or tonify (tone). While some people doubt the existence of acupuncture points, they can be scientifically located with electrical measuring devices. The electrical resistance of the skin is consistently lower at acupuncture points.

Treatment is based on the findings from reading the pulses, which are available at the skin level all along the meridians. However, the practitioner usually takes the organ pulses at the wrist to diagnose the condition of the energy flow in the body.

❚ *Moxibustion*

Moxibustion is most often used in conjunction with an acupuncture treatment, but it can be used alone. Moxa is the name given to a smoldering tinder of mugwort leaves and/or root *(Artemesia vulgaris)*. The moxa is prepared, then shaped into either a cone or stick form before use. The stick is usually held above the skin, whereas the cone is usually placed on top of a thin slice of ginger or garlic root, on a thin layer of salt on the skin, or on the top of an acupuncture needle.

The moxa is lit and allowed to smolder until the patient feels the heat to a comfortable level. Pain is *not* a part of the process. The practitioner always monitors the moxibustion process and removes the moxa before the skin starts to blister.

Moxibustion is used to stimulate the flow of energy between yin and yang points of the physical body, and to bring warmth to a cold and/or congested area. The technique allows the heat generated to penetrate the skin and deeper muscle layers. Heat stimulates the acupuncture points and encourages increased circulation and removal of toxins.

❚ *Shiatsu*

Although the roots of Shiatsu can be traced to China some 3,000 years ago, Tokujiro Namikoshi of Japan revived this technique in 1930. Shiatsu is a form of acupressure and has been described as a dance over and along the meridians of the body in order to balance the chi. The practitioner's body weight rather than muscle strength is used to allow the hand and fingers to penetrate into the meridian.

Pressure is applied rhythmically and perpendicularly. The practitioner uses the balls of the fingers and thumbs as well as the base of the thumb. The pressure is varied according to the body part and the condition being addressed. Eleven positions of the hands and fingers can be used. Eight types of pressure can be applied: steady, sustained, graded, concentrated, suction, slowing, vibrational, and palm stimulation.

Giving attention to specific points along a meridian affects various muscles and joints directly. Muscle tension caused by contracted tendons and muscle fibers can be released by stimulating a point along the meridian that is related to the particular muscle or joint. Specific complaints, such as migraine headache, tension headache, nausea, vertigo, stiff neck, sciatica, and many other complaints can be treated by stimulating associated meridian points.

▌ *Reflexology*

In the early 1900s, William H. Fitzgerald, an American physician, rediscovered the centuries-old Chinese method of foot massage, which he called zone therapy. The points used are nerve endings on the feet that correlate to or "reflex" the entire body.

The zones run longitudinally along the foot, with the head, eyes, and ears being mapped on the tip of the big toe, across the tips of the toes to the little toe. Each foot represents one half of the body. The inside of each foot reflexes the spinal column. The soles, upper parts of the foot, and around the heel and ankle all have reflex points to the organs and skeletal structure.

Treatment consists of using the thumbs to apply firm pressure to specific points. Gentle holding and gentle squeezing of the feet before treatment will familiarize the recipient with the touch, as well as warm the tissue that will be massaged. Once the tissue, tendons, and fluids have been warmed, massage becomes more comfortable and effective. Tender areas will indicate where the greatest concentration of time and energy is needed. Pressure should be firm, but *not* painful. Areas of tightness, swelling, or congestion should be gently massaged to relax the muscle, disperse excess fluid, and break up congestion.

Treating the reflex points cleanses the body. Reflexology can relieve headaches, clear congested sinuses, reduce the pain of menstrual cramps, ease a backache, and reduce swelling in a "trick" knee (a knee that causes chronic problems because of prior injuries). Because reflexology is very easy to overdo, causing rapid detoxification, the usual treatment is only 20 minutes.

▌ ENERGY AND HEALING TOUCH

Healing touch is exactly what the name implies—touch that heals. The practitioner touches the patient to reconnect him or her with healing energy that affects the mind, body, and spirit. There are a variety of forms of healing touch, but Reiki and therapeutic touch are two of the most common in North America.

▌ *Reiki*

Reiki is a system of healing that restores and balances the energy within the body. Reiki means universal life energy; it is defined as the power that acts and lives in all created matter. It is thought that Reiki originated in Tibet centuries ago, but Dr. Mikao Usui of Japan rediscovered the basic system in the mid- to late 1800s.

Reiki balances and strengthens the body's energy, promoting its ability to heal itself. This healing system touches a person on all levels: body, mind, and spirit. Treatment involves a practitioner placing hands on a patient's body or moving the hands over the energy meridians without physical contact. Energy from the practitioner is transferred to the patient, removing blockages and bringing the person back into balance. Treatments are carried out in a quiet environment and last about an hour. Although Reiki is a complete treatment in itself, it can also maximize the results from other treatments, such as massage, chiropractic, physiotherapy, and acupuncture.

I *Therapeutic Touch*

Dolores Krieger, a professor of nursing at New York University, demonstrated in controlled studies in 1972 that touch has positive physiological effects. In placing hands on a patient, concern for the person is communicated.

As with other forms of healing touch, the practitioner must be settled and calm before laying on hands. The intent is to communicate love, support, and caring while touching, holding, or lightly stroking the patient in a nonthreatening manner. The person's sense of privacy and private body space is respected. A skilled practitioner is able to act as a conduit of healing energy, providing a healthy energy field for the repatterning of the patient's weak and imbalanced energy flow.

Therapeutic touch can provide relaxation, reduction of pain, acceleration of healing, and alleviation of illness. It is a beneficial addition to other forms of medical care.

CHAPTER 26

Breathing and Oxygen Therapy

THE LUNGS are one of the organs of detoxification and are the first organ exposed to the toxins we breathe in. The whole respiratory system is constantly exposed to dust, dust mites, molds, pollen, chemicals and pollutants, and microorganisms such as viruses and bacteria. The detoxification methods discussed in this chapter particularly affect and help the lungs and respiratory system by increasing oxygenation and helping to remove carbon dioxide. (For further information on the lungs, see chapter 6, Organs of Protection and Detoxification.)

Sufficient oxygen is necessary for detoxification and cleansing. Oxygen promotes healing, destroys pathogens (harmful microorganisms), and deactivates toxins without injury to healthy tissue or cells.

Breathing

Many civilizations and religions have regarded breath as the most important function of life. The ancient Chinese felt that proper breathing could help them attain immortality. In many languages, the word for breath and spirit is the same. In English, we have separate words, and we do not always make the connection between breath and spirit.

While we no longer feel that it is possible to attain immortality by breathing in a certain way, we do consider breathing an important cleansing method. It can help to cleanse the body physically as well as spiritually, mentally, and emotionally. Learning to regulate our breathing and expand our usual lung capacities is one of the master keys to good health.

The more air we move in and out of our lungs, the healthier we are. The efficient functioning of all our body systems is determined to a great extent by the delivery of oxygen and removal of carbon dioxide. Deep breathing can balance the functions of the entire body, including respiration, circulation, metabolism, digestion, elimination, and glandular function. The body cannot cleanse itself, heal itself, or maintain life without the oxygen supplied by breathing. Deep, easy, and full movement of breath

Dysventilation and Environmental Illness

Dr. L. M. McEwen of London, England reports that many people with environmental illness suffer from dysventilation, in which breathing is shallow and rapid. Some of the most incapacitating symptoms experienced by these people are caused by the chronic cerebral lactic acidosis (an excess of lactic acid in the brain) that results from dysventilation. Once this pattern of breathing is established, it becomes self-perpetuating.

Food and chemical allergies as well as candidiasis can contribute to dysventilation, and asthmatics frequently have this breathing problem. Dysventilation encourages histamine release by the alterations it causes in the immune system. Learning appropriate breathing techniques can speed the recovery of many environmentally sensitive people.

allows relaxation, and increased oxygenation can produce spontaneous emotional release.

Breathing also affects the circulation of lymph. The motions of respiration mechanically pump lymphatic fluid through the body. If breathing is restricted, fluid builds up, causing edema and the buildup of waste products from cellular metabolism. Detoxification cannot take place efficiently if lymph circulation is impaired.

Breathing is the only function of the body that we can perform both consciously and unconsciously. It is controlled by two sets of nerves, the involuntary (autonomic) nervous system and the voluntary nervous system. Many illnesses and health problems arise from an imbalance of the autonomic nervous system. By working with the breath, we can positively affect the autonomic nervous system and many of its involuntary functions.

Breathing is also directly connected to our emotions. Our emotional state affects the speed, depth, regularity, and noise level at which we breathe. Breathing slowly, deeply, quietly, and regularly can calm anger. Clearing anger by changing breathing constitutes an emotional cleansing. In addition, the physical after-effects of anger such as headache, and an increase in blood pressure are prevented. Negative emotions, such as nervousness and impatience, can also be helped by full breathing.

■■ SIMPLE BREATHING EXERCISE

In his book *Natural Health, Natural Medicine,* Dr. Andrew Weil recommends the following simple exercise to relieve anxiety, stress, and emotional upset.

- Sit with your back straight.
- Place the tip of your tongue against the ridge of tissue behind your upper front teeth. Keep your tongue there during the entire exercise.
- Exhale completely through your mouth. You will make a noise as you do so.
- Close your mouth and inhale quietly through your nose to a count of four.
- Hold your breath for a count of seven.
- Exhale completely through your mouth to a count of eight, making a noise as you do so.
- This is one cycle. Repeat the cycle three

Yoga Postures

POSTURE	BENEFITS
Head stand	Increases circulation to the brain, stimulates pituitary gland
Should stand	Improves circulation to the heart, rejuvenates the thyroid
Locust	Strengthens reproductive organs and glands
Cobra	Stimulates kidneys
Bow	Stimulates kidneys
Abdominal lift	Provides natural massages for stomach, colon, intestines, kidneys, liver, gallbladder, and pancreas

more times, for a total of four complete breaths.

Begin this exercise by doing it twice a day. As you become accustomed to it, you cannot do it too frequently. Always keep the ratio at 4:7:8, regardless of the speed at which you are counting.

You may notice a shift in awareness or consciousness after four breaths. This is a sign that you are affecting your involuntary nervous system. The breathing exercise is a tool that is always available whenever you need it. Use it to help you in stressful situations, and to help you fall asleep.

∎∎ YOGA

Yoga is a system of postures and breathing movements that is sometimes also classified as a type of exercise. Yoga has been practiced for over 6,000 years, and many different forms of movement have developed in response to climate, culture, and body constitution. Each form of yoga has a particular emphasis, but incorporates facets of other forms. Some of the more physical types of yoga are:

- *Hatha:* Concentrates on postures and movement, stretching and toning the body.
- *Kundalini:* Concentrates on the spinal column, strengthening and balancing the nervous system and increasing the vital life force.
- *Pranayama:* Concentrates on breathing, strengthening and balancing the respiratory system.

Physical balance, alertness, relaxation, calm centeredness, and harmony are integral to the discipline of yoga. All movements are performed slowly, rhythmically, and with full attention from the center of one's being. A pose is assumed and then held while the practitioner "feels" the body and the energy generated by the position. Breathing fully, quietly, and calmly is also an integral part of holding the position.

Yoga has been described as a methodical manipulation of the body. The postures and routines emphasize stretching and toning, with a gradual advancement of posture difficulty. Poses are sequenced so that both sides of the body are worked, providing a complementary balance.

An integral part of all forms of yoga is an emphasis on the complete breath. Yoga practitioners believe that breath is intimately related to the amount of life energy we have, generate, and store. The breath must be deep, rhythmic, slow, and expansive. At the peak of the inhalation, there should be a slight pause before exhalation, which must also be slow, rhythmic, and deep. All yoga postures are practiced with this manner of breathing.

To learn to perform the complete breath, it is simplest to begin by practicing in stages.
- First, lie on your back and rest your fingertips on your abdomen. Breathe through your nose and expand only your abdomen. Your fingertips should part. Release the breath.
- Next, move your hands to your ribcage. Inhale and expand only your ribcage and diaphragm. Your fingertips should part. Release the breath.
- Next, with your fingers on your collarbones, inhale only in the upper chest. Your fingers will rise with this shallow breath. Release the breath.
- Now, place your hands, palms up, beside your body. Put the three breaths described above together. Inhale, expanding the abdomen, then the diaphragm and chest in a wavelike movement. Exhale in the same way, contracting the abdomen, the diaphragm, and the chest. Continue this pattern, adjusting to your rhythm.

The complete breath increases vitality, soothes nerves, and strengthens abdominal and intestinal muscles.

Many yoga postures reverse the effects of gravity's downward pull on the body's vital organs and glands. Postures that incorporate inversion increase blood supply to the organs and glands.

Discipline in the practice of yoga is not limited to just setting aside a time to exercise. In addition to learning and coordinating the various body postures and breathing, patience with your own performance is necessary. The body experiences changes as each new posture creates the opportunity for growth and expansion, both physically and mentally. There will be days when the body will not perform to the standard of the previous day. This apparent plateau is nothing more than the body preparing to take the next step forward to increased capabilities.

■■ NADI SHODHANA (BALANCED BREATHING)

Dr. Deepak Chopra, author of *Perfect Health* and many other books, suggests a breathing exercise from Ayurveda to balance the breath. Called Nadi shodhana, it is a breathing exercise from Pranayama yoga, and the breath is moved from one nostril to the other, making the respiratory rhythm more regular. It has a soothing effect on the nervous system and balances the left and right hemispheres of the brain.

This exercise should be done for five minutes each morning and evening. If your nose is stuffy, wait until it clears to do the exercise. Perform Nadi shodhana in a quiet room where there are no distractions such as radio or TV. The mucous membranes of your nose may undergo changes when you first begin this exercise, but they will normalize in a few days. Do not hold your breath or count the numbers of seconds each breath takes.

The Nadi shodhana begins each breath on the exhalation. Most Western breathing exercises begin with a deep inhalation. You may notice after doing Nadi shodhana for some time that your breathing pattern is changing. This means you are reaching a more balanced style of respiration.

To perform Nadi shodhana:

- Sit with your spine straight and both feet flat on the floor. Close your eyes and let your mind rest.
- Place your right hand on your nose so that your thumb touches your right nostril and your two middle fingers touch your left nostril.
- Pull your right elbow in close to your body. This keeps your arm from getting tired. Do not lean on a chair or table.
- Close your right nostril with your thumb and exhale through your left nostril. Then inhale through your left nostril.
- Close your left nostril with your two middle fingers and exhale out of the right nostril. Then inhale through the right nostril.
- You do not need to take deep breaths, but you may want to breathe more slowly.
- Alternate nostrils in this manner for five minutes. Then rest your arm in your lap and sit quietly with your eyes closed for one to two minutes.

When some people first begin to practice this exercise, they may feel light-headed. This sensation will go away in time. You may also notice a shift in awareness, or consciousness.

■■ GUIDED MEDITATION

Guided meditation (sometimes called co-meditation), or shared breathing, is an ancient breathing meditation that helps to ease fear and anxiety. It originated centuries ago with Tibetan physician-priests as an aid to clear and quiet the minds of dying lamas. It helps a person to enter a meditative state and stops a racing mind. The breath is considered the pulse of the mind, and the correlation between breath and thought directly affects the autonomic nervous system.

Guided meditation is also a detoxification breathing technique in that it increases oxygenation and lymph circulation, as well as encouraging emotional release and cleansing. It helps people to relax, releases emotional stress, and promotes a deep sense of tranquility.

In guided meditation, one person acts as a guide for the other. It is not necessary to have meditation experience, or to hold any particular religious belief system to participate in this technique. It is a physiological approach that uses the autonomic nervous system to quiet the mind. The deep abdominal breathing of guided meditation affects the hypothalamus gland, which controls the autonomic nervous system. Heart rate, blood pressure, respiration, temperature, anxiety, and stress are all reduced.

The meditation begins with traditional relaxation exercises. The guide helps the

Oxygen as Fuel

Oxygen is to our bodies what gasoline is to our cars. With an abundance of oxygen, our bodies can function properly, fighting off disease and eliminating chemical toxins. We can live without food, water, and sleep for several days, but we can live without oxygen for only a few minutes. Irreparable brain damage occurs after that time.

other person to concentrate on relaxing each part of the body, beginning with the toes and working up to the top of the head. The person has only to lie comfortably with the eyes closed, listen, and breathe. The guide uses counting and visualization to help the person slow the rate of breathing. The voice of the guide enables the other person to ignore distractions and reach the meditative state quickly. There are benefits for the guide also. The guide often enters a relaxed state as he or she focuses on the other's breathing.

In addition to helping with detoxification, guided meditation can assist ill patients and their families. It can help seriously ill patients to cope, and dying patients to approach death peacefully and to die with dignity. It can help the families of seriously ill or dying patients to survive overwhelming situations. When a family member acts as the guide, it also gives the chance to be of practical help, diminishing the sense of helplessness and powerlessness that often

result when an ill person is in the care of health professionals.

Dr. Richard Boerstler discusses guided meditation or comeditation at length in his book, *Letting Go: A Holistic and Meditative Approach to Living and Dying*. He states that, "Comeditation involves both the patient and the caregiver, helping them manage stress and relax. It may even bring such deep peace that the immune system is favorably affected."

Oxygen Therapy

Oxygen is an odorless, tasteless, colorless gas found in elemental form in the atmosphere. The oxygen in the atmosphere comes from the metabolic activity of green plants and is found in almost all plant and animal substances. With the exception of anaerobic bacteria, viruses, and fungi, oxygen is essential for maintaining life in all organisms on earth.

Air inhaled into the lungs supplies oxygen to the body. Red blood cells carry oxygen from the lungs to all parts of the body. After releasing the oxygen, they pick up carbon dioxide from the blood plasma and return it to the lungs where it is exhaled from the body.

All biochemical processes in the body require oxygen. Almost all oxygen consumption occurs on the cell membranes. Two-thirds of the body's oxygen consumption is used to burn fuel in the production of adenosine triphosphate (ATP), which is the primary molecule that accepts energy from the breakdown of the fuel. Once ATP has been broken down to adenosine diphosphate and a phosphate group, it donates its energy to the cells of the body. If our cells stop producing sufficient ATP, they become disorganized and are unable to function properly.

Oxygen is also necessary to the body's chemical reactions. It is consumed in both the processes of oxygenation and dehydrogenation of chemical compounds, changing their composition to be more useful to the body. In addition, white blood cells use oxygen to kill the bacteria they have ingested. Toxic compounds are converted to harmless derivatives through oxidation reactions.

Oxygen deficiency, or hypoxia (oxygen starvation at the cellular level), can lead to disease. Normal oxygen reserves can be depleted by a number of factors. Poor diet, alcohol abuse, and lack of exercise greatly reduce the amount of oxygen available to the cells.

The extra oxygen required for digestion after overeating depletes oxygen. The excess foods produce excess metabolic products that must be detoxified, also requiring extra oxygen. Mineral deficiencies reduce the production of digestive and detoxification enzymes. This increases the production of toxins, thus increasing the need for oxygen.

Xenobiotics (foreign chemicals) and pollution can decrease our oxygen stores, as can the use of pharmaceuticals. Helpful "free radical" forms of oxygen are depleted during infections, as they fight microorganisms.

Physical trauma can reduce circulation and oxygen supply to cells and tissues throughout the body. Damaged tissue is frequently oxygen deprived after an injury. Emotional stress produces adrenalin and adrenalin-related hormones that utilize more oxygen. The shallow breathing associated with depression and negativity also leads to oxygen deficiency.

Without sufficient oxygen, all organs and body systems are negatively affected.

- *General health:* Illness, poor stamina, fatigue, and toxicity can result as cells turn to sugar fermentation as another source of energy. Cellular metabolism becomes dysfunctional, and cells lose their immunity, becoming vulnerable to infection.
- *Digestion:* The production of gastric secretions requires calcium, water, and oxygen. Low gastric secretions and resultant poor food assimilation can lead to overeating in an attempt to obtain enough nutrition.
- *Circulation:* Vitamin C cannot be assimilated properly, causing the breakdown of collagen and the hardening of veins and arteries. Hardening of the arteries in older people leads to strokes and degeneration of the brain.
- *Liver function:* The liver, the major organ of cleansing and detoxification, cannot repair its cells.
- *Blood function:* The function of white blood cells is slowed and clumping of red blood cells increases.
- *Healing:* The body is unable to cleanse or repair itself.

Oxygen is an important aid in cleansing the body. Extra oxygen is used by the body to oxidize or burn up toxins. If oxygen therapy is given consistently and for long enough, the body can cleanse itself of all toxins. Chemicals and other substances will be detoxified and anaerobic microorganisms will be unable to live in the oxygen-rich environment.

Oxygen therapy may be administered

Oxygen and Allergic Reactions

Oxygen clears allergic reactions. Inhalation therapy that involves breathing oxygen using a mask for between 5 and 15 minutes at 5 to 6 liters a minute will clear almost any allergic reaction, regardless of the type of symptom caused and the trigger for the reaction.

by inhalation or in a hyperbaric oxygen chamber. Other forms of oxygen, including hydrogen peroxide, ozone, and stabilized oxygen, are also useful for detoxification and some are available to patients without a prescription.

■■ INHALATION THERAPY

Oxygen is given as an inhalant to treat such respiratory problems as asthma, bronchitis, emphysema, and pneumonia, in which lung function is impaired and the body does not receive sufficient oxygen. Oxygen therapy eases the labored breathing caused by these disease processes. The concentration of oxygen available to the lungs is increased, thus increasing the amount of oxygen available to the body and helping to compensate for impaired lung function.

Oxygen will also help to destroy any harmful anaerobic microbes that might be present, without harming helpful aerobic microorganisms. Anaerobic microbes may be viral, bacterial, or fungal.

Used as an inhalant to clear allergic reactions, oxygen plays a very important cleansing role. It helps to stop any allergic reaction, regardless of the symptoms. There does not

have to be difficulty in breathing for oxygen to be of benefit, as it has a biochemical effect, reversing the allergic and inflammatory cascade. In reactive or inflammatory processes, hemoglobin (the oxygen-carrying protein in red blood cells) releases more oxygen to the cells fighting the reaction or foreign substance. Providing more oxygen to these active cells also allows an increase in ATP release, which accelerates the process of detoxification.

Use the following method for the therapeutic inhalation of oxygen for any problem.

- If a mask is used, oxygen should be administered at the rate of 5 to 6 liters per minute. If a cannula (nasal tube) is used, the rate should be 2 to 3 liters per minute.
- Use the oxygen for 15 to 30 minutes to clear an allergic reaction. If the reaction has not stopped, extend the time another 15 to 30 minutes.
- Do not use oxygen continuously for more than 5 hours, as it can dry out mucous membranes.

Ceramic masks and special tubing are available for people who do not tolerate plastic masks and tubing. An oxygen tank and oxygen for emergency use can be obtained by prescription from a physician familiar with your condition.

■■ HYPERBARIC OXYGEN THERAPY

In hyperbaric oxygen therapy, oxygen is administered under pressures greater than atmospheric pressure (barometric pressure) at sea level. Very little oxygen is dissolved in the blood at normal barometric pressure. Under increased pressure, enough oxygen dissolves to meet the normal requirements of the body. The body then uses the oxygen dissolved in the blood rather than that bound to the hemoglobin in red blood cells, which is less readily available.

Hyperbaric oxygen results in:

- decreased cardiac output and lowered heart rate.
- increased blood-brain barrier permeability, allowing more oxygen to reach the brain.
- improved red cell elasticity, thus improving microcirculation.
- reduced fatigue and increased physical endurance.
- suppressed respiratory reactivity to carbon dioxide.

Hyperbaric oxygen treatments are carried out in chambers in which the pressure can be raised to several atmospheres higher than sea level. Mobile hyperbaric oxygen chambers are now available.

The person receiving treatment remains in the chamber for a prescribed amount of time, depending on the condition being treated. The condition most commonly treated with hyperbaric oxygen is decompression sickness, also known as the "bends." The bends are caused by a rapid reduction of environmental pressure that allows inert gases in the body tissues to form bubbles, causing extreme pain and, in some cases, death. Divers may suffer from the bends if they return to the surface too quickly.

Other conditions that have been successfully treated with hyperbaric oxygen therapy include:

- Poisoning by carbon monoxide, smoke, cyanide, hydrogen sulfide, and carbon tetrachloride.

- Crush syndrome, compartment syndrome, and other acute traumatic ischemia (mechanical obstruction of blood supply). Crush injuries to limbs involving injury to muscle, bone, skin, connective tissue, and nerves respond well to hyperbaric oxygen therapy. It counteracts the effects produced by the lack of oxygen reaching injured tissue.
- Soft tissue infections, osteomyelitis (bone infections), gas gangrene, and other infections. Used at higher pressures, oxygen is a broad-spectrum antibiotic, cleansing the body of anaerobic microorganisms.
- Skin transplants or skin flaps with marginal chance of survival because of circulatory or nutritional disturbances. Hyperbaric oxygen therapy is of particular value for burns, extensive plastic surgery, or skin grafting.

Hyperbaric oxygen has also been successfully used in cases of fat embolism, air embolism during surgery or catheterization, coronary artery occlusion and myocardial infarction (heart attack), and the management of serious neurological disturbances resulting in coma.

■ HYDROGEN PEROXIDE THERAPY

Oxygen is a housecleaner for the body, oxidizing toxins and increasing the production of enzymes that participate in detoxification reactions. One of the simplest sources of healing oxygen can be found in food-grade hydrogen peroxide (H_2O_2), which comes in a 35 percent solution. The more familiar 3 percent hydrogen peroxide found in pharmacies has been altered by the addition of various stabilizers and metals.

Hydrogen peroxide occurs naturally from atmospheric ozone, in rain and snow, and in the running water of mountain streams, where the continuously moving water is naturally aerated. Raw vegetables and fruits contain natural hydrogen peroxide. The body's immune system combines free oxygen with some of the body's water to create hydrogen peroxide as part of its defense against invading pathogens. It is released from human blood platelets and white cells when they are disturbed by particulate matter irritating their membranes.

The increased oxygen provided by hydrogen peroxide helps digestion, aids liver function and repair, slows collagen breakdown, relieves hypoxia (lack of oxygen reaching the tissues), and helps prevent wound infection. It alters the body chemistry to help fight disease, promote tissue repair, promote healing, and improve overall function.

Hydrogen peroxide can reduce the physical stress of chronic infection and disease. It regulates tissue repair, cellular respiration, and growth; stimulates immune function and the energy systems; and increases the production of cytokines, chemical messengers involved in the regulation of body systems. Hydrogen peroxide can also directly destroy bacteria, yeasts, viruses, and parasites, and has been used to treat heart and blood vessel diseases, pulmonary diseases, infectious diseases, immune disorders, Parkinson's disease, Alzheimer's disease, migraine headaches, cancer pain, and blood and lymph node cancers.

■ ORAL ADMINISTRATION

Use only diluted 35 percent pure food-grade hydrogen peroxide and always keep it refrig-

> ### Hydrogen Peroxide Caution
>
> *Thirty-five percent hydrogen peroxide is flammable and can be dangerous. It should always be diluted and handled with care. Rinse immediately and thoroughly with water if it gets on the skin.*
>
> *People with organ transplants CANNOT use hydrogen peroxide. The immune system will be strengthened and will reject the transplant as a foreign body. However, it is safe to use for people who have plastic or metal implants.*

erated. Stir the prescribed amount of hydrogen peroxide into 5 ounces of distilled water, fruit juice, or milk. A bite of orange or banana may be eaten to remove the aftertaste. *Never* mix with carrot juice, carbonated juice, or alcoholic beverages. Enzymes in the carrot juice cause the oxygen to bubble out.

- *Day 1:* 1 drop of hydrogen peroxide per dose
- *Day 2:* 2 drops of hydrogen peroxide per dose
- *Day 3:* 3 drops of hydrogen peroxide per dose
- *Day 4:* 4 drops of hydrogen peroxide per dose

Continue, if you choose, adding a drop per dose each day until day 16. Many people choose to stop at 10 drops per dose. Take up to three doses a day on an empty stomach, one hour before or after a meal or taking medicine. If your stomach becomes upset, stay at that level or go back a level.

Because this is a cleansing process, you will likely have ups and downs as your body gradually releases toxins long stored in the organs. Toxins may be released faster than your capacity to eliminate them, causing symptoms. These symptoms will be temporary, usually lasting three days, as the body tries to maintain homeostasis. If your energy level is already low, you might be uncomfortable for as long as a week. This overload can include skin eruptions, nausea, diarrhea, headache, unusual fatigue, a cold, sinus flare-up, ear infections, or flulike symptoms.

If undesirable cleansing symptoms occur, go off the program for a few days to give the body a chance to catch up with elimination. Then begin where you left off or at a lower level.

For very serious complaints such as emphysema, cancer, and AIDS, it may be possible to ingest as much as 25 drops three times a day for one to three weeks. Then intake should be reduced to twice a day until detoxification is complete. This treatment may take six months or longer. A good maintenance program is 5 to 15 drops per week, depending on the amount of cooked or processed foods in the diet.

Some healthcare professionals prefer to use magnesium peroxide (MgO_2), sometimes called magnesium dioxide. It is an excellent oxygen donor and, used orally, provides the same effect as oral hydrogen peroxide. Magnesium peroxide is more stable, easier to handle than hydrogen peroxide, and tastes better. As its oxygen is released, the magnesium that it leaves behind is a beneficial mineral.

Candida and Ulcer Caution

If you have Candida overgrowth or ulcers, begin the program very slowly. You may experience severe symptoms due to Candida die-off, and ulcers may be irritated. One drop a day for the first week may be your tolerance level.

■ INTRAVENOUS ADMINISTRATION
Hydrogen peroxide in a diluted solution can be administered intravenously for a rapid response in serious infections. It helps to reoxygenate the cells and stimulate the immune system. Viral infections respond more rapidly than bacterial infections. This treatment must be administered by a licensed healthcare professional.

■ TOPICAL CLEANSING
   APPLICATIONS
Hydrogen peroxide has many uses as a topical cleansing agent. Only a few of them are listed below. To make your own safe 3 percent solution, add 1 ounce of 35 percent food-grade hydrogen peroxide to 11 ounces of distilled water.

- *Body spray:* After a shower or bath, dry off, then spray your body with a 3 percent dilution of hydrogen peroxide and let dry. This restores the acid mantle that soap removes.
- *Mouth rinse:* Use a 3 percent dilution of hydrogen peroxide as a mouthwash to fight tartar and plaque.
- *Gum disease:* Add enough 3 percent diluted hydrogen peroxide to baking soda to form a paste, and apply to gums. This mixture fights infection and helps oxygenate gum tissue, promoting healing.

After Hydrogen Peroxide Treatment

Always follow hydrogen peroxide treatment with Lactobacillus acidophilus *replacement. For a discussion of acidophilus therapy, see Beneficial Bacteria in chapter 23, Nutrients.*

- *Facial freshener and acne control:* Apply a 3 percent dilution of hydrogen peroxide on a cotton ball to the skin after washing your face. *Warning:* Be careful to avoid eyes.
- *Nasal spray:* Use 1 part 3 percent dilution of hydrogen peroxide to 1 part distilled water. Use as needed for sinusitis and allergic rhinitis.
- *Wound cleanser:* Pour a small amount of 3 percent diluted hydrogen peroxide over the wound. Thick foaming indicates that infectious material is being killed. Be aware that the damaged tissue will be sensitive. If necessary, you may repeat the treatment several hours later.

OZONE THERAPY

Ozone is triatomic oxygen, a molecule containing three atoms of oxygen instead of the usual two. It is created in nature as solar radiation ionizes oxygen at higher altitudes. Electrical discharges also produce ozone, causing the fresh smell that accompanies lightning and rain.

Copy machines, some printers and appliances, and electric trains have high-voltage discharges that cause ozone to form. Ozone is also produced when nitrous oxides and hydrocarbons react in the presence of sunlight. Refineries, factories, automobiles, and chemical manufacturing plants produce ozone in this way. In these cases, ozone is an air pollutant.

Ozone is more reactive than oxygen and as extra oxygen breaks away from the ozone molecule, it leaves a normal oxygen molecule. Used medically, ozone increases the oxygen available to lesions and tissues, improves wound healing, deactivates viruses and bacteria, and speeds up local metabolism by increasing temperature.

Ozone is unstable and cannot be stored. For treatment purposes, ozone is usually produced by passing air or oxygen through a high-energy field. An ozone-producing apparatus is called an ozone generator. Ozone generators can be used to help detoxify homes and workplaces. Ozone kills molds and oxidizes (breaks down) chemicals so that they are less harmful.

An important cleansing agent, ozone has disinfectant properties and can kill bacteria, viruses, fungi, and parasites. Ozone can be used to purify drinking water, disinfect utensils, and sanitize air. Some municipalities use ozone to treat water supplies and swimming pools. Ozone treatment of industrial wastewater, lakes, ponds, and fisheries is of both economic and environmental importance. Pesticides are difficult to remove from water by reverse osmosis and distillation, but they are reduced by ozone treatment.

In microdoses, ozone has important medical uses. It is used topically to treat skin problems such as fungal infections, poorly healing wounds, and burns. It can also be administered rectally or vaginally to treat

Stabilized Oxygen to Go

It is useful to take a bottle of stabilized oxygen when traveling, both to treat water and to increase oxygenation to your cells. A variety of toxic exposures encountered when traveling can deplete oxygen reserves in the body.

candidiasis and *Herpes*. An ozone bath can provide as much benefit as a hyperbaric oxygen treatment with much less cost and equipment. In high concentrations, ozone is toxic to the epithelium (lining) of the lungs and is therefore not administered medically in nebulizers.

Some physicians use ozone to cleanse bacteria and viruses from the blood. A pint of blood is drawn from the person and placed in a special infusion bottle. Ozone is forced into the bottle and thoroughly mixed with the blood. The ozone molecules give up their third oxygen atom, in a process that inactivates the microorganisms. The treated blood is then returned to the patient. Some practitioners use direct intravascular injections of an oxygen/ozone mixture.

Ozone also has antitumor properties. It is believed that the hydroxyperoxides formed by ozone in the blood seek out and destroy diseased cells. The peroxides react with the weakened cell's membrane lipids, invading and destroying the diseased cell. Hydroxyperoxides have no negative effect on healthy cells, but do oxygenate their environment and enhance circulation.

Ozone has additional cleansing benefits. It:

- activates enzymes involved in oxygen radical or peroxide scavenging.
- accelerates glycolysis (breakdown of glucose) in red blood cells.
- activates the citric acid cycle (the energy-producing cycle of the body).
- increases blood oxygen, blood fluidity, and red blood cell pliability.
- has bactericidal, viricidal, and fungicidal properties.

■■ STABILIZED OXYGEN THERAPY

Stabilized oxygen is a liquid supplement that contains stabilized electrolytes of oxygen. Several companies make stabilized oxygen, and most of them use sodium chlorite ($NaClO_2$), chlorous acid ($HClO_2$), or chlorine dioxide (ClO_2) in solution. (See Sources for companies that produce stabilized oxygen.) When taken orally, the chlorine-oxygen molecule enters the bloodstream intact. In the bloodstream, the oxygen molecule has a greater affinity for hemoglobin and leaves the chlorine, which is then excreted through the kidneys.

Sodium chlorite, chlorous acid, and chlorine dixoide are a rich source of oxygen and are anti-inflammatory, bactericidal, and fungicidal. The oxygen they release is also effective in combating viruses. These substances can reduce the severity and duration of diarrhea and stomach flu. Although chlorine oxides are normally unstable, the manufacturing process has stabilized them. Their half-life in the body is approximately 12 hours, and they do not initiate free radical activity in the body.

There is some concern over using chlorine compounds in stabilized oxygen ther-

Oxygen Treatment for Infections

Developing a bladder infection on a trip, far away from your customary medical care, can be frightening. One woman was introduced to stabilized oxygen after developing the symptoms of a bladder infection while at a meeting across the United States from her home state. Not only did the stabilized oxygen clear her bladder infection, but also her stools became very foul smelling as it cleared intestinal organisms she had not known she had.

apy because studies have shown a higher incidence of bladder cancer among people who drink chlorinated water. There are now magnesium-based (MgO_7) and potassium-based (KO_7) stabilized oxygen compounds available. These compounds have been ozonated and stabilized to release monoatomie oxygen slowly over 12 hours or more to ensure adequate amounts and utilization of oxygen. The magnesium and potassium transport the oxygen through the body. The MgO_7 compound also has a laxative effect on the body that helps loosen intestinal buildup, resulting in the release of waste products and toxins. Both products come in powder and capsule form.

Stabilized oxygen can be used to purify water. It is effective against coliform bacteria, streptococcus, staphylococcus, fungi, and *Giardia lamblia*. (See chapter 15, Plants and Organisms, for further information on these microorganisms.) It can be used to purify mountain water and to keep stored water pure of coliform bacteria. Stabilized oxygen products can be taken with nutritional supplements, and enhance the assimilation of some nutrients.

Stabilized oxygen solutions can be added to mouthwash, vaginal douches, enemas, and skin care products. The oxygenating properties of these solutions help reduce inflammation, remove toxins, and promote healing. For some conditions, the antimicrobial properties are important. Some people use stabilized oxygen solutions in food preservation, water treatment, and vegetable washes as a disinfectant.

Allergy Treatment and Chelation

Allergy Treatment

Allergies are a type of toxin that must be cleansed to restore body balance and to prevent damage caused by repeated reactions. Allergy extracts and hands-on allergy treatments are two excellent methods of accomplishing this type of detoxification.

■■ ALLERGY EXTRACTS

Allergy extracts consist of dilutions of small amounts of antigen that are used for immunotherapy and for cleansing. The antigen is the substance to which the person is allergic and may include foods, chemicals, pollens, terpenes, molds, dust and dust mites, animal danders, phenolics, tobacco smoke, organisms, or chemicals produced in the body. Allergy extracts are used to control allergic symptoms to the substance contained in the extract. A precise dose will prevent allergic symptoms to the substance.

Allergy extracts may be given either by injection or sublingually (under the tongue). Most individuals respond quite well to sublingual administration and, with a few exceptions, injections are not necessary. (Homeopaths do not like any type of injection because they are a puncture wound and create the possibility for loss of vital fluid.)

Symptom control is desirable for the comfort of the allergic person, as well as for the protection of the immune system. If the immune system is constantly stressed by adverse reactions to foods, chemicals, inhalants, or organisms, its efficiency suffers. Over a period of time, the immune system can become weak and damaged, and target organ (the organ usually affected in an allergic reaction) damage can occur. If the immune cascade (a series of biochemical reactions that make up an allergic response) continues, tissue damage follows. The use of extracts protects the immune system and allows it to repair and heal.

Allergy extracts also have a cleansing action. The more dilute extracts are homeopathic in nature and allow the body to release stored debris and toxins related to the aller-

Restoring Your pH

In addition to allergy extracts and hands-on allergy treatment, two very simple measures will help stop allergic reactions. People experience a shift in body pH when they react and become either very acidic or very alkaline. Buffered vitamin C (ascorbic acid in combination with calcium and magnesium carbonate and potassium bicarbonate) will help stop allergic reactions for people who become acidic when they react. Those who become alkaline will clear with ascorbic acid, which helps reduce the alkalinity to restore body pH.

Another simple, but effective buffer that helps with acid/alkaline imbalance, as well as stopping allergic reactions, is ""Magic Brew." Add 1 tsp. salt and 1 tsp. baking soda to a quart of water and sip; some people prefer it chilled. This combination will help stop allergic reactions, clear headaches, soothe an upset stomach, and restore pH.

gens in the extract. The release and excretion of these substances has a cleansing and balancing effect on the body.

❚ FOOD EXTRACTS

Foods to which a person is allergic can be avoided. However, some people are sensitive to many foods and their nutrition would suffer if they avoided all of them. Food extracts allow these individuals to eat problem foods without symptoms and without damage to their immune systems or bodies. Food extracts can also be used to stop acute allergic reactions to foods.

Most people are able to stop taking their extracts over time and have decreased or no sensitivity to the foods treated. If the food allergy is a permanent allergy, they may always have to be careful about exposure to that food. Cyclic allergies, those that come and go according to frequency of exposure to the food, can be eliminated.

Phenolic food compounds are naturally occurring chemical compounds in foods that frequently cause allergies. All foods contain these compounds in varying amounts. Many people must take an allergy extract to these compounds in addition to whole food extracts to control their symptoms and prevent allergic reactions. If there are food residues in the body, whether from whole foods or phenolic food compounds, the food extracts cause them to release, helping to cleanse the body. (See chapter 13, Food, for a detailed discussion of foods.)

Many people are sensitive to the additives, flavors, colors, and preservatives that are added to many foods. Allergy extracts for these compounds allow people to eat food containing these substances without having an allergic reaction. The purpose of the extracts is not to enable sensitive people to eat the foods regularly but to give them the freedom to consume these foods on special occasions. These extracts will also protect them in the event of an unexpected exposure. In addition, they help the body release related compounds, which promotes cleansing and rebalancing.

■ CHEMICAL EXTRACTS

Exposures to chemicals are very difficult for the chemically sensitive person to avoid. We can control most chemical exposures in our homes. However, when we leave our safe homes, we can be exposed to thousands of chemicals under the control of others, such as perfume, fabric softener, hair spray and other toiletries, air pollution, car and diesel exhaust, cleaning compounds, pesticides, and many other substances.

Chemical extracts prevent and relieve reactions to chemicals. They are helpful for chemical exposures encountered at work, at school, while traveling, from hobbies, and while going about daily activities. They allow people to lead a more normal and comfortable life in spite of their sensitivities.

Many chemicals are fat-soluble, and are stored in the fat cells and cell membranes of our bodies. The use of dilute chemical extracts aids in the release and excretion of these chemicals. (See chapter 16, Chemicals and Metals, for a detailed discussion of chemicals.)

■ INHALANT EXTRACTS

Inhalant extracts include extracts for pollens, terpenes, molds, dust and dust mites, animal danders, feathers, and some fibers. We cannot avoid exposure to most of these inhalants, as they are everywhere in our environment, but we can exert environmental controls that help. For example, we can choose not to have pets in order to avoid animal danders and feathers. However, we may still be exposed to them on the clothes or in the homes of other people.

Inhalant extracts give relief from the allergic symptoms caused by these sub-

Perfume Reactions

Perfumes, colognes, and aftershaves constitute a major chemical exposure, and many people are acutely sensitive to them. Headaches, nausea, dizziness, and emotional symptoms such as hostility and depression are among the symptoms suffered by sensitive people when they are exposed to scents.

Allergy extracts for ethanol, benzyl alcohol, and phenol help protect these people from symptoms and reactions to scents. Custom-made homeopathic remedies, specific for popular scents, are also very effective in controlling and preventing allergic reactions.

stances. They also stop acute allergic reactions to the inhalants. Inhalant extracts are the best protection from pollen, terpene, dust and dust mite, and mold allergies. Many times extracts can completely eliminate reactions. By preventing reactions, the immune system is spared from constant stress and can heal. In cases where extracts do not eliminate the reactions, they will still lessen their severity. Inhalant extracts also cause the release of pollen and mold debris or terpenes in the body, aiding in cleansing. (See chapter 15, Plants and Organisms, for a detailed discussion of pollen and mold allergies.)

■ TOBACCO EXTRACTS

Tobacco smoke is a very potent allergen. It is made up of extremely small particles that are distributed throughout a room by air streams and convection currents. Smoke odors and particles cling to walls, furnishings, carpeting, draperies, clothing, hair, skin, and other materials. People who do not smoke are often forced to breathe the smoke of their spouses, children, or coworkers, and tobacco odor and residues are left wherever smoking takes place.

Many people are allergic to tobacco smoke and react to both the tobacco smoke from active smoking and smoke residues in rooms and on smokers. Many smokers are unaware of their tobacco allergy because their constant smoking keeps it masked. (Masking is the suppression of symptoms due to frequent exposure to the substance to which a person is sensitive.) A tobacco extract will prevent symptoms from tobacco exposures that cannot be avoided. (See Air in chapter 14 for a detailed discussion of tobacco and smoking.)

❚ ORGANISM EXTRACTS

Bacteria, viruses, parasites, and fungi can cause infection in humans. Many symptoms of infections are caused by an allergic response to the organism. Extracts for these organisms relieve the allergic symptoms caused by both the organisms and their metabolic products.

The effects of an infection do not stop when the acute symptoms clear. Debris from the infectious organism remains in and on our cells. This debris, which may be fragments of the organism or remaining toxins produced by the organism, will continue to cause allergic symptoms as long as it is in the body. In some cases, an inactive organism, a spore, or cyst of the infecting organism—all of which are allergenic—may remain in the body.

Allergy extracts for organisms reduce or eliminate these symptoms. They also aid in cleansing the body of toxins from both past and current infections. (See chapter 15, Plants and Organisms, for a detailed discussion of organisms.)

❚ BODY CHEMICALS

Chemicals that are produced by the body include hormones, neurotransmitters, enzymes, nutrients, and metabolic products such as lactic acid. An excess or deficiency of these substances becomes an internal toxin. In addition, some people have a sensitivity to their own body chemicals that can cause them to have symptoms. Allergy extracts to these substances can help control symptoms, as well as helping to cleanse the body.

Sensitivity to hormones appears to play a role in premenstrual syndrome (PMS), menstrual cramps, and painful ovulation. Extracts for progesterone, estrogen, luteinizing hormone (LH), follicle-stimulating hormone (FSH), and in some cases, testosterone can help relieve the symptoms of PMS and control menstrual cramps and painful ovulation.

Sensitivity to the hormone insulin may play a role in hyperinsulinemia and diabetes. In many cases, a homeopathically diluted extract for insulin is helpful for people with these conditions.

As discussed in chapter 20, Toxins Produced in the Body, deficiencies and excesses of neurotransmitters, the communication chemicals of the body, can be an internal toxin. Many people appear to be sensitive to their own neurotransmitters, contributing to a wide variety of symptoms including depression, hyperactivity, insomnia, poor memory, sugar craving, and many other symptoms. Allergy extracts prepared from homeopathically diluted neurotransmitters can help relieve these symptoms, as well as cleanse the body. For example, a serotonin extract can help alleviate sleep problems, sugar craving, and rampant appetite. Melatonin helps with seasonal affective disorder (SAD) and insomnia. An extract for dopamine, norepinephrine, and other neurotransmitters can help relieve anxiety and depression.

Some people are sensitive to the nutrients produced in their body, such as the B vitamins produced in the intestines, as well as the nutrients they take as a supplement. Because of this, many people who need nutrients the most are unable to take them. The function of detoxification pathways is dependent on specific nutrients, and if they are not present, detoxification cannot take place (see chapter 5, Phases of Detoxification). Allergy extracts prepared from the problem nutrient will allow most people to clear the sensitivity and be able to take the nutrients. Their bodies then function better in every way, including their detoxification processes.

Allergy extracts can also help relieve symptoms caused by excess substances produced in the body. In chapter 20, Toxins Produced in the Body, the problems caused by excess lactic acid were discussed. An allergy extract for lactic acid can often help relieve these symptoms, particularly muscle pain. It will also help balance a lactic acid/lactate excess, regardless of its cause.

Some people do not efficiently excrete the waste product uric acid, and it builds up in the joints, causing pain. An extract for uric acid is helpful in reducing and controlling the pain in many joints.

▌▌HANDS-ON ALLERGY TREATMENT

Several of the specialized hands-on treatments developed by chiropractors are very effective for treating allergies. These treatments are available from chiropractors, allopaths, osteopaths, naturopaths, doctors of oriental medicine, and acupuncturists who have received training from the originators of these techniques.

▌ BIOSET™

Developed by Dr. Ellen Cutler of Corte Madera, California, BioSet™ assists in building body strength and encourages homeostasis, well-being, and rejuvenation. It consists of four branches of healing. These include specific organ detoxification, muscle or bioenergetic testing for sensitivities and meridian evaluation, enzyme therapy, and an allergy elimination technique to remove allergies.

In addition to treating allergies, this technique can give direction in correcting chronic health problems, as well as providing tools for obtaining and maintaining optimal health. Health problems helped by this technique include attention deficit hyperactivity disorder (ADHD), asthma, chronic fatigue, colitis, ear infections, eczema, emotional issues, headaches, menstrual problems, PMS, sinusitis, vaginitis, and many others.

NAET, developed by Dr. Devi Nambudripad of Buena Park, California, is a healing technique that combines effective facets of allopathy, acupuncture, chiropractic, kinesiology, and nutrition. This technique will eliminate allergies to:

- *Inhalants:* pollens, dust, chemicals
- *Ingestants:* foods, additives, vitamins, drugs
- *Contactants:* chemicals, fabrics
- *Infectants:* viruses, bacteria, parasites
- *Physical agents:* heat, cold, humidity, sunlight, sound
- *Genetic factors:* inherited illnesses
- *Molds and fungi:* yeast *(Candida),* mold
- *Emotional factors:* painful memories, past and present

In addition to allergies, NAET has proven helpful in eliminating and reducing other health problems, including addictions, asthma, bronchitis, cough, constipation, ear infections, fatigue, headaches, hives, menstrual problems, mood swings, psoriasis, sinusitis, vertigo, and many others.

∎ TOTAL BODY MODIFICATION (TBM)

Dr. Victor Frank of Sandy, Utah, developed Total Body Modification. This technique combines kinesiology, chiropractic, and acupressure to treat and relieve physical and emotional problems. Its allergy protocol effectively relieves allergies to foods, chemicals, pollens, dust, dust mites, microorganisms, nutrients, body chemicals, and other substances.

TBM balances and treats physical, mental, emotional, and structural aspects of health with its hands-on techniques. Chiropractic manipulations where indicated are helpful, but many non-chiropractors effectively perform this technique using alternative techniques to substitute for the chiropractic manipulations.

In addition to allergies, TBM is useful for treating headaches, joint problems, lung disorders, endocrine imbalances, endometriosis, hypertension (high blood pressure), sugar imbalance, problems from infectious organisms, and many other conditions.

Chelation

Chelation therapy is a nonsurgical cleansing method that removes toxins, including toxic metals. There are several substances that can be used, depending on the substance to be detoxified. Some chelating substances are used intravenously, and others can be administered orally. A few chelating agents can used intravenously, intramuscularly, or orally.

∎∎ EDTA CHELATION

EDTA chelation involves the intravenous use of a medication called ethylenediamine tetra-acetic acid (EDTA). EDTA is a protein-like molecule that binds to metal ions, making them soluble in blood. This action allows the kidneys to excrete such metals as cadmium, calcium, copper, mercury, lead, and strontium. Chelation allows leaking and damaged cell walls to heal. When cell walls are leaky, excess calcium, sodium, and other elements are able to enter the cell.

EDTA was developed in Germany for

nonmedical purposes and was patented in 1930. The United States patent appeared in 1941. It was used then and is still used by the food industry as a stabilizer in canned goods, salad dressings, and other products. The original medical use for EDTA was as a treatment for heavy metal toxicity. It was first used by the U.S. Navy in 1948 for lead poisoning developed by sailors while painting ships and dock facilities with lead paint. It was also used to remove lead from workers employed at a battery factory. In 1951, it saved the life of a child suffering from lead poisoning, and was reported by Harold F. Walton in the June 1953 issue of *Scientific American*.

By removing excess metallic elements, EDTA improves calcium and cholesterol metabolism and normalizes most of the metallic elements in the body. This helps to prevent the formation of free radicals, which most scientists now believe to be a contributing cause to atherosclerosis and many other diseases. Reducing free radical proliferation allows the natural antioxidant defenses of the body to regain control. (See chapter 23, Nutrients, for a detailed discussion of antioxidants.)

Other conditions in which blood-flow impairment plays a role are diabetes, emphysema, macular degeneration, varicose veins, gallstones, cataracts, osteoporosis, hypertension, cancer, arthritis, Parkinson's disease, psoriasis, muscular dystrophy, and kidney diseases. All these conditions can be helped with a course of chelation therapy.

▮ ATHEROSCLEROSIS

Commonly known as hardening of the arteries, atherosclerosis is a disease of the arterial

> ## EDTA Controversial?
>
> *According to the American College for Advancement in Medicine (ACAM), more than 500,000 people have received over 4 million EDTA chelation treatments in the last 40 years. It is one of the safest medical procedures when used correctly, yet remains a controversial treatment. This is puzzling to many medical professionals, as well as lay people, because there has never been a death caused from chelation therapy when administered by a trained physician. Even though chelation therapy has been safely used for atherosclerosis and other health problems since 1952, the Food and Drug Administration has approved chelation treatment only for lead and heavy metal toxicity.*

walls that affects the whole body, slowly deteriorating the entire arterial system. Often, it is not obvious that damage has been done until a person has a stroke or heart attack, or develops signs of senility.

Atherosclerosis is caused by several factors. Plaque, which is composed of fibrous tissue, cholesterol, and calcium, forms on the interior arterial walls. The passage can become so narrow that the blood flow is eventually blocked. The chelating agent EDTA binds with the calcium, allowing it to be removed from the body. This breaks up the plaque, unclogging the arteries. According to some physicians and researchers, the most important cause of atherosclerosis is abnormal accumulations of metals. Ciga-

Improved Circulation

One man who had a heart attack and triple bypass surgery suffered a second heart attack when one of his grafts failed 11 years later. After a chelation series, he exclaimed to his wife that his feet were warm for the first time in years. The circulation to his extremities had been so poor that his feet were cold year-round. After chelation, the restored circulation throughout his body made his feet seem almost uncomfortably hot.

rette smoking, diets high in saturated fats, high blood cholesterol levels, diabetes, hypertension, and hyperinsulinemia are also associated with an increased incidence of this disease.

Emerging evidence points to hyperinsulinemia as a major cause of elevated low-density lipoprotein cholesterol, which is implicated in atherosclerosis. The problem in these cases is a sugar metabolism problem rather than a fat metabolism problem. In hyperinsulinemia, insulin levels in the blood remain constantly elevated. When insulin levels are high, the pancreas does not release glucagon, which is the hormone that signals the liver to stop making cholesterol. Without glucagon, the liver continues to produce cholesterol, leading to elevated levels.

Once the blood flow through the arteries has been significantly reduced, vital organs become starved for oxygen and other nutrients. Cell walls lose their integrity and allow excessive calcium, sodium, and other metals to enter. When calcium accumulates in the plaque, it forms hard deposits that can be seen on X-ray. Some physicians believe that excess calcium ion concentration can also cause arterial spasms, which further reduce blood flow to vital organs.

While surgery is the usual treatment recommended for coronary arteries blocked by atherosclerosis, it offers only mechanical repair of a localized area of the arterial tree. Chelation therapy improves the flow of blood throughout the entire vascular system. Chelation can be used instead of bypass surgery, or when bypass surgery has failed to give relief.

■ BENEFITS OF EDTA CHELATION

People who have received chelation therapy report:

- improvement in overall appearance and physical performance
- improved memory and concentration
- increased energy and capacity to exercise
- better skin color
- more rapid wound healing
- normalization of blood pressure
- improved kidney function
- disappearance of angina pain
- amelioration of cardiac symptoms
- improved vision
- disappearance of senility
- increased blood flow that warms previously cold parts of the body
- disappearance of leg cramps
- healing of gangrenous limbs
- disappearance of impotence

Objective evidence of the effectiveness of chelation therapy can be provided by a comparison of pre- and post-therapy diagnostic tests.

■ SIDE EFFECTS

As with any therapy, side effects are possible. Temporary vein irritation, mild pain, headache, fatigue, and occasionally fever may occur. These effects tend to disappear with continued treatment. Most patients experience minimal or no side effects.

■■ OTHER CHELATING AGENTS

Several other agents can be used for chelating metals and can be given intravenously or orally. All of these agents are prescription medications.

■ DIMERCAPROL, OR
BRITISH ANTI-LEWISITE (BAL)

BAL therapy is used intramuscularly to treat elemental and inorganic mercury poisoning, but should not be used in organic mercury poisoning because it may cause an increase in mercury levels in the brain. BAL is also used to treat lead and arsenic poisoning.

■ SUCCIMER, OR DMSA
(2,3-DIMERCAPTOSUCCINIC ACID)

DMSA is a derivative of BAL and is less toxic than DMPS. It is given orally to treat both acute and chronic mercury poisoning. It has the ability to enter the cells of all tissues and organs and remove mercury. It is particularly good at pulling mercury and other metals from the head.

DMSA is used to treat lead poisoning. It takes four to five days to remove 5 mg of lead, when there is a total of 50 to 100 mg of lead in the body. Succimer is also an effective alternative in cases of arsenic poisoning if adverse reactions to dimercaprol develop.

■ DMPS (2,3-DIMERCAPTOPROPANE-1-SULFONATE)

DMPS is also a derivative of BAL, and has been used to treat acute and chronic mercury poisoning. Whereas DMSA removes mercury from the head, DMPS works in the lower torso. It forms complexes with heavy metals including cadmium, arsenic, lead, copper, silver, tin, and others, in addition to mercury. When DMPS is given intravenously, large amounts of heavy metals are excreted through the kidneys. It also "cleans" the kidneys of heavy metals. DMPS should not be given to a person who has existing amalgam fillings. It appears in the saliva and dissolves the surfaces of the fillings.

Given orally, DMPS leads to excretion of heavy metals through the stool, but is not as effective as intravenous administration. DMPS can also be given intramuscularly, but is less effective than intravenous administration.

■ PENICILLAMINE

Penicillamine is a degradation compound of penicillin that is a chelating agent. It is given orally and is used to treat less severe inorganic mercury poisoning and lead poisoning, and to remove copper in Wilson's disease, a condition in which there is excess copper in the body.

■■ ORAL CHELATION

When intravenous chelation is used, benefits occur rapidly. Oral chelating agents are available and do help, but work more slowly. Dr. Richard Passwater of Maryland first began using the term oral chelation to refer to nutritional supplements and specific foods that help cleanse blood vessels and improve blood flow.

The following nutrients can act as oral chelating agents to prevent degenerative conditions and alleviate symptoms of existing illness.

- *Vitamins:* Vitamin A, vitamin E, vitamin C, B complex vitamins, B_{15} (pangamic acid), beta-carotene or carotenoids, and bioflavonoids all have chelating properties.
- *Minerals:* The orotate salts of calcium, magnesium, and zinc are excellent chelating agents. The trace minerals chromium, manganese, organic germanium, potassium, selenium, silicon, and vanadium have chelating effects.
- *Enzymes:* Bromelain and papain contribute to chelation.
- *Amino acids:* Chelating amino acids include glutathione, cysteine, glutamic acid, and glycine.
- *Glandulars:* Thymus and adrenal glandulars are helpful for chelation.
- *Food supplements:* Food supplements that function as chelating agents are lactic acid, acetic acid, citric acid, rutin, and lecithin.
- *Foods:* Fiber, garlic, bee pollen, apple pectin, alfalfa, and sea kelp have chelating abilities.

- *Coenzyme Q_{10}:* This nutrient acts as a chelating agent, in addition to lowering blood pressure and improving circulation.

Formulations are available that contain balanced amounts of a selection of the oral chelating agents, and some of them also contain oral EDTA. These formulations may be used alone or as supplementation to intravenous chelation therapy. (See Sources for the availability of these nutrients.)

■■ HERBAL CHELATION

Crataegus oxyacantha (English hawthorn) berries, prepared as an herbal tincture, is a very effective oral chelating agent that helps heart problems. *Crataegus* acts on the heart muscle as well as on plaque in the arteries. It lowers and regulates pulse, strengthens a weak pulse, and reduces chest pain. When combined with cayenne, the mixture slowly reduces cholesterol deposits and provides relief from high blood pressure.

Crataegus can be used regularly, or in conjunction with oral or intravenous chelation. Many people take it daily as a preventive and maintenance measure.

CHAPTER 28

Homeopathy and
Bach Flower Remedies

HOMEOPATHY ORIGINATED 200 years ago in Germany with Dr. Samuel Hahnemann. (See chapter 3, Contemporary Approaches to Detoxification, for further information on the origins and development of this medical discipline.) Today's homeopathic philosophies range from the classical homeopaths, who use only one remedy at a time, to those who use combination or complex remedies, which are mixtures of low-potency doses of the most commonly used remedies for a given condition. The body selects the remedy it needs and excretes the rest. A general overview of homeopathic treatments that are useful for detoxification is presented in this chapter.

Bach Flower Remedies are also discussed in this chapter because of their similarity to homeopathic remedies. Even though the inspiration for these remedies probably was homeopathy, the manufacturing process and prescribing guidelines are different. Both homeopathic remedies and Bach Flower Remedies can be used alone or with other types of treatment.

Homeopathy

Homeopathic remedies are small potentized doses from the plant, mineral, or animal kingdom. They stimulate the immune response, begin the healing response, increase overall resistance to infection, and increase a person's vital force. Any substance that can cause symptoms when given to healthy people can help to heal those who are experiencing similar symptoms. This is commonly known as the Law of Similars, and Hahnemann coined the Latin phrase *Similia similibus curentur*—"Let likes be cured with likes."

Hahnemann recognized that the body makes an effort to heal itself, but may not be strong enough to complete the healing process. It needs a catalyst to stimulate its defenses. Hahnemann used the Law of Similars to individualize the choice of the right catalyst by prescribing a remedy that imitates the defenses of the body.

Homeopathic remedies are significantly safer than conventional drugs. The many and sometimes serious side effects of phar-

Polycrest Remedies

Although there are over 2,000 homeopathic remedies, a small group of about 14 to 20 remedies called polycrest remedies are the most frequently used. They will help symptoms related to many different body systems.

maceuticals are well known. Homeopathic remedies do not have these side effects. The wrong remedy will either have no effect or the person will experience a temporary worsening of symptoms that will clear very quickly. Many of the "successes" of conventional medicine are only temporary and are often harmful, because symptoms return or more serious symptoms develop as the body tries to regain internal balance.

Soluble homeopathic remedies are diluted in water or alcohol. If the remedy is insoluble, it is ground (titurated) in powdered lactose (milk sugar) and then put into solution. Once in solution, all remedies are succussed, not stirred, by hitting them firmly against a leather surface. This potentizes the remedy.

Some alcohol- and ethanol-sensitive people may have to set their homeopathic remedy dose out ahead of time to allow most of the ethanol to evaporate before taking it. It is also possible to put the remedy dose in hot water to speed evaporation. However, there is controversy over this method, as some practitioners believe the heat alters the remedy and its effects.

Remedies diluted in a 1-to-9 ratio are known as a decimal potency and labeled as

X. If this 1-to-9 remedy is diluted in the same proportions 30 times, it is known as a 30X potency. Some common potencies used are 6X and 12X. Remedies diluted in a 1-to-99 ratio are known as centesimal, or C potencies; common C potencies are 6C and 30C. M potencies are diluted in a 1-to-1,000 and LM remedies, which require a higher level of skill in prescribing, are diluted in a 1-to-50,000 ratio. The more diluted remedies have a higher potency, act more deeply, act longer, and require fewer doses to effect a cure.

Any given remedy may be used for more than one condition or problem. The remedy that best fits the person and his or her symptoms should be used. The X potencies are the most commonly available homeopathic remedies and are generally low doses that are repeated 3 to 4 times a day. The C potencies require more skill to prescribe and are usually taken twice a day. M and LM potencies are available only from a homeopathic practitioner.

With homeopathic treatment, acute symptoms are treated first, fundamental or chronic symptoms are treated next, and constitutional remedies, which strengthen the immune system, are given last. As with all medical treatment, discussing and understanding your planned treatment fully with a well-trained practitioner is essential.

Once a person takes the correct homeopathic remedy, he or she will feel better in many ways. If the person wakes up the next day feeling refreshed, this indicates that the vital force is improved and that the remedy chosen is the correct one. Sometimes one dose of a single remedy is enough to bring

Mammogram Remedy

Following a mammogram, one woman felt very ill after the procedure, and on the day after. A dose of Cadmium sulphuratum *cleared the feeling of illness and she rapidly regained her strength and energy.*

about a cure, while other times a series of remedies may be used.

Homeopathic remedies are useful detoxification aids and are suggested as treatment for many different toxic exposures, including radiation, surgery, chemotherapy, and insect or snake bites. Homeopathic remedies reduce the toxic effects of many different conditions, including diarrhea and emotional trauma. They also help to strengthen organs such as the liver, the major organ of detoxification.

The remedies listed below are but a few of the many possibilities. Simple acute conditions can easily be treated with homeopathic remedies by the lay person. Seek the help of a qualified homeopathic practitioner if your health problem is chronic, complicated, or severe.

■■ TRAVEL

Travel involves many exposures, including the mode of travel, the environment, foods eaten, and the people encountered. Travel exposures are discussed in detail in chapter 10.

- Airsickness: *Argentum nitricum, Cocculus indicus, Gelsemium*
- Ear pain: *Chamomilla, Kali muriaticum*
- Ears that will not pop: *Kali muriaticum*

- Jet lag: *Arnica, Cocculus, Gelsemium*
- Motion sickness: *Cocculus, Petroleum, Sepia*
- Nausea, seasickness: *Cocculus, Conium, Euphorbia corrolata, Nux vomica, Petroleum, Tabacum, Zingibar*
- Vomiting: *Carbolicum acidum, Cocculus, Petroleum, Tabacum*

■■ MEDICAL TREATMENT

A detailed discussion of toxins that may be encountered during medical treatment is presented in chapter 11. The following remedies can be used to treat many of these problems and will help to detoxify the body.

■ SURGERY

Multiple toxic exposures occur as a result of surgery. The anesthesia and medications used during and after surgery can cause severe symptoms. The following homeopathic remedies help detoxify the body following these exposures.

- Anesthetic poisoning: *Aceticum acidum, Phosphorus*
- Coma after surgery: *Carbo animalis, Carbo vegetabilis*
- Discomfort of bedridden patient, trauma of respirator: *Arnica*
- Fever after surgery: *Pyrogenium*
- Healing after pelvic surgery: *Hypericum*
- Hematomas (bruises) from intravenous sites, bedsores: *Ledum*
- Prevention of keloids (scar tissue) after surgery: *Graphites*
- Post-operative gas: *China*
- Severe pain after breast surgery: *Staphysagria*
- Surgical shock, post-operative problems, exhaustion after surgery, bone pain, never well since surgery: *Strontium carbonicum*

• Weakness, emaciation, anemia, and vertigo after surgery: *Phosphorus*

❚ RADIATION

Several homeopathic remedies provide cleansing and balancing after both radiation diagnostic (ionizing radiation) procedures and treatment.

• Anemia after radiation: *Ferrum metallicum*
• Exposure to radioactive iodine: *Iodium*
• Nausea after radiation: *Ipecac, Nux vomica*
• Nausea after radiation, antidotes radiation poisoning: *Cadmium iodatum*
• Radiation antidote, never well since X-rays: *Cadmium sulphuratum*
• Weak, emaciated, anemic, vertigo since radiation: *Phosphorus*
• Radiation burns: *Fluoricum acidum, Radium bromatum*
• Radiation poisoning: *Radiatum bromatum, Sol*
• Eczema after X-ray: *Radium bromatum*
• X-ray burns, weakness after X-rays: *Sol*
• Radiation sickness antidote; helps X-ray burns, weakness after X-rays, bone damage, people who are worse after X-rays: *X-ray* (a potentized X-ray)

❚ CHEMOTHERAPY

Many people who develop cancer elect to have chemotherapy, which has many unpleasant side effects. Homeopathic remedies can alleviate side effects and help to cleanse and rebalance the body during and after chemotherapy.

• Anemia: *China, Ferrum metallicum* (acute)
• Bruising, bleeding: *Phosphorus*
• Diarrhea, weakness, some kinds of nausea and vomiting: *Arsenicum album*
• Nausea: *Cadmium sulphuratum* (main chemotherapy antidote), *Ipecac, Nux vomica, Opium, Phosphorus*
• Stomach tonic after chemotherapy: *Hydrastis*

❚ PHARMACEUTICALS

If you take pharmaceutical medication and experience side effects, homeopathic remedies can help.

• Constipation after use or abuse of drugs: *Colocynthis, Nux vomica*
• Diarrhea after antibiotics: *Nitricum acidum*
• Oversensitivity to drugs: *Nux vomica, Pulsatilla, Sulphur*
• Narcotics abuse: *Avena sativa, Belladonna, Chamomilla, Coffea, Lachesis, Nux vomica*
• Ailments from narcotics: *Avena sativa*

❚ VACCINATIONS

A combination of allergy extracts and homeopathy can help avoid problems with vaccinations. (Vaccinations are discussed in chapter 11 and allergy extracts are discussed in chapter 27.) The following remedies can help with side effects:

• Acute antidote for vaccination: *Ledum* (helps also with the puncture wound caused by the injection, and can be given beforehand as a preventive for side effects.)
• Antidotes vaccination symptoms: *Vaccininum*
• Painful injection site: *Hypericum* (can be given beforehand as a preventive for side effects.)
• Skin eruptions after vaccination: *Mezereum*
• Ill effects of vaccination: *Malandrinum, Thuja occidentalis*
• Worse since vaccination: *Carcinosum, Silicea terra*
• Never well since vaccination: *Sulphur*

Belladonna

A crying child with a very red sore throat could not be comforted, and had been crying for some time. After being given a dose of Belladonna, *the child immediately went to sleep in his mother's arms. When he awakened, he began to play again as if nothing had ever affected him.*

- Problems after vaccination: *Thuja occidentalis*
- DPT, worse since: *Diphtherinum*
- MMR, problems after: *Pulsatilla*

▮ DENTAL WORK

Dental procedures are toxic exposures, both from the dental materials and the procedures themselves. Homeopathy offers several remedies that cleanse and balance after dental work.

- Dry socket (a healing problem that sometimes occurs after an extraction): *Ruta graveolens*
- Dry socket with bad taste in the mouth, decayed teeth: *Kreosotum*
- Gum pain after dental procedures, oral lesions: *Calendula*
- Nerve injury, pain from drilling, extractions, or root canal preparation: *Hypericum*
- Tooth extractions, gum surgery, pain from drilling: *Arnica*
- Periodontal disease: *Mercurius solubilis*
- Root canal trauma: *Ledum*
- Sore gums, to control toothache pain until a visit to the dentist can be arranged: *Arnica*
- Toothache with earache and saliva tion, major teething remedy, TMJ pain, bruxism (grinding the teeth): *Plantago major*
- Toothache: *Rhododendrum*
- Toothache, better with warm water: *Magnesia phosphorica*
- Toothache, worse with cold: *Spigelia*
- Tooth decay: *Mezereum*

▮▮ FOOD AND WATER

Toxic symptoms can result from consuming contaminated food or water. The remedies listed below will help clear the symptoms, as well as help the body detoxify from the substance. Food and its possible toxins are discussed in chapter 13. Contaminants of water are presented in chapter 14.

- Acids, alcohol, citrus, or sweets excess: *Natrum phosphoricum*
- Alcohol or spicy food excess: *Nux vomica*
- Food poisoning: *Arsenicum album, Ipecacuanha, Zingiber officinale*
- Water poisoning: *Baptisia tinctoria, Zingiber officinale*
- Diarrhea from contaminated food or water: *Zingiber*
- Coffee headache: *Chamomilla, Nux vomica*
- Fat, ailments from: *Nux vomica, Pulsatilla*
- Sugar poisoning: *Argentum nitricum*
- Meat, adverse reactions from: *Arsenicum album*
- Shellfish poisoning: *Lycopodium*
- Spoiled fish: *Pulsatilla*
- Food allergy: *Nux moschata*
- Egg allergy: *Ferrum metallicum, Natrum muriaticum, Sulphur, Tuberculinum*
- Milk intolerance: *Lac defloratum, Natrum carbonicum, Natrum muriaticum, Sulphur, Tuberculinum, Urtica urens*

- Onions, disagree with: *Natrum muriaticum, Pulsatilla, Thuja*
- Oranges, worse after eating: *Oleander, Pulsatilla*
- Wheat allergy: *Natrum sulphuricum, Psorinum*
- Chocolate allergy: *Sulphur*

❚❚ AIR

Inhalants are the particulate substances that we inhale as we breathe. Many of these substances are potent allergens. Listed below are homeopathic treatments for some common inhalants. Mold and dust are discussed in chapters 8 and 14, and a discussion of animal dander is in chapter 8.

- Animal dander allergy, especially cats: *Tuberculinum*
- Cat allergy: *Dulcamara*
- Dust allergy: *Bromium, Silica, Sulphuricum acidum*
- Mold and mildew allergy: *Blatta orientalis*
- Tobacco abuse: *Caladium*
- Tobacco, aggravation from: *Arsenicum, Ignatia, Nux vomica, Plantago major, Pulsatilla, Spigelia, Spongia, Staphysagria*
- Tobacco, ailments from: *Caladium, Nux vomica*
- Tobacco, headache from: *Ignatia, Natrum aceticum*
- Air pollution: *Sulphuricum acidum*

❚❚ PLANT TOXINS

Plants may be toxic through skin contact or breathing in their pollens or terpenes. The many ways in which plants can affect us are discussed in chapter 15. The remedies listed below will treat toxicity and restore balance.
- Poison ivy or poison oak: *Anacardium, Cle-*

matis erecta, Croton tiglium, Rhus toxicodendron (most important)
- Hay fever symptoms from pollen: *Allium cepa, Ambrosia, Euphrasia, Nitricum muriaticum, Sabadilla, Sinapis nigra, Wyethia*
- Hay fever and allergy that resembles an infection: *Arsenicum iodatum*
- Worse from flowers, pollen allergy: *Allium cepa, Sanguinaria*

❚❚ ORGANISMS

Exposure to and infections caused by microorganisms cause many problems. Organisms release their metabolic products into our bodies as they grow, and these products are toxic to us. Additional substances are released when the organisms die or are destroyed by treatment. Organisms are discussed in chapter 15. The remedies listed below will cleanse and relieve symptoms.

❚ BACTERIA
- Cholera (and cholera preventive): *Camphora, Cuprum metallicum, Veratrum album*
- Diphtheria: *Apis, Diphtherinum, Lac caninum, Phytolacca*
- Dysentery: *Aloe, Cantharis, Capsicum, China officinalis, Colchicum, Colocynthis, Ipecacuanha, Mercurius corrosivus, Mercurius solubilis, Nux vomica, Podophyllum*
- Gangrene: *Anthracinum, Arsenicum album, Kreosotum, Secale* (fingers and toes)
- Strep throat: *Arsenicum album, Belladonna*
- Tetanus (lockjaw): *Cicuta, Hypericum, Ledum*
- Tetanus (preventive for): *Arnica, Hypericum, Ledum*

❚ PARASITES
- Amebic dysentery: *Ipecacuanha*
- Ameba: *Mercurius sulphuricus*

- Hookworm, roundworm: *Chenopodium antihelminticum*
- Tapeworm: *Granatum, Magnesia muriatica*
- Worms (recurrent): *Natrum phosphoricum*
- Worms (all types): *Podophyllum, Ratanhia, Spigelia, Zincum metallicum*
- Worms and parasites (all types): *Cina*

▌ VIRUSES

- Common flu, never been well since the flu: *Gelsemium*
- Fever blisters, chickenpox: *Rhus toxicodendron*
- Toxic flu, came on quickly: *Baptisia tinctoria*
- Toxic flu, high fever, accompanied by delirium: *Pyrogenium*
- Viral infections, feels as if the sufferer "has been run over by a truck": *Arnica*

Scientific studies have shown the homeopathic preparation Oscillococcinum® to be effective against the influenza virus. Engystol® is an immune system stimulant that can help to prevent a viral infection or shorten the course and severity of an active infection.

▌ YEAST AND FUNGI

- Candida in the bowel, digestive problems: *China officinalis* (combats fermentation), *Natrum carbonicum*
- Candida, abdominal distention: *Thuja*
- Candida, craves sweets, gas, bloating: *Lycopodium, Medorrhinum*
- Oral thrush: *Borax*
- Mushroom poisoning: *Absinthium, Arsenicum album, Belladonna, Camphor*

▌ INSECTS

- Any insect bite: *Apis, Cantharis* (bites that burn and blister), *Gunpowder, Tabacum*
- Bedbug: *Ledum*
- Bee stings: *Carbolicum acidum, Plantago, Urtica urens*

- Fleas: *Arsenicum* (if glands are swollen), *Ledum, Pulex*
- Lice: *Staphysagria*
- Mosquito: *Caladium, Staphysagria* (prevents mosquito bites)
- Scorpion and spider bites: *Hypericum, Latrodectus curassavicus* (brown recluse), *Ledum, Tarentula cubensis, Tarentula hispanica*
- Ticks: *Ledum*

▌▌ CHEMICALS AND METALS

We are exposed to many toxic environmental chemicals and metals, which can trigger a variety of severe symptoms. The following remedies will help cleanse from these toxic exposures. See chapter 16 for a detailed discussion of these substances.

- Chemical poisoning: *Arsenicum album, Phosphorus*
- Perfume exposure: *Ignatia*
- Pesticide and chemical poisoning: *Arsenicum album*
- Air pollutants: *Sulphuricum acidum*
- Aluminum toxicity: *Alumina, Bryonia, Plumbum metallicum*
- Cadmium toxicity: *Cadmium metallicum, Cadmium sulfuricum*
- Lead poisoning: *Alumina, Arsenicum, Causticum, Platinum metallicum, Plumbum metallicum, Sulphuricum acidum*
- Mercury poisoning: *Aurum metallicum, Carbo vegetabilis, Hepar sulphuris calcareum, Kali iodatum, Lachesis, Mercurius solubilis, Natrum sulphuricum, Sulphur lotum*

▌▌ NOISE

As discussed in chapter 17, not only is noise a nuisance, but it can seriously damage hearing. Above certain levels, hearing is destroyed. The remedies below are helpful after noise exposure.

- Damage to the ear from chronic loud noise: *Silicea terra*
- Ruptured eardrums and deafness: *Calendula*
- Penetrating noise, worse from: *Asarum europaeum*
- Sudden noise, worse from: *Borax*
- Restore hearing after loud noise: *Arnica*

◼◼ WEATHER

Weather-sensitive people sometimes have great difficulty in alleviating their symptoms. The following remedies can help various symptoms of weather sensitivity. For some people, other treatments may also have to be used to obtain complete relief. See chapter 17 for a detailed discussion of weather.

- Sensitive to heat and cold, "human barometer": *Mercurius vivus*
- Hot weather aggravates: *Apis, Lachesis, Pulsatilla, Sulphur*
- Worse summer, heat aggravates: *Fluoricum acidum*
- Warm wet weather aggravates: *Carbo vegetabilis, Lachesis, Natrum sulphuricum, Sepia, Syphillinum*
- Cold to warm weather aggravates: *Bryonia, Kali sulphuricum, Psorinum, Sulphur, Tuberculinum*
- Warm to cold weather aggravates: *Dulcamara, Mercurius solubilis, Veratum album*
- Cold dry weather aggravates: *Aconite, Asarum europaeum, Causticum, Hepar sulphuricum, Kali carbonicum, Nux vomica*
- Frostbite treatment: *Agaricus muscarius, Plantago major, Zincum metallicum*

- Cold and storms, worse before: *Rhus toxicodendron*
- Storms, worse before and during, worse with barometric changes, sensitive to lightning and thunder, weather-change headache, neuralgia, or toothache: *Rhododendron*
- Worse with cold, change of weather, thunderstorms: *Psorinum*
- Worse with summer heat, change of weather, storms: *Natrum carbonicum*
- Worse with cold and windy, thunderstorms, lightning: *Phosphorus*
- Electrical storms and thunderstorms, worse during: *Phosphorus, Sanicula aqua*
- Thunderstorms, worse before: *Pulsatilla*
- Storms, worse afternoon: *Badiaga*
- Storms, wet: *Lycopodium*
- Foggy weather aggravates: *Hypericum, Rhus toxicodendron*
- Wind aggravates: *Chamomilla*
- Wind, worse when dry, cold: *Spongia*

◼ OVEREXPOSURE TO SUN

The sun emits nonionizing radiation. Several homeopathic remedies are helpful in restoring balance after overexposure to the sun:

- General aggravation from the sun: *Natrum carbonicum, Pulsatilla*
- Headache from sun: *Antimonium crudum, Bryonia, Glonoinum, Lachesis, Natrum carbonicum, Natrum muriaticum, Pulsatilla*
- Rash from exposure to sun: *Camphora*
- Sunstroke or heat stroke: *Amylenum nitrosum, Glonoinum, Natrum carbonicum, Sol, Staphysagria, Veratrum album*
- Sunburn: *Belladonna, Cantharis, Pulsatilla, Sol, Urtica urens*

■ ALTITUDE

Ascending to high altitudes can adversely affect the body and be toxic for many people. They may develop altitude sickness, headache, shortness of breath, frostbite, or snow blindness. The following remedies can help to alleviate these symptoms. Altitude is discussed in detail in chapter 17.

- Altitude sickness: *Carbo vegetabilis, Coca*
- Shortness of breath associated with altitude: *Calcarea carbonica* (elderly people), *Silica*
- Snow blindness: *Kali muriaticum, Sol*
- Worse ascending: *Calcarea carbonica*

■ INTERNAL TOXINS

Internal toxins are those that are either stored in the body or produced in the body, and are presented in chapters 19, 20, and 21. Homeopathic remedies are most helpful for the internal toxins that are produced in the body.

■ TOXINS PRODUCED IN THE BODY

- Acid/alkali imbalance: *Natrum phosphoricum*
- Elevated bilirubin: *Carduus marianus, Chelidonium, Crotalus horridus, Iodium purum, Lachesis*
- Hormone imbalance or sensitivity in the following conditions:
  - Diabetes: *Carcinosum, Helonias dioica, Lacticum acidum, Lycopodium, Phosphoric acidum, Phosphorus, Plumbum metallicum, Sulphur, Tarentula hispanica*
  - Dysmenorrhea: *Belladonna, Cactus, Calcarea phosphoricum, Cocculus, Kali carbonicum, Magnesium phosphoricum, Pulsatilla, Sulphur*

Calming Remedy

Being in a car accident is very frightening, even if you are not injured. One child was bounced around considerably in a wreck and was badly bruised. He was terrified afterward, was sobbing, and could not be comforted. In less than one minute after the administration of an Arnica *pellet under his tongue, he calmed down and went to sleep in his mother's arms.* Arnica *is also helpful in cases of the flu that cause you to feel as though you have "been run over by a truck."*

- Hypoglycemia: *Graphites, Iodium purum, Kali carbonicum, Lycopodium, Phosphorus, Silica, Sulphur*
- Impotence: *Calcarea carbonicum, Lycopodium, Phosphorus, Sepia, Sulphur*
- PMS: *Calcarea carbonicum, Calcarea phosphoricum, Kreosotum, Lachesis, Lilium tigrinum, Lycopodium, Pulsatilla, Sepia, Sulphur*
- Lactic acid excess: *Lacticum acidum*
- Neurotransmitter imbalance or sensitivity, as indicated by the following symptoms:
  - Anxiety: *Aconite, Arsenicum album, Aurum metallicum, Calcarea carbonicum, Lycopodium, Phosphorus, Pulsatilla, Rhus toxicodendron, Veratrum album*
  - Depression: *Aconite, Arsenicum album, Aurum metallicum, Calcarea carbonicum, Hyoscyamus niger, Natrum muriaticum, Phosphoric acid, Pulsatilla, Rhus toxicodendron, Stramonium, Veratrum album*

- Insomnia: *Arsenicum album, Calcarea carbonicum, Hyoscyamus, Nux vomica, Phosphorus, Pulsatilla, Rhus toxicodendron, Stramonium*
- Obsessive compulsion: *Arsenicum album, Hyoscyamus, Nux vomica, Pulsatilla*
- Panic: *Aconite, Phosphorus*
- Rage: *Hyoscyamus, Lac caninum, Lycopodium, Nux vomica, Stramonium, Veratrum album*
- Uric acid excess: *Benzoic acidum, Bryonia, Calcarea carbonicum, Causticum, Colchicum, Lycopodium, Rhus toxicodendron, Spongia, Sulphur*

■■ TOXINS OF THE MIND AND SPIRIT

Several homeopathic remedies help with emotional and physical abuse, as well as accompanying physical trauma.

- Lack of self-esteem, goes from relationship to relationship and career to career: *Lycopodium*
- Sciatica after grief or hysteria: *Ignatia*
- Promiscuity, high sex drive: *Nux vomica*
- Fear, rape by stranger, bruised with emotional shock: *Aconite*
- Rape, acute shock from: *Gelsemium*
- Rape, acute fear after: *Opium*
- Rape, incest, or child abuse: *Medorrhinum*
- Rape, sexual abuse, multiple personalities, hypersensitivity in vaginal area and pain with sex: *Platina*
- Rape, loss of sex drive, development of sexual aversion, then disgust: *Sepia*
- Rape, acute remedy; recurrent bladder infections if a history of rape or incest: *Staphysagria*
- Sexual abuse, chronic, with humiliation and inferiority complex, possibly with multiple personalities or may hear voices with religious overtones: *Anacardium*
- Sexual abuse: *Carcinosum*
- Sexual abuse, deep guilt from, or sexual identity crisis: *Thuja*

Bach Flower Remedies

Developed by Dr. Edward Bach (1886–1936), the Bach Flower Remedies were probably inspired by homeopathy. His remedies are similar to homeopathic remedies in that they are dilute, natural, and gentle, but they do not require potentization nor do they work according to the Law of Similars. Bach used his flower remedies to relieve mental stress and heal attitudes. He believed that the basic cause of disease was disharmony between the spiritual and mental aspects of a human being. Bach considered that his remedies comforted, soothed, and relieved cares and anxieties, bringing the person nearer to the divinity within, enabling divinity within to heal the body.

Bach felt that a good doctor could recognize disease on the basis of moods and attitude before it had physical manifestations; he treated disease while it was still at the energy level. Bach felt that the person, rather than the disease, was the key and that the mental and emotional aspect of the person guided the practitioner to the remedy for the body. He took no notice of the nature of the disease, but treated the individual. As health improved, the disease left.

The Bach Flower Remedy repertoire contains 38 easily understood remedies. These remedies provide the stimulus to bring the mind and spirit into balance, allowing the body to heal. They work well for chronic illness, but can also be used for acute illnesses. Some of the remedies work deeply to treat the root causes of the problem, while others treat superficially, alleviating immediate symptoms. They can cure some illnesses before they manifest physically.

All of the remedies have both positive and negative aspects, and deal with both positive and negative emotions and state of mind. However, because an unwanted condition is usually being treated, the remedies are linked with the negative aspect. Even so, the positive side of the remedy does exert influence on the person. The remedies work well alone, but can be used in conjunction with any orthodox treatment or added to any prescription.

■ PREPARATION OF REMEDIES

The remedies are prepared from flowers picked in the morning several hours after sunup. Twenty-one of the remedies are prepared by the sunshine method, in which the flowers are placed in water and left in the sun for four hours. Seventeen are prepared by boiling the specimen in pure water. A mother tincture is prepared and all subsequent dilutions of the remedy are made from this tincture. Stock bottles are prepared from the mother tincture and contain only one remedy. Treatment bottles are made up from the stock bottles and contain two drops of each indicated remedy.

The dosage is one to four drops from the treatment bottle, in water, four times daily. Up to six remedies can be combined and given at one time. However, fewer remedies are considered to be more effective.

■ SELECTION

Even though the remedies are used to treat illness, the appropriate remedy is chosen on the basis of the emotional and mental status and symptoms of the patient. Twelve of the thirty-eight herbs are for illness that is just beginning or has only lasted a short time. Where illness is merely threatening, six to seven hours should be allowed for the remedy to work. Up to six of the following remedies can be matched to the patient and used in this situation.

Agrimony	Impatiens—
Centaury	pale mauve only
Cerato	Mimulus
Chicory	Rock rose
Clematis	Scleranthus
Gentian	Vervain
	Water violet

Seven of thirty-eight herbs are for those who have been ill for a long time. Remedy selection is determined by the hue of the patient's skin at the time of consultation. If the skin is pale, Olive, Gorse, and Oak are indicated. If the skin is highly colored, Vine, Heather (slender, small, rose-pink), and Rock water are the remedies needed. In this case, allow four or five days for the remedy to work. Wild oat, the seventh remedy, is saved for use in cases in which there is no response to the other herbs.

A combination of herbs called the Bach Flower Rescue Remedy contains a combination of Rock rose, Clematis, Impatiens, Cherry plum, and Star of Bethlehem. It is

Seven Categories of Bach Remedies

EMOTION	REMEDY	SYMPTOMS
Fear	Rock rose	Emergency, panic, terror
	Mimulus	Fear of physical misfortunes, the dark, poverty, pain, illness, misfortune
	Plum	Fear of losing reason; the mind is overwhelmed to the point of breaking
	Aspen	Vague, unknown, undefinable fears
	Red chestnut	Anxious for the welfare and well-being of others
Uncertainty	Cerato	Lack of self-confidence, lack of interest in life itself, asking others' opinion or advice often
	Scleranthus	Inability to choose or to decide between two aspects or things
	Gentian	Easily discouraged
	Gorse	Great hopelessness; nothing more can be done to help
	Hornbeam	Lack mental and physical strength to continue with life's burdens
	Wild oat	Desire for life in its fullest but cannot settle on one occupation
Insufficient interest in the present	Clematis	Dreamy, drowsy, not fully awake, no great interest in the present
	Honeysuckle	Living in the past, memories of lost friend or ambitions that did not come to pass
	Wild rose	Absolutely resigned, makes no effort to seek joy or to improve
	Olive	Extreme suffering, too weary to make any effort, strength is gone
	White chestnut	Undesirable mind chatter, thoughts revolving in negativity
	Mustard	Susceptible to cycles of gloom, despair
	Chestnut bud	Does not learn from experience, observation does not help, but takes a long time to learn life lessons
Loneliness	Water violet	"I want to be alone." Very quiet people, very independent, self-reliant
	Impatiens	Impatient thought and action, everything must be done quickly. Needs to work alone.

EMOTION	REMEDY	SYMPTOMS
Loneliness (cont.)	Heather	Cannot stand to be alone, seeks out anyone for company
Oversensitive to influences and ideas	Agrimony	Supersensitive to argument or quarrel, will desperately try to avoid confrontation, happy and good-natured
	Centaury	Kind, quiet, gentle, most desirous of serving others; become servants rather than helpers
	Walnut	Person is on their path of life, fulfilling their ambitions, but occasionally can be swayed by strong outside influences
	Holly	Sometimes attacked by rage, jealousy, and suspicion without cause
Despondency or despair	Larch	Expect failure because they are not as capable or as good as others
	Pine	Never content with efforts or results
	Elm	Doing good work, following life calling, often for the good of humankind; occasionally have depression, feeling their work is too difficult
	Sweet chestnut	Mind or body feels it has borne all it can; now it must give way
	Star of Bethlehem	Shock of serious news, unconsolable for a time
	Willow	Suffered bad luck or hard times that they feel were undeserved, now bitter
	Oak	Fighters, persevere when everyone else would have stopped
	Crabapple	Feel unclean, become despondent if any kind of treatment fails
Over-care for welfare of others	Chicory	Caretakers, mindful of needs of others and want care recipients near them
	Vervain	Fixed principles and ideas; sure they are right and need to convert others
	Vine	Certain of their own ability and rightness, others should follow their lead
	Beech	Can only see the negative; need to be able to see more good in all, need more tolerance of others
	Rock water	Very strict with themselves, deny themselves because it might interfere with their work

Bach Remedies for Sensitive People

Because all flower essences, including Bach Remedies, are prepared with some type of alcohol, chemically sensitive people may not be able to use them. Pouring the prescribed dose of the remedy into a glass of water and allowing the alcohol to evaporate is helpful for many people.

to speed healing after medical and dental surgery.

It can be administered orally, in water, or by simply wiping a person's lips or skin with the Rescue Remedy. For people who cannot swallow, it can be placed on the pulse points. It can be dropped into food or drinking water for children and animals. Symptoms are often cleared very quickly, and Rescue Remedy can be taken again if needed. It is now available as a cream for topical application to bumps, bruises, sprains, and insect bites.

There are now several manufacturers of "flower essence" remedies that are similar to Bach Remedies. These other flower essence lines are effective for a variety of conditions, but contain more remedies than the original Bach line. They are prescribed according to the same basic guidelines as the Bach Remedies.

helpful for numerous acute health crises, such as allergic reactions, anxiety, hysteria, shock, physical trauma, or accidents. Rescue Remedy was named for its calming and stabilizing effect on the emotions during a crisis, and has also been successfully used

CHAPTER 29

Herbs and Aromatherapy

Herbs

Herbs were used for medicinal purposes long before written history began. One of the first written records dates back to the Sumerians, who described medicinal uses for herbs 5,000 years ago. The first Chinese herb book was written in 2700 B.C., and in 1000 B.C., the Egyptians are known to have been using medicinal herbs. The Old Testament mentions the use of herbs. Before the advent of modern pharmaceuticals, herbs were the main medical treatment for all people.

Today, herbs are still the primary medication for over 4 billion people—two-thirds of the world's population. Most of these people live in developing countries. Herbs are used in North America, but on a more limited basis. However, there is renewed interest in the use of herbs, particularly their role in helping to maintain good health.

Because healing herbs cannot be patented, giving pharmaceutical companies exclusive rights to the herb, these compa-

nies are not interested in them. The collection and preparation of herbs cannot be controlled as easily as synthesizing drugs, making profits less predictable and dependable. Also, access to herbs is sometimes limited and unstable. Instead, researchers isolate their active constituents and chemically alter them slightly to create a unique product. They synthesize a compound that mimics a natural plant compound, which can then be patented as a marketable drug.

Many lay herbalists, as well as innovative physicians and healthcare professionals, have added herbs to their treatment methods. Many botanical remedies have worked consistently and successfully for hundreds of years, and they are a very effective treatment for many conditions. However, with their high terpene and phenolic content, some people sensitize to herbs very quickly, particularly people with chemical and food sensitivities. In addition, herbs imported from other countries are usually sprayed upon arrival, thus contaminating them with

Use with Care

Herbs must be used appropriately and carefully. They are less likely to cause side effects than pharmaceuticals, but they can be very potent. Trained herbalists use them with great care, as improper use can cause unwanted and sometimes dangerous results.

Herbs and prescription drugs can interact. Some herbs can negate the action of prescription drugs, while others potentiate their effect, causing unwanted and uncomfortable results. Consult a trained herbalist if you take prescription drugs and wish to begin using herbs.

plant of which parts, including roots, leaves, bark, or berries, are used for medicine, food, or scent. Herbs are used as medical treatment, food seasoning, nutritional supplements, and dyeing or coloring substances.

The medical action of herbs is subtle. It is not always possible to separate herbs into their specific, isolated components because the herb functions as a whole rather than as a single active ingredient. Although there is an active ingredient, there are also other components that may act as synergists, counterbalances, or buffers. Nature provides a balance of ingredients that the body utilizes for healing.

■■ ACTION OF HERBS

Herbs have many different actions. The following are some of the detoxification actions of various herbs:

- *Adaptogen:* Improve the body's adaptability; help the body deal with stress; support adrenal gland and possibly pituitary gland function; increase the resistance of glands to damage.
- *Anticatarrhal:* Remove catarrah (excess

pesticides. Some imported herbs have been mixed with pharmaceuticals, and some have been mixed with less expensive herbs, diluting their purity.

The information presented in this chapter is an introduction to herbs only. Further research and guidance in the use of herbs is recommended. As with all things in life, good quality, moderation, and balance are of prime importance when using herbs. They are powerful medicines and should have our respect. It is our responsibility to seek information and qualified assistance before acting. Time and small doses of herbs will support our bodies to heal themselves.

■■ WHAT IS AN HERB?

The word "herb" has many definitions. Some consider it a nonwoody plant that dies after it flowers. Others define an herb as any

Herbs and Pregnancy

The following herbs should not be taken if you are, or might be, pregnant:

barberry	goldenseal
black cohosh	green tea
blue cohosh	licorice
cat's claw	passion flower
cinnamon	rhubarb
comfrey	wormwood
feverfew	

mucus) by reducing the secretion or making the secretion more fluid to flush out the infecting organism.

- *Antihelmintic:* Destroy and/or expel worms from the digestive system.
- *Antiparasitic:* Rid the body of parasites.
- *Antipyretic:* Prevent or reduce fevers.
- *Antiseptic:* Destroy pathogenic bacteria.
- *Aperient:* Mild laxative; promote natural bowel movements and functions.
- *Blood purifier:* Cleanse the blood.
- *Carminative:* Expel gas from the intestine.
- *Cholagogue:* Stimulate the flow of liver bile, helping fat digestion; a natural laxative the facilitates cleansing.
- *Choleretic:* Stimulates production of bile by the liver.
- *Depurative:* "Blood cleanser"; restore proper function; usually indicated in chronic inflammation or degeneration (skin, arthritic, autoimmune).
- *Diaphoretic:* Promote sweating and help skin eliminate wastes; some diuretic effects.
- *Diuretic:* Increase blood flow through kidneys and reduce water reabsorption in the kidney nephrons; some have cardio-active

properties (they stimulate the heart) also. People with high blood pressure should not use cardio-active herbs.

- *Expectorant:* Stimulating; chemically irritates the lining of the bronchioles.
- *Hepatonic:* Tone and strengthen the liver, and in some cases increase the flow of bile.
- *Purgative:* Empties bowels.
- *Respiratory relaxing:* Soothe bronchial spasms and loosen mucus.
- *Rubefacient:* Cause dilation of blood vessels and a gentle increase in surface blood flow.
- *Vulnerary:* Healing application for wounds.

■ PREPARATION AND ADMINISTRATION OF HERBS

Plants are composed of root, stem, leaf, flower, and fruit. Some parts of a plant may be more medically active than others. Fresh herbs contain more enzymes, making the herbs more potent and active than those that have been dried. Freeze-dried herbs are also more potent than air-dried herbs. Availability usually determines what form people use, as herbal supplies vary greatly from community to community.

Herbs can be administered in several different forms. The carrier used for administration will partially depend on the solubility of the herb or its parts in water, alcohol, or fat (oil). It is vital to use good-quality herbs and cold-pressed oils, and to prepare herbs in clean glass or lead-free ceramic containers. Herbs should be stored in colored glass or ceramic containers, as exposure to light can destroy their potency.

Some of the common carriers by which herbs may be administered are described below.

Dosage

The doses for herbs must be adjusted according to the needs of the person. Older people and children require smaller doses. Likewise, a slightly built person will need a smaller dose than a very heavy person. People who are normally very sensitive to medications will require small amounts of herbs.

Always begin with the lowest recommended dose. If you experience no problems and are not getting the desired response, build up to the maximum dose. Do not exceed the recommended dose on the label. Some herbs are recommended only for short-term use, such as echinacea and goldenseal.

■ CAPSULE

Capsules are filled with powdered herbs, and the gelatin of the capsule may be of plant or animal origin. Herbal capsules usually contain only the herbs. They do not contain the fillers and binders found in some nutrients and pharmaceuticals that are dispensed in capsules. Capsules allow you to take herbs that have an unpleasant taste, and are convenient when traveling.

■ COMPRESS

A compress is used to apply herbs to an area to reduce pain and inflammation and prevent infection. It may be applied with pressure. (See chapter 30, Topical Detoxification, for more information on compresses.) To prepare a compress, bring 1 or 2 heaping Tbsp. herbs to a boil in 1 cup water. Dip a cotton pad or gauze into the strained liquid. Apply to the body at a safe skin temperature and cover if needed. Change when cool.

Cold herbal compresses can be made by soaking a cloth or towel in an infusion or decoction that has cooled. Wring out the excess liquid and apply to the affected area. Leave in place until warmed by body heat. Repeat if needed.

■ DECOCTION

A decoction is a tea usually made from roots, seeds, berries, and barks that contain the mineral salts and bitter components rather than vitamins and volatile components. More heat is required to release these parts of the herb. A decoction is prepared by soaking the herb, then boiling it in water for 5 to 20 minutes. The mixture is then strained, and may be taken hot or cold.

■ EXTRACT

Extracts are prepared by soaking the herb in water, vinegar, or oil, depending on the solubility of the herb, for 4 to 15 days, shaking the container twice daily. Vitamin E can be added as a preservative.

Extracts prepared with cold water will

Buckthorn

A child who missed days and days of school with a stomach ache was found on examination to have intestines full of stool. Her stomach aches were caused by profound chronic constipation. Buckthorn (Cascara sagrada) gently relieved the constipation and ended her stomach pain.

preserve the most volatile ingredients and extract only minor amounts of mineral salts and bitter components. Soaking herbs for a cold-water extract requires only 8 to 12 hours. Extracts are not as strong as tinctures (see below).

■ INFUSION

Although the terms infusion and tea are used interchangeably by some herbalists, they are not the same. Infusions are steeped much longer and as a result are stronger. Infusions are made from flowers, leaves, and stems and may be hot or cold. To prepare a hot infusion, pour 2 cups hot liquid over 1/2 to 1 ounce powdered herbs. Cover tightly to prevent evaporation and steep 10 to 20 minutes before drinking.

Cold infusions are made by placing the herb or herb parts in water in a clear glass container and placing them in the sun to steep. Steep for an hour, or until the desired strength is obtained.

■ OINTMENT

An ointment is intended to hold herbal ingredients in a Vaseline or non-petroleum jelly or oil on an area for an extended time. To prepare an herbal ointment, use Vaseline, non-petroleum jelly, or oil as a base. Add 1 or 2 heaping Tbsp. herbs and bring to a boil. Stir and strain. Allow to cool to a safe skin temperature before using.

■ POULTICE

A poultice is used to apply warm mashed, ground, or powdered herbs directly to the skin to draw out toxins or embedded objects, or to relieve pain and muscle spasms. (See chapter 29, Topical Detoxification, for specific poultices.) It has to be replaced frequently to preserve the warmth.

Herbal Antibiotics

Many sensitive people are unable to take antibiotics, but there are times when they may need to do so. Bladder infections, abscessed teeth, or strep throat are conditions that require treatment. The combination of echinacea and colostrum or goldenseal and colostrum will act as an effective herbal antibiotic for some people.

To use a poultice, clean the skin surface with a tolerated antiseptic, such as Zephiran, then oil the skin before applying the poultice. Moisten the herbs with a warm liquid such as water, apple cider vinegar, herbal tea, liniment, or tincture. Spread 1/4 to 1/2 inch thick, and apply to the skin directly, or between a layer of gauze.

■ TINCTURE

Used topically or in liniments, a tincture is prepared by steeping the herb in alcohol. Warm wine or apple cider vinegar can be used, but this produces a solution rather than a true tincture.

To prepare a tincture, combine 4 ounces powdered or cut herbs with 2 cups alcohol (vodka, brandy, gin, run, bourbon, or Everclear—a liquor that is 90 proof ethanol). Shake daily, and steep for two to four weeks. Let herbs settle completely, then pour off the tincture, straining out the herbs through cheesecloth or an unbleached coffee filter.

Drinkable tinctures are made by using 1 ounce powdered herbs to 5 ounces alcohol. Use ethanol or Everclear for the alcohol. To drink, put 10 to 30 drops of the tincture in

Herbs for Cleansing and Strengthening Organs

ORGAN	HERB	ACTION
Liver	Burdock root, yellow dock	Cleanses, restores function
	Licorice root	Cleanses and heals
	Oregon grape	Cleanses
	Dandelion	Cleanses, increases production of bile
	Siberian ginseng, ginseng	Detoxifies and protects liver from effects of drugs, improves function
	Cayenne	Lowers cholesterol, increases blood flow
	Milk thistle, rosemary, turmeric	Protects liver against toxins
	Blessed thistle	Heals the liver
	Fennel, goldenseal	Promotes liver function
Colon/intestines	Buchu	Decreases inflammation
	Buckthorn, cat's claw, chlorophyll, flax, ginger, licorice, sarsaparilla	Colon/intestinal tract cleanser
	Damiana, yellow dock	Stimulates contractions, improves function
	Fenugreek, mullein	Laxative
Kidneys	Bearberry, bilberry, birch, corn silk, dandelion, gravel root, horsetail, hydrangea, nettle, juniper, kava kava, sarsaparilla, yarrow	Diuretic
	Cayenne, fennel, yellow dock	Promotes kidney function
	Burdock root, ginger, licorice root	Detoxifies through kidney
Lungs	Lungwort	Respiratory problems
	Lobelia	Bronchial smooth muscle relaxant and expectorant
	Black radish, chickweed, gingko biloba, lobelia, mullein	Relieves bronchial congestion, aids circulation
	Echinacea, ephedra, goldenseal, horsetail, juniper berries, licorice root, skunk cabbage, slippery elm bark	Relieves asthma

ORGAN	HERB	ACTION
Lungs (cont.)	Astragalus, myrrh	Antibiotic
	Pau d'arco	Antibiotic, reduces inflammation
	Ephedra	Relieves bronchial spasms
	Fenugreek	Reduces flow of mucus
	Siberian ginseng	Cleans bronchial passages, reduces inflammation
	Horsetail	Anti-inflammatory and expectorant, strengthens lungs
	Blue vervain, Iceland moss, nettle	Mucus congestion
	Feverfew, licorice	Increases fluidity of mucus in lungs
Skin	Alfalfa, burdock, cayenne, dandelion root, echinacea, marshmallow, Oregon grape, tea tree, wild strawberry, witch hazel, yellow dock	Treats acne
	Burdock, calendula, dandelion root, oat straw, onion, Pau d'arco, red clover	Cleanses boils
	Alfalfa, black walnut, calendula, comfrey, dandelion, horsetail, rose hips, yellow dock	Clears up bruises
	Burdock root	Increases circulation to skin
	Aloe vera, barberry, calendula	Kills organisms on skin
	Aloe, arnica, calendula, comfrey, dandelion, echinacea, St. John's wort	Cleanses and treats wounds
Lymph	Bayberry, bearberry, echinacea, goldenseal, lemon balm, lobelia, oatstraw, wild cherry bark, sage, thyme, yellow dock	Cleanses
Blood	Blessed thistle, burdock root, dandelion, echinacea, Pau d'arco, red clover, sage, yellow dock, yerba maté, yucca	Cleanses
	Bayberry, blessed thistle, cayenne, cedar, cinnamon, elder, eucalyptus, garlic, gentian, ginger	Improves circulation
	Elder	Strengthens blood

Herbs to Treat Specific Conditions

CONDITION	HERB	ROUTE OF ADMINISTRATION	ACTION
High blood pressure	Celery, garlic	Oral	Reduces blood pressure; improves circulation
Dysentery	Bayberry, blackberry garlic, marshmallow, prickly ash bark, slippery elm bark, turmeric	Oral	Combats diarrhea, stomach problems
Amebic dysentery	Barberry	Oral	Purges bowels; stimulates intestinal movement
Lead poisoning	Garlic	Oral	Sulfur removes metals
	Apple, pectin	Oral	Source of fiber, which helps remove metals
Free radical excess	Cat's claw, chaparral, elder, ginger, milk thistle, turmeric	Oral	Antioxidant; free radical scavenger
Bacterial infections	Buckthorn, goldenseal, licorice root, pau d'arco, rosemary, tea tree	Oral	Antibacterial; counters infection
Canker sore	Myrrh	Topical	Combats bacteria in mouth
Viral infections	Balm, boneset, cedar, chamomile, cinnamon, echinacea, ginger, ginseng, goldenseal, licorice root, lobelia, St. John's wort, slippery elm bark	Oral	Antiviral; anti-inflammatory; helps with diarrhea, nausea
Fungal infections	Alfalfa, black walnut, cedar, cinnamon, Pau d'arco	Oral	Antifungal

CONDITION	HERB	ROUTE OF ADMINISTRATION	ACTION
Candidiasis	Barberry, chamomile, cinnamon, dandelion, echinacea, garlic, goldenseal	Oral	Antifungal
	Tea tree, thyme	Topical	Antifungal; relieves scalp itching and flaking from Candidiasis
Urinary tract infections	Cranberry, rose	Oral	Acidifies urine; prevents bacteria from sticking to bladder wall
Parasitic infection	Black walnut, buckthorn, clove, gentian, parsley, rhubarb, senna	Oral	Helps rid body of parasites
Giardia lamblia	Barberry, bayberry, echinacea, elecampane, garlic, goldenrod, turmeric	Oral	Antibiotic action; relieves digestive problems
Intestinal worms	Black walnut bark, garlic, parsley, rhubarb, wormwood	Oral	Expels worms
Premenstrual syndrome	Alfalfa, angelica root, asparagus, black cohosh, blessed thistle, celery, cramp bark, dong quai, false unicorn root, rosemary, strawberry lleaf, valerian root	Oral	Balances hormones; relieves cramps and hot flashes, menstrual irregularities

CONDITION	HERB	ROUTE OF ADMINISTRATION	ACTION
Gangrene	Garlic	Oral	Combats infection
Insect bites	Aloe vera, calendula, comfrey, echinacea, goldenrod, lobelia, marsh tea, mint, parsley, plantain, skullcap, wild hyssop, witch hazel	Topical	Anti-inflammatory
Poison ivy/ poison oak	Aloe, black walnut, grindelia, gumplant, jewelweed, lobelia, mugwort, Solomon's seal, sumac, sweet fern, white oak, witch hazel	Topical	Relieves blisters, rashes
Burns	Aloe vera, bayberry, blackberry leaves, goldenseal, horsetail, slippery elm, sumac leaves, sweet gum, white oak bark	Topical	Heals burns
Eczema	Chaparral, dandelion, goldenseal, myrrh, Pau d'arco, red clover, yellow dock root	Topical	Relieves and heals eczema
Rashes	Calendula, chamomile, chaparral, dandelion, elder flower, tea tree oil, yellow dock	Topical	Relieves and heals rashes

one glass of water or juice and take two to three times daily.

■■ DETOXIFYING WITH HERBS

The focus of cleansing with herbs is to promote healing by eliminating toxins from the organs and systems of the body. This purification process begins by using aromatic and bitter herbs that initiate purging of body systems. Herbalists then revitalize the systems with toning, soothing, and strengthening herbs.

Thousands of herbs have medicinal properties. Herbalists know the strengths and weaknesses of these herbs and can dependably predict their action on a given person. There are around 100 herbs that are commonly used, but most herbalists regularly use fewer than 25 herbs.

Aromatherapy

Aromatherapy is a branch of herbal medicine that makes use of scents for treating various health problems. Scents or aromas

> ### Dental Work
>
> *For canker sores, infected gums, sore tongue, or tonsillitis, a goldenseal mouth rinse is helpful. Combine:*
> *1 cup warm water*
> *¼ tsp. salt*
> *¼ tsp. goldenseal powder*
> *For people who tolerate it, a little cayenne pepper in this mixture is also helpful. Use as needed to control pain and soothe the tissues.*

from the essential oils of plants affect the way people feel. These oils can cause mental, emotional, and physical changes, both positive and negative. Researchers have found that scents affect mood, and that people in a good mood are more productive. Some fragrances can counter the negative effects of stress. Calming oils not only promote calmness, but also a general sense of well-being, while stimulating oils can produce heightened energy.

Aromatherapy had its beginnings over 5,000 years ago in Egypt. Egyptian men would place a cone of solid unguent on the top of their heads. During the day, the unguent would slowly melt, covering their head and body with perfume. The Egyptians also used essential oils in cosmetics, embalming, medicines, and religious ceremonies. Aromatherapy later spread throughout the Mediterranean countries. Both the Greeks and Romans used plant and flower essences in connection with their public baths.

> ### Surgery
>
> *Post-surgery trauma is helped by the following herbal combination, using equal amounts of each herb. It can be used as a tea or taken in capsules. Use two to three times daily, for up to a month after surgery.*
>
> | | |
> |---|---|
> | Buckthorn bark | Prickly ash bark |
> | Burdock root | Red clover |
> | Kelp | Sarsaparilla root |
> | Licorice root | Stillingia |
> | Oregon grape root | |

Essential Oils During Pregnancy

Pregnant women must check with a healthcare professional before using essential oils. The following essential oils are permissible during pregnancy, with a physician's approval, after the first trimester:

Bergamot	*Lemon*
Chamomile	*Mandarin*
Coriander	*Neroli*
Frankincense	*Orange*
Geranium	*Rose otto*
Ginger	*Sandalwood*
Grapefruit	*Spearmint*
Lavender	*Ylang ylang*

An Arabian physician known as Avicenna (980 to 1037 A.D.) invented the process of distillation, making it possible to prepare very pure essential oils from plants that could previously not be used. Distillation is a purification process that is able to separate a mixture. When the mixture is heated, each substance in it boils at a different temperature. As it boils, each substance is condensed to a liquid and collected. Although cold-pressed oils had been used in rituals and healing prior to this time, they were not as pure. The discovery of distillation laid the foundation for modern aromatherapy, because pure essential oils could be obtained from many more plants.

The *Vedas*, a 2,600-year-old text from India, contains the recording of Ayurveda, a medical system practiced in India for over 4,000 years. In it, the therapeutic properties of numerous aromas are classified. Later works, including Nicholas Culpeper's 1651 book, *The Complete Herbal*, detailed medicinal properties of hundreds of herbs. Salmon's *Dispensatory of 1696* contains a recipe for an "apoplectick balsam." The same book also contains an herbal recipe for treating the loss of memory. By the turn of the 18th century, essential oils were being widely used in medicine, both internally and externally.

In 1937, the term aromatherapy was coined by Rene M. Gattefossé, a French research chemist. He became convinced of the value of essential oils as the result of a laboratory accident in which his right hand was burned. He instantly immersed it in pure lavender oil and discovered that the hand healed very quickly without infection or scar. Jean Valnet, a physician inspired by the work of Gattefossé, used essential oils extensively for treating battle wounds in French military hospitals during World War II. In 1961, he published *Aromatherapie*, later published in English as *The Practice of Aromatherapy* (1977).

■■ PREPARATION AND ADMINISTRATION

In aromatherapy, essential oils extracted from the flowers, fruits, leaves, stems, or roots of a plant or tree are used therapeutically. The oils are found in tiny oil glands or sacs that are concentrated in various parts of the plant. These oils carry the taste and scent of the original plant. Essential oils are odorous and highly volatile. Their chemical composition constantly changes according to the location, time of day, and the season. Soil

Essential Oils for Sensitive People

Sensitive people may have difficulty tolerating essential oils. For some people, diluting the formulas to one-fourth strength or less is helpful. Other people who are sensitive to phenolics and terpenes may not tolerate essential oils at all.

conditions, climate, and cultivation also affect their odor and chemical constituents.

Several types of oils are used in aromatherapy. These include:

• *Base or carrier oil:* a natural oil such as almond, corn, olive, or sunflower that is unrefined or cold-pressed and is used to dilute essential oils.

• *Essential oil:* aromatic oil prepared by distillation and composed entirely of volatile molecules.

• *Infusion oil:* made by macerating fresh plant material in a high-quality vegetable oil.

Most essential oils are clear, and they are soluble in alcohol, ether, and base or carrier oils. Some of them are not as soluble in water, but a water solution will be as effective as other preparations. Essential oils may be administered orally, topically, or by inhalation. Inhalation allows the treatment of respiratory conditions, as well as promoting the calming or mood-lifting properties of the aroma.

Use 6 to 12 drops of essential oil in $1/2$ to 1 gallon of water for topical application or inhalation. Awareness of the aroma will fade

with continued exposure. Essential oils are used in massage, in compresses, and in baths. For massage, use 10 to 30 drops of essential oil per ounce of olive or almond oil. For baths, put 5 to 10 drops of essential oil in a bathtub of water. Oral administration requires expert medical supervision, and the oils must be diluted and combinations precisely formulated.

Essential oils affect many body systems, and many conditions can benefit from aromatherapy. The lightest, fastest-acting essential oils are useful in cases of lethargy, apathy, or depression. They counteract physical heaviness and can be used in situation of shock caused by physical or emotional trauma. Medium-density essences affect the metabolism and functions of the body. The heavier oils, gums, and resins act on the mucous membranes and are valuable for treating chronic conditions. Nervous conditions respond well to these essences.

Be sure that you purchase good-quality essential oils that have not been diluted. True essential oils are extremely concentrated, and dilution is mandatory before using them.

■ ESSENTIAL OIL FORMULAS

The following formulas are only a sample of the great number that are available. See Suggested Reading for recommended books on aromatherapy.

■ COLD SORES
1 Tbsp. St. John's wort infusion oil
1 Tbsp. mullein infusion oil
$1/4$ tsp. wheat germ infusion oil
$1/4$ tsp. carrot seed infusion oil
400 IU vitamin E

10 drops Melissa essential oil
5 drops geranium essential oil
5 drops tea tree essential oil
3 drops rose essential oil
2 drops bergamot essential oil

Add the infusion oils and vitamin E to a dark glass bottle. Then add the essential oils, shake well, and label.

Saturate a cotton swab and apply to the skin lesions four times a day. It is also very effective applied to the skin when it begins to tingle, before blister formation. Wash hands well after applying the oils.

■ POISON IVY, OAK, AND SUMAC
1/4 cup apple cider vinegar
1/4 cup witch hazel lotion
1/2 cup cold water
2 tsp. baking soda
2 drops chamomile essential oil
2 drops geranium essential oil

Mix vinegar, witch hazel, and water in a bowl. Mix the baking soda and essential oils in a separate cup. Add to the vinegar mixture and blend well. Soak a clean cloth in this solution.

Apply the cloth to the affected skin and place plastic wrap over it. Replace when the cloth becomes dry or warm. Treatment time should be 15 to 20 minutes. Use three or four times per day to relieve itching and promote healing.

■ JET LAG
4 parts lavender essential oil
2 parts lemon essential oil
1 part rosemary essential oil
1 part bergamot essential oil

Mix the oils in a small, dark glass bottle. Inhale a few drops from a tissue while traveling.

Aromatherapy for Cleansing and Strengthening Organs

ORGAN	ESSENTIAL OIL	ACTION
Body balancer	Bergamot, geranium, lemon, juniper, rose otto	Balances according to needs, cleanses, depurative
Liver	Lavender, lemon, rosemary, rose otto, peppermint	Cleanses and strengthens liver, stimulates bile flow
Colon/intestines	Black pepper, rosemary, rose otto, sweet marjoram	Relieves constipation
	Coriander	Relieves diarrhea
Kidneys	Cedarwood, juniper, Scotch pine	Diuretic
Lungs	Cedarwood, cypress, eucalyptus, frankincense, orange, rosemary	Relieves bronchitis
	Chamomile roman	Clears respiratory allergies
	Juniper	Treats infections
	Sandalwood	Treats respiratory disorders
Skin	Bergamot, cedarwood, cypress, eucalyptus, geranium, juniper, lavender, neroli orange blossom, peppermint, Roman chamomile, rose otto, Scotch pine, sandalwood	Treats acne, other skin problems
	Lavender, sweet marjoram	Clears bruises
	Geranium, lavender	Treats burns and scalds
	Cedarwood, geranium, lavender, Roman chamomile, sandalwood	Treats eczema
	Cedarwood, eucalyptus, frankincense, geranium, lavender, lemon, patchouli, tea tree, ylang ylang	Treats wounds, cuts, and scrapes
Blood	Angelica, fennel, juniper, rose otto	Combat impurities in the blood

Aromatherapy to Treat Specific Conditions

CONDITION	ESSENTIAL OIL	APPLICATION	ACTION
Anxiety	Bergamont, chamomile, clary sage, frankincense, juniper berry, lavender, melissa, neroli, rose otto, ylang ylang	Baths, massage, skin, and as a room perfume	Sedative, dulls nervous sensibility, lightly hypnotic
Depression	Basil, bergamot, citrus, clary sage, lavender, neroli, sandalwood, vetiver ylang ylang	Baths, massage, skin, and as a room perfume	Antidepressant, restorative, adrenal stimulant, nervous system regulator
Poor circulation	Black pepper, coriander, cypress, ginger, juniper, lavender, lemon, orange, rosemary, rose otto, sweet marjoram, vetiver	Baths, foot/hand bath, massage	Improves circulation, produces warmth, raises body temperature
Hypertension	Clary sage, lavender, lemon, marjoram, ylang ylang	Baths, massage, personal perfume, vaporizer	Hypotensives (lower blood pressure)
Constipation	Black pepper, rosemary, rose otto, sweet marjoram	Baths, massage (especially over abdomen)	Strengthens peristalsis, supports digestion and elimination
Endocrine problems	Camphor, chamomile, clary sage, marjoram, rose, sandalwood, ylang ylang	Massage oil, aromatic baths, mood-enhancing room scents, personal perfumes	Balances hormones or acts as quasi-hormone
Infections	Frankincense, lavender, rosemary	Baths, infusion, tincture, decoction, lotion	Stimulate white blood cell production

CONDITION	ESSENTIAL OIL	APPLICATION	ACTION
Premenstrual syndrome	Chamomile, clary sage, cypress, frankincense, geranium, juniper, lavender, marjoram, neroli, rose otto, sandalwood, vetiver, ylang ylang	Baths, dry inhalation, massage (full body), personal perfume, vaporizer	Analgesic, anti-depressant, anti-inflammatory, antispasmodic, sedative
Bacterial infection	Clary sage, eucalyptus, garlic, lemon, onion, Scotch pine (all essences are bactericidal but these are particularly effective)	Effusion, essential oil, inhalation, skin lotions	Antibacterial
Viral infections	Black pepper, cypress, eucalyptus, ginger, marjoram, peppermint, Scotch pine, tea tree	Baths, foot bath, inhalations, massage oil (chest rub), room perfume, and fumigant	Antiviral
Cystitis	Bergamot, cedarwood, chamomile, eucalyptus, frankincense, juniper, lavender, pine, sandalwood, tea tree	Compresses on lower back, sitz baths, ordinary baths, massage	Antiseptic, antispasmodic, diuretic
Fungal infection	Myrrh, lavender, patchouli, tea tree	Facial oils and/or skin tonics, facial sauna, body massage, baths, essential oil ointment	Antifungal
Insect bites or stings	Eucalyptus, lavender, tea tree	Apply essential oil or essential oil ointment	Antivenomous and antitoxic

CHAPTER 30

Topical Detoxification

Topical ways of detoxification include the cleansing of skin lesions or other skin problems, as well as pulling toxins out of the body through the surface application of substances that draw and detoxify. Some applications are capable of stimulating the immune system and increasing white blood cell count.

Compresses, Poultices, and Packs

When used for cleansing the body, compresses, poultices, and packs stimulate circulation, cause sweating that excretes toxins, and draw out impurities. These noninvasive treatments can help to rid the body of many different toxins and infections.

Caution: Occasionally, sensitive people may develop a rash after a particular treatment. If this happens, do not use that treatment again.

▌▌COMPRESSES

A compress is a soft pad of gauze or cloth applied to a body part with varying degrees of pressure. Compresses can be used to control bleeding, to reduce pain and inflammation, or to prevent infection.

▌ICE OR COLD

Cold compresses soothe pain and reduce swelling. They are removed or changed when they warm to body temperature.

Ice or cold compresses can be used for bursitis, strains, sprains, sore throat, arthritis, inflammation, fever, headaches, hemorrhoids, and swelling.

▌HOT

Warm or hot compresses stimulate the circulation of blood and lymph, and heat cold joints. They are removed or replaced when they cool to body temperature.

Heat compresses can be used to relieve the pain of earaches, cystitis, diverticulitis, flatulence, old injuries, and headache.

▌ALTERNATING HOT AND COLD

Alternating hot and cold compresses applied over the affected area will help flush fluids in the area, pulling out waste products with the cold (contractive) phase, and bringing in fresh fluid (blood and nutrients) with the hot (expansive) phase.

Eye Compress

A special compress can be made for the eye by putting cotton in the bowl of a wooden spoon, wrapping it with cotton cloth or gauze, and tying it into place. The eye compress can then be dipped into hot or cold water. Express the excess water between layers of a folded towel and apply the compress to the eye. It may be used for 20 minutes out of every hour. For sties it may be used for 20 minutes every hour for three to four hours, until the stye either opens or subsides.

Heat helps for any condition in the front of the eyeball, such as infection. Cold relieves pain and congestion caused by a black eye or an insect bite to the eyelid.

Sore and inflamed eyes can also be helped by herbs. Dip the spoon compress in a decoction or infusion of an herb, such as goldenseal, aloe, anise, fennel, eyebright, or meadowsweet, and apply to the eye. Herbal compresses may be used hot or cold.

Use the hot compress for three to four minutes and follow with cold for thirty to sixty seconds. Repeat three to five times, always ending with cold. This treatment will help many conditions, including inflamed ovaries, nephritis, hepatitis, hemorrhoids, glaucoma, and sinusitis.

■ EPSOM SALTS
Dissolve 1 cup Epsom salts in 1/2 gallon hot water and apply as a compress to draw out boils or any type of infection. Leave on until the compress cools. Repeat if needed.

■ HERBAL
Specific herbal compresses can be used for bruises, swelling, hematomas, and pain. Compresses are made by diluting herbs in water. See chapter 29, Herbs and Aromatherapy, for instructions on making an herbal compress.

If used warm, allow to cool; if used cool, leave on until warmed by body heat. Repeat as necessary to obtain relief.

■ ESSENTIAL OILS
A cloth soaked in water to which 6 drops of essential oils have been added can be used for spot treatment of injured areas, such as wounds, sore muscles, joint aches and pains, or skin problems.

Make a hot compress with hot water, but allow it to cool to a safe skin temperature before using, then leave in place until it cools to body temperature. For a cold compress, use ice-cold water and leave in place until it warms to body heat. Repeat at intervals as needed. (See Aromatherapy in chapter 29 for recommendations of essential oils for specific conditions.)

■■ POULTICES

A poultice is usually described as a hot, moist preparation that may be applied to any part of the body. Poultices are used to relieve pain and congestion, reduce inflammation, promote absorption or resolution of an abscess, diminish tissue swelling and tension, soften crusted lesions, encourage muscle relaxation, stimulate healthy granulation (the formation of new tissue), and deodorize or disinfect.

Poultices

CONDITION	POULTICE
Cancer pain	Charcoal
Arthritis	Cabbage or comfrey leaf
Abdominal pain	Charcoal
Sore throat	Charcoal
Neuritis or neuralgia	Mullein or mustard
Bursitis	Green cabbage leaf or comfrey leaf
Inflammation	Charcoal or elderberry
Phlebitis	Papaya, mullein tea, or comfrey
Abcesses	Charcoal or goldenseal
Boils	Charcoal or flaxseed
Ear and eye infections	Charcoal
Superficial wounds	Aloe vera juice, charcoal, comfrey
Bruises	Comfrey or hyssop
Sprains	Charcoal
Varicose veins	Mullein
Warts	Comfrey root or leaf, or chickweed
Insect bites	Charcoal, plantain or lobelia

Poultices differ from a compress in that no pressure is used, and whole substances, such as herbs or clay, are usually used rather than a watered solution. The moist heat of a poultice can penetrate into the body for almost an inch and in some cases up to 3 inches. The poultice should always be slightly larger than the organ it is treating.

A poultice can be left on all night. Most poultices are applied warm and should not be reheated. When the poultice cools, discard it.

∎ CLAY

Clays have excellent drawing power for pulling toxins out of the body. Clay can be used in poultices, as a clay-water paste, or in a clay-glycerine mixture.

To make a clay poultice, sterilize the clay in a 350°F oven until heated through before mixing with the water or glycerine. Apply the paste to the skin and cover with cotton cloth; keep moist. Clay poultices may be left on for 6 to 10 hours. After removing the poultice, rinse the skin thoroughly and pat dry. Allow 1 to 2 hours before reapplying the poultice.

Clay poultices are effective for boils, corns, callouses, hemorrhoids, insect stings, ringworm, acne, gangrene, skin sores, and ulcers.

∎ CHARCOAL

Charcoal poultices are extremely effective against insect venom, such as spider bites and bee stings.

Charcoal combined with water and ground flaxseed (as a thickening agent) makes an excellent poultice that can be used almost anywhere on the body's surface. Use 3 Tbsp. ground flaxseed combined with 1 to 3

Charcoal Therapy

Charcoal is a superb cleaning material. Because it is very porous, charcoal has a large surface area to adsorb (attract and hold) toxins. For example, 1 quart of pulverized charcoal can adsorb 80 quarts of ammonia gas. Charcoal will adsorb chemicals, drugs, gases, body wastes, and foreign proteins. Activated charcoal is the best form for detoxification and cleansing.

Finely pulverized charcoal has the most cleansing power. Charcoal capsules and tablets help, but their efficiency is below that of powdered charcoal. While it is possible to make your own charcoal, in terms of purity and effectiveness, it is better to

purchase it at a health food store or drug store. Never use briquet charcoal intended for charcoal grilling, either internally or externally. This charcoal contains undesirable fillers, as well as chemicals to make it ignite rapidly.

Charcoal can be used both topically and orally for detoxification. Used topically, charcoal adsorbs harmful chemicals and microorganisms on the skin. No harmful effects have ever been reported from topical use. However, charcoal should not be placed on freshly broken skin. If the lesion extends through the skin into the dermis, it may result in tattooing of the skin.

Tbsp. charcoal and 1 cup water. Let set for 20 minutes or heat gently to thicken.

Spread the charcoal mix approximately 1/4 inch thick over a square of white paper towel or cotton cloth. Cover with another paper towel or cloth. Apply to the affected area and cover with plastic, then a towel, and leave the poultice in place for 6 to 10 hours. After removing and discarding the poultice, rub the skin gently with a cold, wet cloth.

Mini-poultices are effective for ant, mosquito, and chigger bites. They will also detoxify poison ivy eruptions. Apply charcoal to a piece of gauze or a Band-Aid. Dip the damp gauze into charcoal powder, or rub a charcoal tablet on the dampened gauze or Band-Aid until it is black. Place the poultice over the injury.

A second type of charcoal poultice uses equal parts of charcoal powder and olive oil.

Apply to the bite or sting on a paper towel or cotton cloth thoroughly saturated with the mixture. Cover with plastic and hold in place with adhesive tape. Leave in place for several hours.

■ CORNSTARCH

A poultice of cornstarch and fresh lemon juice, or cornstarch and witch hazel, alleviates the itching of mosquito bites. Mix in equal parts and apply to the bite with a large Band-Aid or a paper towel or cotton cloth held in place with adhesive tape for 30 to 60 minutes. Repeat as necessary.

■ HERBAL

Herbal poultices are made from crushed herbs or a paste of herbs, moistened and applied directly to the body or between a layer of gauze. The poultice should be 1/4 to 1/2 inch thick. Hold it in place with adhesive tape or an elastic bandage, and leave it on at

Castor Oil Packs

In addition to their excellent detoxification properties, castor oil packs have many other uses with surprising results. They have been used over the thymus to increase T-cell counts. One woman, troubled by adhesions because of many surgeries to her intestines, used castor oil packs once a week on her abdomen. During a subsequent surgery, her surgeon was amazed at the decrease in her adhesions.

least 3 hours or overnight. (See Herbs in chapter 29 for information on preparing herbal poultices.)

■ MUSTARD

Although called a plaster, a mustard plaster is actually a poultice. Many people remember mustard plasters from their childhood, sometimes with less than pleasant memories. However, correctly applied, a mustard plaster can be very helpful in relieving congestion and increasing circulation.

To make a mustard plaster, stir 1 Tbsp. dry mustard into 4 Tbsp. flour. Add enough warm water to make a paste thin enough to spread, but not thin enough to run. Place a clean cloth on a warm plate and spread the paste over the surface, but not extending over the edges. Place a clean cloth over the patient's chest so that there is a layer of cloth between the poultice and the patient's skin. Put the poultice in place and cover with a piece of plastic to prevent soiling the patient's clothing and bedclothes. Place a towel over the plastic and carefully pin through the clean cloth to hold the poultice in place.

Leave the poultice in place for 20 minutes only. The skin can blister if the mustard plaster is left on the skin longer. Remove it sooner if the patient complains of stinging and burning or if the skin becomes quite red. After removing, wipe the skin with a tissue or cloth dipped in a tolerated oil, such as mineral or cooking oil, to remove the mustard traces. Cover the area with flannel or a towel and leave overnight.

■■ PACKS

A pack treats the whole body or a body part by wrapping it to provide cover, containment, or therapy. For detoxification purposes, packs are used to hold a treatment in place or to provide a cold or hot application to a larger area of the body.

■ COLD PACK

Cold packs are administered with a cotton cloth that has been saturated with ice water, wrung so that it is not dripping, and placed on the treatment area. Always be sure there is a layer of dry cloth between a cold pack and the skin. A cold pack is replaced when it warms to body temperature.

Both hot and cold applications may be wrapped with another dry cloth to hold them in place.

■ HOT PACK

Hot applications are usually given with a cotton cloth that has been dipped in very hot water. Place the cloth over the treatment area and replace when it cools to body temperature.

Always check the temperature to be certain it is tolerable before placing the pack.

Packs for Specific Conditions

CONDITION	TYPE OF PACK	APPLICATION
Celiac disease	Castor oil pack	Over abdomen
Diabetes	Castor oil pack	From lower ribs to pubis
Liver pain	Hot castor oil pack	Over the liver
Immune depression	Hot castor oil pack	Over the thymus
Diverticulitis	Castor oil or cold pack	Over the pelvic area
Fever	Cold pack	Over the pelvic area
Tonsillitis	Cold pack	Around the throat
Cystitis	Hot pack	Over the pelvic area
Tendonitis	Hot castor oil pack	On affected tendons

∎ CASTOR OIL

Castor oil packs can be used on the liver to aid detoxification and on the thymus gland to strengthen the immune system. They have a drawing power as deep as 4 inches into the body. Use undyed or white cotton cloth or wool flannel (wool flannel is preferable) to saturate the oil for application to the body. Soak the flannel in cold-pressed castor oil. The castor oil *must* be cold-pressed, as heat processing destroys its therapeutic properties. Wring the cloth so it is still wet, but not dripping.

Apply the cloth to the affected area of the body and cover with plastic. Cover the plastic with a towel and place a heating pad or hot water bottle over the towel. If you use a heating pad, it should be as warm as it can be tolerated. You may have to refill the hot water bottle if it cools off too quickly. Leave the pack on for 1 to 1¹/₂ hours. Wash off any remaining oil with a water and baking soda mixture.

Some healthcare practitioners feel that the cloth can be stored in a covered pan or Ziploc bag and reused numerous times before it is washed. Others feel that one or two uses before washing and reusing are appropriate. The number of safe uses can be partially determined by the degree of toxicity being treated.

∎ CLAY

Clay has antibacterial properties and attracts toxins in much the same way as does charcoal. Clay packs may be used to reduce edema and to resolve boils. Clay has deep drawing power and will draw toxins and excess fluid out of the body through the skin. Clay packs help infections, both superficial and deep, and can help reduce pain and swelling. There are many clays suitable for packs, such as Indian Healing Clay, green clay, and bentonite clay. These clays and others are available at health food stores.

To make a clay pack, mix the clay until it is soft and has no lumps. It should be the consistency of a heavy ointment or cream cheese. Apply to the affected area to a 1/4 inch thickness. Cover with a damp cloth. Leave on for 30 to 60 minutes. Rinse off with water and pat skin dry. If the pack causes a rash, do not repeat.

Medicated Soaks

Soaks containing skin-soothing substances in the water can be used as topical means of detoxification. Soaks are similar to detoxification baths, but are concentrated on the affected area rather than the whole body. (See chapter 22, Saunas, Baths, and Hydrotherapy, for further information.)

▮ BAKING SODA

Soda soaks and baths are alkaline baths that are slightly anesthetic. They are soothing for drug reactions, poison ivy, itching eczema, hives, insect stings, heat rash, sensitivities to plants or chemicals, sunburns, and other general skin reactions and problems.

Use 1 cup baking soda to a tub of water at approximately 94° to 98°F. The soaking water should be dipped up with a cup so that it continually bathes all portions of the affected skin. Use the soak for 30 minutes to an hour. Allow the excess water to drip from the skin and then pat dry.

▮ STARCH

Used for the same skin irritations as baking soda, starch soaks consist of 1/2 cup starch stirred into a clean dishpan or bucket of hot water. Baths consist of 1 cup starch stirred into a shallow tub of water. The temperature should be at 94° to 98°F and the water must be stirred to keep the starch suspended.

Use a cup to dip the water onto all affected skin surfaces. Soak the affected part or stay in the tub for 20 to 30 minutes, then allow the skin to air dry, or pat dry gently.

▮ EPSOM SALTS

Dissolve Epsom salts in hot water for soaking infected fingers, hands, toes, and feet. Use 1 cup Epsom salts to 1/2 gallon of hot water. Soak for 30 minutes to draw out infections. Repeat several times during the day.

▮ OATMEAL

Oatmeal soaks and baths are soothing for poison ivy, eczema, hives, and any itching affliction.

For a bath, tie 1 pound uncooked oatmeal in a large piece of gauze and hang it under the bath spigot so that the water runs through the oatmeal. Use hot water so that it will soften the oatmeal and extract the starch. After the tub is filled, put the bag of oatmeal in the bath water or use it to sponge the surface of the body. One heaping cup of uncooked rolled oats ground fine in the blender can be substituted for the bag. Stay in the bath for 20 to 30 minutes and finish by gently patting skin dry.

To soak a hand or foot, use a dishpan or bucket of hot water and stir in 1/2 cup uncooked rolled oats ground in the blender.

CHAPTER 31

Organ Cleansing

Organs that participate in detoxifying the body are the liver, colon, kidneys, lungs, and skin. During times of stress and acute overload, cleansing procedures will help restore optimal function of these organs. In addition, before beginning any detoxification program it is imperative to be certain that these organs are functioning adequately. If any one of them is not performing well, there will be blockages in the detoxification process that will result in increased symptoms.

Although they are not organs, the lymph system and blood participate in detoxification. In many people, they are overloaded and in need of cleansing, which will improve both their detoxification efficiency and the health of the person.

Methods for cleansing the organs of detoxification are presented in this chapter. In addition, nutrients that aid organ cleansing are listed in chapter 23, Nutrients, and helpful herbs and essential oils are listed in chapter 29, Herbs and Aromatherapy.

It is helpful to consult a healthcare practitioner before beginning an organ cleanse to be certain your body is ready for and can handle these procedures. It is particularly important that the kidneys are capable of processing the increased load they will have to excrete, and most people will need to do the kidney cleanse first.

Liver

The liver is a major organ of digestion and assimilation, with many functions. The liver:

- detoxifies and eliminates xenobiotics (foreign chemicals).
- processes fats with the bile it produces.
- metabolizes hormones produced by the body.
- filters the blood.
- is the most important organ for the elimination of toxic wastes.

The liver requires large amounts of vitamins and minerals to function, but is able to store them in order to have a reserve. It can

Organ Cleansing Before Detox

Cleansing the organs that participate in detoxification before beginning any procedures that increase toxic load is imperative. This is clearly demonstrated in people who have their mercury amalgams removed without first determining whether their liver can handle the increased need for detoxification. Several patients who rushed into mercury amalgam removal became much worse because their bodies could not process the mercury and other toxins released.

Laboratory tests that indicate the efficiency and status of the detoxification pathways are available and provide useful information in planning treatment. (See chapter 5, Phases of Detoxification, for a discussion of the available tests.)

store enough vitamin A to last for four years, and enough vitamin D and B_{12} to last for four months.

All of the foreign chemicals to which we are increasingly exposed every day must be processed by the liver. Drugs, although they may be given for medicinal purposes, also stress the liver and must be detoxified by it. Using a complex system of enzymes, the liver transforms fat-soluble toxic chemicals into water-soluble compounds. They can then be released and eliminated from the body through the kidneys and gastrointestinal tract. An overburdened liver eliminates only part of the toxins, storing other toxins in its cells. These cells can store toxins for months, even years, eventually causing irreversible damage to the liver.

The liver processes estrogen produced by the body, as well as that taken in estrogen hormone therapy. If the liver cannot process the estrogen adequately, an excess results, increasing the risk of endometriosis; high blood pressure; premenstrual syndrome; inflammation of blood vessels; and breast, uterine, and vaginal cancer. In contrast, excess testosterone increases levels of aggressiveness, mood swings, and sexual energy. Dysfunction of reproductive cycles can result if the liver is unable to process the sex hormones properly.

The adrenal glands produce many hormones, including cortisol, aldosterone, androgens, and norepinephrine. The liver also processes all adrenal hormones, including the adrenalin produced by the adrenal glands in response to stress. Excesses of any hormones contribute to emotional imbalances, as well as stressing the liver; anger and depression may indicate poor liver detoxification functions.

The liver's sinusoids (filtering channels) allow it to filter the blood. These sinusoids are lined with special cells that engulf foreign debris, bacteria, and toxic chemicals.

When the body has an excess of toxins and waste materials, the liver cannot metabolize and detoxify them all. This results in unmetabolized toxins throughout the body and can lead to disease. Other organs involved in detoxification can help reduce the load for the liver. The health of these organs helps the liver retain its own health and ability to function. (See chapter 6, Organs of Protection and Detoxification, for more information on the liver and kidneys, and below for a discussion of the importance of kidney health.)

An overworked or poorly functioning liver is indicated by:

- poor or painful digestion, and soreness in the liver area with moderate fingertip pressure
- gas, constipation, a feeling of fullness, loss of appetite
- unexplained fatigue, listlessness, lethargy
- unexplained weight gain
- weak ligaments, tendons, and muscles
- food and chemical sensitivities and numerous reactions
- poor hair texture and slow hair growth
- skin itching and irritation, "liver spots," large bruises, yellow tint to the skin
- skin problems such as acne or psoriasis
- frequent headaches not related to tension or eyestrain
- emotional excesses, anger, moodiness

Diet, exercise, and lifestyle all influence liver health. The following suggestions will help to strengthen, support, and improve liver function.

∎∎ LIVER STRENGTHENING MEASURES

∎ DIET

Consume 30 to 60 grams of high-quality animal or vegetable protein a day. (However, a low-protein diet is recommended for people with significant liver disease.)

To increase enzyme activity, eat foods containing sulfur, such as garlic, onions,

---

Remedies for Strengthening and Cleansing

Many homeopathic, herbal, and aromatherapy remedies are helpful for both strengthening and cleansing the organs. See the charts in chapters 28 and 29 for remedies that aid specific organs.

---

and broccoli. Eliminate refined sugars, as they can lower enzyme activity.

Eat small portions of light, easy-to-digest foods, such as steamed vegetables, raw salad greens, and semi-sweet fruits (apples and pears). The moderately bitter taste of green vegetables such as endive, collard, dock, and dandelion activates the flow of bile. Also eat whole nuts and seeds. Drink roasted chicory and dandelion "coffee," adding ginger, cardamom, or fennel to taste.

Fats provide sources of energy but are hard to process. However, small amounts of unsaturated fats are essential for health. Lower your fat intake by eating less food cooked in oils or fats and avoiding margarine and shortening. Use virgin, cold-pressed olive oil in teaspoonful amounts over food (cold-pressed oil is more resistant to oxidation).

Eat sparingly and eat your larger meal early in the day. Allow at least 12 hours between the evening and morning meals. After 7 PM, take only a little herbal tea or a small amount of fruit.

∎ NUTRIENTS

Take vitamin, mineral, herb, amino acid, and bioflavonoid supplements to protect the liver. Phosphatidyl choline (a component of lecithin) can improve the health of membranes surrounding the microsomes, where enzymes are produced in the liver.

Use antioxidants, such as vitamins C and E, beta-carotene, zinc, and selenium. (See chapter 23 for a full discussion of nutrients.)

■ EXERCISE

Exercise before breakfast to keep eliminative channels open (the skin, lungs, kidneys, and colon). Exercise also increases oxygen metabolism, and high oxygen concentration is required for enzyme production, as well as for detoxification. Take a moderate walk after meals and try to release worry and anger.

■■ LIVER CLEANSING

■ LIVER MASSAGE

Massage helps to cleanse the liver. While lying flat on your back, using your flat fingertips, *gently* massage the liver area with clockwise circular motions. If soreness persists or if there is marked tenderness, you should consult a qualified professional.

■ LIVER FLUSH

Liver flushes stimulate the elimination of stored toxic wastes from the body, increase bile flow, and improve liver function. Christopher Hobbs, an herbalist from Santa Cruz, California, suggests this liver flush in his book, *Natural Liver Therapy:*

Mix fresh-squeezed orange, grapefruit, and lemon or lime juices to make 1 cup of liquid. The mixture should taste sour. Add 1 to 2 cloves of fresh garlic and a small amount of fresh ginger juice. (Grate the ginger on a vegetable grater and squeeze the fibers in a garlic press.) Stir in 1 Tbsp. of olive oil and drink.

> ## Maintaining Liver Health
>
> *The following procedures are helpful to maintain liver health. Use one or two of them weekly.*
> - *Take 1 to 3 Tbsp. of fruit pectin powder in water or fruit juice to increase fiber and to help absorb toxins.*
> - *Put 1 tsp. of bentonite clay in a glass of water, stir, leave in the sun for a few hours, then stir and drink. This helps remove toxins from the digestive tract, which in turn helps the liver.*
> - *Squeeze half a lemon into a quart of spring or distilled water (do not add honey) and drink. The sour taste cools and cleanses the liver.*

Follow the liver flush mixture with the following tea:

1 part fennel	1/4 part burdock
1 part fenugreek	1/4 part licorice
1 part flax	

Use 1 ounce of the herb mixture to 20 ounces of water and simmer for 20 minutes, then add 1 part peppermint. Steep for 10 more minutes.

For additional soothing properties, add 1/2 part marshmallow root (sliced and shredded) to the initial herb blend.

■ COFFEE ENEMA

One of the best liver cleansers is a coffee enema. Coffee enemas were listed in folk literature for years as a method of helping the body rid itself of toxins and accumulated waste products. They were listed in the Merck Manual until 1977, when they were removed for lack of space. After pharmaceuticals became the main focus of medicine in the 1920s, coffee enemas were seldom used. In the past 10 to 15 years, however, their usefulness has again been recognized. Dr. Sherry Rogers discusses them in detail in her book, *Wellness Against All Odds*.

A coffee enema is a low-volume enema that stays in the sigmoid colon, the S-shaped last section of the large intestine. A special circulatory system exists between the sigmoid colon and the liver, called the enterohepatic circulation system. When the stool reaches the sigmoid colon, it is full of decomposed material and toxins. These toxins are sent directly to the liver for detoxification rather than being circulated throughout the body.

The caffeine in the coffee is the active ingredient in a coffee enema. Given rectally, it helps detoxify the liver and emulsifies fat. While coffee enemas do promote cleansing of the intestines as well as the liver and gallbladder, they are used primarily to clean the liver and gallbladder.

A coffee enema:

- increases the peristaltic action of the intestines, and speeds up the emptying of the bowel.
- makes the toxins accumulated in the bile ducts empty, allowing other toxins in the body to filter into the liver for detoxification.
- increases the emptying speed of the liver ducts holding detoxified materials, speeding the detoxification process.
- encourages the removal of gallstones in the bile.
- stimulates the production of the enzyme

> ## Coffee Cleanse
>
> *While the idea of coffee enemas is strange to some people, and even repugnant to others, they can be extremely helpful. One important use for these enemas is to combat the toxicity produced by chemotherapy.*
>
> *Used on a regular basis, they will help people with high toxic burdens to detoxify. In addition, they can be used on an acute basis to clear allergic reactions, particularly those triggered by chemical exposures.*

glutathione-S-transferase, which makes the liver detoxification pathways function.

- breaks down accumulated fat in the liver cells.
- clears chemical overloads and chemical reactions.
- helps the body cope with chemotherapy and side effects caused by toxic overload from destruction of cells.

Minerals and electrolytes are not washed out by coffee enemas. The important nutrients have already been absorbed higher in the bowel, long before the food residue reaches the sigmoid colon.

Unsulfured molasses is used in the coffee enema to aid with retention and increase detoxification efficiency.

▮ *Materials Needed*

- a large stainless-steel or glass pot
- a Pyrex measuring cup with handle and pour spout
- tolerated water, as pure and free of chemi-

Coffee Sensitivity

Many people who are sensitive to coffee or do not tolerate caffeine are reluctant to try coffee enemas but, because the coffee stays in the sigmoid colon, and the caffeine only enters the entero-hepatic circulation system, it is safe for most people.

cals as possible. Do not use treated tap water from a city water supply.
• fully caffeinated, drip-grind organic coffee
• unsulfured molasses
• an enema bag
• if you have hemorrhoid problems, a soft rubber French catheter to fit over the hard plastic nozzle of the enema bag

❚ *Preparing the Enema*

Bring 1 quart of tolerated water to a boil in the stainless-steel or glass pot. Add 2 flat Tbsp. of coffee and continue to boil for 5 minutes. Turn off the heat and leave the pan on the burner. Add 1 Tbsp. of unsulfured molasses. Cool to a tepid temperature that feels comfortable to the touch. *Never* use the coffee mixture hot or steaming.

Strain, then pour half the coffee mixture into the measuring cup, being careful not to let the coffee grounds go into the cup. Put the enema bag in the sink and clamp off the tubing.

Pour the coffee mixture into the enema bag, then release the clamp long enough to allow the liquid to run to the end of the enema tube. Hang the enema bag 24 to 30 inches above the floor. A doorknob makes a good hanger. *Do not hang it any higher,* or fluid will be forced too high into the intes-

tine. Cover the area on which you are going to lie with old towels to prevent staining.

❚ *Taking the Enema*

First half:

Lie down on the floor and gently insert the nozzle or catheter. If you need lubrication, use only food-grade vegetable oil, K-Y jelly, or vitamin E. Do not use Vaseline or other petroleum jelly products, which are toxic.

Release the clamp and let the coffee mixture flow slowly in. Clamp off the tubing as soon as there is any sensation of fullness.

If you can do so, retain the enema for 10 minutes. Do not force yourself to hold it if an uncomfortable feeling develops.

Clamp the tubing and remove the nozzle or catheter, and empty your bowel.

Second half:

After emptying the bowel, repeat the procedure with the remaining half of the coffee mixture. If you cannot hold half of the enema mixture, take three or four small enemas.

When the gallbadder's bile duct empties, you will hear or feel a squirting under the right ribcage, or in that general area. Once you feel this, you should not take any more enemas that day.

If, after a week of daily enemas, you have not felt or heard the gallbladder release its bile, you may need to:
• increase the strength of the coffee 1 tsp. per quart at a time, but do not exceed 2 Tbsp. per cup.
• take slightly larger volume enemas with each half.
• take three enemas of 2 cups each or less.

Coffee enemas can be used without the

unsulfured molasses if tolerance is a problem. However, after taking the enemas for several weeks, you will probably be able to safely add it.

Most people do not feel "wired" or hyper as a result of coffee enemas. Should you feel this way, or if you have palpitations or irregular heartbeats after a coffee enema, reduce the amount of coffee by half for a few days to a week. Caffeine blood levels have been checked on people who felt they were "wired" after a coffee enema, and caffeine was not detectable in their blood.

Coffee enemas can be used as often as needed. The usual frequency for detoxification purposes is around three times per week. Some people may need to use them daily if their toxic load is high.

■ OTHER CLEANSING METHODS

Castor oil packs are extremely beneficial in cleansing the liver. For instructions on the use of a castor oil pack, see chapter 30, Topical Detoxification.

Several commercially prepared liver cleansing and support products are also available. We have found complex homeopathic products, such as PHP Liver Liquescence, which encourages liver drainage, to be extremely helpful for liver support and repair.

Gallbladder

The liver creates bile, a bipolar molecule (one end of the molecule is water-soluble and the other end is fat-soluble) that helps to emulsify fats, enabling the fat globules to be more easily broken down by enzymes from the pancreas. The bile produced by the liver is stored in the gallbladder, a pear-shaped

Gallstone Caution

People who have gallstones should not take coffee enemas. These enemas cause the gallbladder to empty, and if there are large gallstones present, they can block the bile duct as they leave the gallbladder.

sac on the underside of the liver. Because the liver and gallbladder are interconnected, the health of one affects the other.

■■ GALLSTONES

When the liver secretes too much cholesterol or bile becomes highly concentrated in the gallbladder, the cholesterol content becomes too high for the amounts of phospholipids (a type of fat molecule containing a phosphate portion from phosphoric acid) and bile salts. As a result, gallstones can form. Bile pigment crystals and calcium can harden the stones, which seem to form around a bacteria or other contaminant that serves as a "seed" to begin growth.

The typical North American diet promotes gallstones because of its high fat content. Many people have a gallstone that may or may not cause symptoms. If the stone is

Gallbladder Pain

Intense abdominal pain that radiates to the upper back is usually a sign that gallstones are present, and professional evaluation and help are needed. Do not undertake a gallbladder cleanse if you have this type of pain.

not calcified, it may not show up on X-ray. A gallbladder cleanse is helpful for many people. However, if you have symptoms suggestive of gallstones (nausea, abdominal pain, and clay-colored stools), have an ultrasound to determine the size of the stones. If they are too large to pass, do not do this cleanse. See your healthcare practitioner for advice.

Indications that a gallbladder cleanse is needed are:

- nausea after fatty meals, oily taste in the mouth or throat, revulsion to fatty foods
- poor digestion and soreness in the liver and gallbladder area with moderate fingertip pressure

■■ GALLBLADDER STRENGTHENING MEASURES

A diet favorable for gallbladder health is moderately high in animal or vegetable protein and low in refined carbohydrates, such as sugar and white flour. It should also be low in or contain no animal fat and red meat, fried foods, margarine, or commercial oils. Avoid spicy foods, soft drinks, coffee, and chocolate.

Take a B complex vitamin and lecithin, along with 400 to 800 IU of vitamin E daily. Soybeans and eggs are rich in lecithin, but some people may need a lecithin supplement in addition. The amino acid taurine helps keep the bile fluid.

■■ GALLBLADDER CLEANSE

Before you start a gallbladder cleanse, your bowels must be clean. Take an herbal laxative such as *Cascara sagrada* (buckthorn) or senna for two to three days before your cleanse. Also take three to four capsules of

---

Tea to Aid Fat Digestion

Poor digestion of fats may be accompanied by nausea and soreness in the gallbladder area. To help this condition, prepare as a tea:

1 part milkthistle seed
1 part artichoke leaves
1 part dandelion root
½ part mugwort
½ part skullcap
Use 1 ounce of the herbal combination in 2 cups of water. Simmer for 20 minutes. Remove from the heat and let stand for 10 minutes. Drink up to ½ cup three times a day.

---

hydrangea or hyssop twice a day for about a week before this cleanse to reduce any gallstones in size and number.

Use a juice fast for two days (see chapter 24), then follow the protocol below:

Day 1: Do not eat on this day. Drink the following amounts of pure, organic, preservative-free apple juice.

8 AM	1 glass (8 ounces)
10 AM	2 glasses
12 noon	2 glasses
2 PM	2 glasses
4 PM	2 glasses
6 PM	2 glasses
8 PM	2 glasses

Day 2: Do not eat on this day. Follow the same routine as on Day 1. At bedtime, drink 4 ounces of cold-pressed or extra virgin olive oil. (You may wash down the oil with hot lemon or apple juice.)

As a rule, this decongestion formula

starts to work on the second day. You may find small stones and/or green mud in the fecal matter. The malic acid in the apple juice helps to break down stagnant bile.

A cleansing, warm water enema may be necessary during the cleanse to alleviate nausea created by ingesting a large amount of oil at one time. This flush may be repeated in two months.

Colon

The gastrointestinal (GI) tract is one of the most important systems for removing toxins from the body. Toxins are contained in undigested material, or are secreted from the blood into the gastrointestinal tract. Here they are detoxified, eliminated from the body, or reabsorbed into the bloodstream. Toxins are sent from the intestines to the liver for detoxification. (See chapter 6, Organs of Protection and Detoxification, for further discussion of the GI tract.)

The colon acts as both the collector and eliminator of waste from the body. If the colon becomes sluggish and overworked, it cannot function properly. Poor diet, stress, use of laxatives, lack of exercise, and infrequent bowel movements all affect the function of the colon. As undigested food and wastes accumulate, they harden and adhere to the walls of the colon, making elimination even more difficult. Toxins from accumulated fecal matter are reabsorbed into the system, causing fever, earache, sore throat, headache, and many other symptoms. Such material also interferes with the absorption of nutrients from the colon.

This condition encourages the growth of unfavorable strains of bacteria, fungi, and parasites. The metabolic products of these organisms can spread from the colon into the body. An imbalance in bowel flora is known as intestinal or bowel dysbiosis. (Supplementation with *Lactobacillus acidophilus*, a beneficial bacteria normally present in the colon, will help re-establish balance. See Beneficial Bacteria in chapter 23 for a discussion of acidophilus treatment.)

Allergy extracts for pathogenic bowel bacteria help to cleanse the colon and relieve allergic symptoms caused by these organisms. Homeopathic bowel nosodes (remedies prepared from an organism or diseased tissue) are helpful for intestinal dysbiosis. Bowel nosodes are prepared from stool cultures. They are so dilute that the actual organism is not in the remedy. Bowel nosodes are taken orally and are prescribed by homeopaths based on the percentages of organisms found in the stools of patients or on clinical indications.

▮▮ COLON CLEANSING

Indications that a colon cleanse would be helpful include:

- *Constipation:* Unless you have at least one bowel movement a day and can evacuate your bowels quickly, you may need a colon cleanse.
- *Body and breath odor:* Any unpleasant body or breath odor, or a coated tongue, can be indicative of a high toxic accumulation in the colon.
- *Chronic health problems:* Many problems such as acne, allergies, arthritis, fatigue, gas, migraine, and recurrent bladder and vaginal infections may be caused or aggravated by a toxic colon.

Colon cleansing is a controversial method of detoxification and cleansing. There seems to be no middle viewpoint; people are either very much in favor or violently opposed. Those who favor colon cleansing feel that the health of the body reflects the health of the colon. They further believe that colon cleansing, either with enemas or colonics, is necessary for good health.

Those opposed to colon cleansing feel that it is an invasive treatment and that there is no medical reason to irrigate the colon. Homeopaths feel this method causes the loss of vital body fluids. Opponents of colon cleansing believe that proper diet, along with sufficient water and exercise, should allow you to move your bowels regularly. When the bowels function well, their natural physiological action should keep them clean.

Any cleansing method should be approached with caution, as you determine the appropriateness of a particular treatment for you. Very allergic people should be especially careful. You will have to make your own decision based on your own research.

Fasting is sometimes advocated before a colon cleanse. During a fast, your eliminative organs begin to remove concentrated and old, hard wastes, although they will not be able to eliminate all the accumulated material.

■ ENEMAS

Colon cleansing may be accomplished by administering an enema, which flushes the lower intestines. Substances used in enemas include water, coffee, herbal tea, mild soap solution, meat broth, chicken soup, wheat-grass juice, barley juice, chlorophyll, oils, or other nutritional substances. The fre-quency of enema use depends on the person's philosophy and tolerance. Some people take enemas once a month for preventive health maintenance. Others take a series of enemas seasonally.

■ *General Instructions*

Fill an enema bag with warm distilled or other tolerated water, or other liquid. Warmth allows the intestines to relax and expand.

Hang the bag 24 to 30 inches above the floor. A doorknob makes a good hanger. Cover the area on which you are going to lie with old towels.

Lying on the floor, lie on your left side or assume a knee-chest position (face down, supporting your weight on your knees and upper chest) to help water go through the colon.

Always lubricate the end of the rectal nozzle with vitamin E, food-grade vegetable oil, or K-Y jelly. Do not use petroleum jelly, which is a toxin.

Insert the tube or nozzle just inside the rectum. For a French catheter, as water begins to flow, gently insert the tube further—but never force it. The maximum tube insertion is 3 to 6 inches.

At the first urge or cramp, remove the tube and allow elimination.

Follow the warm enema with a cool water enema to stimulate peristaltic action and to soak off more material. When the intestinal muscles contract, more encrusted debris breaks off and leaves the body.

■ *Enemas for Specific Conditions*

• *To stimulate the liver, kidneys, spleen, and pancreas:* Add $^1/_2$ tsp. cayenne to an enema bag of water. This enema will also help stop

Restoring Bacteria

After taking an enema, always take some form of acidophilus, yogurt, buttermilk, or kefir to replace the natural beneficial bacteria of the colon. The colon cleanses will remove both harmful and beneficial organisms from the gut. Take acidophilus powder for at least five days after the cleanse.

bleeding that sometimes occurs with tissue irritation during rapid elimination.

- *To help eliminate parasites and Candida:* Blend 1 or 2 crushed garlic buds in 1 quart of tolerated water. Strain. Add enough tepid water to fill the enema bag. Repeat once a day for three days.
- *To clear allergic reactions:* Use 60 grams (8 level Tbsp.) of *buffered* vitamin C per quart of tolerated water. Allow the enema to run in very slowly and retain the fluid as long as you can comfortably do so. *Caution:* Never use ascorbic acid in an enema, as it is irritating to the colon.

▮ COLONICS

Some colon therapists advocate the use of high colonics, using specialized equipment to deliver the cleansing solution into the colon and to pump it out. This treatment cleans the entire colon.

Great care must be taken to clean the equipment between clients. If the equipment is not properly sterilized, parasites can be passed from one person to another.

▮ CLAY AND FIBER CLEANSE

A colon cleanse using a fibrous material, called psyllium, and clay can remove years of accumulated, caked-on material. Because it is taken orally and moves through the GI tract naturally, many people feel this is a safe, non-invasive method of cleansing the colon.

Psyllium attracts moisture into the bowel, which causes the psyllium to expand, filling the intestine. The clay absorbs toxins and helps carry them out of the colon. As it passes through the intestines, it drags out stored wastes. Do not exceed three colon cleanses per year, and wait at least two months between cleanses.

▮ *Materials needed:*
- bentonite clay (liquid solution)
- psyllium husks
- pint jar

▮ *Preparing the Cleanse*

Mix 1 Tbsp. of the liquid bentonite in the pint jar with 4 ounces of tolerated water. (If you cannot find a liquid bentonite solution, you may make your own by dissolving 2 ounces of bentonite clay in 1 quart of tolerated water. Shake well and allow to stand for 12 hours.) Then add 1 Tbsp. of psyllium husks. Cover and shake well.

▮ *Taking the Cleanse*

Drink the mixture quickly after you shake it. The longer it stands, the more it will clump. Follow with 8 ounces of pure, tolerated water. Drink this mixture three times a day, between meals, for 3 to 4 days. Take no food 2 hours before or for 2 hours afterward. Drink at least eight 8-ounce glasses of water a day.

This mixture can be constipating for some people. Should you become constipated, take extra vitamin C and magnesium (see chapter 23, Nutrients, for guidance). Some people may also need to use a plain

413

water enema, or the coffee enema described under Liver Cleansing, above.

Some people feel abdominal discomfort during the first day or two of the cleanse when the psyllium has expanded in the bowel. Many people pass particles of varying size and shape. Some report long casings that may be mucosal debris and dead cells from the intestinal lining.

❚❚ EXERCISE

Many people who have constipation do not exercise enough. Research tells us that our bowels will not move unless we move. Exercise helps keep abdominal muscles healthy and muscle tone optimal. Simple walking is very beneficial, but the following activities are particularly helpful to combat constipation:

- hill climbing
- climbing a ladder or stairs
- tennis
- rowing, with chest held high, and giving the trunk a strong backward movement
- medicine ball bouncing, to give the trunk muscles vigorous action
- chopping, digging, swinging, mowing
- folk and square dancing
- horseback riding

❚❚ FIBER

Fiber, sometimes called roughage or bulk, helps to relieve constipation. It absorbs water in the large intestine and makes stools larger, softer, and easier to pass. Food fiber is soluble and is best for your body. High-fiber foods include grains and bran, fresh fruits with skin on, dried fruits, raw vegetables, legumes, nuts, and seeds. Peeled, cooked, or

Movement and the Colon

Movement during exercise creates a series of light shocks, which encourage reflexive movements of the colon. The active play of children is a perfect example of this concept. Skipping, hopping, and jumping movements are especially beneficial. They initiate contractions of abdominal muscles and vigorous diaphragm movements, creating an accordionlike action in the intestines.

puréed fruits and vegetables have less useful fiber than those eaten raw.

By increasing high-fiber foods in your diet, fiber supplementation is not usually necessary. If you need to take a fiber supplement, start with small amounts and increase your water intake. You may experience some cramping, diarrhea, or gas at first. Fiber supplements can lead to dehydration, and minerals will be lost with the water. They can also decrease the absorption of dietary protein.

❚❚ FLUID

Many people are constipated or have difficult bowel movements because they do not consume enough liquid. Liquids, particularly water, keep stools soft. When liquid intake is too low, stools become small and hard. Coffee, tea, and caffeinated soft drinks can deplete the body of water because caffeine acts a diuretic.

There is controversy over how much water you should drink ordinarily. Many physicians say six to eight glasses per day, but some homeopaths feel that this much water overworks the kidneys. Certainly you should always drink when you are thirsty, and the bulk of your fluid intake should be water. During detoxification procedures, it is important to drink extra water.

■ LAXATIVES

Commercial laxatives can make a constipation problem worse. They are physically addictive and their frequent use can lead to vitamin and mineral deficiencies. Laxatives can weaken the GI muscles and decrease the effectiveness of peristalsis. Over a period of time, bowel movements become difficult without a laxative.

There are more natural options that will not harm your body. Ground psyllium seeds are a concentrated source of fiber, which has laxative properties. Psyllium is available at health food stores.

If you take vitamin C to bowel tolerance levels every day, you will not be constipated. Even if you do not take these amounts, extra doses of vitamin C help relieve constipation. (For further information on vitamin C, see chapter 23, Nutrients.)

Extra magnesium also relieves constipation. Magnesium is the active portion of Epsom salts and Milk of Magnesia. However, these laxatives are harsh to your body. Simply increasing your magnesium supplementation should clear constipation.

■ ORAL CHARCOAL

Taken orally, charcoal is an excellent cleanser for the gastrointestinal tract. Charcoal removes the odor from intestinal gas,

and it also helps indigestion, peptic ulcers, or other forms of gastrointestinal distress. It is generally tolerated well orally, and the only reported side effects have been bowel irritation in extremely sensitive individuals with bowel inflammatory problems.

Charcoal should not be taken continuously for years. It can be used intermittently for long periods of time, and regularly for several months. Some people are concerned that charcoal might adsorb nutrients, although there are studies that show it does not. It adsorbs mineral acids, alkalis, and salts poorly; for this reason, it does not adsorb nutrients. Food and bile interfere with charcoal's effectiveness, yet its adsorption capacity is still rapid. Charcoal works better in an acid than an alkaline medium.

Charcoal can be taken orally in the following ways:

- *Slurry:* Charcoal stirred into water forms a slurry. The usual oral dose of charcoal is 1 Tbsp. of powder stirred into a glass of water, taken mid-morning or mid-afternoon.
- *Tablets and capsules:* Intestinal gas and bloating can be treated with four capsules or eight tablets of charcoal taken three to four times per day, between meals. This treatment also helps with malodorous stools and bad breath originating both from the mouth and gastrointestinal tract.

Oral charcoal can prevent toxins from building up in the blood when the liver is not functioning well. The respiratory tract medication, Theophylline, has a narrow therapeutic range and overdoses are a common occurrence. People taking this drug should keep charcoal on hand to treat these overdoses.

Charcoal Slurry for Poisoning

In cases of poisoning, a charcoal slurry is more effective than induced vomiting or stomach lavage (pumping the stomach) to remove poison. Vomiting brings up only 30 percent of the poison. It is totally safe to use in acute poisonings; no contraindications are known.

Charcoal is the most important antidote for poisoning by acetaminophen, alcohol, amphetamines, aspirin, chlordane, cocaine, cyanide, gasoline, iodine, kerosene, Malathion, morphine, narcotics, nicotine, pesticides, phenol, and radioactive substances. For caustic agents such as lye, large amounts of charcoal are given. Larger amounts of charcoal must also be used to adsorb gasoline, lighter fluid, kerosene, and cleaning fluids. Mushroom poisoning can be treated with charcoal powder capsules or tablets even as long as 24 hours after consuming the mushroom.

In most cases, the effectiveness of charcoal is determined by the dosage and by how quickly it is given after a toxic exposure. The first dosage should be 8 to 10 times the estimated weight of the toxin. Subsequent doses should be twice the estimated weight of the toxin.

Charcoal forms a stable complex with toxins and does not subsequently release them for reabsorption into the bloodstream. The toxins are then excreted with the charcoal in the feces.

Kidneys

Our kidneys are a filtration system that constantly filters toxins and waste materials from the blood. The health of all the other organs is dependent on the proper functioning of the kidneys. If they are burdened with bacteria, calculi (stones), and accumulated toxins, they cannot filter the blood or regulate the body functions for which they are responsible.

When toxins are released from the tissues into the bloodstream, the kidneys must filter them for removal from the body. If the kidneys are unable to remove these additional toxins, they will be redeposited in the tissues. No detoxification will have been accomplished, and the kidneys may be overstressed and damaged.

Dehydration from the lack of sufficient water and fluids constitutes the most common stress to the kidneys. Kidney health is also affected by other factors, including diet, exercise, cardiovascular disease, stress, genetic weakness, infections, and kidney stones.

■■ KIDNEY STONES

Kidney stones and gravel (small stones) develop when calcium and other minerals crystallize in the collection ducts of the kidneys. They can cause a blockage anywhere in the urinary canal. This can impair the flow of urine, setting up conditions that encourage bacterial growth.

Proper diet, exercise, and adequate consumption of fluid can keep kidney stones from forming, but once they have formed, measures must be taken to rid the body of them.

∎∎ KIDNEY AND BLADDER INFECTIONS

Infections anywhere in the urinary tract can damage the kidneys if they are prolonged or left untreated. Lower back pain, unusual fluid retention, pain with urination, frequent unexplained chills, fever, or nausea may be a signal that you are on the verge of a bladder infection and are in need of a kidney and bladder cleanse.

Most urinary tract infections are caused by bacteria from the colon, making colon health and proper hygiene vital to the health of the urinary tract.

∎∎ KIDNEY CLEANSING MEASURES

For the kidney to be healthy, infections must be cleared and any stones dissolved. A kidney cleanse must remove all irritating chemicals, metabolic waste, and crystal deposits. It must also replace damaged cells with new healthy tissues.

∎ WATER

Drink eight to ten 8-ounce glasses of bottled or tolerated water every day during the cleanse. Make water your only beverage. Juices, caffeinated drinks, and sodas *do not* substitute for water.

After the cleanse, continue to drink eight 8-ounce glasses of water daily. Water helps detoxify the kidneys, as well as diluting the urine, preventing concentrations of the minerals and salts that can form stones.

∎ DIET

Diet has a major influence on kidney health.

Kidney Cleanse First

Because other organ cleansings, particularly for the liver, put the kidneys under stress, they should always be detoxified or cleansed first. (See chapter 6, Organs of Protection and Detoxification, for further information on kidneys.) Before beginning any type of detoxification program, be certain that your kidneys are functioning properly by undertaking a kidney cleanse.

Avoid acid-forming foods such as caffeine-containing foods; salty, sugary, and fried foods; and soft drinks, which adversely affect the filtering ability of the kidneys. Also avoid mucus-forming foods, including all dairy products, heavy grains, starches, and fats. This will relieve irritation and inflammation and inhibit sediment formation.

Do not consume kidney irritants such as alcohol and excessive protein. The release of insulin following sugar consumption increases the level of calcium in the blood, which can contribute to the formation of kidney stones. Rhubarb and raw spinach must also be avoided, as they encourage the formation of stones.

Consumption of citric acid also helps prevent the formation of kidney stones. Drink the juice of a fresh lemon in a glass of warm water every morning, both during and after a kidney cleanse. Lemons inhibit kidney stone formation because of their citric acid content. Lemonade should not be substituted for plain lemon and water, because it usually contains a high level of sugar.

Kidney Gravel and Stones

To help pass gravel and stones, drink the following tea:

Birch leaves	Speedwell
Chicory	Witch grass

Combine the herbs in equal parts and steep 1 tsp. of the mixture in ½ cup of boiling water. Take 1 to 1 ½ cups per day, sipped throughout the day.

■ NUTRIENTS

The prevention of kidney stones is an essential factor in the health of the kidney. Zinc is an important inhibitor of crystallization. Take 50 to 80 mg of a zinc supplement and balance with 2 to 3 mg of copper. Use these amounts routinely if you are prone to kidney stones.

A raw kidney glandular, which is a concentrated form of animal kidney, strengthens the kidneys. It should be prepared from a young, organically raised, free-range animal that has not been given hormones.

■ HERBS

The herbs ginkgo biloba and goldenseal in extract form increase circulation to the kidneys and have antioxidant and anti-inflammatory properties. Apples are considered to be a healing herb for the kidney and serve as a purifier, cleanser, disinfectant, and toner.

The following herbal cleanse is recommended by Daniel B. Mowrey, in his book *The Scientific Validation of Herbal Medicine*. As well as cleansing and detoxifying, it treats urinary tract infections.

Caution: People who have nephritis or who take diuretics frequently should not use this formula, since it acts as a diuretic. Avoid high-sodium foods while using this formula.

Combine equal amounts of the following herbs and put into capsules. Take 5 to 8 capsules per day:

Bearberry leaves	Gravel root
Buchu leaves	Juniper berries
Cayenne	Kelp
Cleavers	Parsley
Cornsilk	

■ EXERCISE

Exercise daily. Sedentary people have a high level of calcium in their blood. Exercise forces the calcium into the bones, lessening the risk of kidney stones, as well as promoting the elimination of toxins through increased circulation and sweating.

■ OTHER CLEANSING MEASURES

Take saunas or hot baths to increase sweating, which causes the excretion of toxins and excess fluid through the skin, sparing the kidneys. Essential oils in the bath water will help relieve kidney stress. Use 8 to 10 drops of two of the following: cedarwood, chamomile, eucalyptus, geranium, lemon, juniper, or sandalwood.

Homeopathic remedies that support the kidney or a complex homeopathic remedy, such as PHP Kidney Liquescence, will assist a kidney cleanse. (See chapter 28 for a discussion of homeopathic remedies.)

Lungs

Asthma has increased by one-third in the last decade. Hospitalizations for asthma have increased five-fold for children and doubled for adults in the last 30 years. As pollution has increased in North America, all respiratory problems have increased. The lungs are taxed more and more with the substances contained in the air we breathe.

■■ LUNG CLEANSING MEASURES

If you have a chronic cough that brings up phlegm, a constant runny nose, bronchitis or wheezing, or severe sinusitis, a lung cleanse should be helpful for you. (Lung function and detoxification physiology are discussed in chapter 6, Organs of Protection and Detoxification.) People who have problems with fluid retention may not be able to do this cleanse.

■ DIET

Drink 8 to 12 glasses of water, juices, herb teas, and broth daily. Avoid dairy and dairy products, which can cause congestion. Eat fresh fruits, high-chlorophyll vegetables, sea vegetables, and non-gluten grains such as millet or brown rice. These are alkalizing foods and should be eaten in a ratio of about 4 to 1 over acid-forming foods. Chlorophyll-rich foods such as chlorella, spirulina, and barley green will enhance lung cleansing, in addition to increasing oxygenation and helping to clear respiratory infections. Pitted fruits such as apricots, peaches, and plums are "lung-friendly" foods because of their flavonoid content.

■ NUTRIENTS

Antioxidants are particularly important for lung function. Be certain to include vitamins A, C, and E in your nutrients as well as selenium, cysteine, and CoQ$_{10}$.

Take an anti-infective such as garlic, olive leaf extract, or colloidal silver if you have bronchitis or similar lung symptoms. Proteolytic enzymes taken between meals

will reduce inflammation, and quercetin between meals has a powerful antihistamine effect. (See chapter 23, Nutrients.)

■ HERBAL TEAS

Try one of the following teas to relieve congestion and inflammation.

  1 part lance-leaf plantain
  1 part lungwort
  1 part mullein flowers
  2 parts speedwell

Mix the herbs in the indicated proportions and steep 1 tsp. of the mixture in 1/2 cup boiling water. Sweeten with honey and sip 1 to 1 1/2 cups over the course of a day.

  Hemp nettle
  Shave grass
  Witch grass

Mix the herbs in equal parts. Use 1 heaping tsp. of the mixture to 1/2 cup cold water. Bring to a boil for 1 minute, then steep for 1 minute and strain. Sweeten with a little honey, if desired. Sip 1 to 1 1/2 cups over the course of a day.

■ ENVIRONMENTAL MEASURES

Be vigilant about your environment and avoid all forms of tobacco smoke. Try to avoid exposures to dust or dust mites, molds, pollens, terpenes, and chemicals.

Be particularly careful in your home and, if you are not already doing so, avoid cleaning compounds and toiletries that have a scent of any kind. (See discussion of safe products in Part VII, Prevention, chapter 36). Use an air cleaner and, if necessary, wear a charcoal filter mask at home and at work.

■ OTHER CLEANSING MEASURES

Breathing exercises are very helpful in lung

detoxification, as is physical exercise. (See chapter 26 for breathing exercises.) A brisk daily walk during which you breathe deeply will accelerate your cleanse.

A chest rub of essential oils or inhaling steam to which essential oils have been added will thin and stop excessive mucus production. Oregano, tea tree, and eucalyptus oils singly or in combination will help. For a chest rub, put 15 drops in 1 ounce of a base oil and rub on the chest. (See chapter 29, Herbs and Aromatherapy, for further information.) For steam inhalation, put 6 drops in 1 quart of hot water and breathe the fumes.

Homeopathic remedies that are supportive of the lungs are helpful in a cleanse. PHP Lung Liquescence, a complex homeopathic remedy, helps to cleanse and heal. (See also the list at the end of the chapter for remedies that support the lungs.)

Skin

The blood vessels, lymphatic vessels, vasculature of the hair follicles, enzyme systems, the detoxification capability of the sweat glands, and other factors make the skin important in the detoxification process. When functioning properly, the skin protects other organs, such as the heart, liver, kidneys, and gastrointestinal tract, from overwork.

When other detoxification organs are not functioning properly, the skin tries to compensate by releasing toxins through sweat, rashes, or abscesses. In people who have chronic kidney disease, the sweat glands can become damaged from overuse, excreting toxic wastes that would normally be excreted by the kidneys. (The role of the skin in detox-

ification is discussed in detail in chapter 6, Organs of Protection and Detoxification.)

It has been said that the skin is a mirror of what is happening in our bodies. It is our largest organ of detoxification, as well as our largest organ of absorption. It will absorb both nutrients and toxins, including perfume and skin care products. Stress, hormone imbalances, poor diet, and nutrient deficiencies all affect our skin's health. Fortunately, old, dying skin cells are sloughed off daily, and the skin is able to renew itself. If your skin has any of the following signs, however, you may need a skin cleanse.

- Sallow skin, age spots, acne, and uneven skin texture can be signs of poor liver function.
- Wrinkles, dry skin, and sagging skin indicate free radical activity that damages collagen and skin elasticity.
- Puffy eyes, dark circles under the eyes, and crusty lids signal an overload of fluid wastes.
- Skin sores, rashes, and bumps signal an overload of wastes that are not being excreted.
- Oily, scaly, itchy, chronically chapped, or red skin are definite signs of toxic overload.

■■ SKIN CLEANSING MEASURES
■ DIET

Proper diet can improve your skin and overall appearance. Eat fresh fruits and vegetables and eliminate sugar, fried foods, margarine, shortening, hydrogenated oils, and dairy products. Eat foods high in fiber to keep the colon clean, which will help keep the skin clean.

Eat zinc-rich foods such as egg yolks,

fish, meat, liver, grains, beans, and pumpkin and sunflower seeds, as a low-zinc diet can cause skin flare-ups. Zinc has antibacterial properties and is also necessary to the oil-producing glands of the skin.

Eliminate coffee and alcohol, as they affect circulation to the skin. Also avoid processed foods, which are high in sugar, salt, and fat. Saturated fats promote inflammation.

■ WATER AND TEAS

As with the other organ cleanses, it is important to drink 8 to 10 glasses of tolerated water to flush toxins through the kidneys. This helps to prevent toxins from having to exit via the skin as blemishes or rashes. Herbal teas also help the skin. Alternate between dandelion, goldenseal, myrrh, pau d'arco, and red cloves. *Caution:* Do not use goldenseal on a daily basis for more than a week and do not use during pregnancy.

■ *Skin Support Tea*

    Elder leaves and flowers
    Elecampane root
    Ground ivy
    Juniper berries
    Witch grass root

Mix the herbs in equal parts and steep 1 tsp. of the mixture in 1/2 cup boiling water. Sip 1/2 to 1 cup daily, unsweetened. Use daily over several months.

■ *Speedwell Tea*

    2 parts speedwell
    1 part black elder leaves
    1 part English walnut leaves
    1 part pansy

Mix herbs in the indicated proportions. Steep 1 tsp. of the mixture in 1/2 cup boiling water. Sip 1 to 1 1/2 cups daily, unsweetened.

Clear Complexion Juice

The following juice mix helps clear skin problems. When taken several times a week, it also acts as a blood purifier.

Beet juice   Celery juice
Tomato juice
Mix 2 oz. of each juice together and drink two or three times a day (for a total of 12 to 18 ounces per day).

■ NUTRIENTS

Antioxidants are essential for skin health. Be certain to take vitamins A, C, and E, as well as bioflavonoids. Vitamin E protects against ultraviolet light damage and bioflavonoids improve the skin's blood supply. Essential fatty acids, such as evening primrose oil, help prevent dehydration and wrinkling. Protease, an enzyme, will help to heal some skin disorders. MSM helps repair damaged skin and enhances tissue pliability. (Nutrients are discussed in detail in chapter 23.)

■ OTHER CLEANSING MEASURES

Dry brushing is important for a skin cleanse. It removes the top layer of old skin, helping to remove mucus residues and uric acid crystals. Use a natural bristle or a soft surgical scrub brush. Begin with the soles of your feet, and using a rotary motion, brush every inch of your skin except the nipples. Follow the brushing with a cleansing shower or bath.

Massage therapy will help improve skin tone by increasing circulation. Essential oils help to detoxify, nourish, tone, soothe, and support skin function. Essential oils that as-

Charcoal Powder

Charcoal powder can be placed directly on the skin to reduce swelling by absorbing excess fluid and the products of inflammation. It will also adsorb toxins, bacteria, carcinogens, products of allergies, and wound secretions. Charcoal powder will remove odors from skin ulcers if it is placed directly on the ulcer or in a dressing over the ulcer. It will also remove odors from casts.

sist in a skin cleanse include lavender, geranium, sandalwood, and neroli. Add 15 drops of one oil, or a combination, to 2 ounces of a base or fixed oil and rub on the skin (see Aromatherapy in chapter 27).

Lymph and Blood

The lymph system and the blood are not organs, but play an important role in detoxification. In many people, they are overloaded and are not functioning efficiently, affecting both the health of the person and the detoxification capabilities. Cleansing methods for the lymph and blood can be very helpful.

There is no one lymph organ. The lymphatic system is composed of the lymph glands and nodes, the spleen, thymus, and tonsils. It is considered by some to be a secondary circulation system because it collects tissue fluid through a system of vessels and ducts and returns it for recirculation. Lymph circulation plays an important role in detox-

ification. It carries the wastes that the cells excrete through the body to the bloodstream, where they can then be detoxified and eliminated. The lymph contains white blood cells and antibodies to combat infections, and the lymph nodes help to remove infective organisms.

The liver produces most of the body's lymph, and the spleen, which is the largest mass of lymph tissue, destroys worn-out red blood cells and acts as a reservoir for fresh red blood.

Blood plasma is known as lymph once it flows beyond the capillary walls. Red blood cells cannot fit through the pores in the capillary walls and continue to circulate through the capillaries and veins. The lymph bathes all of the cells of the body and delivers the oxygen and nutrients carried by the blood to the cells.

Breathing, muscular contraction, and movement supply the pumping force for the lymph system. If we do not exercise and breathe deeply, lymph does not circulate properly in our bodies. If the blood continues to release lymph and it is not pulled back into the lymph vessels, it builds up, causing puffiness or edema. The lymph in a sedentary person can stagnate in the body, resulting in an inefficient immune system and poor or reduced detoxification capacity.

You would benefit from a lymph cleanse if you:

• are pale and extremely thin.

• have poor immunity with frequent colds.

• are uncharacteristically soft and pudgy with cellulite.

• are under chronic stress and your memory

is suffering. (A congested lymph system increases the toxic load of the body and affects mental function.)

■■ LYMPH CLEANSING MEASURES

■ DIET

Poor diet adversely affects the immune system and the lymphatic system. Sugar and alcohol inhibit white blood cell activity. Sugar consumption (the amount of sugar in a sweetened soft drink) will stop white blood cell activity within 30 minutes and normal activity will not return for four to five hours.

To strengthen immune response, eat foods that are high in essential fatty acids, such as salmon, fresh tuna, and sea vegetables. It is also important to eat adequate amounts of protein and fresh fruits and vegetables.

■ NUTRIENTS

Supporting lymph nutrients include vitamins A, C, E, and B complex, beta-carotene, iron, zinc, and selenium. The enzyme protease is a lymph and immune booster. (See chapter 23 for a detailed discussion of nutrients.)

■ HERBS

Echinacea extract and astragalus extract are deep lymph-cleansing herbs. Echinacea also reduces lymphatic congestion and swelling. Red root is a powerful lymphatic cleanser and is synergistic with echinacea. Ocotillo flushes lymph congestion.

■ EXERCISE

Regular exercise is critical for lymph flow in the body. Rhythmic aerobic exercise, such as walking, dancing, or "step" exercise, is help-ful. Begin each exercise session with deep breathing and stretching.

Set a specific time to exercise and choose an activity you enjoy. The exercise should be convenient for you and one you can do at almost any time.

Be sure to shower after your exercise session to wash off the toxins excreted in your sweat.

■ OTHER CLEANSING MEASURES

Massage therapy and manual lymph drainage are helpful in encouraging lymphatic circulation. Acupuncture and acupressure can also be useful.

Alternating hot and cold showers will stimulate lymph circulation, as will breathing exercises. (See chapters 25 and 26 for a discussion of exercise, bodywork, and breathing.)

The essential oils of geranium, juniper, and black pepper will assist a lymph cleanse when rubbed on the skin. Use 15 drops of oil in 1 ounce of a base or carrier oil. Eight to ten drops of these essential oils are also supportive of the lymph system when added to bath water.

Complex homeopathic remedies such as PHP Lymph Liquescence are helpful in cleansing and supporting the lymphatic system. (See also the list at the end of the chapter for remedies that help to cleanse the lymphatic system.)

■■ BLOOD

Blood is a thick liquid made up of red blood cells, which transport oxygen; white blood cells, which combat microorganisms; platelets, which participate in clotting; and plasma, the fluid in which these cells are transported. White blood cells also circulate in the lymph. The heart acts as a pump to push blood through the arteries, veins, and capillaries of the circulatory system.

Blood is essential for life and performs many important functions for the body. It supplies oxygen to all of the cells of the body, and transports hormones, as well as vitamins, minerals, protein, and other nutrients. In addition, the blood warms and cools the body, seals off wounds, and fights and removes microorganisms. It also removes waste materials, including dietary and environmental toxins and dead cells.

If toxins build up in the blood, a person's health suffers, and disease can result. Blood toxicity plays a role in many immune deficiency diseases. For example, large amounts of toxins and pollutants are found in the blood of patients with chronic fatigue, fibromyalgia, lupus, and other serious chronic degenerative conditions. The body has a detoxification system for continuously purifying the blood, but it can become overloaded with a high toxic burden.

A blood cleanse is needed when you:

- have dark-colored blood, rather than bright red.
- have black or dark spots on the gums, and bad breath.
- experience unusual insomnia, memory loss, or unexplained depression.
- have a chronic cough.
- experience difficulty with hand and eye coordination.
- have increased, unpleasant body odor.
- have unusual, severe reactions to foods and odors.

❚❚ BLOOD CLEANSING MEASURES

❚ DIET

Diet is important in cleansing the blood. Follow a juice diet for three days, unless you have a degenerative disease. A juice diet or fast is not recommended in these cases because the toxins released by a fast may be more than the body and blood can detoxify. (See chapter 24, Diet, Fasting, and Juicing, for further information.)

After the fast, eat only very pure foods, including as much organic food as possible, and avoid canned, frozen, and processed foods. Do not eat food that contains any additives, including colors, flavors, and preservatives. Avoid sugar, sodas, artificial sweeteners, and fried foods.

❚ WATER AND TEAS

In addition to pure, tolerated water, drink bottled mineral water throughout the day to hydrate and alkalize the body. Mild herb teas, such as sarsaparilla and pau d'arco, can improve body chemistry and enhance blood cleansing, as can chlorophyll.

❚ NUTRIENTS

Nutrients will help with a blood cleanse, particularly the antioxidants, which clean the blood and strengthen white blood cells. Buffered vitamin C in small doses throughout the day will cause a rapid improvement. Take enzymes to help with digestion, particularly protein digestion. Enzymes break down organisms and incompletely digested protein in the blood, enabling them to be destroyed by the immune system. Probiotics are important for building blood and improving digestion. (See chapter 23, Nutrients, for a discussion of nutrients that are important for the blood and the immune system.)

■ OTHER CLEANSING MEASURES

Many herbs, including red clover, dandelion, burdock, yellow dock, echinacea, and Oregon grape root, cleanse the blood and are discussed in chapter 29, Herbs and Aromatherapy.

Essential oils, such as rosemary, cypress, and vetiver assist in blood cleansing. Use 15 drops of each oil in 1 ounce of base or carrier oil and rub on the skin. Eight to ten drops of each of these oils may also be used in bath water.

Aerobic exercise increases the level of oxygen in the blood, which assists with blood cleansing.

Massage therapy will increase circulation, and detoxification baths also help cleanse the blood.

Some people improve with an enema at the beginning and end of their blood cleanses, which prevents new toxins from entering the bloodstream.

■■ ADDITIONAL METHODS FOR
CLEANSING AND
STRENGTHENING ORGANS

The homeopathic remedies listed below will help treat and give support to the major organs that participate in detoxification. These remedies are only a few of those that are helpful for the indicated organs. Remedy selection must be made on the basis of the symptoms and needs of each person.

- Blood: *Arsenicum album, Crotalus horridus, Ferrum, Lachesis, Pyrogenium*
- Intestines: *Alumina, Bryonia, Carbo vegetabilis, China, Colchicum, Lycopodium, Nux vomica, Opium*
- Kidney: *Apis, Berberis vulgaris, Cantharis, Equisetum hyemale, Natrum muriaticum, Phosphorus*
- Liver: *Carduus marianus, Chelidonium majus, Kali carbonicum, Magnesia muriaticum, Natrum sulphuricum, Nux vomica, Phosphorus, Sulphur*
- Lung: *Arsenicum album, Blatta orientalis, Ipecacuanha, Kali carbonicum, Natrum sulphuratum, Silica, Spongia tosta, Tuberculinum*
- Lymph: *Apis, Carbo animalis, Conium, Gelsemium, Hepar sulphuratum, Iodum, Kali muriaticum*
- Skin: *Arsenicum album, Calcarea sulphuratum, Graphites, Mezereum, Petroleum, Psorinum, Rhus toxicodendron, Sulphur*

Many times drainage remedies are need to help cleanse and strengthen the organs of detoxification, as well as the other organs of the body. Sluggish circulation in these organs or in any tissue, causes buildup of cellular waste that severely impacts organ or tissue function. This buildup of waste metabolites prevents nutrients from entering the cells, further affecting function. Efficient drainage is essential to enable the detoxification organs to function optimally, excreting toxins and metabolic waste, and cleansing the body.

Helpful drainage remedies contain low-potency homeopathic remedies, sarcodes (remedies made from healthy tissue), nosodes (remedies made from diseased tissue), herbs, minerals, trace minerals, vitamins, plant bud extracts, flower essences, and other substances. Several companies have formulated excellent drainage remedies that assist in detoxification, increasing its efficiency. (See Sources.)

CHAPTER 32

Energy Balancing

THE METHODS OF detoxification discussed in this chapter all involve the use of energy to help cleanse and restore balance. Color, light, electrical and magnetic energies, and sound are differing forms of the same source of energy. We perceive this energy in varying ways because of the difference in the vibrational frequency and wavelength that stimulates a particular receiving organ within our bodies.

Color and light therapy utilize the vibrations, wavelengths, and frequencies inherent in those forms of energy. Gem therapy taps into the energy and vibrations built into crystals by nature. Electromagnetic and magnetic therapy are powerful treatments because their energy can penetrate into the body. The success of sound therapy is attributed to the vibration, frequency, and energy of the sound.

The energy therapies play an important role in detoxification and balancing, because their effects are unique and unlike any other methods available to us. Most of medicine is concentrated on the "physical body," with little thought given to the "energy body." These techniques help to correct and cleanse problems with our energy, to bring our bodies back into balance, and to maintain optimal health.

Color Therapy

Color permeates every aspect of our lives. Plants and animals are often named for their color—blue spruce, red-winged blackbird, and yellow jackets. People are described by the color of their hair, eyes, or skin. Athletic teams have special team colors. We like to wear colors that are pleasing to us and flattering to our own coloring. We want our foods to be a color that is appetizing. We even associate our moods and emotions with color. We see red when we are angry; depression is black; and our moods can be blue.

It should not be surprising that color has therapeutic value, and that we unknowingly use color therapy daily. We instinctively use color therapy when we choose the color of our clothes, our cars, and the colors of the walls, floors, and furnishing of our houses.

We use a type of color therapy when we paint locker rooms and restaurants red. Red in the locker room stimulates the team members, and in the restaurant makes us feel we have spent more time there than we actually have. Industry has found that muscular reaction time is quicker under a red light, which has useful applications for assembly lines.

Employee morale, efficiency, accident rates, and absenteeism in industrial or business settings are affected by the color of the walls. In schools where the walls are painted light yellow or light blue, absenteeism and discipline problems are lower. Bubble-gum pink has a physical, rather than a physiological, effect and will calm frayed nerves in minutes.

Specific colors affect mood, blood pressure, breathing rate, and pulse rate. These values increase with yellows, oranges, and reds, and decrease with greens, blues, and black.

Ancient civilizations used color in their worship and for healing. The Egyptians used colorful gems and light in their religious ceremonies, and their priests developed a color science. The Chinese believed color was the healing reconciliation between yin and yang, the male and female principles. They related colors to the five elements, the seasons, and organs, and still use these relationships today. Color therapy is also a part of Ayurvedic medicine, which is over 4,000 years old. Ayurveda teaches that colors res-

Response to Red

Color affects us in many ways. One little boy with terrible eczema triggered by food allergy could not wear red. His eczema immediately became worse if his mother dressed him in any shade of red, regardless of the fabric content.

onate with specific chakras, which are energy centers in the body. Color helps to energize, cleanse, and rebalance chakras that are abnormal or blocked by toxins and disease.

The ancient Japanese hung red drapes in the rooms of smallpox victims to prevent skin pitting. In the 14th century in Europe, red light treatment was used for the same reason. Smallpox, lupus, and other skin problems were successfully treated in the late 1800s and early 1900s with the Finsen light, which is red. During this time period, European psychologists utilized rooms with red or bright yellow walls for depressive patients and blue or green walls for hyperactive patients. Today we use light in the blue range to treat infant jaundice.

The spectrographical analysis of light shows that, in addition to the seven visible colors—red, orange, yellow, green, blue, indigo, and violet—there are other colors inherent in "white light" as we know it. Ultraviolet and infrared are at either end of the light spectrum. Thus we are exposed to a greater variety of "colors" than we often realize. Warm colors of the visible spectrum are red, yellow, and orange, while green may be considered a neutral color. The cool colors of the visible spectrum are blue, indigo, and violet.

∎∎ HEALING WITH COLOR

Color therapy involves the use of color for physical, emotional, and spiritual benefits. The properties of color are unalterable and will have an effect on every type of living organism. Both colored and white lights have the ability to directly affect tissues, organs, and biological functions in specific and precise ways. For example, responses of the retina to color have an effect on the nervous system, and healthy tissue absorbs color differently than does diseased tissue. Some colors stimulate hormone production, and others inhibit it.

Colored light acts as both a wave and as a particle. The vibrational energy from color activates organs, glands, and systems of the body. Each organ and cell within our body resonates to a specific color, intensity, hue, and brightness. Enzymes in the body can be activated or deactivated by colored light. The movement of substances across cell membranes is also affected by colored light. Color vibration and frequency have the ability to cool or heat and can create chemical reactions within the body that will alter its temperature.

Each color has its own specific energy that characterizes it. This energy, administered with a colored light, is imparted to whatever the light touches. Color can be reflected, absorbed, or passed through objects. The skin acts as a filter, and as the color wave continues into the body, it is absorbed by the body fluids. The part of the color ray that passed through the skin is now available to the body. Interaction between the color and the receiving cells and organs causes therapeutic results.

Color healing re-establishes color balance in the body by releasing tension caused by color starvation. Errors in thinking, feeling, nutrition, posture, and poor habits and lifestyle cause this starvation. Color healing renews vital energy and balances the body.

Color may be applied therapeutically in many ways. Color tinctures may be prepared and used to supply missing colors or to treat the chakra in which there is a problem. Direct lighting can be shone through color filters onto treatment areas, and is probably the most common method used. Hydrochromatic therapy uses color-solarized water prepared by exposing water in colored glass containers to the sun. Breathing air charged with the energy of a particular color is known as color breathing. The natural colors of food can be used to supply healing color, as can gemstones. A very simple way to supply therapeutic color is to wear eyeglasses with lenses of different colors for several hours a day.

When healthcare professionals use color therapy for healing, they consider the color or colors needed, where to apply it, and the proper sequencing and timing of color changes. It is easy to oversimplify color therapy and to minimize its treatment possibilities. Treating correctly with color therapy requires extensive knowledge of both colors and the disease processes they will help. For the best results in treating disease and imbalances, consult a therapist skilled in the use of color.

Color therapy is usually administered using colored lights. Some examples of color therapy treatment are:

- *Asthma:* red, yellow, or orange on the chest and upper body
- *Colds:* red if no fever; orange if the person has hypertension; green on the head and blue on the chest if fever is present
- *Kidney stones:* orange on the lower back, groin, hips, thighs, and feet
- *Liver:* blue over the fifth rib on the right side in the midline
- *Wounds:* violet directly on the wound
- *Bruises:* magenta, locally

Color therapy is usually applied once or twice a day for an average of about 7 minutes. Changes resulting from the treatment take time, and a common tendency is to overtreat. Do not use colored light therapy while eating or sleeping. The position of the body is not important as long as you are comfortable. External auditory, visual, and olfactory stimuli do not play a role in color therapy, but treatment is more efficient in an environment free from most stimuli.

Light Therapy

A discussion of light therapy cannot be entirely separate from color therapy, because color therapy involves the use of light. Many wavelengths are used in light therapy today, and many treatments can be done at home. Detoxification, cleansing, and balancing, as well as a number of health problems, can be helped with light therapy. Proponents of

---

Emotional Detox

Some types of color therapy can be used to help detoxify emotional issues. A combination of color over a blinking light source is very effective for accessing this type of problem. However, this method must be used only by a skilled therapist.

---

light therapy feel that it is just as important to pay attention to the amount and type of light the body receives, as it is to watch diet and exercise.

■■ FULL-SPECTRUM LIGHT

The oldest light therapy is exposure to the sun. Our bodies are nourished directly by sunlight or indirectly by eating foods, drinking water, and breathing air that has been energized by sunlight. Sunlight is full-spectrum light, containing all of the wavelengths of light. It triggers the hypothalamus gland to produce neurotransmitters, which are the communication molecules of the nervous system. Neurotransmitters govern most body functions, including body temperature, blood pressure, breathing, digestion, sexual function, moods, the immune system, the aging processes, and the circadian rhythm.

Full-spectrum light therapy is still used today, in the form of exposure to the sun or exposure to full-spectrum lights. It helps to treat depression, insomnia, hypertension, PMS, and migraines. When full-spectrum lights are used in schools and workplaces,

New Light Therapies

Dr. Jacob Liberman, author of Light-Medicine of the Future, *and director of the Aspen Center for Energy Medicine in Aspen, Colorado, writes that new applications for light therapy are constantly being developed. He feels we are entering a "light age," where lasers will replace scalpels, phototherapy will replace chemotherapy, prescription colors will replace prescription drugs, and needles of light will replace* acupuncture needles. Our homes, schools, and businesses will be open to the sunlight, as well as illuminated with full-spectrum light.

These applications can be used to improve physical health, as well as psychological and spiritual well-being. Many of the light therapies being developed can be used at home and will provide an alternative to more invasive therapy.

absenteeism caused by illnesses is significantly reduced. Schools also report that hyperactivity and behavior problems are reduced and academic performance is improved with the use of full-spectrum lights. Full-spectrum lights are available in both incandescent and fluorescent bulbs.

■■ BRIGHT LIGHT THERAPY

Bright light therapy is used to treat seasonal affective disorder (SAD), a chronic depression that occurs in the winter and affects over 36 million North Americans. Symptoms of SAD develop within the same 60-day period each year. (See Weather in chapter 17 for further information.) In addition to the depression that is its major symptom, people crave carbohydrates, feel better when they eat them, and gain weight. Even though they sleep more, they are always tired, have little interest in sex, feel overwhelmed, have difficulty concentrating, avoid friends and family, and suffer from frequent infections and muscle aches. More women than

men are affected, and SAD seems to run in families.

It is generally agreed that SAD is related to the decrease in light that accompanies the change in season and the corresponding increase in the production of the hormone melatonin. A high-intensity white light ranging from 2,000 to 5,000 lux (sunlight is 50,000 lux) helps to decrease depression in people who suffer from SAD. Exposure to the bright light daily for a specified amount of time decreases melatonin production and the symptoms of SAD.

Bright light therapy also has other applications. It is used effectively for reducing bingeing in people with bulimia, an eating disorder characterized by episodes of overeating followed by self-induced vomiting, purges, or fasting. Long and irregular menstrual cycles can frequently be regulated with this therapy. Bright light therapy can help normalize sleep for people with delayed sleep-phase syndrome, in which people fall asleep at progressively later times each night and thus have trouble getting up in the morning.

■■ ULTRAVIOLET LIGHT

Ultraviolet light has many uses in light therapy. Dr. Niels Finsen of Denmark won the Nobel Prize in 1903 for his work in "photobiology." Among his achievements was the treatment of tubercular skin lesions with ultraviolet light.

Today a part of the ultraviolet wavelength is used to treat systemic lupus erythematosus. Ultraviolet light is used in combination with a light-sensitive drug, psoralen, to treat vitiligo, a skin depigmentation problem, and psoriasis, a chronic skin disease. In hemoirradiation, blood drawn from a patient is exposed to ultraviolet light, then reinjected. This inactivates body toxins, kills bacteria, restores chemical balances, and increases oxygen absorption. Hemoirradiation has been successfully used to treat many conditions, including asthma, blood poisoning, infection, cancer, and symptoms of AIDS.

■■ COLD LASER THERAPY

Cold laser therapy, also called soft or low-level laser therapy, uses a low-intensity laser to stimulate a series of enzymatic and bioelectric reactions that promote the natural healing process of the body at the cellular level. The use of this laser increases microcirculation, the synthesis of collagen, the production of neurotransmitters, and pain relief. It will also reduce inflammation and balance energy in the acupuncture meridians. Some physicians use cold laser instead of acupuncture needles to stimulate acupuncture points. Cold laser has applications in dentistry, particularly to treat infections under teeth.

Treatment may be applied by a health-care professional or can be self-applied now that pen-sized, low-level lasers are available. This type of laser is found in electronics equipment shops, sometimes for use as a pointer.

Caution: Eyes can be temporarily or permanently injured by the lasers. Never shine them into the eyes.

Gem or Crystal Therapy

Gemstones are high-quality crystals that contain electromagnetic energy and emit frequencies and vibrations. They are able to resist distortion or alteration of their own vibration when in the presence of another, differing vibration. Crystals are capable of acting as amplifiers, and were used as the original radio receivers.

Today, gemstones and other crystals are used in technology, as well as in healing. Both natural and artificial rubies are used in lasers, sometimes for microscopic surgery. Quartz crystals are used in computers for memory chips, in capacitors to modify circuits, as oscillators to control radio frequencies, and as condensers to store energy. Crystals are also used in watches, transducers, ultrasound devices, communication equipment, solar cells, and information storage devices.

Gemstones have been used in various ways for many thousands of years. In the book of Exodus, the Bible mentions jewels on the breastplate of judgment, for which

God gave Moses the design. Twelve jewels, for the twelve tribes of Israel, were combined in four rows on this breastplate. The jewels included a sardius, topaz, carbuncle, emerald, sapphire, diamond, ligure, agate, amethyst, beryl, onyx, and jasper. The breastplate was created as a holy garment for Aaron, the high priest.

Royalty has always surrounded itself with gems and jewels, and monarchs in many countries have long collected gemstones for protection. The stones were worn on crowns and in decorative jewelry. Jewels were also used on swords, thrones, goblets, and other personal effects.

Ancient cultures wore talismans and amulets as part of medical prescriptions. Specific stones were chosen to bring about desired effects. American Indians used gems and crystals for both diagnosis and treatment. Gemstones are still used today for healing purposes. Practitioners worldwide use gem therapy, which is frequently combined with color therapy.

■ CRYSTAL SYSTEMS

The gemstones used for therapy are natural crystals grown within the earth. The vibrations and frequencies they emit have the potential to affect the body, mind, and spirit.

The symmetrical arrangements of atoms in gems comprise seven crystal systems. Each system has its own outer shape, luster, colors, cleavage, hardness, type of fracture, tenacity, specific gravity, and optical properties. Each gemstone or crystal of a given chemical formula will have the same angles between facets, regardless of the size of the crystal. All gems belonging to the same sys-

Classes of Gems

Real gems, which have been cut and polished, are of the highest quality and are the most potent for medical use. Polished but uncut gems are more potent than rough gems, which have not been polished or cut and may be irregularly shaped. Imitation gems made of glass are unfit for medical use.

tem share properties. In addition, each type of gem has its own slight variations that give it unique energetic properties and qualities.

■ HEALING WITH GEMS

The intention of gem therapy is to balance the body physically, mentally, and emotionally. Gemstones are used in healing both for their specific vibratory and color frequencies. The selection of stones and colors must take into consideration both the qualities and frequency of the stones, as well as the condition of the body to be assisted.

The body responds to gemstones because of the principles of resonance, harmonics, and vibration. As physics has demonstrated, all things are in a state of constant vibration. In this state, a defined range of harmonics and vibration is inherent to each object. Gemstones resonate with similar patterns within the biocrystalline network in the human body—the network of cellular elements in the body that have liquid crystal or quartzlike properties. This network includes cell salts, lymphatics, fatty tissue, red and white blood cells, and the pineal gland. The vibrations of gemstones stimu-

Healing Actions of Crystals

CRYSTAL SYSTEM	SPECIFIC GEMS	ACTION OF GEMSTONES
Triclinic: thrice inclined crystals that form a triad with all angles less than 90°	Turquoise and rhodonite	Bring things to a completion.
Monoclinic: singly inclined crystals	Azurite, jade, malachite, and moonstone	Pulsing action and growth, helping to clear inner obstructions.
Orthorhombic: lozenge-shaped crystals	Peridot, topaz, and alexandrite	Help bring perspective to issues; identify the irrelevant and magnify consciousness, problems, thoughts, and energy.
Tetragonal: elongated rectangular crystal	Zircons, chalcopyrite, and wulfenite crystal	Absorb negativity yet emit positive energy; are transmutation stones with balancing action, able to convert energy.
Hexagonal: six-sided cubic crystals that are more complex	Emeralds, beryls, aquamarines, apatites	Give off energy; can be used for energy balancing, healing, communicating, and storing energy.
Isometric: cubic crystals of a basic or fundamental nature	Diamonds, garnets, fluorites	Assist in repair of damaged cellular structures; have a basic type of energy patterning.
Trigonal: three-sided crystals	Bloodstones, carnelians, agates, amethysts	Continuously give off balanced energy; can balance any type of energy.

late energy centers within the electromagnetic systems in our bodies.

It is believed that gemstones assist in the healing process because they transmit their extremely stable resonance into the biomolecular level. At this level, the gemstone energy finds a sympathetic resonance. This activity might be compared to the action of a tuning fork that causes a piano string tuned to the same frequency to vibrate without being touched. Similarly, gemstones activate a vibrational response in dormant energy fields within the body. Healing proceeds from the biomolecular level to the cellular level and throughout the physical body.

Gemstones are also used to regulate the flow of energy in and around the body. Blockages of the vital energy in the body can cause disease and other physical problems. Balance is restored to the energy system when energy blocks are removed and the flow of free energy is increased. In Ayurvedic medicine, gemstones are placed on parts of the body corresponding to chakra points (the energy centers of the body), to remove blocks and restore balance.

Some people report distinct balancing and cleansing effects when using gemstones. Some people are able to tell when a given stone is or is not helpful for them. One woman was unable to wear a necklace her grandmother had given her. The stone in the pendant was the wrong frequency for her and she did not feel well when she wore it.

Gemstones should always be cleansed before they are used for therapy, to remove old vibrational energy. Use one of the following methods to cleanse crystals:

- Run cold water over the crystal and place it in the sun for 30 minutes, then shine with a white cotton cloth.
- Pack the crystal in sea salt for three to four hours.
- Place the crystal in spring or distilled water with several drops of pennyroyal flower essence for 5 to 10 minutes.

Gemstones may be carried on the person, worn as jewelry, held in the hand, placed next to the person, laid directly on the body, or placed in a person's home.

Practitioners may treat with remedies or tinctures of gemstones. These are prepared by placing the clean stone in vodka or another form of alcohol used to make tinctures. (See chapter 29, Herbs and Aromatherapy.) Allow the stone to remain in the alcohol, preferably in the sunlight, for seven days, shaking each day. If the tincture has been made using an ingestable alcohol, 6 to 12 drops daily of the tincture taken orally will impart the characteristics of the stone. Otherwise, the tincture should only be used externally.

Skilled practitioners of gem therapy are able to assist with a variety of conditions in people who seek their help. Some gemstones that are helpful for specific conditions are:

- *Amethyst:* calming effect for tension headaches, nightmares
- *Coral:* stomach and liver problems
- *Diamond:* eye problems, lung problems
- *Emerald:* heart trouble, high blood pressure
- *Rose quartz:* soothes the heart
- *Ruby:* stomach pains, problems with the blood
- *Yellow sapphire:* throat problems

Electromagnetic and Magnetic Therapy

Our bodies have chemical, electrical, and magnetic properties. Every chemical bond has a magnetic and electrical field associated with it. These interrelated electrical and magnetic properties can become imbalanced.

■■ ELECTROMAGNETIC THERAPY

Many people suffer from an electromagnetic imbalance that affects their sleep, their ability to wear a watch, their response to storm and weather fronts, and their ability to use electrical equipment of many kinds, including computers. Symptoms of an electromagnetic imbalance are discussed in chapter 18.

There are several ways to correct an electromagnetic imbalance. Grounding techniques help to relieve electromagnetic imbalances. One of the simplest techniques involves turning clockwise (to your right), working up to 21 turns per day. Spot an object as you turn to prevent dizziness. If performed regularly, over a period of time, electromagnetic balance will be restored. Allowing the bare feet to touch the earth and lying on the grass are two more simple, but effective, techniques.

People who live in mobile homes should be certain that the buildings are adequately grounded. The electrical wiring runs the length of both sides of the structure, and the sides and roof are nearly always metal, causing problems for electrically sensitive people. These sensitive individuals may require additional grounding over that provided by the manufacturer. This can be accomplished by driving a copper pipe two feet into the

Teslar Watches

In our experience, many patients with electromagnetic imbalances have improved significantly by wearing a Teslar watch. However, the bodies of some patients were so imbalanced and toxic that they could wear the watch for only a few minutes each day, gradually increasing the time until they could wear it all day.

Several patients spontaneously detoxified very rapidly when they began to wear their watches. Their sleep was affected and they had skin eruptions until their balance and levels of toxins improved. A few patients have not been able to wear Teslar watches at all.

ground and attaching a copper wire to both the pipe and the metal frame or siding of the mobile home.

Wearing a Teslar watch can be beneficial in restoring electromagnetic balance. This high-quality watch contains a chip that connects the clocking mechanism and the battery in a magnetic frequency that resembles the natural field of the earth. It is weaker than the earth's field, but because the watch is worn against the skin, its effects reach the whole body. The watch offers protection from electromagnetic pollution caused by extremely low frequencies, including fields generated by electrical appliances, comput-

Electromagnetic Imbalance

A patient announced one day that she had had "radio static" in her ears for years. She feared that people would think she was crazy. This "static" was a symptom of an electromagnetic imbalance. Six diodes in her pocket made this woman feel, as she put it, "that her cells were holding together" for the first time in many years. When she tried to put the diodes down, she burst into tears and sobbed that she was "falling apart." She felt calm and composed again after restoring them to her pocket.

We wondered how she was going to take them off long enough to take a bath. She informed us that baths made her feel sick, but that she felt wonderful in the shower! This response to baths and showers is another symptom of electromagnetic imbalance.

ers, televisions, electrical wiring, and electric motors. It also eases stress and bolsters stamina. People suffering from multiple allergies frequently improve when wearing a Teslar watch. Jet lag can be significantly reduced or even eliminated by wearing one. (See Sources.)

Wearing diodes, a copper-colored composite of specifically prepared natural elements, also helps electromagnetic imbalances. Diodes help to maintain energy levels along acupuncture meridians, to hold the body in its correct frequency, to hold energy patterns and polarity in balance, and to counteract harmful external electromagnetic energies. The number of diodes needed varies from person to person and it is best to seek professional guidance. Some people feel better when they wear their diodes 24 hours a day. Others become too energized if they wear them at night. (See Sources.)

Tachyon beads are also helpful for electromagnetic imbalances. These beads are made of special materials that emit photon (light) energy in a wavelength from 4 to 16 millimicrons. This short wavelength helps maintain proper cellular metabolism and organizes the water molecules in the body to allow increased oxygen flow and absorption of important nutrients. Tachyon beads are available in head and wrist bands, as well as individual beads. (See Sources.)

Electromagnetic energy has also proven useful in the treatment of some injuries, including bone fractures that will not heal. Dr. Robert O. Becker, author of *The Body Electric* and *Cross Currents*, discovered that a flow of electrical current to the injury site is necessary for bone healing. An externally applied, small amount of current facilitates the healing of fractures by stimulating cells to regenerate and tissue to repair.

Transcutaneous Electrical Nerve Stimulation (TENS) units have proven very helpful in controlling chronic pain. These units apply electrical current to the affected nerves, causing conduction to be blocked and pain to be relieved. A variety of unit types are available, using various electrical waveforms, frequencies, pulse shapes, and current density. They are also sometimes used as electrostimulators in acupuncture treatments. *Caution:* TENS units should not be used by people with pacemakers except under the advice of a physician.

■ MAGNETIC THERAPY

Not only are we surrounded by magnetic fields, from the earth, solar storms, and those created by electrical appliances, but the human body also produces weak magnetic fields that are generated by the chemical reactions in the cells and the ionic currents of the nervous system. Magnetic therapy can be used to help diagnose, as well as treat, physical and emotional disorders. Magnets can be used to treat electromagnetic imbalances and many other conditions.

Although we think of magnetic therapy as being new, physicians have been using natural magnets for thousands of years. For example, Galen (approximately 129 to 201 A.D.) found that application of a natural magnet to various areas of the body would relieve pain. Ancient cultures, including Arab, Chinese, Egyptian, Hebrew, and Indian, used magnets for healing. Austrian physician Franz Anton Mesmer, who was greatly ridiculed at the time for his theories on magnetism, laid the foundation for magnetic healing in the 1700s.

Extensive work on healing with magnets has been done since that time, particularly in Japan in the late 1950s by Dr. Kyoichi Nakagawa, director of the Isuzu Hospital in Tokyo. Dr. Nakagawa believes that the time people spend inside buildings and cars reduces their exposure to the natural geomagnetic fields of the earth, interfering with health.

Caution with Magnets

Because weak magnets can affect the electromagnetic fields of the body, and even small changes in the fields of the body can cause adverse symptoms, magnetic therapy is best used under the supervision of a qualified health-care professional. People with pacemakers should not use magnetic therapy except under the advice of a physician.

Magnets should never be used on the abdomen during pregnancy, and a magnetic bed should not be used for more than 8 to 10 hours. To prevent interference with peristalsis, do not apply a magnet to the abdomen for at least 60 to 90 minutes after a meal, and never apply the positive magnetic pole to your body unless you are under direct medical supervision.

Negative magnetic energy (the north pole) facilitates healing, while positive magnetic energy (the south pole) interferes with healing. In his *Biomagnetic Handbook*, Dr. William Philpott of Choctaw, Oklahoma, states that negative magnetic energy:

- oxygenates tissues
- fights infections
- reduces fluid retention
- supports biological healing
- reduces inflammation
- normalizes acid-base balance
- encourages deep sleep
- relieves pain
- promotes mental acuity
- reduces or dissolves fatty deposits

• reduces fat and calcium deposits in the circulatory system

Dr. Philpott also describes treatments for many conditions, using only magnets. For example, placing the negative side of a magnet toward the top of the head helps reduce stress and induce sleep. Many of the treatments he describes have a cleansing and balancing effect. A major effect of magnetic therapy is to increase the circulation of oxygenated, nutrient-rich blood, which is essential to healing and detoxification.

Magnetic therapy is also useful for healing broken bones. Broken bones behave as two separate magnets that repel each other. Placing a magnet over the fracture site helps the fractured ends to come together smoothly. The negative magnetic energy also speeds healing by pulling nutrients and oxygen into the injured tissues. Magnetic fields increase blood flow more effectively than electrical current because magnetic wavelengths have greater penetrating power into the body. They can penetrate through nerves, fat, and bones, whereas electrical stimulation can penetrate less than half an inch.

Today's medical magnets are made from various materials and include ceramic, plastiform, and neodymeum magnets that hold a permanent charge. Some of them are flat and flexible, and others are hard ferrite-type magnets. The flexible magnets can be molded into a variety of shapes and attached to an injury or pain site on the body.

Magnets have been incorporated into blankets, mattresses, pillow head supports, and beds; wrist, elbow, and knee joint supports; shoe soles; inner soles; vests; and a variety of jewelry. They have even been incorporated into acupuncture needles. Treatments last from a few minutes to overnight. They may be applied several times a day, or used continuously for days or weeks at time.

Sound Therapy

Consider the old expressions, "Music has charms to soothe a savage breast" and "Music alone with sudden charms can bind the wand'ring sense, and calm the troubled mind." These expressions from the writings of William Congreve (1670–1729) refer to the ability of sound and music to function as a healing tool. This ability has been recognized and utilized for thousands of years, and is well documented in ancient literature.

The effects of sound and music are still widely recognized today. Red Auerbach, former head coach of the Boston Celtics basketball team, has stated that "Music washes away from the soul the dust of everyday life." We now call this phenomenon sound therapy, and it is successfully used in the modern world in hospitals, corporate offices, schools, and psychological treatment programs. Sound therapy is effective in reducing stress, alleviating pain, lowering blood pressure, slowing breathing, improving movement and balance, promoting strength and endurance, soothing restless babies and agitated people, and overcoming learning disabilities.

Sound can influence brain wave frequencies, alter skin temperature, help regulate corticosteroid hormone levels, reduce cancer pain, reduce stress in heart patients, and control the severity of muscle tremors. Because of these properties, sound is being used more frequently in hospitals, hospices, dental offices, and in psychotherapy. Sound therapy can reduce the amount of anesthesia needed in surgical and dental procedures, as well as reducing pain and improving mood. It has proven useful in caring for cancer, AIDS, and Alzheimer's patients.

■ TONING

Used for years at the Institute for Music, Health, and Education in Boulder, Colorado, toning involves making elongated vowel sounds and allowing them to resonate through the body. It is similar to and may have had its origins in chanting a mantra.

Toning is a simple way to release stress, improve the ability of the ear to listen, improve the speaking and singing voice, and balance the mind and body. With toning, the brain waves synchronize and balance within three to five minutes, which increases the sense of physical and emotional well-being. Different parts of the brain will be benefited by different tones, and toning has been described as massaging the body internally. Toning produces energizing, calming vibrations within the body.

■ SIGNATURE SOUND

Sharry Edwards, a teacher, lecturer, and researcher in Denver, Colorado, has developed an alternative medicine sound therapy. According to Edwards, all people have a distinctive "signature sound," which corresponds to their physiological and psychological states.

Missing frequencies in the voice are indicators of physical or emotional distress. Emotional states can be recognized from the

> ## Sound Therapy
>
> *Sound therapy can include simple techniques that you may already do for yourself. For example, listening to marches or "peppy" sounding music when you are depressed, soothing music when you are angry or upset, or baroque or classical music when you need to concentrate or to memorize something are all varieties of elementary sound therapy.*

missing notes and octaves. Providing the missing frequencies can allow the body to repair itself, even from supposedly incurable diseases. A Self-Management Auditory Device (SMAD), developed under the supervision of Edwards, supplies the missing tones.

■ INFRATONIC QGM MACHINE

Developed in China by Lu Yan Fang of the National Electro Acoustics Laboratory, the Infratonic QGM machine simulates the infratonic sound made by the hands of Qigong masters. (See chapter 25, Exercise and Bodywork, for a discussion of Qigong.) This production of chi energy produces many therapeutic benefits, including headache relief, increased circulatory functioning, alleviation of depression, and muscular relaxation.

The QGM machine is currently awaiting FDA approval for therapeutic use in the United States.

Cymatic therapy uses a computerized instrument to transmit resonant frequencies into the body, establishing equilibrium. The sounds pass through healthy tissues, but reestablish healthy resonance in unhealthy tissues. Cymatic therapy does not heal, but helps re-equilibrate the body so it can heal itself without pain, drugs, or surgery.

Cymatic instruments have been utilized in the United States since the late 1960s and training is required to use them. There are no side effects and the only people who should not use this method are those who have pacemakers.

CHAPTER 33

Detoxification for Mind and Spirit

Toxins of the mind and spirit must be detoxified, just as physical toxins must be cleansed. These toxins will remain as an "obstacle to cure" unless they are removed, because the body cannot completely heal if the mind and the spirit are ill. A healthy mind and a healthy spirit are essential for a healthy body. Many people overlook this aspect, working hard to heal their bodies, but never attaining full health.

Some people consciously and subconsciously handle toxins of the mind and spirit by keeping them suppressed rather than dealing with them and detoxifying them. They bury the toxins so deeply that they appear to become totally unaware of their presence. Keeping them suppressed requires a tremendous amount of energy, however, leaving very little energy for healing either the body or the mind.

Because of the different nature of mind and spirit toxins, the detoxification techniques required will differ from those used for other types of toxins. Some of the techniques discussed in this chapter require professional help, and others are self-help techniques. All will require time and commitment.

Counseling and Psychotherapy

Sharing your feelings with family, friends, and church members or pastor may not be enough to help you through trauma. Professional guidance may be necessary, and counseling and psychotherapy are important cleansing tools to help resolve problems and reduce stress loads.

Two major fields have developed to understand human behavior: psychoanalysis and behavioral psychology. Austrian neurologist Dr. Sigmund Freud (1856–1939) developed psychoanalysis. He emphasized the interconnection between biological and environmental influences on a person and described the mind as composed of the conscious, unconscious, and preconscious. The conflict between the conscious and unconscious affects behavior and is the focus of

Choosing a Therapist

Choose a competent, licensed therapist and take particular care in your choice. In many areas, anyone can work as a counselor or therapist, without proper training or license. The person you choose should be someone to whom you can easily talk, as well as someone who has had experience in dealing with the particular problems you have.

therapy. Examining personal history is an important part of the therapy, to bring unconscious conflicts into consciousness.

Behavioral psychology uses objectively measurable experimentation to study the relationship between behavior and the environment. This discipline believes that both adaptive and maladaptive behaviors are acquired from learning experiences, with genetic endowment also playing a role. Problem behavior is the focus, and is treated with classical conditioning, using positive and negative reinforcement and other techniques.

Most psychiatrists and psychologists use one of these approaches in their treatment. A psychiatrist is an M.D. or a D.O. who has received specialty training in psychiatry beyond basic medical school training. A psychologist may have either a Ph.D. or an M.A. in psychology. In most states and provinces, psychologists with a master's degree practice under the supervision of a Ph.D.

Psychologists, generally speaking, use fewer pharmaceuticals in their treatment methods, because they are not licensed to prescribe drugs. Should a prescription be necessary, psychologists enlist the help of a physician, who prescribes the medication. Both psychiatrists and psychologists teach tools and skills that can be incorporated into daily life.

Counseling is not limited to verbal discussion. Other treatments can help cleanse emotional trauma. These include:

- *Art therapy:* Simple art materials provide a means to restore, maintain, or improve physical and mental health. This therapy is used to both assess and treat, providing a person with means for nonverbal communication and expression.

- *Dance therapy:* People become more aware of their feelings by experiencing movement. It restores the integration of body and mind, rebuilding a sense of identity and self-esteem. It can aid verbal psychotherapy, physical therapy, and medical therapy.

- *Dream therapy:* Dreams and the dream state are utilized for physical and emotional healing. It involves both dream interpretation and active participation in the dream process. Dreams may warn of oncoming health problems, suggest diagnosis and treatment, accelerate the healing process, and contribute to overall health.

- *Gestalt therapy:* Treatment of the person as a whole being is emphasized, focusing on the person's immediate experiences rather than the past or future. It employs role-playing to promote the person's growth process and to develop the individual's full potential.

- *Guided imagery:* The power of the mind is used to evoke emotional and physical responses, such as reducing stress, alleviating fear, reducing anxiety, reducing heart rate, stimulating the immune system, and reducing pain. It can be applied in almost any medical condition, including toxic overload.

Neuro Emotional Technique and Other Hands-On Treatments

Neuro Emotional Technique (NET) is a treatment that has many applications. Developed by Dr. Scott Walker, a chiropractor from Encinitas, California, NET helps release emotions held in the body tissue memory. Therapists who practice any type of hands-on treatment have long known that memories from the past are stored in the tissues. These memories can be released during bodywork. Other therapies may not be totally successful as long as the tissue memories are present.

NET involves the use of basic muscle testing, acupressure treatment, and homeopathics to achieve complete healing. It allows the removal of emotional blocks that prevent the regaining of health and the reestablishing of emotional balance in a nonthreatening way. It does not take the place of counseling, but can assist the counseling process.

Other hands-on treatments developed by chiropractors that treat tissue memory and emotions include Total Body Modification (TBM), developed by Dr. Victor Frank of Sandy, Utah; Nambudripad's Allergy Elimination Technique (NAET), developed by Dr. Devi Nambudripad of Buena Park, California; and BioSET, developed by Dr. Ellen Cutler of Corte Madera, California. Specialized procedures in these methods also allow the removal of stored tissue memories. (See chapter 27, Allergy Treatment and Chelation for a description of these techniques.)

Journaling

Journaling is an excellent self-help technique. It can involve writing in a journal either daily or at times of need. Happy experiences can be recorded by remembering and reliving. During times of distress, journaling offers an outlet for emotions. It can also be a means to analyze problems and to determine causes and effects. Journaling often allows a new perspective and release of misperceptions. It can help you to better know yourself and your mind.

Journaling allows you to have active participation in dealing with emotional issues, and it provides a safe way to feel and experience the emotions of the moment. It serves as a catharsis for pent-up emotions. You can express grief or disappointment, or vent anger in a nonviolent way.

Journaling can also have physical benefits. A study in the April 1999 *Journal of the American Medical Association* examined the effect on the chronically ill of writing about stressful events. A group of patients with asthma and rheumatoid arthritis was divided into two groups, with one group writing about stressful events, and the other simply writing down their plans for the day. Four months later, those patients who wrote about stressful events showed physical improvements, while those who wrote about daily plans had no change in their physical condition. Numerous other studies have confirmed that people who write about trau-

Therapeutic Letters

Although it usually takes the form of recording events, thoughts, or feelings in a journal, journaling can also mean writing a letter that is never mailed. Sometimes burning or tearing up the letter can represent a symbolic completion or laying aside of an issue.

Letters to the deceased are an excellent way of dealing with unfinished business. Anger, emotional pain, or frustration can be freely expressed with no threat of reprisal. A letter to a deceased person can also express love, pain of loss, and loneliness. This assists the grieving process with a ritual of acknowledgment and completion, often resulting in forgiveness and peace of mind.

these simple guidelines. Always date your entries so that when you look back you can observe cycles, patterns, and trends. Write quickly so that your internal censor cannot stifle your intentions. Do not "grade" yourself on grammar, spelling, or word usage. Mistakes may be your subconscious asking for attention. Write what you feel to be the truth, and write when you have the desire to do so. Keep what you write, even though you may feel you never want to read it again. In the future it may be what you need to hear, and it can serve as a "mileage post" for your progress.

Art Therapy

Art therapy utilizes various forms of art for therapeutic purposes. Simple art materials provide a means to restore, maintain, or improve physical and mental health. This therapy is used to both assess and treat, providing a person with a means of nonverbal communication and expression. Artwork can unleash emotions as it bypasses the rigid ego and controlling intellect, allowing freedom of expression. People can use the creative process to reconcile emotional conflicts, increase self-awareness, and increase personal growth.

Art therapy can be as simple as applying colored pens and pencils, crayons, or ink to paper, creating designs or pictures. It can also take the form of making craft projects; doing fiber art such as knitting, crocheting, or tatting; or creating needlework, such as cross stitch, latch hook, or embroidery. The artwork can be kept or symbolically destroyed, depending on the creator's needs. A

matic experiences and difficult emotions feel better and have stronger immune function.

When you write, you transfer thoughts, feelings, and energy out of your mind and body onto paper, where they will be stored for you. You may look at them at another time, or never refer to them again. To prevent journaling from becoming emotionally overwhelming and a task rather than a help, use a page or a time limit for your writing during a given session. If you feel yourself becoming too intense, take breaks, stretch, look out the window, get a drink, and then go back to your writing.

To get the most out of journaling, follow

person does not have to be an artist to benefit from this type of therapy.

Laughter and Attitude

Laughter can be a very powerful healer for emotional trauma and abuse. Aristotle (384–322 B.C.) felt that laughter was a "bodily exercise precious to health." Norman Cousins, the author of *Anatomy of an Illness*, discovered in the course of his two serious illnesses that "love, hope, faith, laughter, confidence, and will to live have therapeutic value." He was able to recover by emphasizing positive emotions and actions, including laughing.

Laughing causes positive changes in brain chemistry by releasing endorphins, and it brings more oxygen into the body because of the deeper inhalations. It enhances cardiovascular flexibility and increases metabolism and muscle activity, including the heart muscle. Laughter releases anger, fear, guilt, and anxiety. It can rebalance the chemistry of stress and tension, altering neurotransmitter levels, increasing oxygenation, and releasing endorphins. A good laughing session can completely change your attitude and increase your "spirit quotient."

Dr. William Fry, professor emeritus at Stanford University Medical School and an expert in humor physiology, feels that humor may have benefits similar to exercise. Mirthful laughter is a total body activity that affects all the major physiological systems of the body.

Laughter gives us both psychological and spiritual benefits, in addition to the physical effects. It enlarges our perspective,

Therapeutic Handwork

Many times, needlework, such as crochet, knitting, or embroidery, can help a person cleanse toxins of the mind and spirit. Going through a traumatic event brings up many toxins that must be removed, as well as wounds to the spirit that must be healed.

One woman learned to crochet while going through her divorce. The rhythm of the stitches was soothing to her, and having to count them and concentrate on the pattern kept her from obsessive thoughts about her problems. She found working with the colors a "balm to her soul." In addition, she felt that she was able to transfer many of her toxic thoughts and wounds out of her mind, body, and spirit as she crocheted.

allowing us to cope with stress, pain, and problems. Tapping into laughter restores our sense of personal power so that we do not feel like victims. Every time we laugh, we heal.

Laugh therapy can include:
- reading comedies, cartoon books, or joke books
- watching comedies or cartoon videos
- listening to humorous programs and recordings
- telling jokes and amusing experiences, and listening to others do the same
- thinking of amusing experiences
- watching animals or children at play
- visiting with people you enjoy

Hugs for the Soul

Hugs—both given and received—touch the soul. They involve a transfer of energy and give both people an emotional boost. Jo Lindberg of Tustin, California, founder of the Hugs for Health Foundation, states that hugs are the best form of emotional and physical therapy. She feels that we need four hugs a day for survival, eight for maintenance, and twelve for growth.

• planning enjoyable activities for the future
• smiling as much as possible—a smile is a precursor to a laugh and increases feelings of happiness.

Hug Therapy

The importance of touch to human health was discussed in chapter 25, Exercise and Bodywork. The skin is our largest organ, and it needs care and touching. Research has revealed that caring touch can strengthen the immune system, lower high blood pressure and cholesterol, reduce stress, induce sleep, and calm hyperactive children.

Kathleen Keating of Center City, Minnesota, developed a program of Hug Therapy and has written two books on the subject: *The Hug Therapy Book* and *Hug Therapy 2*. She states that hugs convey a sense of safety, security, and trust. They increase self-worth and impart strength and healing. Hugs are important during both happy and sad times.

Susan Franke, a nurse at Shadyside Hospital in Pittsburgh, Pennsylvania, uses Hug Therapy on her floor in the hospital. She reports that it eases tension, imparts a feeling of belonging, and helps fill empty spaces in the lives of her patients. Hugs dispel loneliness, help overcome fears, build self-esteem, and open the door to acknowledging and expressing feelings. Hugs can also help to fight insomnia, relieve pain, and reduce depression.

You can both initiate and participate in Hug Therapy. Hugging requires no special training, but does require both a sender and a receiver. Always ask for permission to hug and be aware that hugging is not for everyone. Hug therapy is compassionate, not passionate—caring and comfort should be communicated, not the needs or desires of the hugger.

If you need a hug, ask for one, and let your hugger know you appreciate the understanding and acceptance. Sharing is an important aspect of a healing hug.

Changing Focus

Being turned completely inward and focusing only on themselves can be a symptom of a toxic mind and spirit for some people. They have come to view themselves as victims and always concentrate on their own situation and what they view as their needs. Selfishness and negativity become a way of life for them.

Our bodies have miraculous powers to heal, but sometimes our own negativity shuts down this healing capacity. Positive, hopeful attitudes can be cleansing, and give the body and mind healing messages. They increase our confidence in our coping ability, as well as our self-esteem. Focusing on "rights" rather than "wrongs" reinforces positive thoughts and behaviors and stops circular thoughts (repeating same thoughts over and over) and behaviors. Positive attitudes help you to look forward with hopes rather than dwelling on illness or past unhappiness.

Many times concentrated, conscious effort is necessary to change the focus of a life. Detoxification methods to accomplish this change frequently involve reaching out to others as well as becoming involved in the lives of others. Thinking of and helping others directs thoughts away from an inward focus. Reaching out to others and being concerned for them helps neutralize negativity.

Getting out of the house and being around people anywhere, even at a shopping center or grocery store, can be a first step. "People watching" is the beginning of refocusing on others rather than on yourself.

Volunteer work at a hospital, nursing home, charity, church, or youth organization such as Big Brothers or Big Sisters forces a person to look at other people and their needs rather than their own. Working with animals in a shelter brings rewards and "warm fuzzies" in many ways that help direct attention outward.

Simple activities, if consistently practiced, will gradually help to create a more positive attitude. Activities might include:
• making an effort to smile at people, acknowledging their presence in a positive way, regardless of where you are. Nodding as you smile, or even speaking, can make both of you feel better.
• noticing other people, and finding something about them to compliment or a way to make a positive comment to them.
• inquiring about others' health instead of telling them about yours.
• inquiring about others' families and loved ones, and truly listening to what they say.
• discussing others' projects and interests first, rather than yours.
• remembering what others say and asking for an update the next time you see them.

Becoming passionately interested in and learning more about a subject can also change focus and reduce negativity. Libraries and the Internet contain a wealth of easy-to-access information about almost any subject. Clubs and interest groups allow you to meet and interact with people who share similar interests. Finding common ground or interests to discuss, rather than talking about yourself and your problems, will also help to change focus.

Spirituality

If you have had a crisis of spirituality and faith, cleansing and balancing must be accomplished to restore it, or your health and your quality of life will suffer.

Whether you are suffering from a crisis of spirituality and faith or you feel you have lost your faith, exploring different religions and belief systems can allow you to regain your faith or to find new strength and faith in another religion or belief system. People who have never had a religious background or a particular belief system may find stabil-

Symbolic Ceremonies

Completing a class, reaching a goal, or learning a new skill can be symbolic of a new beginning, leaving old habits and an old life behind. Even something as simple as a new outfit, changing a room arrangement or decorations, or discarding objects that remind you of negative events or people can effect positive changes.

Separation ceremonies can allow you to release negative events and distance yourself from negative influences

or people. The ceremony can be one of your own devising, and one that is meaningful to you. A ceremony might involve writing messages to a person or simply stating behavior or circumstances from which you are separating. The message can then be burned or destroyed in some way, as a symbol of breaking the connection. Separating from negative influences or people can change your spiritual direction.

ity and a spiritual home through their explorations.

To restore, preserve, and protect your spirituality, the following actions are helpful:

• practicing regular prayer or meditation
• counseling with clergy or spiritual leader
• attending a church, synagogue, temple, mosque, or religious organizational meeting of your choice
• reading inspirational materials of any type
• listening to or performing soul-restoring music
• watching spiritual or religious television programs
• listening to religious or spiritual radio programs
• attending self-help groups and participating in the bonding and caring of the group
• respecting yourself, your higher power, and all living things
• finding and observing beauty in all things and appreciating the smallest perfection of form and expression

• cultivating a sense of joy and gratitude toward life itself and each day's new experiences

Ceremonies and symbols that acknowledge and celebrate the transitions of life can cause dramatic changes, helping to cleanse the mind and heal a spiritual crisis.

Special prayers and meditation can help heal both mentally and physically. Several studies have shown that prayer, both their praying and having others pray for them, helps people regain their health. The prayers of others can help even when people are unaware that someone is praying for them. Studies have shown that patients whose physicians pray for them improve more rapidly and have fewer problems and complications.

You must allow time to nurture and care for your spiritual being. This is not something that just happens, but requires attention and effort on your part. A healthy spirit encourages a healthy body and increases immensely the possibilities of a rich, happy life.

Forgiveness

One of the most important aspects of cleansing and balancing emotional trauma is forgiveness. To heal completely, a person must forgive the one who caused the trauma and, in addition, forgive the act itself. A person must also forgive himself or herself for any real or imagined wrongdoing in the situation. With time and work, this can be done, even in cases of the most severe trauma or abuse.

If you feel you cannot forgive the person or the act, it may help to give this task to your higher power. Write the name of the person and/or the event on a piece of paper, ask your higher power to do the forgiving, and throw the paper away or burn it. Do not attempt to take the burden back, because you have given it to your higher power to carry for you. Over time, many people find that forgiveness has become possible without their conscious awareness of the healing process.

Once total forgiveness has been achieved, people can shed the burden of being a victim and be released from the suffering they have carried in their mind and body.

CHAPTER 34

Detoxification Methods for Children

WHEN A CHILD has a health problem, we recommend that parents consult a qualified healthcare practitioner to make or confirm a diagnosis, to clarify a confusing or unclear diagnosis, to rule out complications, and to deal with any life-threatening emergency. Any sudden or unexpected change in a child's condition should immediately be investigated.

Parents who learn about natural medicines are able to be more involved in their child's healthcare. They become more sensitive to their child's physical and emotional temperament and can recognize early warning signs of illness. Because parents are the guardians of their child's health, they must also monitor the child's exposures to toxins, as well as helping to determine the need for and overseeing detoxification procedures.

Children are exposed to toxins daily, and if the natural detoxification processes in their body cannot handle the load, they can develop bioaccumulation. Children with toxic overloads need detoxification and cleansing just as adults do. Many of the same methods used for adults can be used for children. However, differences in physiology and responses to toxins require that some detoxification methods be modified for children. These methods and the necessary modifications are discussed below.

Saunas, Baths, and Hydrotherapy

Heat depuration helps to mobilize chemicals in children's fat cells. Children have used saunas safely in Sweden and Finland for hundreds of years, with shorter exposure times and lower temperatures than for adults. If a child does use a sauna, monitor the heart rate, which should not exceed the suggested maximum pulse (220 minus child's age $\times$ 0.85 = maximum pulse). Twenty minutes is the maximum sauna time for a child.

Detox baths are also an effective detoxification method for children. Plain water baths, Epsom salt baths, and apple cider vinegar baths have all been used safely, with beneficial results.

Children do well with hydrotherapy, with

the exception of cold baths, which should not be used. A full-body cold pack is also not recommended for children.

Nutrients

Because children often do not eat a balanced diet, supplementation with nutrients is recommended. A good multivitamin/mineral is helpful for many children. For children who cannot swallow capsules or tablets, chewable vitamins, and to a limited extent, liquid vitamins, are available. Reading labels carefully is essential as many of them contain added sugar to make them more palatable. Healthier versions containing fruit juices or molasses are preferable.

Vitamin doses are usually recommended at one-third to one-half the adult dosages, depending on the child's body weight. This can be estimated using a typical adult body weight of 120 to 140 pounds. Children may take extra nutrients for special needs, but there are limits that should not be exceeded.

For children, no more than 5,000 to 10,000 units a day of vitamin A are recommended, as it can be toxic in excessive doses. However, beta-carotene is the precursor of vitamin A, and it is not toxic at all. The only side effect from beta-carotene is a yellow or orange tint to the skin, known as carotenemia. This does not cause any clinical symptoms and can be reversed simply by reducing or stopping the excess intake of beta-carotene. Babies who eat large amounts of carrots, squash, and sweet potatoes have a tendency to develop carotenemia.

Vitamin B_3 (niacin) is frequently used in sauna programs. It may cause transient tingling or flushing if taken in excess amounts.

Breathing Steam

Steam inhalation from a steamer or a bathroom with a hot shower running can aid breathing during viral infections. This method has been used successfully for children with croup for many years. The heat reduces swelling and eases breathing.

A small dose, such as 100 mg, can be used and built up as tolerated. If children take larger doses of vitamin B_3, their liver enzyme levels should be monitored.

Vitamin B_6 is safe for children in doses from 25 to 100 mg a day. It has been reported to cause peripheral neuropathy (numbness in the extremities) when used in excessive doses, such as 1,200 to 2,000 mg a day for extended periods of time.

Vitamin C has been recommended in doses of 20 mg per pound of body weight per day, but can be taken by children in doses close to bowel tolerance level. Doses close to bowel tolerance are encouraged for children with allergies.

Excess amounts of vitamin D (over 400 IU in non-deficient states) can cause excessive calcification of bones or organs of the body, but rickets (a disease caused by vitamin D deficiency) is more common in children. Premature babies are prone to develop rickets, and various diseases of calcium metabolism can also cause rickets.

Vitamin E is an antioxidant, and can be used safely in proper doses to combat excess free radicals. No more than 400 IU of vitamin E daily should be given to children.

Special nutrient combinations are helpful to prevent and treat metal poisoning in children:

- *Aluminum:* Selenium supplementation is helpful for aluminum poisoning. When children are given selenium, doses have to be monitored closely and should not exceed 125 micrograms a day.
- *Cadmium:* Children eating a diet high in whole grains and vegetables will ingest extra vitamin C, thiamin, and zinc, which decreases cadmium absorption and retention. They will also get adequate amounts of copper, fiber, and vitamin E. Because most children do not eat enough of these foods, a multivitamin is recommended. Pectin is found in fruits and helps protect against cadmium poisoning.
- *Lead:* Extra vitamin C, thiamine, and zinc (15 to 20 mg a day) helps protect children against lead toxicity and deposition.
- *Mercury:* Children can take extra nutrients, including vitamin C, glutathione, calcium, iron, magnesium, manganese, and zinc, to help combat mercury poisoning.

Diet, Fasting, and Juicing

A wholesome diet is very important to a child's health and for detoxification. Although fast foods and processed foods are appealing to many children, these foods are high in fats, salt, sugars, additives, and preservatives, and are low in nutrition. Peer pressure and advertising hype seem to draw children to this type of food.

Creative cooking and serving can help combat these pressures. In most cases, an acceptable and healthy substitute can be made at home or obtained at a health food

Not for Children

Complete fasting, where nothing is taken orally, should not be undertaken by children of any age. Older children can tolerate short fasts in which fasting drinks are used. Older children have fasted for religious reasons without adverse effects, but this type of fast is usually only from sunrise to sundown. Children who have insulin-dependent diabetes or any serious disease should not fast.

store. However, you must read labels even at a health food store, as its place of purchase does not guarantee the quality of a food.

Some children do well on a macrobiotic diet, particularly when the whole family participates. A macrobiotic diet is wholesome and free from chemicals, simple sugars, saturated fats, and processed food. On the macrobiotic diet, children will:

- eat more complex carbohydrates and fewer simple sugars.
- eat vegetable protein instead of animal protein.
- reduce the intake of fat and have less saturated fat in their diet.
- have a better balance between vitamins, minerals, and other nutrients.
- use fewer artificially processed and chemically treated foods.
- use more foods in whole form than in refined or partial form.
- increase the amount of foods eaten with natural fiber.

Studies show that children on a balanced

vegetarian diet grow adequately and remain healthy.

Cleansing diets are helpful for children, and can be used on a short-term basis. A child will self-select a diet of from one to three puréed fruits or vegetables from cleansing diet choices offered by the parent.

Exercise and Bodywork

Children can do many forms of exercise, including walking, running, swimming, bike riding, aerobic dancing, and cross-country skiing. However, children should not be forced to exercise. They seem to be motivated most effectively if their parents exercise regularly and serve as positive role models. Children should be encouraged in the aerobic exercises that they enjoy, rather than the activities in which the parents want them to participate.

Dr. Kenneth Cooper of Dallas, Texas recommends that children *not* begin a disciplined long-distance aerobic program until at least 10 years of age. This allows time for their bones and muscles to become fairly well developed. He recommends that children should be tested for physical fitness in the fourth grade, and by the seventh grade a regular aerobic exercise program at least three times a week should be part of a child's lifestyle.

Bodywork is helpful for children, and gentle stroking massage techniques are recommended for all ages. Massage techniques have been used effectively even with premature babies, resulting in better neurological development and weight gain.

Massage stimulates the skin, which in turn increases cardiac output, promotes res-piration, and develops the efficiency of the gastrointestinal tract of infants. It has positive benefits for many hormone levels, promotes bonding, and eases tension and physical discomforts. Massage also teaches babies ways to relax their bodies when stressed.

Parents can use simple bodywork techniques on their children at home. The physical contact of gentle massage is beneficial to both the parents and the child. For maximum benefit, parents must be relaxed as they massage their children.

Use natural cold-pressed fruit and/or vegetable oils for massaging infants and children. Apricot kernel and almond oil are two recommended oils. Baby oils have a petroleum base (mineral oil), which is distilled from crude petroleum and is toxic.

The use of essential oils for parental massage of children and babies can be very effective, but these oils should be diluted with a base or carrier oil, such as almond oil. For babies under one year old, use only the plain almond oil. For children over one year, add one drop of essential oil to 25 ml of almond oil. (See Aromatherapy in chapter 29 for further information.)

Other types of bodywork that are safe for children are:

- *Acupressure:* Helps to release tension in specific areas.
- *Acupuncture:* Safe, but the child should be old enough not to be frightened by the acupuncture needle.
- *Manual lymph drainage:* Very effective, but should be done with less pressure and for a shorter time than with adults.
- *Reflexology:* Can be very relaxing, especially

if a child is too excited to fall asleep at bedtime.

- *Shiatsu:* The gentle finger pressure improves muscle tone and circulation.
- *Therapeutic Touch:* Helpful for children of all ages and can be used to calm crying babies.

Rolfing is not recommended for young children. For all types of treatment, it is important for children to be comfortable with the practitioner. If they are nervous, they may giggle or act silly, rather than relaxing, and so lose the benefits of treatment.

Breathing and Oxygen

Breathing exercises are safe and effective, and can be used with all age groups. When children are old enough to understand the directions, these exercises can be both fun and helpful for them. Infants automatically do abdominal breathing, which is said to be the ideal way to breathe. Children can perform yoga when they are capable of understanding the directions. Guided meditation can help calm a troubled or disturbed child, enabling relaxation and helping the child to sleep.

Oxygen therapy can be used for children who have diseases such as asthma and pneumonia. It can also be used with premature babies, but must be monitored carefully. If the oxygen level in the blood is too high, premature babies can develop retinopathy of prematurity (an eye disease), which can lead to blindness. The more premature a baby is, the higher the risk for this disease.

Hyperbaric oxygen therapy has been used for children with carbon monoxide poisoning, most commonly caused by leaking gas stoves and improper ventilation. Carbon monoxide poisoning can also occur in children who ride in the back of a pickup truck. Hyperbaric oxygen may be used for older children who have decompression sickness (the "bends"). It may also be used for treating other conditions, such as tissue injury, at the discretion of the physician.

Hydrogen peroxide should not be taken orally by children or given to them intravenously. It can be used topically on small areas of skin. Hydrogen peroxide can be safely used for skin or nail fungal infections. Hydrogen peroxide can also be used as a diluted mouthwash when children are old enough to be able to gargle.

Ozone can be used topically for children in a bath, but should not be used by them in any other manner. Stabilized oxygen therapy can be used for localized skin care in children, but should not be given internally.

Allergy Treatment and Chelation

Neutralizing doses for foods, pollens, molds, danders, and chemicals can be given sublingually or by injection. Sublingual extracts are very effective for children and there is no danger of anaphylaxis (allergic shock). Sublingual allergy extracts can be used safely even for infants. Traditional injectable allergy extracts must be administered in a physician's office, as there is a risk of anaphylaxis. These shots are usually not tolerated well by children until age five or older because of the frequency of the injections.

Children respond well to extracts and hands-on treatment for pollens, terpenes, mold, dust, dust mites, and animal danders.

Allergy extracts and hands-on allergy treatment can be used to treat and detoxify bacteria, viruses, parasites, and fungi in infants and children. They can also be used to cleanse and balance neurotransmitter sensitivities and imbalances.

All of the hands-on allergy treatments described in chapter 27 can be safely and effectively used for infants and children.

Chelation therapy for atherosclerosis is not used in children. Atherosclerosis is thought to be rare in children, but it has been found in autopsies of 18- and 19-year-olds. Chelation therapy has been used in children for metal poisoning, particularly lead poisoning. Intravenous EDTA and intramuscular BAL help remove lead from the kidneys. Succimer (DMSA) was approved for use in children in 1991, for treatment of lead poisoning, and it can be given orally.

DMSA has also been used as an oral chelation agent for mercury poisoning. For mercury poisoning, children can be treated with BAL, penicillamine, or DMSA.

Homeopathy and Bach Flower Remedies

Homeopathy is extremely safe for newborns, infants, and children. For babies, a poppy seed–sized pellet can be placed in the mouth and will rapidly dissolve. Even if children spit out a homeopathic remedy, they receive a dose if it touches their mouth. For infants and children, a 6X dose is usually recommended. In acute conditions, 30C doses may be used. However, for an acute condition or an emergency, any available strength would be acceptable.

Caffeine, camphor, menthol, and pepper-

Safe Skin First Aid

Homeopathic gels such as Calendula can be applied to open wounds and burns, including sunburn. Arnica gel is very helpful for bruises and tissue injury but should never be applied in any form to broken skin.

mint, including peppermint toothpaste, can cancel or antidote homeopathic remedies.

Homeopathic remedies to treat organisms such as bacteria, viruses, parasites, and fungi are well tolerated by infants and children. Children who need to detoxify from medications, surgery, radiation, chemotherapy, vaccinations, and dental work can also be helped with homeopathic remedies.

Children are more frequently bitten by venomous insects and arachnids than are adults. They respond well to the homeopathic remedies listed in chapter 28 for treatment of insect bites.

Bach Flower Remedies are very effective for children and are valuable in dealing with children's emotional difficulties. To choose the remedy, the child's state of mind is assessed and physical symptoms are not considered. Both the negative and positive aspects of the emotions are taken into account.

Children should be treated before complex emotional patterns are established. The response to Bach Flower Remedies varies in acute and chronic cases. In acute cases, such as temper tantrums, changes will occur rapidly. In chronic cases, a child may be more in touch with his or her emotions, and may be able to help choose the proper remedy. How-

Herbs for Children

When choosing herbs for children, taste is important. The sweeter-tasting herbs will be more readily accepted. Once a child tastes a strong herb, he or she may be reluctant to take another dose. Onion and garlic syrups and glycerin have been used as herbal vehicles to improve the taste.

ever, an improvement in the child's condition may take more time.

A dropper bottle of 20 to 30 ml is filled with spring water or boiled tap water, and two to three drops of each Bach Flower Remedy is added. For children, it is recommended not to give more than four remedies at a time. Two to four drops of this dilute form can be given directly under the tongue, or added to food or drink four times a day.

The lips of a breast-feeding infant can be moistened with the remedy. A small quantity of a dilute Bach Flower Remedy applied to the bottom of the feet will be absorbed immediately, and a few drops on a tissue or cotton ball placed next to a child's nose will also give an adequate dose. Children respond more rapidly to treatment than adults, and do not have to be treated as long or as often.

Herbs and Aromatherapy

The many herbs that can be used safely for children should be chosen with care. For the untrained person, consultation with an expert in herbs is recommended, as some herbs have a very narrow range of safety. In many cases, these herbs have also been pre-pared as homeopathic remedies, and for children the homeopathic remedies are recommended. Rarely, a child may be sensitive or allergic to a particular herb. If a child shows an unusual reaction after taking an herb, stop the treatment and consult an expert.

For children, the standard dose of a dried herb is one-quarter to one-half the adult dose, either in a capsule or as an infusion. For chronic conditions, the dose is three times a day, and for acute conditions, the herbs may be taken every two to four hours. The dose for infants is 1 tsp. daily of an infusion tea or decoction. A breastfed infant will ingest herbs taken by the mother.

Tinctures should never be given undiluted because the alcohol can burn a child's mouth. Tinctures should be mixed in 2 to 3 ounces of tolerated water, stirred, and slowly sipped by the child. The herbal tincture dose for children is two to four drops in water three times a day. For infants, one drop in water three times a day is recommended.

Aromatic herbs, which contain volatile oils that give them an agreeable odor and stimulating qualities, can be put in a vaporizer for inhalation.

Because a child's skin is more porous than an adult's, herbs can be absorbed through their skin:
- A tincture can be rubbed into the skin of the abdomen at three times the dose recommended above.
- A tincture can be rubbed on the bottoms of the feet at the recommended dose.
- An herbal preparation may be put in the bath water at 10 to 20 times the normal dose.

Children have a stronger response to aromatherapy than do adults. The neural pathway to their brain is shorter than in adults, so that they respond more rapidly to scents. A small amount of dilute essential oil on a tissue or a cotton ball placed next to the child's nose for a few minutes will give rapid absorption. A child can also be treated by simply inhaling the fumes of a bottle of dilute essential oil. However, essential oils should never be used directly on the face of a child under 10 years of age, and only qualified aromatherapists should use essences for infants.

The aromatherapy baths discussed in chapter 29, Herbs and Aromatherapy, can be used for children, but with only three drops of essential oil to an averaged-sized bath.

Topical Detoxification

Compresses, packs, and poultices are a useful, effective treatment for children. Children usually do not need to use these treatments for as long as an adult would. However, garlic poultices (garlic crushed and mixed with oil) can be used overnight on the sole of the foot for coughs.

Cold and hot compresses can be used for children, but the temperature must be carefully monitored.

Mustard plasters can be used on children if the amounts of materials used in the plaster are reduced. For children, use 1 Tbsp. powdered mustard to 8 Tbsp. flour, and for infants, 1 Tbsp. mustard to 12 Tbsp. flour. Remove the plaster at the first sign of redness or discomfort. (Directions for making and applying mustard plasters are in chap-

> ### Flaxseed for Colon Health
>
> *Enemas are considered too harsh and invasive for children. Grated flaxseeds can be added to a drink or given as a purée to help with constipation and colon cleansing. Flaxseeds are essentially tasteless, whereas flax oil has a definite taste and is less readily accepted by children.*

ter 30, Topical Detoxification, under Compresses, Packs, and Poultices. Also see this chapter for information on topical detoxification methods for many health needs.)

Calamine lotion and colloidal oatmeal packs or soaks can be used for children who have poison ivy, oak, or sumac rashes. Soda and starch soaks are also helpful.

Charcoal therapy is very effective for children. Mini poultices are helpful for injuries, and topical charcoal poultices will help to relieve the pain of earache. (See chapter 30 for further information on the topical use of charcoal.)

Organ Cleansing

Children who are in need of detoxification may need organ cleansing prior to beginning detoxification measures. However, strict organ cleansing regimens are not recommended for children.

Diets containing adequate amounts of fresh fruits and vegetables will help cleanse organs, as will omitting all dairy products from the diet. Lemon juice in water will help cleanse the liver, and is safe for children to take.

Baths and aromatherapy will also contribute to organ cleansing in children. Homeopathic remedies, both single and complex, can greatly aid organ cleansing.

In cases of poisoning, children can safely drink the charcoal slurry recommended in the Colon Cleanse in chapter 30.

Energy Balancing

Children enjoy color therapy. They will choose the color that they prefer, and it frequently is the one that they need and that will help them. Useful materials are crayons, colored pens, toys, clothes, construction or origami paper, marbles, or colored stones.

Children also enjoy gem therapy and it works well for any age. Children can choose polished stones that they like and carry them in a pocket or in a special pouch. The gemstones can be worn as jewelry or used on the chakras (energy centers) also.

Sound therapy can be helpful, as well as fun, for children. Marching or dancing to music are favorite activities. Singing touches the mind and spirit and can change moods, calm emotions, and make children more receptive to listening and learning.

Children should not sleep next to electrical appliances. If possible, a child's bed should face north or east. We have found some children who have consistently awakened very irritable in the morning, but improved when the position of their bed was changed. Other children have improved when a magnet was placed under the pillow. Lay the magnet on the bed, under the pillow, and place the north side of the magnet toward the child.

Both diodes and tachyon beads are effective for children. However, because they tend to lose them, they may have to be placed in a small pouch or purse and pinned in a pocket or under the waistband of the child's clothing. (See Electromagnetic Fields in chapter 32 for more information.)

Detoxification for Mind and Spirit

Toxins of the mind and spirit have no age boundaries or limits. Unfortunately, most children experience toxins of the mind and spirit because of the way they are treated or because of toxic mental and emotional exposures.

Art therapy and color therapy can be very effectively used to help children cleanse this type of toxin. Laughter and hugs can help to heal many wounds.

Guided play therapy can substitute for formal counseling for younger children. Older children generally respond well to counseling.

PART VII

Prevention

THE OLD ADAGE, "An ounce of prevention is worth a pound of cure," is particularly true for toxic body overload. However, in this case the adage could go further: "An ounce of prevention is far preferable to a pound of cure." At times, detoxification can be both difficult and painful, and it is easier to prevent the buildup of toxins than to rid the body of them. It is also better for the health of the body to prevent the accumulation of toxins in the first place, than to stress the body with toxins and their symptoms.

There are many methods of prevention that can help lessen or even eliminate the need for detoxification. In some instances, prevention methods and detoxification techniques are the same. Many prevention methods involve creating a cleaner lifestyle. The changes you are advised to make may seem overwhelming at first. When you get used to them, however, they will seem quite natural and you will begin to wonder why you ever lived any other way. You will wonder why everyone does not live the same way. You may have to be careful not to become so evangelical about the benefits of cleaner, healthier living that you become annoying to your friends and relatives!

CHAPTER 35

Food and Water

Food

The basic "rule of thumb" for preventing diet-related problems is to eat clean foods that have been purchased wisely and stored and cooked properly. The information presented in this chapter will teach you how to purchase the best foods, store them under optimum conditions, and cook or prepare them in the healthiest fashion. Methods of preventing food poisoning are also discussed.

▌▌ QUALITY FOODS

Quality, organic foods contain more nutrients than chemically fertilized food grown in depleted soils. Contrary to a February 2000 ABC 20/20 report, organic food is healthier for those who eat it, as well as for the environment. The program stated that farmers who use pesticides and chemical fertilizers produce more food per acre, allowing more efficient use of land. The investigation attempted to prove that organic food does not contain more nutrients and has no health benefits. The program also tried to establish that organic farming practices are unsafe and have contributed to serious health problems in people who consumed organically grown produce, containing harmful bacteria from the manure used as fertilizer.

However, while both "chemical" farmers and organic farmers use manure as a fertilizer, certified organic farmers are required to compost it. Composting reduces bacterial hazards because the heat produced during composting destroys bacteria. As well, certified organic farmers are prohibited from using raw manure for at least 60 days before harvesting crops for human consumption. In contrast, manure use is not regulated or inspected on industrial farms. These farms often fertilize with sewage sludge, which can contain heavy metals and other toxic substances. Organic farms do not use sewage sludge. Organic farmers adhere to the same health and safety standards as other farmers and food producers, and, in addition, must obey very strict standards enforced by organic certifying agencies. Inde-

Prevention through Diet

Diet can help prevent food allergies. Eating a variety of foods, rather than the same foods over and over, prevents overexposure to foods, as well as preventing a cumulative effect from consuming offending foods. It helps to preserve tolerance for foods to which you are not sensitive. A varied diet also prevents overtaxing enzyme systems, allowing them to continue to function efficiently.

pendent agents regularly inspect organic farms to ensure that farmers are following the guidelines.

For the best nutrition, eat high-quality, fresh, organic fruits, vegetables, whole grains, and meat. Organic fruits and vegetables contain nutrients needed for optimum health and detoxification, as well as the food enzymes needed to help digest them. Whole grains have not been processed, which can remove nutrients and fiber. Meat from organic, free-range animals will not contain hormone and drug residues.

Limited amounts of honey and molasses can be substituted for sugar, or use herbal sweeteners. Reduce salt intake by seasoning with herbs.

This type of diet promotes the proper balance of intestinal flora and decreases the transit time—the time it takes digested food to pass through the small and large intestines. Prolonged transit time allows intestinal waste to be reabsorbed into the blood and recirculated. See chapter 24 for a review of good dietary habits, as well as a description of diets that will aid detoxification and prevent the buildup of toxins.

▌▌ PURCHASING FOOD

Most of us shop at supermarkets, which carry literally thousands of items. Some areas have health food stores and health food supermarkets that also carry numerous products. Knowing basic information about foods allows you to make healthy choices when you shop. The information that follows in this chapter will help you become a more informed shopper.

▌ STAPLES

Although staples have a long shelf life, buy only what you can expect to use within the time recommended for each product. Date your purchases and use the oldest items first. Buy only fresh-looking packages and check for signs of insect infestation. Be suspicious of breaks or tears in the packaging.

Dusty cans and packages may indicate old stock. Cans should be rust free. Carefully inspect dented cans and buy only those that will still stack. Never purchase a bulging can or one with a split seam.

▌ FRUIT

When purchasing fruit, it is important to know whether it was picked before it reached maturity. Many fruits will never ripen if they are picked too early. Select fruit that is firm and has a sweet scent. Avoid fruit that is moldy, decayed, or damaged. Do not purchase fruits with breaks in the skin, bruised spots, moldy patches, or "off" odors.

Because most fruits have a short life, purchase only what you can realistically eat in a few days. Otherwise, you will have to preserve the fruit by freezing, juicing,

Foods to Avoid

Some foods should be avoided as preventive measures and during detoxification. Avoid sugar, salt, white flour products, saturated fats, uncultured dairy products, fried foods, alcohol, caffeine, soft drinks, artificial sweeteners, and vinegar, except apple cider vinegar.

*Avoid processed foods to which flavors, colors, and preservatives have been added. Flavors can make poor-quality food taste better, and colors make it look better. The flavors and colors used are frequently artifi-*cial. Artificial colors tend to be both toxic and allergenic. Preservatives extend the shelf life of food by preventing or retarding spoilage.*

Even enriched and fortified foods can be problematic. These are foods from which nutrients have been removed during processing, then added back in. The quality and quantity of the added nutrients never totally equals that of the nutrients removed, and usually the balance of nutrients is destroyed.

canning, drying, making jam or jelly, or pickling.

At home, sort through your fruits and discard any that are decayed or damaged. Prepackaged fruit may contain bad individual items that you were unable to see. Always handle fruit gently.

Frozen fruit is available at the grocery store. It retains most of its nutrients because the fruit is frozen immediately after being picked. However, most frozen fruit has sugar added to preserve the natural sweetness of the fruit. Unless the package feels completely solid, do not buy it. Also, if the package is stained, it probably has been thawed and refrozen. Do not purchase these fruits.

Fruit may also be purchased canned, and several grades of canned fruit are available. Grade A or "fancy fruit" has been picked and canned at the proper stage of ripeness and will have the best appearance. Grade B is less perfect in appearance, but the taste will be acceptable. Canned fruit is packed either in a sugar syrup or in its own juice. Fruit packed in its own juice will taste less sweet, but will allow you to avoid consuming additional sugar. Canned fruits have lost most of their vitamins and all of their enzymes because of the heating involved in the canning process.

■ VEGETABLES

Vegetables contain less sugar than fruits, as well as less acid and more starch, giving them a less intense flavor. To keep vegetables fresh and preserve their nutrients, the activity of their natural enzymes is usually suppressed by cooling. Microbes attack freshly picked vegetables, and cooling inhibits them as well. Different gases and chemicals are used by growers and shippers to alter the function of enzymes and stop the action of microorganisms. Refrigerated warehouses and trucks retard plant metabolism and slow aging. High humidity prevents wilting.

Choose vegetables with bright, rich color and firm texture. Avoid those that already

Colors of Eggs

Be aware that different breeds of poultry lay eggs of different colors and that color has no effect on the flavor, freshness, nutritional value, quality, or texture of the egg.

show signs of decay and spoilage, such as discolored patches, spots, and bleached surfaces.

If you cannot obtain a sufficient variety of fresh vegetables, both frozen and canned vegetables are available. Frozen vegetables are preferable to canned ones in most cases. Vegetables are canned or frozen immediately after harvest, but canning alters the food slightly and lowers its vitamin and mineral content. Some canned vegetables, such as tomatoes and sweet potatoes, are more appealing canned than frozen.

There is a large variety of frozen vegetables from which to choose. However, many bags of frozen vegetables at the grocery store will be frozen in a hard block. This means that they have thawed a little and refrozen, but they are still safe to eat.

▌ EGGS

Fresh eggs are the best egg choice, but unless you have chickens or ducks, or can buy eggs directly from a farmer, very fresh eggs will not be available to you. A fresh egg has a compact, orange-yellow yolk that is a half dome centered in a dense cohesive white.

Supermarket eggs are graded according to their freshness by candling. In this process, the egg is held up to an intense light and the freshness is determined by the size of the air pocket. Grade AA is the freshest, and grade B, most of which go to restaurants and institutions, are older. The date on the carton is the date the egg was packaged, and in areas that require a "sell by" date, as much as two weeks may be allowed from the packaging date. Eggs are also packaged according to size, including jumbo, extra large, large, medium, and small.

To help assess the quality of the eggs you are buying:

- Be certain that they do not have breaks or cracks that can allow microorganisms to invade.
- Look for dirt on the shell. All eggs should be washed, and the shells should be clean.
- Pick up the eggs. Fresh eggs feel heavier for their size, and stale eggs will "slosh" when you shake them.
- Look at the shape of the egg. Misshapen eggs may reduce the protection afforded the yolk by its position in the white and its distance from the air pocket.

▌ DAIRY PRODUCTS

Dairy products include milk, buttermilk, cream, butter, cheese, ice cream, sour cream, yogurt, and kefir. All these products come from the milk of farm animals, including cows, goats, and sheep.

Milk contains protein, fat (sometimes called butterfat), lactose (milk sugar), and water. Unless it has been homogenized (forced under pressure through a very fine screen that breaks up the fat into minute globules evenly distributed through the milk), the fat in the milk will rise to the top as cream.

All milk sold in stores is pasteurized,

which does not make it sterile, but kills the disease-causing bacteria. The bacteria that is left does not cause illness, but will eventually multiply and cause the milk to spoil. All milk is labeled with a date code and should be purchased by this date. Be certain the milk is cold and the container shows no evidence of spillage.

Types of milk available include:

- pasteurized, homogenized cow's milk with varying amounts of fat, including whole milk, with 3 to 3.8 percent fat; lowfat milk, 0.5 to 2 percent fat, and skim milk, less than 0.5 percent. Some dairies add stabilizers and emulsifiers to milk, and "protein fortified" indicates that nonfat milk solids have been added.
- fresh goat's milk, which is ultrapasteurized, giving it a longer shelf life.
- buttermilk, made when special bacteria are added to fresh skim milk. Part of the milk sugar converts to acid, making the milk thick and tangy tasting.
- dried milk, which is a powdered concentration of pasteurized skim milk. Check the date codes and clean packaging.
- evaporated milk, made from fresh, unpasteurized whole milk. Sixty percent of the water is removed, and the concentrate is heated, homogenized, canned, and heated a second time to sterilize it. Vitamin D is added and sometimes other nutrients and chemical stabilizers are added. Cans of evaporated milk usually do not have a dating code.

Cream is milk containing 18 to 40 percent butterfat, and it is classified by its fat content. Half and half is about 11 percent fat, light cream is 18 percent fat, and heavy, or

Margarine

Margarine, which is sold as a butter substitute, is made from vegetable fats and contains no cholesterol. Some margarine contains whey and other dairy elements, but it is not a dairy product. Margarine does not contain as much saturated fat as butter, but the fats in margarine are in a chemical form called the "trans" form, which the body cannot use. Margarine also contains many additives, and is not recommended for a healthy diet.

whipping, cream is 36 percent or higher in fat. Note the dating code before purchasing, and buy only chilled, clean containers.

Butter is cream that has been whipped so that the butterfat in the cream separates from the liquid. It is washed in cold water and kneaded into a solid form. Butter is available salted, unsalted, and whipped, which is full of tiny air bubbles. Choose butter that has a sweet aroma and is cold, firm, and in a clean, unbroken package.

Cheese is made from cow's, goat's, and ewe's milk. As cheese ripens, natural enzymes and microorganisms determine its flavor and texture. Hundreds of different cheeses are made, including hard, firm, soft, semisoft, blue, and processed cheeses.

When you buy cheese, be aware that natural cheese should be kept in the store's refrigerator. Examine each piece of cheese for the presence of unwanted mold. Avoid signs of drying, such as cracked and darkened edges. Cheese that is greasy on the surface

Processed Cheese

Processed cheeses are not natural cheeses, and have been heated and pasteurized to stop the natural ripening processes. Other ingredients may be blended into processed cheese for additional flavor, softer texture and longer shelf life. At best, these products are a cheese substitute. Many contain significant amounts of sugar.

may have been warmed and chilled too many times. Note the date code and choose packages that are clean, not sticky, and tightly sealed.

Several frozen desserts are made from milk products, including ice cream, ice milk, custards, frozen yogurts, and sherbets. The term ice cream indicates that the product was made from the best-quality milk and has high butterfat and milk solid content. Most frozen desserts are whipped to incorporate air, making the ice cream light and smooth. This keeps it from turning into a frozen block. Do not purchase frozen desserts unless they are completely solid and the package is clean. Sticky or frosted packages have been partially thawed. Most frozen desserts purchased at a grocery store will be very high in sugar. Health food stores carry frozen desserts made with alternative sweeteners, including honey, as well as with dairy alternatives such as soy and rice.

Yogurt, sour cream, and kefir are products made from milk. Yogurt is made from milk to which *Lactobacillus bulgaricus* and *Streptococcus thermophilus* are added. These beneficial bacteria convert milk sugar to lactic acid, which thickens the milk and gives yogurt a pleasant tartness. Read the labels carefully because manufacturers often add sugar, fruit, colorings, and chemical stabilizers. The healthiest yogurts contain active bacterial culture.

Sour cream is made from pasteurized, homogenized cream to which a combination of souring bacteria is added. These bacteria create the tangy flavor and stiff consistency. Check the sour cream label for extra ingredients such as stabilizers and sweeteners, and for the date code.

Kefir is made from acidophilus milk to which yeast is added. Depending on the water content, it is sold as a thick drink, or as a thick mixture similar to sour cream. The drink frequently contains sugar and flavors.

For all these products, check the date code and purchase only clean, well-chilled containers.

▪ MEAT AND POULTRY

Eat only quality, clean meats and poultry. Purchase organic meat or meat from range-raised animals if it is available to you. Avoid meats from animals raised on feed to which hormones, antibiotics, and drugs have been added.

The following guidelines will help you purchase quality meat.

- Beef should be lean and a uniform, bright, light to deep red on the outside and dark purple on the inside. The bones of younger animals will be porous and red and those of older animals will be white and flinty. The fat should be creamy white.
- Lamb is meat from young sheep, usually less than a year old. The darker the lean

meat, the older the animal. The bones of older lambs will be drier, harder, and less red than bones of younger animals. The fat should be firm and white.

- Pork from young animals is grayish-pink, while lean meat from older animals will be rose-pink in color. The fat should be creamy white and firm, and the bones soft and tinged with red.

Poultry is very perishable and must be purchased with care. Chicken can be purchased either whole or cut up. Many stores carry packaged chicken parts and the consumer can buy a package of favorite chicken parts. Whether whole or cut up, the chicken should look moist and rounded. If the skin is on the meat, it should not be mottled or transparent, and should also be unbroken.

Although chicken is monitored for the presence of drugs more carefully than meat, buying and eating organically grown chicken is a better guarantee of avoiding the chemicals that are given to chickens as they are raised for market.

Turkey is usually sold frozen, unless it is ordered in advance or purchased directly from the farmer. Never buy frozen poultry, particularly turkey, in a bag that is leaking. This can mean it has partially thawed, which is dangerous for all poultry. If you are not buying free-range, organic turkey, read labels on frozen turkey for information on additives.

Turkey parts are also available and may be packaged fresh or frozen. Rolled turkey roasts are made from boned, tied turkey meat, either all white or dark and white mixed. Read labels to avoid a similar-looking product made from cooked, processed tur-

Frozen Fish

Frozen fish is acceptable, but should be used within a month. The "fishy" odor of fish increases with age. Frozen fish should have no fishy odor. Never refeeze any fish or other seafood after it has thawed.

key meat, which contains additives.

Ducks, geese, guineas, and Rock Cornish game hens are usually sold as whole birds, and unless the store is a specialty store or it is near a holiday, they will be frozen. Note the date code, and do not purchase these birds if the bags are leaking, stained, or sticky. Read the label for additives.

■ SEAFOODS

It is important to know the history of any fish that you purchase. Be aware that many fish are dipped in formaldehyde just after they are caught to prevent the growth of microorganisms. Be certain that the fish you purchase are fresh and unadulterated. Look for fish with bright, clear eyes that may protrude a little. As fish becomes old, the eyes turn cloudy and become sunken. The skin should be shiny, and the color should not be faded. The gills should be deep red, and there should be no red patches on the belly. Serve fresh fish as soon as possible, preferably the same day it is caught.

As a rule, do not buy fish from your local supermarket on Sunday. Fish is usually delivered Monday through Friday and anything left on ice after Saturday has been kept too long. Check the delivery dates for your store and plan your purchases accordingly.

Use the following guidelines when purchasing shellfish. Always be aware of local closures before harvesting shellfish yourself or buying from a vendor.

- Clams in the shell should be alive when you purchase them. If the shell is tightly closed or shuts down when you tap on it, the clam is alive.
- The shells of live oysters will also be shut tight. Select oysters that have a fresh scent but feel heavy for their size.
- Mussels are best in fall and winter. Their shells should be tightly shut and you should discard any whose shells remain closed after cooking. However, an abrupt temperature change before cooking can cause the shell to open. If the upper and lower shell will not slide across one another, the mussel is still alive.
- Live crabs are best. Crabs contain potent enzymes that start to decompose their flesh when they die. Cooked, frozen, or thawed crab should be eaten the day of purchase.
- Lobsters also contain these enzymes and should be purchased live and have energetic leg movement. A healthy lobster will curl its tail under when it is picked up. Precooked lobster tails should be curled, which means the lobster was alive when it was cooked. Whole, frozen, uncooked lobsters are available; they should be frozen solid with no trace of odor.
- Scallops will be purchased shucked and should be white, translucent, and smell fresh.
- Shrimp and prawns sold in the shell usu-

ally have their heads removed. For shelled shrimp and prawns, the skin should be translucent and they should have only a mild odor.

▮▮ STORING FOOD

Storage of all foods is very important in preventing problems that develop from consuming spoiled or contaminated food. It is also vital for preserving and maintaining the nutrient content of food, as well as taste and texture. There are optimum storage conditions for each food, in addition to time constraints.

▮ FRESH FOOD

With the exception of berries and cherries, wash and dry fruits before you put them away. Store all ripe fruit in the refrigerator. Unripe fruit should be kept at room temperature, away from sunlight. Never store fruit or fruit juices in galvanized containers. The acid from the fruit will dissolve the zinc, which is poisonous. Fruits and juices may develop a metallic taste if stored in iron, tin, or chipped enamel containers.

Fresh fruit can be frozen, but it must first be washed, pitted, peeled, or sliced. Most fruit must also be treated with ascorbic or citric acid to prevent darkening and have sugar added to help preserve the natural sweeteners in the fruit. Honey may be used instead of sugar, but its crystallization properties are different from those of sugar and may slightly change the frozen fruit. Berries can be frozen individually on a tray and then bagged. Frozen berries do not need sugar added. Blueberries can be frozen individually or in rigid containers.

Store vegetables in the vegetable crisper

drawer in your refrigerator to protect them from the dry air of the refrigerator. Storing unwashed vegetables in plastic bags will help give sufficient humidity. Some vegetables do not keep well in the refrigerator, including onions, potatoes, and tomatoes. They are best stored at 50°F in 80 percent humidity.

To freeze vegetables, they must first be washed, peeled, trimmed, and cut into uniform pieces. They must also be blanched in boiling water just long enough to destroy the enzymes that would age them, even in the freezer. Frozen vegetables will keep for 10 to 12 months if stored at 0°F or less.

■ REFRIGERATED FOODS

Chilling foods in the refrigerator can extend their storage life and prevent food spoilage. Cold temperatures slow the activity of enzymes and microorganisms. Meats, poultry, and fish should be kept in the coldest part of the refrigerator. Do not open prepackaged meats purchased from self-serve counters before cooking. Many people have handled these packages and opening the containers before cooking provides opportunity for contamination. Be careful to store meats so that their juices cannot leak and contaminate other foods.

Place foods in the refrigerator so that air can flow around each container easily. Cover all foods, as refrigerator air tends to dry out food and it will absorb food odors. Clean your refrigerator regularly with a baking soda solution or tolerated soap (rinse well) to cut down on food odors. Baking soda, either in the specialized boxes now available for refrigerators or simply in an open dish, will significantly reduce odors.

Food stored in the refrigerator will even-

During a Power Failure

Food in the refrigerator will stay cold during a power failure for about six hours if you do not open the door. Placing bags of ice on the upper shelves will keep food cold longer. Place pans beneath the bags to hold melted water. As long as the temperature has remained below 45°F, the food will be safe to eat. A refrigerator thermometer is helpful to monitor refrigerator function at all times, not just during a power failure.

tually grow mold. Most foods will keep adequately in a cold refrigerator (34° to 40°F) for a week. Beyond that time, they should be discarded. Do not eat food that has molded and remove spoiled foods immediately to avoid contaminating your refrigerator. (See the refrigerator chart below for storage times of common foods.)

Remove any stuffing before storing cooked poultry in the refrigerator or freezer. Stuffing will keep in the refrigerator for only two days, but can be frozen for one month. Cooked poultry should be stored immediately and not left at room temperature for more than a few minutes. Cooked poultry will keep for three to four days in the refrigerator.

Cooked meat should be refrigerated immediately after a meal. After it has cooled thoroughly in the refrigerator, seal it tightly with foil or in a container and refrigerate for up to four days. If you are not going to use the meat within that time, freeze it.

Refrigerator Storage Chart

FOOD	RECOMMENDED STORAGE TIME AT 37°F	HANDLING HINTS
Fresh fruit:		
Apples	1 to 2 weeks	Discard bruised or decayed fruit.
Berries, cherries	1 to 2 days	Store in moisture-resistant bag
Citrus	1 week	or wrap, or in crisper.
Melons	1 week	Wrap uncut melons to prevent odor spreading to other food. Wrap cut surfaces.
Vegetables:		
Asparagus, corn in husks, green or wax beans, mushrooms, shredded cabbage, salad greens, tomatoes	1 to 2 days	Keep in crisper or moisture-resistant wrap or bag.
Beets, cabbage, celery, carrots, radishes	1 to 2 weeks	Remove leafy tops. Keep in crisper or moisture-resistant wrap or bag.
Lettuce, head (unwashed) (washed and drained)	5 to 7 days 3 to 5 days	Store in moisture-resistant bag, wrap, or lettuce keeper away from other vegetables and fruit.
Unshelled peas, limas, spinach	3 to 5 days	Keep in crisper or moisture-resistant wrap or bag.
Butter	1 to 2 weeks	Wrap or cover tightly. Keep only a two-day supply in a butter dish.
Buttermilk	3 to 5 days	Cover tightly, shake before serving.
Cheese:		
Cottage, ricotta	5 days	Keep packaged tightly in
Cream, neufchatel	2 weeks	moisture-resistant wrap.
Hard and wax-coated:		If mold develops on the outside
Unopened	3 to 6 months	of hard cheese, trim it away.
Opened	3 to 4 weeks	
Sliced	2 weeks	
Parmesan and Romano (grated and opened)	2 months	Refrigerate after opening.

FOOD	RECOMMENDED STORAGE TIME AT 37°F	HANDLING HINTS
Cream	3 days	Cover tightly.
Milk:		
Homogenized, reconstituted dry milk	5 days	Keep containers tightly closed. Do not return milk from serving container to original container.
Evaporated (opened)	4 to 5 days	
Condensed (opened)	4 to 5 days	
Sour cream	2 weeks	Keep covered.
Yogurt	7 to 10 days	Keep covered.
Eggs in shell	2 to 3 weeks	Store covered with small end down to keep yolk centered.
Meat (beef*, pork, lamb):		
Chops	2 to 3 days	Store prepackaged meats in original store packaging. If packaged by butcher, remove from original packaging and wrap in waxed paper to allow surface to dry.
Ground meat	1 to 2 days	
Roasts	2 to 4 days	
Steaks	2 to 3 days	
Variety (liver, heart, etc.)	1 day	
		*Because it has a high proportion of saturated fats, large cuts of beef will keep in a very cold refrigerator for as long as 8 days.
Poultry:		
Chicken (fresh whole)	1 to 2 days	Do not open prepackaged containers or wrapping before storing.
(fresh cut up)	24 hours	
Ready to cook duck or turkey (frozen)	2 days	
Seafood:		
Fish	1 day	Follow directions for meat.
Shucked clams, oysters, scallops, shrimp	1 day	Store in coldest part of refrigerator.
Clams, crab, lobster in shell	2 days	
Cooked shrimp and prawns	3 days	Store in plastic bag in coldest part of the refrigerator.

Keep It Shut!

A fully loaded freezer will stay cold for up to two days after a power failure if you do not open the door. After the power is back on, carefully examine all foods stored in the freezer. Foods that contain ice crystals are safe to refreeze. Meat should have a hard central core of ice.

Throw out any fully or partially thawed foods with suspicious color or odor. Discard any thawed vegetables packed in butter or cream sauce. Use all refrozen foods within two weeks.

Leftover canned vegetables should be removed from the can and stored in a closed container in the refrigerator. They will keep for three to five days. Leftover cooked vegetables can be stored in the refrigerator in a closed container for three to five days.

Cooked fish will keep in the refrigerator for three or four days in a tightly covered container. Reheating cooked fish causes it to become dry, but it can be prepared in a sauce or served cold in a salad. After opening, remove fish from the can and store in a tightly covered container in the refrigerator for three to five days.

Cooked clams can be kept in the refrigerator for three to four days, covered. Raw shrimp and prawns can only be kept refrigerated for several hours.

Eggs must be stored below 40°F at all times. At room temperature, they will age as much in one day as they will during a week in the refrigerator. Eggs should be stored covered, as their porous shells absorb odors.

Their original carton is the best storage container. Never use the open egg racks in the refrigerator door, as they are too warm, as well as uncovered. If eggs are clean and unbroken, they can be stored in the refrigerator for four to five weeks after purchase. After five weeks, their flavor and texture will have suffered, but they are still safe to eat and are best used for baking. Throw away cracked eggs unless you use them immediately in baked or thoroughly cooked foods.

■ FROZEN FOODS

The best freezer temperature is 0°F or below, with a maximum temperature of 5°F. Keep a thermometer in your freezer to check the temperature regularly. If your freezer cannot keep ice cream rock hard, the temperature is above the top limit. If your freezer is above 0°F, safe storage times must be reduced. One year is the top limit that foods should be kept in the freezer at the appropriate temperature. Foods begin to lose nutrients after this time, and flavors and textures begin to deteriorate. Some foods should be stored only a few months.

If frozen food dries out, it can develop freezer burn—discolored, papery patches on the food. Even though the food is safe to eat, freezer burn ruins the taste and texture. Packaging must be airtight to prevent freezer burn.

Purchase only frozen foods that are frozen solid, and place them in your freezer as soon as possible. Thaw and cook according to the package directions. Cooked foods should never be refrozen once they have been thawed.

Remove stuffing before storing poultry in the freezer. Coated with gravy, poultry will

Freezer Storage Chart

FOOD	RECOMMENDED STORAGE TIME AT 0°F	HANDLING HINTS
Meat:		
Beef	6 to 12 months	Trim away excess fat and freeze in airtight packages or containers
Ground beef	2 to 4 months	Freeze in airtight packages or containers.
Pork	6 months	Freeze in airtight packages or containers.
Ground pork	3 months	
Lamb (large cuts)	6 to 9 months	Overwrap with suitable freezer wrap.
Ground lamb, chops, stew meat	3 to 4 months	
Poultry:		
Chicken	1 year	Must be well wrapped.
Chicken parts	6 to 9 months	
Seafood:		
Fish, lean	6 months	Freeze in original wrap up to 2
Fish, fatty	2 to 3 months	weeks, wrap with freezer wrap for longer periods.
Clams, raw	3 months	Shuck and freeze raw in natural liquid, adding light brine to cover the meat. Fill container ½ inch below the rim and seal. Cooked clams become rubbery in the freezer.
Crab, cooked	3 to 4 months	Scrub shells, boil or steam, remove meat from shells and freeze in airtight rigid container. Cover with light brine and leave ½ inch headroom.
Lobsters (raw)	3 to 4 months	Follow directions for clams.
Mussels (raw)	3 months	
Oysters	3 to 4 months	
Scallops (cooked)	3 months	Must be poahced, frozen and tightly sealed.
Shrimp and prawns (raw)	4 to 6 months	Rinse in light brine and freeze in rigid container with no headroom.

FOOD	RECOMMENDED STORAGE TIME AT 0°F	HANDLING HINTS
Seafood: (cont.)		
Shrimp and prawns (cooked)	1 to 2 months	Pack in rigid containers without headroom and seal airtight.
Fruit (home frozen or purchased frozen):		
Berries, cherries, peaches, pears, pineapple	12 months	Freeze in moisture- and vapor-proof container.
Citrus Fruit	6 months	
Vegetables:*		
Home frozen	10 months	Freeze in moisture vapor-proof container.
Purchased frozen	8 months	Leave in original container if intact. Put original container in Ziploc if not. *Cabbage, celery, salad greens, and tomatoes do not freeze successfully
Dairy:		
Butter	6 to 9 months	Store in moisture- and vapor-proof container or wrap.
Whipped butter	Do not freeze	Emulsion will break and product will separate.
Buttermilk, sour cream, yogurt, and kefir	Do not freeze	Product will separate and become grainy.
Cream—light, heavy, half and half	2 months	May not whip after thawing. Thaw in refrigerator.
Whipped cream	1 months	Freeze firm in spoonfuls, store in plastic bag. Thaw in refrigerator.
Milk	1 month	Allow room for expansion. Thaw in refrigerator.
Cheese (soft)*	3 months	Thaw in refrigerator.
Cheese (hard)	6 weeks	Cut and wrap in small pieces, color may become mottled. Thaw in refrigerator.
Cheese roquefort, blue	3 months	May be crumbly after thawing. *Do not freeze ricotta, cottage cheese, creamed cheese or neufchatel.

Storing Flour

Whole-grain flour that contains the germ and bran must be stored in the refrigerator or freezer in lightproof, tightly sealed containers. It cannot be stored in the pantry. Wheat and triticale will keep for one year, and other whole-grain flours will keep for two to three months in the refrigerator or freezer. Measure the amount of flour you need, then return the container to the refrigerator or freezer. Allow the flour to warm to room temperature before using.

last for six months in the freezer. Without gravy, it should be kept no longer than one month.

■ PANTRY STORAGE

Many staples have a long shelf life, but will eventually spoil. Care must be taken in storing them properly so that they will last for the anticipated shelf life. Store staple foods in closed cupboards away from stoves, dishwashers, dryers, and other sources of heat. Heat, including direct sunlight, shortens the storage life of all food. Also avoid too much light and too much moisture. Never store food under the sink or near any other open plumbing. Water dripping on cans can rust them, and it can penetrate packages of dry foods and spoil the contents.

Cans of fruits and vegetables can be kept on a cool, dry shelf for up to one year. After that time they will still be safe to eat, but will not be as nutritious or taste as good. Citrus fruits and juices, and mixed fruit salads will keep for only six months. Canned fish can be stored unopened for a year.

Flour is commonly stored in cupboards or pantries. It does not spoil in an immediately obvious way, but it can absorb moisture from the air and will not give consistent results in baking. The fat in the flour can become rancid, imparting the flavor and odor of rancid fat to foods. The protein can degenerate and lose nutritive value. Flour should be stored in airtight containers. If kept cool, dry, and dark, it will keep for six months to a year. In warm, humid climates it will keep for only six months.

■■ FOOD PREPARATION

Food preparation can make the difference between having a healthy meal and having one that can add to your toxic burden. For example, oven broiling or baking produces a healthier dish than frying, which adds saturated fats to the food. Charcoal broiling deposits a coat of polycyclic aromatic hydrocarbons (PAHs) on the food. Smoking foods over an open fire exposes them to carcinogenic chemicals in the smoke, including benzo[a]pyrene. (See Solvents in chapter 16, Chemicals and Metals, for a discussion of PAHs.)

Although they are very convenient, there is much controversy over preparing food in the microwave. Some scientists feel that all food prepared in the microwave is changed in ways that are harmful to us. Others feel that microwaves are safe for rewarming food, but not for cooking raw foods, particularly meats. Microwaving particularly changes milk products, and baby bottles should never be warmed in the microwave.

Pantry Storage Chart

FOOD	RECOMMENDED STORAGE TIME AT 70°F	HANDLING HINTS
Baking powder	18 months or expiration date on can	Keep dry and covered.
Baking soda	2 years	Keep dry and covered.
Cereal:		
(unopened)	6 to 12 months	Refold package liner tightly
(opened)	2 to 3 months	after opening.
Cornmeal	12 months	Keep tightly closed
Cornstarch	18 months	Keep tightly closed.
Gelatin	18 months	Keep in original container
Honey	12 months	Cover tightly. If crystallizes, warm jar in pan of hot water.
Molasses:		
(unopened)	12+ months	Keep tightly closed.
(opened)	6 months	Refrigerate to extend life.
Mayonnaise (unopened)	2 to 3 months	Refrigerate after opening.
Oils:		
(unopened)	6 months	Keep tightly closed. Refrigerate after opening.
Pasta	2 years	Store in airtight container after opening.
Salad dressings:		
(unopened)	10 to 12 months	Keep tightly closed. Refrigerate after opening.
Tea:		
Bags	18 months	Put in airtight container.
Loose	2 years	
Canned foods (unopened)	12 months	Keep cool.
Fruits, dried	6 months	Keep cool in airtight container, refrigerate if possible.

FOOD	RECOMMENDED STORAGE TIME AT 70°F	HANDLING HINTS
Vegetables, dried	1 year	Keep cool in airtight container, refrigerate if possible.
Catsup:		
(unopened)	12 months	Refrigerate for longer storage.
(opened)	1 month	
Mustard:		
(unopened)	2 years	
(opened)	6 to 8 months	May be refrigerated, stir before using.
Spices and herbs:		
(whole)	1 to 2 years	Store in airtight containers away from sunlight and heat.
(ground)	6 months	
Nuts:		
(in shell)	4 months	Freeze for longer storage.
(shelled)	2 weeks	Unsalted and blanched last longer than salted.
Dried peas and beans	12 months	Store in airtight container in cool place.
Yeast, dry	Expiration date on package	Store in cool place.

If you use a microwave oven, it should be checked yearly for leakage using a well-calibrated meter. If the door gasket is damaged, replace it before using the oven again. The dose and the time of microwave exposure that can cause problems are unknown. Do not stand in front of microwave ovens while they are in operation; stay at least four feet away.

Steaming vegetables allows retention of more nutrients than boiling. With boiling, the nutrients that are not destroyed are left in the water, which is usually discarded. Food enzymes are also destroyed with heat. Eating raw vegetables allows the benefit of the food enzymes. Eating raw fruits allows the benefits of food enzymes that help to process the sugar fruits contain. These enzymes have been destroyed in juices, and natural juice has a high sugar content.

Stir-frying, either in a wok or a skillet, is a healthful way to prepare either vegetables or vegetables and meat. The high heat and short cooking time locks in the nutrients

477

Caution Against Aluminum Poisoning

Foods and food preparation can contribute to aluminum poisoning. Avoid using baking powders made with aluminum, as well as salt that contains aluminum compounds to prevent caking. Do not cook acidic foods (such as tomatoes) or alkaline foods (such as grains) in aluminum pots and pans. Cook only in stainless-steel, glass, or ceramic cookware.

and keeps the bite-sized food intact. Foods do not become limp and lose their appeal. If an oil is used, the food becomes coated with the oil as it is stirred. This makes it less allergenic for some people. However, cooking the food for too long can increase the number of free radicals that are produced. Water may be used instead of oil to reduce calories and avoid free radicals.

When making a salad, tear greens at the last minute. This keeps them crisp and prevents the loss of vitamin C that occurs when the torn cells release ascorbic acid oxidase, an enzyme that destroys vitamin C.

See chapter 24, Diet, Fasting, and Juicing, for more information on healthy eating and detoxification. Detoxification techniques for diet are also useful prevention techniques.

■■ FOOD POISONING

Proper food handling is the key to preventing food poisoning caused by organisms in food that subsequently multiply in the body.

Inadequate storage, cooking temperature, or cooking time can contribute to this type of food poisoning. Food must be thoroughly cooked in order to destroy organisms. Foods kept at low temperatures on warming tables are also susceptible to contamination. The careful handling of raw meats and proper cleansing of utensils such as knives and cleavers is critical. Thoroughly clean any knives, particularly those used for cutting poultry, and clean cutting boards thoroughly after each use. Eggs, poultry, beef, pork, baked goods, milk and milk products, vegetables, dried coconut, and cocoa are common offenders in this type of food poisoning.

Food poisoning is also caused by organisms that produce toxins. Controlling the temperature of foods is the single most effective method of preventing this type of food poisoning. Promptly refrigerating food prevents the growth of toxin-producing bacteria. It must be refrigerated before the incubation period of the bacteria, which is less than four hours. Meats, cooked ham, smoked fish, milk, cream-filled bakery goods, and home-canned foods are susceptible to this type of contamination. (See chapter 13, Food, for a detailed discussion of food poisoning.)

To help prevent food poisoning, use the following measures:
• Wash your hands frequently while you are cooking. Wash them before you begin to cook, and after handling raw meat, poultry, seafood, or egg shells.
• Wash cutting boards and cabinet tops. Use bleach diluted in water if they have been in contact with raw meat, fish, or poultry.
• Keep surfaces clean and take measures to

Cooking Frozen Foods

Temperature during food preparation is just as important as the temperature at which the food is held and stored after its preparation. Any frozen foods or frozen ingredients used in preparing foods should generally be thawed in the refrigerator, not at room temperature. Many foods can be cooked directly from the frozen state.

For most cooking methods, poultry can be cooked from the frozen state. Only poultry that you are going to roast must be thawed before cooking. It should be thawed in the refrigerator or under cold water (50°F). After thawing, cook poultry promptly.

eliminate flies and crawling insects from the kitchen.

- Use kitchen utensils for only one job at a time and wash them between tasks. Use different spoons to stir raw and cooked foods.
- Sanitize all dishes and other kitchen equipment with detergent and extremely hot water or run them through the dishwasher.
- Keep foods clean with proper washing and storage. Wash all produce and store foods at the proper temperature.
- Heat foods to the proper temperature both when cooking and reheating. Be sure foods are cooked thoroughly and allow extra cooking time for frozen or partially frozen food.
- Keep hot foods hot. Heat foods to at least 150°F and maintain at that temperature.

- Chill foods rapidly by putting them in the refrigerator immediately. Cooling hot foods to room temperature before putting them in the refrigerator allows them to remain in the danger zone (45°F to 140°F) too long.
- Keep cold foods cold. Be sure your refrigerator maintains a temperature of 40°F or lower.
- Handle home-canned foods with care. Discard cans and bottles that leak or bulge, or that have mold on the seal or on the contents. Also discard those with tiny bubbles in the contents and those that have an "off" odor. Do not taste suspicious food, and dispose of it in such a way that it does not contaminate your kitchen or give your children or pets access to it.

Water

The role of water in detoxification has been described in previous chapters. Clean water is essential for both detoxification and prevention of health problems. Prevention of illnesses caused by contaminated water can also reduce the necessity for detoxification procedures.

It is vital to use safe water for drinking, cooking, brushing teeth, and washing fresh foods. Some very sensitive people may also need filtered water for bathing if chlorine or fluoride is a severe problem. Showering and bathing can expose people to more of the harmful chemicals in tap water than drinking it, because they are absorbed through the skin and inhaled in the steam from the water. The American Chemical Society states that exposure to chemicals by breathing the air in and around the shower is up to 100 times greater than by drinking tap water.

Treating Food Poisoning

- *"Magic Brew" will help control the nausea and headaches that accompany food poisoning. Mix 1 tsp. sea salt and 1 tsp. baking soda in 1 quart of tolerated water and sip as needed. It may be more soothing cold.*
- *Herbs that can relieve symptoms of food poisoning include angelica, barberry, bayberry, burdock, catnip, chamomile, cinnamon, echinacea, garlic, goldenseal, mint, and mullein.*
- *See Food and Water toxins in chapter 28, Homeopathy and Bach Flower Remedies, for homeopathic remedies to treat specific types of food poisoning.*

❚❚ PURIFICATION METHODS

Frequently, additional purification treatment is required at home. Treatment possibilities are:

- *Boiling water:* Destroys organisms and removes chlorine and volatile chemicals. Heavy metals and nitrates remain in the water. Do not use aluminum pots to boil water because this will add aluminum to the water.
- *Filtering water:* Removes many contaminants. Portable, single-faucet, and whole house filters are available. Carbon block filters are more efficient than granulated carbon and are the most common type of filter available. They remove pesticides, chloroform, organic chemicals, bad taste and odor, some organisms *(Giardia lamblia),* and chlorine. Charcoal filters do not remove heavy metals, salts, minerals, nitrates, fluorides, or bacteria. These filters must be changed regularly to prevent the growth of bacteria and mold in the carbon medium. Some people are sensitive to the carbon medium, which can cause stomachache and headache.
- *Distillation:* Water is boiled into steam, then condensed and collected, to remove salts, asbestos, organisms, minerals, heavy metals, and nitrates. It will also remove viruses and bacteria. Distillation does not remove chlorine, organic chemicals, or vocs. The apparatus is more complicated to use than other water purification methods, and is also noisy and gives off heat.
- *Reverse osmosis:* Reverse osmosis filters are arranged in a series with a sediment filter, reverse osmosis filter, and an activated carbon cartridge. Water is forced under pressure through the filters, which removes particulate matter, some organic chemicals and pesticides, asbestos, nitrates, heavy metals, fluorides, and chlorine compounds. It does not remove chlorine, all organisms, all chemicals, or all pesticides. Reverse osmosis units are dependent on water pressure for proper operation and their efficiency decreases with time.
- *Hydrogen peroxide:* Purifies water by killing organisms, but it will not remove chemicals. Add seven drops of 35 percent food-grade hydrogen peroxide per gallon of distilled water. This method is also acceptable for the water of pets.
- *Ultraviolet (uv) light chambers:* Kills microbes and is best used in combination with carbon block filters. Some organic

Metals in Water

Some water contains dissolved metals. Drinking water may have lead in it, usually from the lead solder used to seal joints in older plumbing. To avoid lead that may have leached out in water, run the water from the faucet for a few minutes every morning before drinking the water. Observe this same practice if you have been away, or if a fountain or water source has not been used over a weekend. As the plumbing needs repairs, have the old joints replaced without the use of lead solder. Lead in water can contribute to hypertension, mental deterioration, impotence, birth defects, and learning difficulties.

Drinking water may also contain aluminum. Since it is not an essential metal, it is advisable to minimize your aluminum ingestion because neurological disorders are associated with cumulative doses of aluminum. Check to see if your local water contains high levels of aluminum, and avoid drinking it if it does.

compounds are altered to less harmful compounds but this method is ineffective if the water is turbid or slightly clouded.

• *Copper-Zinc Alloy (KDF):* Uses an electro-chemical process called redox to remove chlorine and its byproducts, heavy metals, and some surface contaminants. It does not remove bacteria, viruses, *Cryptosporidium*, and most organic chemicals.

■■ BOTTLED WATER

Drinking water and distilled water can also be purchased, but you will need to thoroughly investigate the quality of water you are buying. Some companies that sell water do not always offer the quality of water that they claim. Even though bottled water appears to be safe, to be certain, ask the bottler for information on mineral, bacteriological, and chemical content. Also contact your local health department for data on the purity of a particular brand.

Sensitive people should inquire about the source of spring water, since ground water in some areas is chemically contaminated.

Store water in glass or ceramic bottles, rather than plastic containers, which leach plastic components into the water.

When you travel, you will need to assure the quality of the water you consume. Taking bottled water with you or buying it as you travel is one option.

For "city" traveling and hotel and motel trips, portable water filters are available that will fit in your suitcase. Some are shaped like pitchers, while others look like a thermos bottle. You simply pour the water to be treated into the portable filter. The filters in these containers will generally lower the chlorine content. Some of them also remove "scale and scum," which are dissolved minerals. Others claim to remove lead and copper. While they are not as efficient as the larger filters, they do improve the quality and taste of the water.

Never drink untreated spring, stream, lake, or river water when you are on a camping or hiking trip, especially standing water or water that flows through cow feed-lots or pastures. Most untreated water will contain harmful organisms. There are three methods to remove organisms in water on a hiking or camping trip, or even when traveling away from home.

- *Boiling:* Water must be boiled from 5 to 10 minutes, then cooled to a comfortable drinking temperature. This is time-consuming, and finding fuel can be a problem.
- *Iodine crystals or tablets:* The easiest and least expensive way to purify water. This method absolutely kills microorganisms, but the resulting taste of the water is not good.
- *Filters:* Portable ceramic water filters are effective for removing organisms. Most pumps can process a quart of water in one to two minutes. The filters are bulky and can be expensive. However, the extra effort required to carry the filter and use it is worthwhile.

Indoor Environment

WE HAVE MUCH more control over indoor pollution than over outdoor pollution. It is essential that we control indoor pollution to prevent exposure to toxins and the immediate damage they can cause, as well as the bioaccumulation of toxins in our bodies. Many times, simple measures well within our ability to effect can prevent serious health problems.

The indoor environment includes our home, school, workplace, and any building we happen to be in. Although we may not be able to control indoor air pollution in the workplace or in buildings where we shop or visit, we certainly can control it in our homes. Environmentally clean, safe homes help to prevent toxic exposures and allow us to maintain our health after detoxifying.

In this chapter, we have tried to present comprehensive prevention methods for controlling indoor environments. Use only those that apply to your situation.

Home Environment

Because of the number of hours we spend in our homes, the home environment is very important to our health, particularly the air quality. A clean environment helps us to detoxify naturally from the toxic exposures of our workdays. You can conduct your lifestyle to provide an environment that will allow your body to detoxify and prevent toxic bioaccumulation.

▌▌AIR

Air quality in the home is an important factor in maintaining a clean environment. Consider each of the following categories for controlling air pollution in your home and use the safest alternatives possible.

The use of an air cleaner can significantly improve air quality in a home and will prevent the harmful buildup of chemicals, inhalants, and microorganisms. Most air cleaners remove particles such as dust, dust mites, pollen, mold, bacteria, and viruses with the use of two filters. One, a metal mesh, removes the larger particles, and a HEPA (High Efficiency Particulate Accumulator) filter removes the very small particles.

Activated charcoal filters will remove

Controlling Air Pollution in the Home

SOURCE OF POLLUTION	ITEMS	POLLUTANTS	SAFER ALTERNATIVES
Building materials for construction or repair	Plywood, particle-board, paneling, chipboard	Formaldehyde	Hardwoods, sealants to seal out the formaldehyde
	Paint	Mold retardants and fungicides, VOC emissions	Paint with mold retardant and fungicides left out, low VOC paint
Furnishings	Carpets and drapes	Toxic chemicals, including formaldehyde	Hardwood, brick, or tile floors (some less toxic carpets are available), 100 percent washable cotton drapes
	Upholstered furniture	Fabric, padding, spot and stain protection emit chemicals and collect dust	Hardwood, glass or metal furniture. Vacuum furniture regularly to prevent dust buildup.
Cleaning supplies	Commercial cleaners	Scents and harmful chemicals	Hot water, baking soda, and lemon juice
	Disinfectants	Harmful chemicals, leave residue to which bacteria can become resistant	Bleach, alcohol, ammonia, hydrogen peroxide, may not tolerate if chemically sensitive
	Commercial air deodorizers, air fresheners, or disinfectants	Harmful chemicals	Vanilla flavoring on a cotton ball, fresh grated lemon rind in open dish, zephiran (disinfectant available at drug stores)

SOURCE OF POLLUTION	ITEMS	POLLUTANTS	SAFER ALTERNATIVES
Laundry supplies	Fabric softeners, liquid and dryer sheets	Harmful chemicals	½ to 1 cup baking soda in rinse water softens, ¼ cup vinegar in wash water prevents static cling. Hang clothes outdoors unless mold and pollen counts are high.
	Detergents	Harmful chemicals, scents	Unscented detergents, ceramic laundry disks. Masking scents may be used in detergents and fabric softeners, so are not truly unscented.
Personal care products	Soap, deodorant, hair care items, makeup, perfumes, after shaves	Harmful chemicals, scents	Unscented body soaps, deodorants, shampoos, other hair care products, makeup. Avoid perfume.
Tobacco use	All tobacco products	Carcinogenic chemicals	Do not smoke and do not allow anyone else to smoke in your home or car.
Heading systems and appliances	Gas appliances and heaters	Carbon monoxide, nitrogen dioxide	Use carbon monoxide monitor, replace filters often.
	Wood stoves and fireplaces	Carbon monoxide, creosote, smoke fumes	Clean chimney regularly, burn dry wood, no synthetic logs or newspapers.

Dehumidifiers

People who live in damp climates will have a more difficult time achieving moisture control in their homes. If you live in a humid climate, investing in a dehumidifier may be of great benefit to help control mold levels in your home. Be sure to clean and check it regularly.

chemicals, including formaldehyde. However, some very sensitive people may not tolerate the charcoal used in the filter and may have to investigate whether charcoal from other sources will be safe for them. A final filter of glass beads can reduce these problems.

Household appliances and heating systems can be major contributors to indoor pollution. Gas stoves give off both carbon monoxide and nitrogen dioxide. Have gas stoves, furnaces, and hot-water heaters checked regularly for gas leaks and carbon monoxide levels. As a safety precaution, install a carbon monoxide monitor. Clean or replace furnace filters regularly. Oil furnaces, stoves, and appliances must also be inspected regularly. Keep all vent pipes free of soot and obstructions. Good ventilation and properly working stoves will decrease indoor air pollution.

Whether you use a fireplace or a wood-burning stove, clean and inspect chimneys yearly. Creosote buildup has an unpleasant odor and can cause chimney corrosion, as well as causing a chimney fire. Do not vent a wood and oil heater, or wood and gas heater, into the same chimney flue. Burn only dry wood, which burns more cleanly and more efficiently than wet wood. Do not burn synthetic logs, newspapers, garbage, plastic, or treated wood, all of which give off toxic fumes.

To avoid carbon monoxide poisoning, never idle cars in the garage with the door closed. The wall and doorway separating the garage from the house should be airtight to prevent carbon monoxide from entering the house.

■■ PLANTS

While plants in the home environment can add beauty to a home, they can also cause problems. Mold frequently grows in the soil after plants are watered. (See mold control below.) Terpenes in plants can cause problems for people with terpene sensitivities. It is best to avoid houseplants with a scent, and do not bring cut flowers or a live Christmas tree into the house.

Some plants are poisonous if ingested. Children and pets sometimes eat plants, both household and outdoors. Many plants contain a wide range of substances that may cause symptoms as mild as a stomachache or skin rash, to more serious reactions. (See chapter 39 for a discussion of plants and children.)

■■ ORGANISMS

■ MOLDS

Mold is the most serious indoor organism we normally encounter. Because molds can cause many different types of problems, mold control is an important part of managing the indoor environment. (See Organisms in chapter 15 for a discussion of mold.)

- Control dampness in order to control molds.
- Avoid any material that smells musty, because mold produces the odor.
- Keep all plumbing in good repair and fix leaks promptly. If the mold contamination is too great in the area surrounding a leak, the moldy materials will have to be replaced.
- Clean up completely after any flooding or seepage, and correct the cause of the problem.

Be certain there is good ventilation in all parts of your house, particularly in the bathroom, laundry room, and kitchen. Use exhaust fans in these rooms to vent excess moisture to the outside. After showering or bathing, dry off shower walls, the floor, and fixtures with a towel to decrease the amount of standing water in the bathroom. Allow clothing and towels to dry completely before putting them in a laundry hamper. Always vent the clothes dryer to the outside, and do not leave wet clothes in the washer. Keep the lid of the washing machine open when not in use to provide air circulation and prevent mold growth.

Clean the drip pan of self-defrosting refrigerators regularly and check the door seal for mildew. Clean garbage cans regularly to prevent mold growth. Wash dirty dishes after each meal to avoid mold growth on food remains.

Discard moldy items, including old newspapers, books, or magazines; old furniture; bedding; carpet; clothing; and pillows.

Mold Allergies

The hives suffered by one exquisitely mold-sensitive patient made her look as if she had been battered. Her face swelled, particularly her lips, giving them a "turned inside out" look, and her eye on the affected side would almost swell shut.

She was very careful with her exposures and diet, but continued to have occasional outbreaks of hives, particularly when it rained or snowed. Adding 500 mg of quercetin, twice a day, between meals stopped her outbreaks.

Use stringent dust control procedures, as they also help to prevent mold growth. Avoid old dust, as it will be full of mold.

Air cleaners will remove mold spores, which are the reproductive cells of molds. Monitor indoor humidity and use mold plates to determine the amount of mold contamination in your home. (See Sources.)

Air conditioners, particularly "swamp coolers," may be the site of mold growth because of their damp pads. Change these pads frequently.

Houseplants can help clean and humidify indoor air, but can also be sources of mold. Impregnon or taheebo tea (both available at health food stores) added to houseplant water will retard mold in the potting soil of plants. Because mold grows on tree bark, do not store fireplace logs inside the house.

Humidifiers

Some people who live in dry climates use humidifiers to add moisture to the air. Humidifiers frequently grow mold and disperse the spores into the air. Avoid using a humidifier if at all possible, and if you must use one, clean it frequently.

There are chemicals available for humidifiers that prevent mold growth, but chemically sensitive people may not tolerate them.

A pot of water in the room or on a stove will add moisture to the air.

For mold cleanup, soap and hot water, bleach, Zephiran (in a 17 percent aqueous solution), and borax are helpful. Chemically sensitive people should avoid bleach, and some individuals may not be able to tolerate borax. Heat from a hair dryer will dry mold into a powder that can be brushed off. However, the spores remain viable unless the temperature is extremely high.

Wear a mask and gloves for any type of mold cleanup, and wash your clothing, hair, and body afterward. If you are extremely mold sensitive, have someone else do the mold cleanup.

Ozone generators will kill mold in hard-to-reach places. Because ozone is a gas, it will penetrate all parts of the house. However, people, plants, and animals must not be in the house while the generator is in use, or for one hour after it has been turned off. By that time, any ozone in the air will have deteriorated into oxygen. Some ozone gen-erators have timers that allow you to set the generation time. Twenty-four-hour timers available at hardware stores can be connected between the generator and the power source for generators that have no timer.

❚ VIRUSES AND BACTERIA

Viruses and bacteria are other organisms that can be part of the home environment. Viruses are usually present when a member of the household has an infection. Unless preventive measures are taken, the infections caused by these organisms can spread to all members of the family. The spread of bacteria in a household originates from infections such as strep throat and other bacterial diseases, or from food poisoning. Food poisoning is caused by bacteria, but is not contagious. People in the same house will not get food poisoning unless they eat the same contaminated food. (For a detailed discussion of food poisoning, see chapter 35, Food and Water.)

Use the following measures to prevent the spread of these common viruses:

• *Colds and flu:* After being exposed to someone who has a cold or the flu, avoid touching your eyes or nose until you wash your hands with soap and water. Do not share food, drinking glasses, eating utensils, or eyeglasses with the sick person. Disinfect contaminated articles and equipment that is shared with others and cover all open wounds. Do not kiss anyone with a cold or flu during the first three days of the infection. If you are the one with the cold or flu, cover your nose and mouth when you sneeze or cough. Replace your toothbrush once you are better.

• *Herpes:* To prevent the spread of oral herpes

(cold sores), do not kiss anyone, share towels, razors, drinking glasses, eating utensils, or finish the food of anyone with an outbreak. Wash your hands thoroughly after touching a blister, and replace your toothbrush after the cold sore has healed. To prevent the spread of genital herpes, use latex condoms routinely. Wear white cotton underwear to bed during an outbreak and launder after each wearing. Avoid sexual activity during an outbreak to avoid reinfection and to reduce trauma to inflamed tissue.

There are many different bacterial infections. However, some infections, such as a bladder infection, are not contagious. Use the following measures to prevent the spread of these common bacterial infections:

• *Strep throat:* Do not kiss anyone, share towels, razors, drinking glasses, eating utensils, or finish the food of anyone with strep throat. Disinfect contaminated articles and equipment that is shared with others. Replace your toothbrush when you recover from the infection.

• *Impetigo:* This skin disease is caused by *Staphylococcus aureus,* or Group A streptococci. Adults seldom contract impetigo, but it can spread easily among children. It begins with skin redness, which develops into fluid-containing small blisters that gradually crust and erode. It is highly contagious and must be treated with oral or topical antibiotics. Do not touch the affected skin without immediately washing your hands. Cover the area with antibiotic cream before going to bed, and change and wash the bed linens frequently. If it spreads

to areas on the body other than the face, wash the clothes after one wearing.

■ DUST, DUST MITES, AND
ANIMAL DANDER AND HAIR

Dust and dust mite control is important for preventing symptoms in the sensitive person. Unless the person is extremely sensitive, the following measures will be sufficient to prevent problems:

• Dust the house regularly, particularly the bedroom, using a damp cloth.

• Eliminate drapes and blinds. Replace with washable curtains and clean them regularly.

• Wash all bedding in hot water.

• Remove dust-catchers, such as pennants, pictures, trophies, books, models, and dried or silk flower arrangements from the bedroom.

• Do not allow stuffed animals in the bedroom.

• Do not store items under the bed.

• Use an air cleaner with a dust filter and change the filters or clean them as needed.

• Vacuum upholstered furniture and carpet regularly. If dust mites are a problem, dispose of the vacuum cleaner bag immediately after each use.

• Do not allow birds, animals, or reptiles in the house.

It is best if animals are not kept in a home with an extremely sensitive person. However, this is often not a practical option with a family pet. Simple measures help to prevent most problems with animal dander and hair in the home.

• Do not allow animals in the bedroom, and never sleep with an animal.

• Bathe cats and dogs regularly.

Plant Cleansers

Studies done by NASA show that spider plants and banana plants can remove formaldehyde from the air. Several plants in a room will significantly lower the levels of formaldehyde.

- Do not groom animals in the house.
- Use an air cleaner to remove animal dander and hair from the air.

▮▮ CHEMICALS

Unless we take special measures, our homes can be the source of numerous chemical exposures. Many easy-to-make changes can dramatically lower chemical levels in a home.

▮ VOLATILE ORGANIC CHEMICALS

A systematic chemical cleanup of your home is the best way to remove volatile organic chemicals (vocs). Remember that molecules of these substances can slowly escape, even from a tightly closed bottle.

Never store the following products inside the house:
- pesticides
- paints, paint removers, lacquers, adhesives, waxes, solvents, and shellacs
- cleaning products with an odor or scent of any kind
- air fresheners and aerosol sprays
- dry-cleaned clothes that have not aired outside for a month
- perfumes, aftershaves, nail polish, nail polish remover
- scented cosmetics, soaps, lotions, and deodorants

▮ SOLVENTS

Because of their extreme toxicity, preventing exposure to solvents is of utmost importance. Whenever possible, use nontoxic substitutes instead of solvent-containing materials. If you must use a solvent, follow these guidelines to minimize exposure:
- Use solvents only in a well-ventilated area.
- Wear protective clothing, such as a long-sleeved work coat and long pants.
- Use gloves, a mask, and goggles or safety glasses.
- Plan your procedure ahead of time to minimize the length of exposure.
- Run an air cleaner if one is available, and change the filters afterward.
- Take a bath or a shower immediately after you finish working with the solvent.
- Immediately wash or throw away protective clothing.
- Never store solvents inside your home.

▮ *Formaldehyde*

Formaldehyde usually represents a chronic exposure from building materials, or from cleaning supplies, disinfectants, and cosmetics. Read labels and avoid formaldehyde as much as possible. Keep in mind that all paper, which is processed with formaldehyde, can be a significant exposure.

Air cleaners containing sufficient activated charcoal will help to remove formaldehyde from the air. If you are very sensitive to formaldehyde, wear a charcoal mask while shopping, as newly manufactured products contain high levels of formaldehyde.

If you are repairing or building your home, select building supplies with care. Sealing particleboard, plywood, chipboard, and paneling can reduce high formaldehyde

> ## Treatments for Solvent Exposure
>
> *Allergy extracts for formaldehyde, phenol, and ethanol are available. They block and prevent allergic reactions to these solvents and help them to be released from the fat cells. Because of their toxicity, many other solvents cannot be diluted for extracts.*
>
> *Homeopathic preparations prepared for the specific solvent can be safely used for the more toxic solvents.*

levels. Because each coat of sealant seals only 50 percent of outgasing, six coats are required to obtain a seal of 98 percent. While sealants do significantly reduce formaldehyde levels, some sensitive people are unable to tolerate them.

❙ *Phenol*

Phenol is frequently encountered in cleaning supplies. Lysol contains phenol, as does PineSol. It is preferable to avoid using products containing phenol, but if you must use them, wear gloves and a mask.

Avoid perfumes and medications that contain phenol as a preservative.

❙ *Ethanol*

Ethanol is a common denominator in many petrochemical and hydrocarbon environmental exposures, including car exhaust, gasoline, perfumes, liquors, gas, stoves and furnaces, wood smoke, cleaning agents, and airport fumes. Avoid these exposures whenever you can.

Do not wear perfume, limit or avoid alcoholic beverages (ethanol is the alcohol in liquor), and select cleaning supplies with

care. Wear a mask to prevent reactions for exposures you cannot avoid.

❙ ASBESTOS

If your home contains any asbestos, do not undertake renovations without assistance. People working on parts of a house may accidentally dislodge asbestos particles into the air. Never try to remove asbestos; it is a job for trained professionals. Asbestos is not a problem until it begins to flake or crumble, and painting over it will usually stop the problem.

❙ RADON

If radon levels in your home are high, instigate repairs to lower the levels. Seal cracks, cover exposed earth, and improve ventilation. Many areas have professionals who specialize in radon control.

❙ PESTICIDES

Do not use pesticides in your house or on your lawn, or store them in your home. Use nontoxic pest control methods to control insects and other pests and keep your home as pest-free as possible. Integrated pest management is a holistic approach to pest control that employs a variety of methods to minimize the potential for adverse effects on health and the environment.

- Decide when the pest level is intolerable. Zero tolerance may not be necessary for every pest.
- Use physical barriers, such as screens, caulking, and structural repairs that deny pests entry into your home or to their hiding and breeding spaces.
- Inspect your house regularly to identify pests and infested areas.
- Use mechanical controls, such as traps, to catch and kill some pests.

Cockroach Control

- *Sprinkle a boric acid and sugar mixture on surfaces where roaches are likely to crawl.*
- *Make roach traps, using a jar wrapped with masking tape, and half-full of beer or a few boiled raisins. Smear a band of petroleum jelly inside the jar below the rim to prevent roaches from crawling out. Dispose of captured roaches in hot, soapy water.*

- Use products that contain sex attractants or hormones to confuse the pest, arrest its development, or interfere with breeding.
- If you use boric acid to kill insects, be sure that children and pets do not have access to it, as it can make them ill.
- If you have to use a chemical poison as a last resort, use one with low toxicity and use it cautiously. Reduce exposure to humans and pets by putting it only in cracks and crevices, or in closed traps. Treat only infested areas.

There are specific measures you can take inside your house to help control and reduce pests. Make these measures part of your daily routine.

- Keep the inside of your house clean. Vacuuming removes insects, larvae, and eggs.
- Use proper food storage methods, so that pests cannot eat your food. Use closed containers and keep them clean on the outside.
- Sweep up crumbs, clean under the stove, and keep dishes washed. Immediately wipe up crumbs and spills in the kitchen and food storage areas.
- Rinse and dry the sink to discourage insects that like water.
- Cover pet food and water overnight.
- Rinse recyclables before storing.
- Throw away cardboard boxes in which you have brought groceries home from the store. Cockroaches or other insects may be hiding in them.
- Use covered wastebaskets in your home.
- Carry out the garbage as often as possible. Make sure that garbage cans have tight-fitting lids and are cleaned regularly.
- Keep basements and storerooms neat and clean. Stack items 12 inches above the floor to discourage insects and rodents.

Silverfish Control

- *Vacuum bookshelves and books frequently.*
- *Examine secondhand books and old papers before bringing them into the house.*
- *Check lined draperies for silverfish between the lining and drapery.*
- *Make a trap for silverfish by wrapping a jar with masking tape and baiting the jar with flour. Smear a band of petroleum jelly inside the jar below the rim to prevent silverfish from crawling out.*
- *Sprinkle boric acid, flour, and sugar on a piece of paper and place it in a corner or on a window ledge.*

Make a nontoxic insecticide by mincing garlic and covering with mineral oil for 24 hours. Add 1 Tbsp. of the garlic and oil mixture to 1 pint of water and ½ tsp. of dishwashing liquid. Stir well. Mix 3 Tbsp. of this mixture with 1 pint of water and strain. Use in a spray bottle to kill household and garden pests such as cockroaches, aphids, houseflies, mosquitoes, and whiteflies.

Make an insect repellent spray by adding 1 tsp. of the garlic and mineral oil mixture to 1 pint of water with the juice of one slice of lemon. Stir well and strain into a sprayer. Spray it on your body to repel mosquitoes and flies.

Flea Control

- *Comb pets daily for fleas.*
- *Vacuum your house frequently and empty the dust from the vacuum, being careful to bag and burn it, or bake it in the sun.*
- *Have upholstery and carpets steam cleaned.*
- *Wash bed linens every two days (eggs take two days to hatch).*
- *Use brewer's yeast in pet food to help protect some animals.*
- *Wash your dog's fur with lemon infusions to repel fleas. Cut four lemons into eighths. Cover with water and bring to a boil, then simmer for 45 minutes. Cool, strain, and store in a glass container. Brush into the fur, allow to dry, and brush again.*
- *Make light and water traps by filling a shallow dish with water and detergent. For one month, place a lamp over the dish and leave the light on all night.*

Clothes Moth Control

- *Seal as many openings into the house and attic as possible.*
- *Clean closets and stored clothes regularly.*
- *Vacuum all the cracks, the backs of furniture, and under the furniture.*
- *If pollen and mold counts are not high, hang clothing outdoors to air, and brush your clothing regularly.*
- *Freezing clothing, pressing with a steam iron, dry-cleaning, and heating your clothes in an oven at 140°F will kill all stages of insect life.*
- *Store clothing carefully, sealing it in plastic bags or clean cardboard boxes.*
- *Mint, tansy, bay leaves, rosemary, lavender, cloves, spearmint, and cedar will repel moths.*

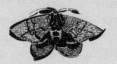

To repel common plant pests, spray with a bar soap and water solution. As an alternative method, mix two cloves of garlic and half an onion in a gallon of water and let it sit overnight. Use as a spray or to wash the leaves of the plants.

Work Environment

There are many different work environments, each with its own exposures. Because space does not permit a discussion of

493

Termite Control

- *Check that doors and windows of your house are adequately flashed.*
- *Attics and crawlspaces should be adequately ventilated and walls fitted with vapor barriers.*
- *Use silica aerogel dust in wall spaces to kill insects that crawl over it.*
- *Arrange an annual termite inspection of your home.*

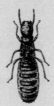

all work environments, the following section is limited to industrial and office exposures.

■■ INDUSTRY

Preventing toxic exposures in the workplace is of paramount importance. However, prevention can be difficult in an industrial setting because workers frequently have little control over their working environment, and exposures to chemicals and other toxins may be numerous.

■ CHEMICALS

The following preventive techniques are helpful to prevent chemical exposures:

- *Ventilation:* Properly placed exhaust fans, chemical hoods, and adequate air exchange will help lower levels of toxic chemicals. Local exhaust systems or hoods should be used in areas where solvents are used. Hoods remove contaminated air, ducts carry it away, and air-cleaning devices purify the air. A hood must be close to the source of contamination to be effective.

Fans also help to remove contaminated air from the room and replace it with fresh air.

- *Air quality:* Even with adequate ventilation, activated charcoal filters in an air cleaner may be necessary to remove chemicals from the air. Change the filters frequently to prevent the release of toxins from saturated filters.
- *Masks:* Charcoal masks or respirators can protect workers exposed to chemicals. In heavily contaminated areas, it may be necessary to wear a mask with an air tank. When not in use, the masks should be kept in an airtight container to prevent toxic contamination inside the mask.
- *Protective clothing:* Goggles or safety glasses, gloves, jackets, coveralls, hats, and special shoes may be necessary for protection from harmful chemicals. Although they do not offer protection from chemicals, safety helmets are necessary to protect the head on some job sites.

■ TOXIC METALS

Toxic metals are used in many manufacturing processes, as well as for other purposes in industry. To avoid toxic metal poisoning, wear protective clothing if you work in a factory or industry where there is possible exposure. This includes gloves, masks, suits, and safety glasses or goggles.

Because cadmium poisoning is difficult to treat, prevention is very important. Adequate zinc levels help to protect against cadmium poisoning. In addition, amino acids, calcium, copper, fiber, garlic, iron, manganese, sulfur, vitamin C, vitamin E, N-acetyl-l-cysteine, kelp, and foods from the cabbage family decrease cadmium absorption and retention.

Worker Safety

Every employer is required to follow strict guidelines to ensure worker safety. If your company does not provide safety clothing, or if working conditions are unsafe in other ways, you should first approach your employer. Make suggestions for correcting problems in your workplace. If your employer does not correct the problems, in the U.S. you have the option of calling the Occupational Safety and Health Administration (OSHA), or a similar government agency that works to ensure the safety of workers. In Canada, federal government employees should contact the Labour Division of Human Resources Development Canada; other workers should contact their provincial or territorial Department of Labour and ask for its occupational health and safety division.

If you feel that your workplace is not safe or that chemicals are not handled properly, you may need to change jobs temporarily if the working conditions and/or building are too toxic. Your health is your most valuable possession, and guarding it must be your first concern.

Calcium, iron, magnesium, manganese, selenium, and zinc protect against organic and inorganic mercury poisoning. Vitamin C, glutathione, and cysteine may ameliorate mercury toxicity. Garlic, which has a high sulfur content, will help chelate mercury.

Zinc (60 mg daily) and vitamin C (2,000 mg daily) have been used successfully to reduce lead levels in workers in a battery factory. Copper, iron, and thiamine also have protective effects against lead poisoning.

▮▮ OFFICE

The prevention of exposures in the office is far preferable to dealing with adverse symptoms later. The following measures can prevent or reduce office exposures:

▮ AIR QUALITY

Use an air cleaner in your immediate work area. Be certain it contains activated charcoal, which removes chemicals from the air. The air cleaner should also remove particles, such as dust, dust mites, mold, pollen, bacteria, and viruses. Change the filters regularly to prevent the release of toxins from saturated filters.

Do not allow anyone to smoke in your work area. It is best if smoking is not allowed in the building at all, or only in specially ventilated smoking rooms.

▮ CHEMICALS

Use a fan to increase ventilation and reduce chemical levels in your work area. Proper ventilation and local exhaust systems will help reduce odors from copiers and computers, as well as reduce the chemical levels in the building.

Wear a mask if there are occasional chemical exposures over which you have no control. It should contain activated charcoal to help remove chemicals. Extreme exposures may require a respirator with specialized filters.

In some settings, such as a medical

office, you may need to wear gloves, a jacket, or a workcoat to protect your skin and your clothing. Goggles or safety glasses may also be necessary.

In many offices, pesticides are applied regularly to control insects. To prevent these exposures, integrated pest management can be implemented in offices. (See Pesticides discussion earlier in this chapter. Some modifications will be necessary for the office setting.)

Use low- or nontoxic office supplies, such as white glues, low-toxicity correction fluid, and adhesives. Avoid the use of carbonless paper. Remember that paper is a formaldehyde exposure, and old paper and books can be moldy.

Educate and enlist the cooperation of coworkers who use and wear scented products or use fabric softener, to minimize or eliminate their use.

Talk to the janitorial staff about using less toxic cleaning products if those being used are not safe. You may have to investigate and suggest safer alternatives.

■ MOLD

Mold exposures in offices can exacerbate mold sensitivities in office workers. Problems with HVAC units, leaking roofs, poor ventilation, humid climates, potted plants, atriums, and other factors contribute to mold growth in an office setting. Many of the mold control measures discussed earlier in this chapter will help control and reduce mold growth in the office.

■ ELECTROMAGNETIC FIELDS

Shielding and grounding of electrical equipment and computers and computer screens

---

Sound is too loud if:

- *you must shout to be heard above the background noise.*
- *the person next to you can hear the music from your headset.*
- *you cannot hear someone speaking less than two feet away.*
- *speech is dulled or muffled after you leave a noisy area.*
- *you have pain, ringing in your ears, a feeling of fullness, or pressure in your ears after noise exposure.*

---

will reduce worker exposure to electromagnetic fields.

Noise

Noise can be a toxin in the home, at work, and during leisure activities. In order to preserve your hearing and avoid permanent hearing loss, it is essential to use prevention methods whenever possible.

Anyone who is regularly exposed to loud noise, newborns with a family history of hearing impairment, infants and toddlers with chronic ear infections, and people over 40 are considered at high risk for hearing loss. People at high risk should have their hearing checked once or twice a year. People at low risk should have their hearing tested every five years. All children should visit an audiologist before starting school.

There are three principles of hearing protection: Reduce noise at the source; interrupt the path between you and the source; and protect your ears with earplugs or headsets. To prevent hearing loss, follow these guidelines:

- Wear ear protection during noise exposure at work or at play.
- Divide noisy chores into small jobs and give your ears a rest between jobs.
- Purchase quiet products; conduct a noise level test before buying.
- Pay special attention to noise-making toys. If the toy is too loud when held at arm's length, it will be much too loud for your child.
- Never use more noise to drown out background noise, such as music from your headset to drown out transportation sounds.
- Use sound-absorbing mats under loud appliances or machinery, and install "soundproof" ceiling tiles in rooms where noisy activities take place.
- Stagger the use of household appliances so that they do not run at the same time.
- Select the location of your home carefully. Try to avoid airport flight paths, high-speed freeways, rapid transit routes, and heavy truck routes. Check with your local zoning board for possible future developments.

For a do-it-yourself hearing test, hold your hand next to your shoulder as though you are taking an oath. Rub your thumb and forefinger together. If you cannot hear a distinct rubbing sound, you may have some high-frequency-range hearing loss. Be sure to check both ears.

Electromagnetic Fields

Because electromagnetic balance can be difficult to re-establish, prevention of an im-

balance is of great importance. The following simple precautions can help to minimize problems.

- Choose a home that is over 200 yards away from transformers or high-voltage wires.
- Locate your bedroom as far away as possible from the entry of the electric current into your house.
- Keep a minimal number of electric appliances in your bedroom.
- Do not use electric blankets, heating pads, or the heater in waterbeds.
- Position the head of your bed to the north (best) or east (next best).
- Check your microwave for leakage, and stay at least four feet away when it is operating.
- If you have fluorescent light fixtures, use full-spectrum bulbs.
- Use a screening shield over your computer screen.

Art and Leisure Activities

Nearly all art supplies contain chemicals and are potentially hazardous to health. However, with careful handling and prevention measures, the harmful effects can be minimized. When you choose an art technique, study all of the materials that are needed and determine their safety and possible harmful effects. Study the Material Safety Data Sheets (MSDS) available from manufacturers of the products. These sheets detail the extent of the hazard, the name of the hazardous components, safe handling instructions, and proper first aid, as well as sources of further information about the product.

Analyze your work habits. Remember

497

that safety takes longer and do not allow yourself to take short cuts. Never skip a precaution to save time. Put on gloves and protective clothing whenever you handle potentially hazardous materials. Clean up spills immediately and never eat in your studio or work area. Wash your hands without fail at the end of a work session.

The area in which you work must have several basic features in order to assure your safety. A source of running water is essential. You will need it to clean up spills, to wash your eyes or skin if hazardous materials contact them, and to wash up after work. The electrical supply must be sufficient for any equipment you will need to use. Adequate ventilation is a must if you are working with materials that release vapors of any kind. In addition, if your work releases vapors that can affect neighbors, you may need a special vent.

Fire extinguishers, sprinkler systems, smoke detectors, a first aid kit, and a telephone are all essential safety equipment. Be sure your fire extinguisher can extinguish a fire caused by the type of materials you are using. Sprinkler systems are very important if you are working with combustible materials, and smoke detectors give early warning. Minor injuries can be treated quickly with a first aid kit, and a telephone allows you to get help or notify the proper authorities in case of an emergency.

Outdoor Environment

THE OUTDOOR ENVIRONMENT is an important part of our total environment. Like the indoor environment, it contains toxins that contribute to our total toxic load. Even though we cannot control this environment as we do our indoor environment, there are measures we can take that will help minimize its toxicity.

Air Pollution

Natural events, such as forest fires, dust storms, floods, and volcano eruptions, contribute to outdoor air pollution. Nothing can be done to prevent these phenomena. However, we do have some measure of control over many other contributors to outdoor air pollution. The prevention and reduction of outdoor air pollution is critical, but can be extremely difficult to accomplish because the entire society has to cooperate to improve air quality. The following measures will help lower and control pollution levels:

• reducing the use of fossil fuels, which are major contributors to air pollution
• controlling emissions from cars, buses, trucks, and trains so that the exhaust emitted contains low levels of pollutants
• controlling factory, industrial, and refinery emissions into both air and water
• controlling industrial and household solvent use and disposal
• controlling wood burning in homes by limiting burning days when air pollution levels are high
• controlling garbage and trash disposal and burning

When we are outdoors and pollution levels are high, wearing a mask can help reduce the contaminants we inhale, preventing respiratory and other problems. Using an air cleaner in our cars also helps reduce our intake of toxins. Both the mask and the automobile air cleaner should remove particulate matter and contain activated charcoal to remove chemicals.

Plants

Plants affect people in several ways. The pollen that many plants produce is an allergen, as are the terpenes that are present in

After Exposure to Skin Irritants

After exposure to poison oak, poison ivy, or poison sumac:

- *Wash the affected skin with rubbing alcohol to remove the oil that causes the skin reaction.*
- *Apply calamine lotion to help reduce the itch and absorb oozing from the rash.*
- *Use colloidal oatmeal mixes, or make your own by finely grinding oatmeal in a blender or food processor. Add ½ cup of the ground mixture to a tub of bath water.*
- *A charcoal poultice is useful in detoxifying poison oak or poison ivy (see chapter 30, Topical Detoxification).*

plants year-round. Many plants also contain toxic substances that are skin irritants.

■ POLLENS AND TERPENES

Just being outdoors will increase your exposure to pollens and terpenes. During pollen season, wear a mask when outdoors to help filter out pollens. Terpene-sensitive people may have to wear a mask that also contains activated charcoal.

When you go inside after being outdoors, wash your hair to remove pollen and wash out your nose with saline nose drops. BHI Allergy, a complex homeopathic preparation, will reduce or eliminate allergic symptoms. Freeze-dried stinging nettles, quercetin, and vitamin C are also helpful for preventing allergic symptoms to pollen.

Terpene-sensitive people are bothered by plants with any sort of scent, whether sweet or pungent. Even though they cannot tolerate plants or cut flowers in the house, many of these people can still enjoy flower gardens, if they plant flowers with little or no scent. Snapdragons, cosmos, pansies, nasturtiums, asters, larkspur, nierembergia, and portulaca are flowering plants with little scent. Ragweed-sensitive people may not tolerate asters. Impatiens and lobelia have no scent and appear to have no pests.

■ SKIN AND EYE IRRITANTS

Wear long sleeves and long pants when outdoors in an area where poison oak, poison ivy, or poison sumac may be growing. Wear gloves to protect your hands and do not touch your eyes. If you are extremely sensitive and there is a high probability you have touched these plants, throw away your clothing. Otherwise, wash it immediately. Keep in mind that simply touching contaminated clothing can affect your skin.

Never burn these plants, or clothing contaminated by them. Inhaling the smoke can damage the lungs of sensitive people.

Mold

Mold and mold spores abound outdoors. Many molds grow in the soil and any movement of the soil sends mold spores into the air. Raking, burning, or jumping in leaves also stirs up molds. Hay, straw, peat moss, compost, and sawdust are all sources of outdoor mold, as are stored fireplace logs.

Walking through weedy fields or vacant lots, playing under shrubbery or climbing trees, going into deep woods and caves, doing clean-up chores in the yard, and mowing the grass are also mold exposures, and should be avoided by the sensitive person.

The following measures will reduce the amount of mold in your immediate outdoor area, and will also reduce the amount of mold that enters your house:

- Keep the exterior of your home free of leaves and debris.
- Remove vines on the outside walls of the house.
- Remove shrubs resting against the walls of the house.
- Clean leaves and debris from gutters on and around the house.
- Eliminate areas of standing water, and remove obstacles that create constant shade.

Pesticides

We are exposed to pesticides outdoors because of their use on crops, on lawns, and in gardens. Avoiding exposure to pesticides is the best prevention technique, because pesticides are extremely toxic and can cause irreversible damage with high exposure. (For

Mosquito Control

- *Eliminate any areas of standing water.*
- *Be sure flat roofs drain well.*
- *Be certain door and window screens fit well and have no holes.*
- *Use bug control lights about 100 feet from the house or outdoor living area.*
- *Erect a habitat to attract blue martins or swallows, which eat large numbers of mosquitoes.*

a detailed discussion of pesticides, see chapter 16. For a discussion of pesticide control in the home, see chapter 35.)

You can control the pesticide exposure in your own home and yard, but unfortunately we have little control over what our neighbors use. Many people apply premixed pesticides and chemical fertilizers to their entire yards with a hose and nozzle. It is worthwhile to talk to your neighbors about safer alternatives. If they will not stop using chemical products, ask them to warn you before they apply pesticides or spray their yards. Arrange to be gone while the pesticides are being applied and for several days afterward.

Pesticides are more dangerous to us than are the insects they are intended to kill. Nontoxic methods of pest control can be used outdoors instead of pesticides. This does require more effort, but you can have a home and yard with very few insects. The following measures will help control insects and prevent exposures to pesticides:

- Choose plants that are insect and disease

Flea Control

- *Do not let dogs roam around the neighborhood.*
- *Do not allow stray animals on your property.*
- *Make sure the outside of your house is in good repair to keep flea-carrying rodents from entering.*
- *If the problem is severe, you can overwater or dry out the yard to kill fleas.*

Ant Control

- Cut plants away from the house.
- Do not overwater the garden.
- Seal entry holes with petro-latum, putty, or caulking.
- Destroy ant nests outdoors by pouring boiling water or hot paraffin into the nests.

resistant and well suited to the planting site.

- Prevent dampness next to the house foundation. Moisture attracts insects both inside and outside the house.
- Be sure that plants do not hug the outside walls of your house.
- A clear strip of concrete or sand against the foundation will act as a barrier for crawling insects.
- Keep your yard well groomed and clean up plant litter and dead branches.
- Use biological controls, such as bacteria, microscopic worms, and beneficial insects to control pests.
- Use traps baited with food, sex attractants, or ultraviolet light to control a variety of insects.

Approach wholesale killing of outdoor insects with caution. They are part of a complete ecosystem which must be balanced. Birds and other animals depend on insects for food, and larger animals depend on these smaller animals for their food. Control the pests on your plants and take steps to prevent them getting into your house, but do not try to make your yard or neighborhood insect-free.

If you cannot avoid pesticide use, take the following steps to minimize your exposure:

- Choose any chemical poisons you must use with care, considering the impact on children, pets, other non-target species, and natural resources.
- Wear protective clothing , including long sleeves, long pants, gloves, a mask, and goggles or safety glasses.
- Launder or throw away the clothes you wore immediately after use.
- Shower and shampoo your hair immediately after working with or being around pesticides.
- Store pesticides outside your home; it is best not to keep any pesticides on your property.
- Undertake a detoxification program to rid your body of pesticide residues if you have had a pesticide exposure of any kind. (See Chemical Problems chart in Part VIII, Detoxification Programs.)

Termite Control

- Be sure the lot drains away from the house.
- Make sure there is a foundation of concrete or concrete-filled block under all wood portions of your house.
- Clear all wood debris away from the house, particularly from the fill dirt from under the porches and steps.
- Avoid wetting stucco and wood siding.
- Fill all cracks around the house.
- Keep gutters and down-spouts in good repair.

■ GARDENING AND LAWN CARE

Carefully planning your lawn or garden can help to prevent pests and the need for pesticides. Planning can also minimize the need for chemical fertilizers. The first step is to optimize soil conditions to promote healthy plants. Soil needs a consistent supply of water and nutrients, and protection from water and wind erosion.

Mulching will insulate soil from extreme temperatures and protect it from erosion. Mulches of leaves, shredded cedar bark or other barks, wood chips, peat moss, or mushroom manure will decompose and resupply humus (brownish-black decaying plant and animal matter). Humus is the major source of nutrients for soil microorganisms and plants, and also helps keep soil from becoming too hard. Although peat moss and humus are beneficial for the soil, both represent significant mold exposures.

Regular maintenance is critical for avoiding the use of chemicals in your garden, lawn, trees, and shrubbery. Proper watering, fertilization, cutting, and pruning will help to maintain healthy plants.

Use natural fertilizers, such as compost and manure, instead of chemical fertilizers. Bonemeal or rock phosphate will add phosphorus, which is needed for strong root and bulb development, and flower and fruit set. Wood ashes will strengthen woody plant parts and enhance plant immune systems against disease. Blended, balanced organic fertilizers are available at many gardening centers.

Weeds sprout faster than grasses and will grow under conditions that are difficult for grasses. Bare patches and compacted soil

Compost for Humus

If you have the space, a compost pile is the best source for humus. It can be composed of vegetable waste from the kitchen, leaves, grass clippings, and soil. Make the compost pile by stacking 2- to 3-inch layers of the materials. Keep it damp at all times, and turn and mix it every two to three months. It takes a year to properly decay and prepare a compost pile. The process can by shortened by adding packets of naturally occurring bacteria that can be purchased at nurseries.

Adding compost each year to a garden or lawn will provide adequate nutrients for the plants so that they are vigorous, healthy, and more disease resistant. It then becomes unnecessary to use pesticides and chemical fertilizers.

favor weed growth; a healthy lawn has a thick turf that crowds out most weeds. Manually pull out weeds to reduce the need for herbicides. Proper mowing at regular intervals helps to control some weeds. Boiling or hot water can also be used to control weeds, especially in sidewalk cracks.

Corn gluten, a byproduct of the corn-milling process, is an effective weed killer for dandelions, crabgrass, and other weeds. Corn gluten is a dry powder that is applied on driveways or other areas where plant growth is not wanted. It forms a barrier to keep plants from emerging. It will also keep grass from germinating, however, and should not be used where you want to sow

Garden Wear

Wear gloves and protective clothing when you work in the yard or garden. Long pants and sleeves will prevent sunburn, scratches, and puncture wounds. Gloves will protect your hands from injury, as well as protecting them from exposure to toxic substances.

A mask will protect you from the pollen and mold spores that are released into the air when working with plants and the soil. Mowing the grass also spreads mold, dust, pollens, and grass fragments, and increases terpene content of the air. If you are terpene sensitive, your mask should protect you from both particles and chemicals.

grass. Corn-sensitive people may have difficulty using this product.

Grubs can be controlled with the bacteria *Bacillus popilliae* (milky spore disease), which will in turn control moles that feed on grubs. The *Bacillus popilliae* spores are mixed with water and used to drench the soil, killing the grubs. Some workers applying this agent can sensitize to it.

Removing diseased portions of plants or even an entire tree is preferable to spraying with a pesticide. Hydrogen peroxide can also be used to treat diseased trees. Spray the trees with one part 35 percent food-grade hydrogen peroxide to 32 parts water. Other plants grow better when sprayed with one ounce of 35 percent food-grade hydrogen peroxide diluted to a 3 percent solution per

quart of water. Spray all parts of trees and other plants.

Change your garden site every few years to prevent disease. Rotate the crops within the garden yearly to help prevent disease and depleting the soil of specific nutrients.

Plant insect-repellent plants in with your vegetables to avoid the use of chemical insecticides and fungicides. Frequent cultivation, removal of garden debris, mulching, rotated plantings, importing praying mantis and ladybugs, and planting disease-resistant varieties are a few of the natural methods of insect control that can be used. Use the natural insecticide recipe given in chapter 36 to treat plants for garden pests such as aphids and slugs.

Weather

No matter how much we might wish it, we cannot control the weather. However, we can try to plan around it, to prevent its adverse effects on us. Some severely weather-sensitive people may be given medication such as antidepressants, but many are helped by the following nontoxic preventive measures:

- *Negative-ion generators:* These help people who suffer from the effects of positive ions. Some air cleaners have negative-ion generators built into them.
- *Water:* Many people who are bothered by the positive ions generated by dry weather work in closed buildings where office machines produce high levels of positive ions. A break beside a fountain or other running water will be refreshing because running water produces negative ions.
- *Showers:* The negative ions produced by showers will help weather-sensitive people.

- *Vacations:* Weather-sensitive people should plan their vacations carefully. Waterfalls, rivers, and seashores can help minimize the effects of weather.
- *Lights:* The daily use of special high-intensity lights will help controls Seasonal Affective Disorder Syndrome (SADS). Allowing extensive light to enter windows and installing a skylight will help, as will using white paint on walls.
- *Diodes and magnets:* Wearing diodes, magnets, and tachyon beads help electromagnetically imbalanced people withstand weather changes and storms more comfortably.
- *Allergy extracts:* Extracts for serotonin and/or melatonin will help people who suffer from SADS or exposure to positive ions.
- *Natural fibers:* Some weather-sensitive people are bothered by synthetic fibers. Wearing natural fibers helps these individuals.

Altitude

Mountain climbers are at risk for altitude sickness, but simply traveling to altitudes higher than those at which you normally live can also cause problems. Several techniques can be used to prevent problems with altitude.

- *Climb slowly:* Physicians advise one day of acclimatization for each 2,000 feet you ascend.
- *Pace your activities:* When you arrive at a high altitude, allow yourself one day to rest before beginning strenuous activities.
- *Reduce your salt intake and drink more water:* This will help reduce edema (swelling).
- *Eat more carbohydrates:* Carbohydrates

make it easier to obtain more oxygen from your metabolism at higher altitudes.
- *Avoid sleeping pills and alcoholic beverages:* They can affect breathing and impair the ability to acclimate.
- *Sleep at lower altitudes if possible:* The altitude at which you sleep determines the severity of altitude sickness.

If you develop severe altitude sickness symptoms, descend to a lower altitude as soon as possible.

The snow and ice often encountered at high altitudes, as well as at lower altitudes in winter, can cause snow blindness. Wearing sunglasses or protective goggles is a necessity for preventing snow blindness. Should you forget your protective eyewear, you can cut makeshift goggles from cardboard. Punch small holes or slits where the lenses should be. Fasten these "goggles" to your head with rubber bands or a cord.

Radiation

The prevention of sunburn is very important to skin health. When you cannot avoid exposure to the sun, use clothing and hats or a tolerated sunscreen to protect against ultraviolet radiation. Remember that you can sunburn even on cloudy days.

Exposure to sunlight is essential for health. Sunlight can decrease high cholesterol, high blood pressure, and blood sugar levels. It can help to build immunity to infectious diseases and provide vitamin D. However, many people sunbathe to develop a tan. Most physicians no longer advise tanning because of the possibility of skin damage and problems this can cause later in life. If you sunbathe, exert extreme caution so that

Sunburn Treatments

If you do get a sunburn, aloe vera gel and Calendula *gel or ointment are very soothing and healing.*

you do not sunburn. Generally speaking, dark-skinned people can tolerate more sun than light-skinned people can. Red-headed and blond people should be extremely cautious.

To sunbathe for health reasons, begin by sunbathing for two minutes on each area—front, back, and sides. Gradually increase the time by one minute each day. *Never allow yourself to sunburn.* As soon as your skin feels uncomfortably hot, you are burning. Don't wait until your skin turns pink to get out of the sun. When you sunbathe again, if your skin feels hot again, decrease the time of exposure.

Beware of reflecting surfaces when you are exposed to the sun. Snow reflects 85 percent of the ultraviolet light, dry sand 17 percent, and grass and water around 3 to 5 per-

cent. Snow or sand can cause you to sunburn very rapidly. In addition, wet skin sunburns more easily than dry skin.

Clean skin is best for sunbathing. Fats and oils, such as those in suntan creams, oils, and lotions, can stimulate the formation of cancer cells when applied to the skin. Sunscreening agents also filter out many of the therapeutic and healing effects of sunlight. Para-aminobenzoic acid (PABA), which is in many of these products, can cause genetic damage to DNA when exposed to sunlight. Many sensitive people are allergic to PABA.

Electromagnetic Imbalance

Several measures help prevent developing an electromagnetic imbalance when you are traveling or outdoors:

• Go barefoot as much as possible. Standing on damp grass or in running water can relieve many symptoms of imbalance.
• Lie in the grass when weather permits.
• When traveling, get out of the car periodically and walk to re-establish ground contact.

CHAPTER 3 8

Medical Treatment

SOMETIMES MEDICAL treatment is necessary, no matter how careful we have been with our health and lifestyle. When your health problems necessitate treatment, you should first investigate all available possibilities. For example, excellent homeopathic remedies are available for many different health problems. Herbs may provide an effective treatment possibility for some people. Nutrients can prevent and treat many different health concerns. While results are sometimes slower from alternative treatments, they can be as effective as standard treatments.

If you need to have standard medical treatment, there are prevention methods and techniques that will minimize or eliminate toxic effects from these treatments. These methods will require preparation on your part. Chapter 11, Toxins from Medical Treatment, describes the toxins that can be encountered during various medical procedures. The information provided in this chapter will enable you to approach your treatments as an informed medical consumer, and to prevent many problems.

Surgery

Regardless of the medical condition and the reason for the surgery, you will encounter toxins both in the hospital and the operating room. If properly approached, exposures to these toxins can be minimized and the toxic after-effects of the surgery and medications can be cleansed.

∎ HOSPITAL ARRANGEMENTS

Many preparations and requests can be made before surgery to lower your toxic exposures. Although most U.S. hospitals are nonsmoking, many allow patients to smoke in their rooms and have special smoking areas for patients and visitors. If at all possible, insist on a "no-smoking" private room. If you must share a room, insist that your roommates be nonsmokers. In Canada, smoking is only permitted in outdoor areas of hospitals.

If you have allergies to flowers, plants, or molds, talk to the nurses on the floor where your room will be. They can ensure that live plants will not be placed in your room. You can request that no scented products be used in your room by the hospital or your room-mates. Extremely sensitive people may need to request that nurses and aides not wear perfumes, scented hand lotion, scented de-odorant, or scented hair spray.

If cleaning supplies are a problem for you, schedule a talk with the hospital's housekeeping department. Request that they do not use bleach, disinfectants, deter-gents, soaps, or room deodorizers in your room while you are in the hospital. Ask that hot water and baking soda be used instead. If they are willing, you could provide a cleaner that is safe for you.

An air cleaner is helpful in maintaining the purity of the air in a hospital room. If you want to use an air cleaner, ask whether it needs to be inspected by anyone before you use it. Some hospitals require that the plug and wiring of any electrical appliance used in a hospital room be inspected first. Also, if you want to use your own bedding, you must discuss it with the housekeeping and laun-dry staff.

Talk to the hospital dietitian and discuss any food allergies or dietary requirements that you may have. Do not cause confusion by giving too many restrictions; just list the most important problems. You may request that whole, unprocessed foods be served, and ask that your snacks be fresh tolerated fruits. Inspect each meal to be sure it does not contain foods you must avoid.

Discuss any medical problems you have, such as asthma, diabetes, and allergies, with your physicians. Find out what medications and anesthetic they plan to use. If testing is available to you, have these substances tested before your surgery to determine which ones are safe for you and to find safe alternatives. If you are latex sensitive, re-quest that the surgical team wear non-latex gloves.

Discuss any medications you are taking, including allergy extracts. You will be unable to take these substances while you are in the hospital unless the physician puts a specific order in your chart. Ask the physician to write this order and have him or her also in-clude any vitamin and mineral supplements you might need. You may want to request that oxygen be available to you in your hospi-tal room, along with an order in your chart that you may use it when you feel it neces-sary. Oxygen helps to clear allergic reactions, as well as to cleanse your body of toxins.

Your admitting physician or an environ-mental physician can assist if you experi-ence difficulty having your requests met.

▮▮ PREPARING FOR SURGERY

For several weeks before your surgery, avoid all substances to which you are allergic, as well as toxic exposures. You want to be as strong as possible when you enter the hospi-tal. Increase your intake of vitamin C to bowel tolerance level. It will strengthen your immune system, promote healing, and lessen pain. However, do not take it the night before surgery, as vitamin C can lessen the effects of anesthesia. Resume taking it after surgery as soon as approved by your physi-cian. (See chapter 23, Nutrients, for a discus-sion of vitamin C).

Researchers from the University of Chicago have found that alkaloids in mem-bers of the nightshade family, including po-tatoes, tomatoes, peppers, and eggplants,

Support After Surgery

If possible, arrange for family or friends to sit with you during the first two days and nights after your surgery. Their support is important, and they can watch for and prevent exposures while you are unable to be vigilant. Be certain they are aware of all the foods and substances you need to avoid.

can inhibit the metabolism of anesthetics and muscle relaxants used during surgery. This can cause drug reactions, as well as prolonged adverse reactions. Avoid these foods for at least a week before surgery and a full month if possible, as these foods contain long-lasting compounds.

Stop taking vitamin E two days before the surgery and do not take it for five to six days afterward. High amounts of vitamin E could potentially contribute to excessive bleeding during and after surgery.

Stop taking herbs 10 to 14 days before surgery, as some herbal remedies can affect the way your body reacts during surgery. St. John's wort can magnify the effects of some anesthetic drugs. Korean, American, and Chinese ginseng, but not Siberian ginseng, can raise blood pressure and heart rate, putting you at increased risk for a heart attack. Ginkgo biloba and feverfew can interfere with the blood-clotting process, causing you to bleed more.

Take coenzyme Q_{10} and organic germanium up to the day of the surgery, and continuing after surgery. Both these supplements act as buffers against the effects of

hypoxia (oxygen deficiency) during surgery. They also combat the free radicals released by damaged tissue.

■ RECOVERING FROM SURGERY

After surgery, move around as soon as your surgeon gives you permission. This will prevent fluid from collecting in your lungs, which can cause such complications as pneumonia. Muscles, nerves, bones, and body functions can suffer even after short periods of inactivity. Begin by walking slowly, and increase the speed and length of your walks as your strength permits. Most hospital halls have rails along the walls. You can hold on to these if necessary while you take your strolls.

Be careful of your diet after surgery. Avoid empty-calorie foods, and eat quality food, concentrating on fresh fruits and vegetables, as well as meats and fish, if you normally eat them. Eat several small meals throughout the day, rather than eating a lot at one sitting. Your digestive organs require large amounts of energy to digest large meals, and your energy needs to be available for healing your body.

Allow yourself to rest. Our bodies heal while we rest and sleep. Do not push yourself to recover too quickly. Everyone has his or her own speed of recovery. Give your body and your immune system the time needed to recover from the stress and exposures of surgery.

Radiology

While diagnostic tests and treatments involving radiation are sometimes necessary, cleansing afterward is very important for the

Nutrition After Radiation

Nutritional therapy is helpful in preventing problems from radiation treatment, as well as in cleansing the body after radiation therapy. It also helps to repair tissues. Antioxidant vitamins are particularly important because they combat the free radicals released by damaged tissue.

Take the following nutrients both before and after radiation therapy:
- *vitamin A*
- *vitamin B5*
- *vitamin B15*
- *vitamin C*
- *vitamin E*
- *selenium*
- *cysteine*
- *glutathione*
- *methionine*
- *coenzyme Q10*
- *organic germanium*
- *N-acetyl cysteine (NAC)*

(See chapter 23, Nutrients, for further information and recommended doses.)

Avoid unnecessary X-rays, but be aware that comparing older X-rays to recent views can be of diagnostic help.

Before you have X-rays or radiation treatments:
- Pick the best facility and find out when the equipment was last inspected. All states and provinces require periodic inspection and certificates of compliance are issued.
- Ask about the light-box equipment used to read the X-ray. The new SmartLight increases light intensity for viewing films and allows radiologists to see smaller abnormalities, increasing rates of early detection.
- Be certain that the technician taking your X-ray is a registered technologist, or R.T.
- Be certain that the radiologist reading your X-ray is board certified. Some emergency rooms do not have a radiologist on duty and most doctors are not as skilled at reading X-rays as a radiologist. Ask that your X-ray be read by a radiologist as soon as one is available.
- Follow instructions exactly and stay as still

body. There are measures that help prevent radiation damage, as well as measures that help remove the harmful effects of radiation exposure.

To prevent damage to the immune system during diagnostic X-rays to the head and neck, be certain that the technician covers your thymus with a lead shield. The thymus, which is behind the breastbone, is an important part of the immune system. If the technician does not provide the lead shield, consider not having the X-ray until the proper shield is provided.

Be certain that any X-ray proposed for you is vital to the success of your treatment.

Herbs for Radiation

The following herbs help to protect against radiation damage. They should be taken after treatment.
- *algin*
- *echinacea*
- *celery seed*
- *fennel*
- *chaparral*
- *ginseng*

Homeopathic remedies that can help with specific side effects are listed in chapter 28, Homeopathy and Bach Flower Remedies.

as possible. Remove any jewelry and avoid makeup containing metallic glitter.
- Make sure the radiologist has your latest X-ray, and if possible, any previous X-rays taken for the same problem. Comparing X-rays to identify changes can be critical.
- Be sure the radiologist is aware of your physical problems, to assist in interpreting the X-ray.
- If there are any doubts about the interpretation, have a second radiologist read the X-ray.

Chemotherapy

Before having chemotherapy treatment, it is wise to investigate the less toxic chemotherapy agents of alternative medicine. One of these agents might be more effective and less damaging than the standard chemo-

Counteracting Chemo Side Effects

If you must have chemotherapy, nutritional supplements are important to help prevent its side effects. The antioxidant nutrients in particular help combat the free radicals released by damaged tissue. Take the following nutrients before and after chemotherapy:
- *vitamin A*
- *vitamin B1*
- *vitamin C*
- *coenzyme Q10*
- *organic germanium*
- *beta-carotene*
- *vitamin E*
- *selenium*
- *N-acetyl cysteine*

See chapter 23 for further information and recommended doses.

Preventing Cancer

Preventing cancer is the best defense, and early detection is the next best defense. Lifestyle changes may be necessary to decrease your risk of developing cancer. For example, a diet high in fiber and cruciferous vegetables exerts a protective effect, as does eating garlic, tomatoes, soy, grapes, citrus fruits, licorice root, green tea, and hot peppers. Decreasing your intake of fats; meats; carcinogenic chemicals in foods, including additives, colors, flavorings, and preservatives; smoked foods; and coffee and black tea can decrease the risk of cancer.

People should not smoke and should also avoid secondhand smoke. Stress reduction, avoidance of toxins in both the home and workplace, and reduction of exposure to electromagnetic fields can also help prevent cancer.

therapeutic agents. There are also other alternative cancer treatments that may be helpful. (For a full description of alternative cancer treatments, see Recommended Books, *Finding the Right Treatment*.)

If you have chemotherapy treatments, coffee enemas can help prevent or reduce side effects. (See chapter 31, Organ Cleansing, for directions.) Homeopathic remedies that can help with specific side effects are listed in chapter 28, Homeopathy and Bach Flower Remedies. The herbs astragalus and fennel will help to protect the immune system and increase stamina.

Using and Storing Medicines Safely

- *Do not take or give a medication when you are not alert or cannot see clearly.*
- *Keep all medicine out of the reach of children.*
- *Do not store medication near a dangerous substance that could be taken by mistake.*
- *Store medication in its original container, which identifies it and gives dosage information.*
- *Discard any outdated medication.*

Medications

People who live a healthy lifestyle usually have few illnesses and rarely need to take medications. With proper diet, exercise, and sufficient rest, many health problems can be prevented.

When you do have to take a medication, be certain that your physician knows of any other medications you may be taking before writing your prescription. In addition, be certain to mention any nonprescription drugs, nutritional supplements, or other products that you take.

Ask your physician about possible side effects of the medication. As a further precaution, ask the pharmacist filling your prescription about possible interactions with any other prescription or nonprescription products you may be taking, as well as about the new medication's possible side effects. Homeopathic remedies that can help with

specific side effects are listed in chapter 28, Homeopathy and Bach Flower Remedies.

Be certain that you fully understand why you are taking the medication, and what its treatment benefits will be. Also ensure that you understand the correct dose, the directions for taking it, and what to do should you inadvertently miss a dose. Be certain that you have no conditions that preclude your taking the medication. Sensitive people will also need to know the types of binders, fillers, and excipients used in the manufacture of the drug.

It is important to take the prescription according to the directions, and for the prescribed number of days. Stopping too soon may cause a relapse.

Vaccinations

Making the decision of whether or not to vaccinate their child can be a very difficult one for parents. If you decide to have your child vaccinated, preventive measures can minimize the side effects, which can include soreness and redness at the injection site, fever, irritability, seizures, limp episodes, and persistent crying. An allergy extract or a homeopathic remedy specific to the vaccination can often prevent problems and side effects. Give the remedy or extract for one week before and for two weeks after the vaccination. Homeopathic remedies for side effects of vaccination are listed in chapter 28, Homeopathy and Bach Flower Remedies.

Nutritional preparation for immunizations can also help prevent side effects. In the 1960s to 1980s, Dr. Lendon Smith, a pediatrician from Portland, Oregon, gave 100 mg of vitamin C, 500 mg of calcium, and 50 mg of vitamin B$_6$ the day before, the day of, and the day after vaccinations. He found that this regimen eliminated the problems that often accompany vaccinations, even the DTP (diphtheria, tetanus, and pertussis) vaccine.

Dental Work

Prevention plays a double role in dental work. It is probably the most important measure to avoid dental problems and the toxic exposures that some types of dental work involve. Brushing and flossing after each meal and at bedtime are musts. Prevention techniques can also prevent problems from occurring when you must have dental work done.

For homeopathic remedies to help with dental problems or side effects from dental work, see chapter 28, Homeopathy and Bach Flower Remedies. For gum pain and periodontal disease, aloe vera, which has antibiotic properties, can be applied topically. Anti-inflammatory herbs that can be taken orally include chamomile, echinacea, goldenseal, myrrh, and rose hips. Cloves, hops, and myrrh can all be used topically to relieve a toothache.

Begin by carefully investigating the ingredients of your toothpaste. Most commercial toothpastes contain glycerine and corn syrup or saccharine. These substances cause problems for some sensitive individuals. Acceptable substitute toothpastes are available at health food stores. Baking soda also makes a good substitute for commercial toothpaste. Sodium lauryl sulfate, contained in most toothpastes, causes canker sores for

Nutrition for Healthy Teeth

Proper nutrition will not only contribute to your general health, but will also aid in maintaining good tooth and gum quality, lessening the need for extensive dental work. Calcium and magnesium contribute to healthy tooth enamel and strong root and bone structure. Vitamin C, organic germanium, and coenzyme Q$_{10}$ are important both in restoring and maintaining gum integrity. However, do not take vitamin C for 24 hours before a dental appointment, as it can reduce the effectiveness of dental anesthetics.

some people and may not be listed on the toothpaste label.

A capful of a 3 percent dilution of 35 percent food-grade hydrogen peroxide mixed with several pinches of baking soda and a little water makes a safe mouthwash. Vitamin C (ascorbic acid) dissolved in water also makes a good mouthwash. Always rinse thoroughly with water after using any mouthwash, but particularly vitamin C, to avoid damage to tooth enamel.

All dentists and dental hygienists normally wear latex gloves. For latex-sensitive people, gloves made of vinyl should be used. Make arrangements several weeks before your appointment for the dentist and hygienist to wear vinyl gloves while working on your teeth.

You may request a substitute polish of plain pumice and water when having your teeth cleaned. This will allow you to avoid the colorings and flavorings in standard polishes.

Avoid having study models made if possible. There are no problem-free alternatives for the impression materials. Minimizing your exposures to these compounds is the only way of reducing this toxic exposure.

The dentist may choose from numerous dental materials for all dental procedures. If testing is available to you, have these materials and local anesthetics tested to determine those you tolerate best. Being certain that you tolerate the materials being used for your dental procedures can prevent many complications and symptoms afterward.

■■ AMALGAM REMOVAL

For many people, having amalgam fillings removed is a positive step toward improving their health. Some people feel better as each amalgam is removed and replaced with a compatible filling material. Others feel better with time, as their bodies detoxify the mercury. Some people experience little or no improvement.

Charges, both positive and negative,

Alternatives to Anesthetics

Hypnosis and acupuncture can be effective alternatives to local anesthetic. Acupuncture anesthesia is generally accomplished by placing one needle in the foot, two needles in each hand, two in each ear, and two or three in one cheek. The needles are inserted just below the surface of the skin, and you should feel little or no sensation upon insertion. This should be done 15 to 20 minutes before your dental appointment.

Hypnosis requires a few practice trials with a hypnotist. The hypnotist will work with you 15 to 20 minutes before your dental appointment so that you will be prepared before dental procedures are begun.

X-Ray Cautions

Do not allow any more X-rays to be taken than are absolutely necessary. Be certain that a lead apron is placed over your vital organs, particularly the thymus, which is under the breastbone. If the vinyl-wrapped X-ray film is a problem for you, request paper-wrapped film.

---

build up on amalgam fillings. Dentists can measure these charges with a special instrument. It is important that amalgams be removed in the proper order, depending on the charges and their magnitude. Those with a higher charge, whether positive or negative, should be removed first. The use of a rubber dam and oxygen during the removal phase will greatly reduce inhalation of mercury vapors.

It may take several months, or even a year, for the body to detoxify after amalgams have been removed and replaced. Nutrients, including B vitamins, vitamin C, magnesium, selenium, zinc, cysteine, glutathione, methionine, and MSM, are helpful in reducing the effects of the mercury that is released when these fillings are removed.

CHAPTER 39

Children

Just as children have special responses to toxins because of physiological differences caused by their age and size, they also have special prevention needs for some toxins. For others, the same prevention methods can be used for both adults and children. It is important that special precautions are taken for children. Their health throughout life will be better if they never become toxic and have to undergo cleansing.

Parents will have to organize prevention methods for their children. Even if the children are not willing, it is important for parents to be firm. Peer pressure can cause children to balk at a healthier lifestyle. However, some children are able to relate improved health to the measures taken to prevent problems and are more cooperative. Over time, children will incorporate healthier choices as they become old enough to assume more responsibility for their health.

In addition to taking care of their child's health, it is critical for parents to take care of their own health. Many parents cannot adequately take care of their children because of their own poor health. We have seen many children who have not received adequate care for their health problems, some of them serious and acute, because their parents were too ill themselves to organize a health program for their children.

Food

Because they are growing and developing, diet is of extreme importance for children. Diet tips for detoxification and improvement of health should be followed by children as well as adults. (See diet tips in chapter 23.)

Children learn their eating habits from adults. If adults eat in a healthy manner, their children are likely to do so. Do not feed children "junk" food or nutritionally empty fast food. Insist that your child eat a variety of foods, which help to prevent and control food allergies.

Minimize or eliminate your child's sugar intake. Many of the foods children like and tend to eat, including fruits, contain hidden

Addictive Sugar

Sugar is an extremely addictive substance. Controlling a child's sugar intake will help to prevent the development of a sugar addiction, which is very difficult to break. One of our adult patients was injured in a car accident and became addicted to morphine because of the many shots she required to control her severe pain. She confessed to us that she was able to give up the morphine shots more easily than she was able to give up sugar.

sugars. Limit juice to 4 ounces a day and offer water instead.

Do not allow your child to eat foods containing artificial sweeteners. Many children consume large amounts of aspartame. With the large numbers of food that contain this artificial sweetener, the total can add up very quickly. Studies have shown that neurological responses in children who have consumed aspartame can be slowed to the point that their ability to hit a baseball is impaired. Thousands of side effects have been documented after aspartame has been ingested.

The safe selection, storage, and preparation of quality food is discussed in chapter 35. Organic food is the best way to ensure that a child consumes nutritious food and does not receive excessive pesticide residues, particularly on produce. A number of non-organic fruits and vegetables contain pesticide residues high enough to be harmful to children, who are more vulnerable because of their small size. However, organic food is not always available. Organic gardening is recommended, both as a fun hobby for the child and for the health of the harvest.

As added protection for children and adults, wash fruits and vegetables thoroughly to remove as much pesticide residue as possible. Wash fruits such as peaches, apples, and pears, then peel them before giving them to your child.

Mothers who are breast-feeding their babies should closely observe the behavior and appearance of the baby after feeding. Fussy, colicky babies with a rash or eczema are almost always reacting to food antigens in the breast milk. The diet of the mother is the source of the food antigens. To prevent the allergic reactions of the baby, the mother must avoid the problem foods, or the baby will have to be treated with food extracts or hands-on allergy treatments.

Water

Children should use safe water for drinking and bathing at all times. (Chapter 14 describes toxins in waters and chapter 35 discusses prevention techniques.) In some areas, dissolved metals and minerals in water can make it unfit to drink. Children can also receive a lead exposure from water that runs through older plumbing. Run the water for a few minutes in the morning to decrease the concentration of lead from plumbing solder. Run water from drinking fountains for a few minutes before allowing children to drink. In some regions, particularly in mining areas, dissolved minerals in the water may make it unsafe. Filtering the water can help remove metals and minerals, but if the levels are very high it may still be unsafe.

In areas with unsafe water, or on trips to other countries, children can use bottled water. Do not give them ice cubes or let them brush their teeth with tap water.

Be certain that your child drinks enough water. As discussed in earlier chapters, most children prefer other beverages to water, and if the weather is hot, children can become dehydrated easily. In addition, normal detoxification processes will not take place without sufficient water. Parents should give as much fluid as possible during hot weather. If the child becomes ill and cannot or will not drink fluids, rehydrating intravenous treatment may be necessary.

Swimming is a favorite summertime activity for most children. Swimming pools can contain many toxins, including water purification agents, urine from swimmers who relieve themselves in the pool, laundry and personal care products from the bathing suits and bodies of other swimmers, as well as algae, mold, and other organisms. Be certain your child showers and washes thoroughly after leaving the swimming pool to remove toxins that may remain on the skin. If the swimming pool water dries on the child's skin, many of the toxins will be absorbed. Also caution your child never to drink swimming pool water. Although swimming is supposed to be a safe sport for asthmatics, many children develop asthma after they begin a swimming program, possibly because of exposure to various toxins in the pool water.

Many children swim in natural bodies of water, such as lakes or rivers. This water may be polluted and can cause problems for children. Algae, *Giardia lamblia* and other or-

---

Washing Water Bottles

Many children and adults drink water from the containers in which bottled water is purchased, refilling them time after time from their water faucets at home. To prevent health problems, these bottles should be thoroughly rinsed before refilling, and cleaned with soap and water several times a week.

---

ganisms, and dissolved chemicals such as solvents and pesticides may be present. There may also be domestic sewage, animal excrement, plant residues, agricultural runoff, detergents, and industrial waste in these waters. Do not allow your child to swim in natural bodies of water until you investigate their safety.

Air

Good air quality is very important in preventing respiratory problems in children. Parents have control over air quality in the home and should ensure that it is as safe as they can make it.

There should be no smoking allowed in the home by anyone, whether parents, children, relatives, or visitors. Children from smoking households have more respiratory and behavioral problems. Many patients who have asthma as adults remember their problems beginning as children in a smoking household.

Dust is an important allergen and can trigger asthma in children. To decrease dust and chemical allergens in a bedroom, do not use carpets. Hang washable curtains, and keep clothes in closets with the doors shut. For very sensitive or sick children, remove dust catchers, such as pictures and books, from the bedroom. Stuffed animals should be washable in order to control dust accumulation. Dust the bedroom every day and damp mop the floor frequently.

Run an air cleaner to remove particulate matter from the bedroom.

Cover the mattresses and pillows with barrier cloth for children who have severe dust mite sensitivities. Keep your whole home vacuumed well and insect free. In addition to dust mites, cockroaches and cockroach parts can trigger asthma in a child.

Never allow pets to sleep in the bedroom or with your child. Also, do not keep a pet of any kind in the bedroom.

Plants

Plants can cause problems for children, and many of them sensitize to pollen and terpenes at a very early age. Allergy extracts or hands-on allergy treatments for pollens and terpenes will prevent and control these allergic reactions. They will also allow a cleansing action that will rid the body of any residue. An air cleaner in the bedroom, which will give the sleeping child at least eight hours in a pollen- and terpene-free environment, will also help lower the allergic load and prevent allergic reactions.

Plants pose another problem for children, who sometimes eat them. In North America, household plants are one of the leading causes of accidental poisoning for children under five years of age. It is also a problem for pets, as cats and dogs also tend to eat plants.

To prevent poisonings, if you have children or pets, do not have any of the following plants in your home or yard. They can cause symptoms from a stomachache or skin rash, to death, if enough is ingested.

- azalea
- castor bean
- foxglove
- holly berries
- jimson weed
- lantana
- larkspur
- mayapple
- mistletoe
- oleander
- philodendron
- poinsettia
- poison hemlock
- pokeweed
- rhododendron
- rhubarb leaves
- water hemlock
- dieffenbachia (dumb cane)
- plants of the nightshade family

To prevent plant poisoning:
- keep all plants, bulbs, and seeds out of the reach of young children.
- teach children never to eat anything that is not served to them unless you give permission.
- teach children never to put mushrooms, berries, or any part of a plant in their mouths or feed them to a pet.
- supervise your children's activities, particularly outdoors.
- remove any mushrooms from your yard and dispose of them. Check the yard after each rain.
- know the names and characteristics of all your plants, both indoors and outdoors.
- do not assume that a plant is not poisonous for your child, even if pets, birds, or other wildlife eat it.
- do not assume that cooking will destroy toxic chemicals in plants.

Syrup of Ipecac for Poisoning

Keep syrup of ipecac in your medicine cabinet. It is a nonprescription medication that can be purchased at any pharmacy. Ipecac safely induces vomiting, but should never be given unless your poison control center or physician recommends it. In many cases, a charcoal slurry is more effective than ipecac.

Poison centers operate 24 hours a day and provide immediate advice on treating all types of toxic exposures, as well as poison prevention.

Organisms

Children have very high exposures to many types of organisms in daycare centers and schools. Teaching children to wash their hands thoroughly after they use the toilet and before they eat a meal or a snack can prevent many infections.

Young children also tend to put their dirty hands and objects in their mouths. Teaching them not to put objects in their mouths and to wash their hands whenever they get dirty will help prevent the spread of organisms.

Teach your child to cover his or her mouth while sneezing or coughing, and to wash the hands afterward. Handwashing should also follow nose-blowing and proper disposal of the tissue. Because it can be difficult to have children wash their hands often enough, some people suggest the child sneeze into his or her elbow, to block the sneeze and keep the hands clean.

Do not share your food with your child if you are ill. Likewise, finishing your child's uneaten food can give his or her infection to you.

Chemicals and Metals

Children are particularly vulnerable to chemical exposures in the environment, but there are many prevention methods that will help.

Parents can decrease their use of gas and wood stoves and fireplaces, and strictly control wood-burning in their homes.

Always keep solvents out of the reach of children, and never place them in a familiar container, such as a soft drink bottle. If a child swallows a solvent, do not induce vomiting because of the risk of aspirating it into the lungs. Call your physician or local poison control center for advice.

Parents can use safe cleaning supplies and avoid using air fresheners, solvents, and pesticides. There are air cleaners available that will help to remove chemicals, odors, pollens, dust, mold, bacteria, and viruses from the air. However, the air cleaner must have a sufficiently thick activated charcoal filter to remove chemicals and odors. Be sure to change the filter often.

Safe laundry products will prevent children from absorbing toxins in their clothes through their skin. Remember that liquid and sheet fabric softeners are particularly toxic. Never allow a child to wear a new garment that has not been washed, as clothing is usually treated with a chemical finish, which may include formaldehyde.

Do not let your children play on any lawn that has been freshly treated with lawn chemicals, fertilizer, or weed killer. Children

Protecting Newborns

Be very careful to prevent chemical exposures for newborn infants. Do not paint or lay carpet in a nursery just before a baby is due. Children are extremely susceptible to the toxins given off by paint and carpet. If you must prepare a nursery and the condition of the room is such that you must improve it, make the changes well ahead of your due date, and use low VOC paint. Special nontoxic carpet is now available, or use tile or safe wood flooring with cotton area rugs. These precautions also apply to an older child's room. Because of the many hours babies and children spend in their rooms, exposures to any chemicals in their rooms can be sizable.

tend to roll around on the grass and can receive a large dose of such toxins. Should your child play on a lawn that has just been treated, have the child take a shower, including shampoo, and a detox bath, followed by another shower. Launder the clothes your child was wearing.

Many yards and playgrounds close to busy streets are contaminated with lead that came from vehicular exhaust during the years when lead was allowed in gasoline. If there is any other place for your children to play, do not let them play in such areas. Because children are more sensitive to lead than are adults, it is particularly important to protect them from lead exposure.

Children may receive a mercury exposure when they play with the mercury from a broken thermometer or blood pressure apparatus. Unfortunately, playing with mercury is fun, making it vital to teach your children about the dangers of mercury. It is the only metal that is a liquid at room temperature, and there are other dangers associated with mercury in addition to touching it. It is very volatile and can evaporate into the air if left in an open container. It is safest not to keep any mercury in your house, but if you do, be certain your children cannot find it.

Noise

Select toys with care to prevent damage to your child's hearing. Toys that are too loud for adults can damage the hearing of children. Monitor the volume on TV sets, video games, stereos, and Walkmans. If the volume is too loud, insist that they turn it down.

Premature newborns, newborns with exposure to drugs that are potentially toxic to the ears, and children who have contracted meningitis (an infection of the covering of the brain and spinal cord) should have their hearing tested. Most hospitals now check the hearing of all newborns before sending them home.

Weather

Children are particularly susceptible to temperature extremes. Do not allow your child to play outside in the cold without a coat and hat. Thirty to forty percent of body heat is lost through the head. They should also wear mittens or gloves to prevent frostbite to their hands.

If they play during cold weather in jeans

that get wet, they are in danger of hypothermia. The cotton in the jeans does not dry or wick away moisture, and the child becomes cold very quickly. Wool pants or those made of synthetic fabric are better.

Some children like to play outdoors in a thunderstorm. Not only is there a danger of being struck by lightning, but at high altitudes temperatures can quickly drop and the child can become too cold.

Children can become overheated in hot weather very easily. Keep them indoors during the middle of the day when it is hottest, to prevent the danger of sunstroke. Do not let them sunburn, and be certain they drink enough liquids, especially water.

Radiation and Electromagnetic Fields

Infants and children should not sunbathe. Sunscreens are not recommended until infants are at least six months of age. Even then, it is better to use lightweight cotton clothes and a wide-brimmed hat as protection, because some children are sensitive to sunscreens. Blistering sunburns in childhood are associated with melanoma (a skin cancer) in adults.

Be very careful of your child's exposure to electromagnetic fields. Many children tend to sit too close to television sets. Be certain that your child sits at least four feet away from the set.

Do not allow your child to sleep on a waterbed or under an electric blanket, and there should be a limited number of electrical appliances in the bedroom. The best position for the bed is with the headboard facing north, or east as the next best option.

School Exposures

The following measures are useful to protect your child from toxic exposures at school. Even though these prevention methods are discussed in terms of children, they are also helpful for adults who are attending school.

If your child is sensitive, it is a good idea to supply the classroom with an air cleaner. Make sure that it is checked and the filters changed regularly.

If you have a choice of schools, do not allow your child to attend school in a new building. If there is no alternative, supply the classroom with several spider plants, which effectively remove formaldehyde from the air. Boston ferns, gerbera daisies, dwarf date palms, and bamboo palms also remove formaldehyde. An air cleaner that removes chemicals placed near your child's desk will help your child, as well as the other children in the room. Allergy extracts for chemicals can help sensitive children to better tolerate a toxic classroom.

- *Portable buildings*: If possible, do not allow your child to attend classes in a portable. If you have no choice, plants and an air cleaner are helpful. In addition to chemical extracts, your child may need a mold extract if the portable building contains mold.
- *Animals*: An allergy extract for animal dander will help protect your child. If the child is significantly affected, request that the animal be removed from the classroom.
- *Chemical exposures*: Avoiding chemicals in science and art classes is difficult. Adequate ventilation helps, as do air cleaners. Activated charcoal masks will reduce the level of chemicals breathed. Sometimes it

may be necessary to arrange alternate projects for your child instead of the more toxic lab or art projects.

- *Carpets*: If your child's school has carpets, find out how often they are cleaned. Keep your child home until cleaned carpets are thoroughly dry.
- *Paint*: Ask to be notified when the school is going to paint. If you have a sensitive child, keep him or her home on those days.
- *Asphalt and tar*: Keep your child home when these substances are being applied.
- *Pesticides*: Inquire about the pesticide spraying schedule both indoors and outdoors, and keep your child home on the days that pesticide is being applied. If lawn chemicals are applied to the playground, keep your child home on the day they are applied, and send a note to school asking that he or she not play on the grass for at least a week. Talk to the school about implementing an integrated pest management program (see chapter 36).
- *Cleaning supplies*: Talk to the school about the active ingredients in their cleaning supplies. If there are cleaners your child tolerates, volunteer to donate some if the school is willing to use them. Allergy extracts for phenol, ethanol, and formaldehyde will help with symptoms caused by cleaning supplies.
- *Instructional materials*: Request that materials be prepared ahead of time and allowed to outgas before being used in the classroom.
- *Personal care products*: Having the teacher and students refrain from wearing scented products is the ideal solution for this problem. However, the chances of achieving

universal cooperation are not high. Allergy extracts for perfume, fabric softener, and detergent will help.
- *Lead*: The use of lead in both new plumbing and plumbing repairs is now prohibited. Any school water coolers or plumbing containing lead parts should be replaced.
- *Fluorescent lights*: Request that your school use full-spectrum fluorescent lights.
- *Electromagnetic radiation*: Transfer your child to another school if there are high-voltage powerlines closer than 200 yards. Have your child wear diodes to help combat the effects of electromagnetic radiation (see Sources).

Dental

Dental hygiene should begin as soon as teeth erupt. Until children are six to seven years of age, their toothbrushing should be monitored and/or done by an adult. If children are not too chemically sensitive, they may have their molars sealed with a dental sealant. You should request that your dentist not use amalgam fillings in your child's teeth.

The amount of toothpaste shown on toothbrushes in advertisements contains enough fluoride to be toxic to young children. Use only a very small amount of fluoride-containing toothpaste. Other toothpastes, available at health food stores, are preferable to a fluoride-containing toothpaste. Baking soda on a damp toothbrush makes a good toothpowder.

Some dentists use fluoride treatments for children to prevent tooth decay. There is controversy over the safety of these treatments and whether they are of benefit after age 11. (See Dental Work in chapter 11 for a discussion of fluoride treatments.)

Mind and Spirit

We can help prevent many of the mind and spirit toxins that affect children, through providing unconditional love, sensible discipline, and moral support and teaching. Be consistent, but kind and firm with your discipline. Be certain that discipline and penalties fit the "crime." Do not measure out harsh discipline for simple wrongdoings. Love your child and show your love by providing structure that the child can depend on, in addition to being able to depend on you.

Make time for your child. Laugh and play with your child. Do not be stingy with hugs and other expressions of love. Let your love and kindness show through, even with firm discipline. Guide your child so that he or she develops a positive self-image. Never belittle your child, and be sure to praise when praise is due. Be gentle and instructive with all correction and criticism.

Many children have extremely high stress levels because of the high standards imposed by their parents, by their teachers, or by themselves. Some children attempt to function under a significant stress overload, and suffer for it. Parents should monitor their child's schedule and limit the number of activities in which he or she participates. Emphasize that your child should perform to the best of his or her abilities and that per-

> ### Abuse
>
> *If you suspect that someone is abusing your child, get help immediately. If you are struggling with your own anger, get help. Abused children often grow up to be abusers. Sometimes children will bully another child, which is a form of abuse. Even if the child is not hurt physically, he or she will suffer considerable emotional stress. Teach your child not to be a bully, and teach them skills to cope with a bully. If necessary, talk to the teacher, the principal, or the parents of the bully to have the action stopped.*

fection is not expected, necessary, or even possible. Be certain that your child receives enough sleep. Healing, repair, and growth take place during periods of rest and sleep.

You can take definite positive steps to prevent your child from being affected by spiritual toxins. Teach your child ethics and morals. Reinforce these teachings with spiritual or religious training or exposure. Insist that your child do what is right, and help him or her learn the difference between right and wrong. Teach children by setting an example of appropriate behavior and responses to life situations. Many children get a poor start in life and learn inappropriate responses because they either have no adult model to emulate or have a very poor role model as their example.

PART VIII

Detoxification Programs

IN THIS BOOK we have tried to present a broad overview of toxins, not in an effort to frighten you, but to make you aware of possible exposures in our world today. We have talked about toxins, how we are exposed to them, ways of detoxification, and prevention methods.

When our toxic burden exceeds the levels that our bodies can detoxify naturally, other steps must be taken. We must use detoxification procedures to cleanse and balance our bodies. Such procedures are usually necessary for most people at some time during their lives. In this section of the book, we will show you how to combine various detoxification methods for your individual needs.

Biochemical individuality dictates that each person will need a unique detoxification program. Genetics, age, gender, level of health, emotional status, nutritional status, environmental exposures, exposure patterns, disease, and behavioral and lifestyle factors will cause differences. Even people who are exposed to the same toxin for the same amount of time will respond differently to the exposure. Each person must investigate his or her toxic exposures, both past and present, and fully identify any health problems in order to determine an appropriate detoxification program.

People respond differently to detoxification programs. Many people feel worse initially. If your symptoms are overwhelming and you are experiencing severe headaches, nausea, and extreme fatigue, you are detoxifying more rapidly than your body is able to accommodate. Stop your detoxification procedures until you feel better, then begin them again at a slower rate. If your symptoms are mild and only moderately uncomfortable, continue your program. You will eventually clear and feel better. Remember, if you do not detoxify, it is probable that you will not get better and you will not enjoy good health. Other people begin to feel better immediately, and continue to improve. A few people begin to spontaneously detoxify as their health improves, and continue to detoxify until their body has rid itself of its toxic load.

The detoxification programs in this section are suggestions for some common conditions. This section is not meant to be comprehensive, but to present a few examples of the measures that people with a variety of health problems can use to cleanse and balance their bodies. If you have many symptoms and health problems, you will need to seek the assistance of a healthcare professional to help you plan and carry out your own individualized detoxification program.

Basic Detoxification Measures

These are the initial measures that everyone should follow, regardless of health status. Once you have made these lifestyle changes, read the following detoxification programs to find the one that is most appropriate for you

RELATED CHAPTERS	WHAT TO DO	COMMENTS/CAUTIONS
13, 23, 35	Clean up your diet.	Sources of toxins in foods must be removed for cleansing to take place.
8, 14, 16, 17 18, 36, 37	Clean up your home, both indoors and outdoors, removing all possible toxins.	A safe, clean place to live is necessary for detoxification and to maintain health after detoxification.
9, 36	Clean up your workplace or school.	Detoxification cannot take place without this step. If it cannot be accomplished, you may have to change jobs or schools.
10, 36, 37	Minimize leisure and recreational exposures.	It is important to eliminate as many sources of toxins as possible.
16	Use nontoxic personal hygiene products.	Scented and other toxic personal care products can undo your detoxification efforts.

Simple Detoxification Program
(For people with few symptoms)

This program is for people who are basically healthy and have very few symptoms. They are healthy and want to stay healthy. These steps will help them to prevent toxic bioaccumulation and to maintain or improve their good health.

RELATED CHAPTERS	WHAT TO DO	COMMENTS/CAUTIONS
See page 527.	Do the Basic Detox Measures.	Emphasize diet and environmental cleanup.
23	Take bowel tolerance vitamin C daily.	Powerful antioxidant; aids detoxification and rebuilding.
23	Take a multivitamin/mineral daily.	Nutrients must be balanced to work. Choose a product free of common allergens (wheat, yeast, corn, soy, egg, milk, and sugar).
22	Take detox baths two to three times a week for two months, then once a week.	Mobilizes chemicals from fat cells. Be careful not to overstay the time limit.
25	Exercise regularly.	Critical to detoxification.
26	Do breathing exercises.	Helps oxygenate the body and relieves stress.
25	Have bodywork once a week for two months, then once a month.	Helps to release both chemical and emotional toxins.
21, 28, 33	Investigate mind and spirit toxins and correct problems.	Full health requires a healthy mind and spirit.

Advanced Detoxification Program
(For people with many symptoms)

This program is for people with many symptoms, whose health is suffering. It is essential that these people have the guidance of a healthcare practitioner to help identify their problems, determine detoxification methods, and guide them back to health. In addition to these measures, people with specific health problems should consider the suggestions in the following charts.

RELATED CHAPTERS	WHAT TO DO	COMMENTS/CAUTIONS
See page 527.	Do the Basic Detox Measures.	Emphasize diet and environmental cleanup.
23	Take bowel tolerance vitamin C daily.	Powerful antioxidant, aids detoxification and rebuilding.
23	Take a multivitamin/mineral daily.	Nutrients must be balanced to work. Choose a product free of common allergens (wheat, yeast, corn, soy, egg, milk, and sugar).
23	Add nutrients specific for your health problems.	Some health problems necessitate specific additional nutrients to heal and rebuild.
31	Do an organ cleansing program.	Organs must be cleansed to be able to process toxins. Do the kidney first, then the liver, followed by lymph, colon, lung, and skin.
22	Take detox baths or do a sauna program.	Do supervised sauna treatments. Use detox baths if a sauna is not available.
15	Treat any infections.	Infections are a source of toxins and must be removed.
27	Identify and treat any allergies.	Untreated allergies stress the immune system and play a role in many health problems.
25	Exercise regularly.	Critical to detoxification.
26	Do breathing exercises.	Help oxygenate the body and relieve stress.
25	Have bodywork once a week for two months, then once or twice a month.	Helps to release chemical and emotional toxins.
32	Use energy balancing treatments.	Helps to detoxify and restore balance.
21, 28, 33	Investigate mind and spirit toxins and correct problems.	Full health requires a healthy mind and spirit.

Detoxification Programs for Specific Health Needs

The following programs include detoxification suggestions for some common health problems. There may be other methods that would be helpful. As well, people may have health problems that are not listed. You and your healthcare professional will have to determine which combination of techniques will be best for you.

Allergies

A number of detoxification techniques will help people with allergies. People can have allergies to foods, chemicals, pollens, terpenes and phenolics, molds, dust, dust mites, and microorganisms. All of their allergies must be addressed for complete symptom relief.

RELATED CHAPTERS	WHAT TO DO	COMMENTS/CAUTIONS
See page 527.	Do the Basic Detox Measures.	Pay particular attention to diet and environmental cleanup. Minimizing exposures reduces the risk of allergic responses and toxic overload.
See page 529.	Do the Advanced Detox Program.	Unless you have a heavy chemical load and multiple chemical allergies, saunas may not be necessary. Detox baths may be sufficient.
23	Add specific nutrients.	Consider quercetin, organic germanium, selenium.
27	Take allergy extracts or have hands-on treatment for your allergies.	Extracts will block reactions and allow your immune system to heal. They will also help chemicals release from cells.
25	Exercise regularly.	Can shorten the duration of an allergic inflammatory cascade, and can help clear an allergic reaction.
26	Have oxygen treatments.	Oxygen will help clear any allergic reaction.
31	Use coffee enemas or vitamin C enemas.	These enemas are helpful for clearing reactions, particularly to chemicals and foods.
28	Take homeopathic remedies.	Consult a trained homeopath for suggested remedies if those you try do not help.
29	Use herbal treatments.	Consider dried stinging nettles. Consult a trained herbalist if the herbs you try are not helpful. Sensitive individuals may not be able to take herbs.
28	Take Bach Flower Remedies.	Help with emotional aspects.

Arthritis

Detoxification can be a significant help to people with arthritis, as many different types of toxins play a role in arthritis. A decrease in pain and increased mobility of joints can result from lessening the toxic burden.

RELATED CHAPTERS	WHAT TO DO	COMMENTS/CAUTIONS
See page 527.	Do the Basic Detox Measures.	Pay particular attention to diet.
See page 529.	Do the Advanced Detox Program.	Pay particular attention to organ cleansing.
23	Add specific nutrients.	Consider MSM, EFA, enzymes between meals, CoQ_{10}, vitamins A and E, calcium, magnesium, pycnogenol, cysteine, methionine.
25	Exercise regularly.	Regular exercise will help maintain mobility, and increases muscle flexibility and strength.
25	Have bodywork.	Bodywork can increase circulation and break up toxin deposits in joints.
26	Have oxygen treatments.	Reverses inflammatory cascade.
27	Take allergy extracts or have hands-on treatments for any sensitivities.	Allergy plays a large role in arthritis, particularly food allergies.
28	Take homeopathic remedies.	There are many homeopathic remedies for arthritis. You may need the help of a trained homeopath.
29	Use herbal treatments.	Consult a trained herbalist to select the proper herb.
22	In addition to sauna or detox baths, use hydrotherapy treatments.	Hydrotherapy treatments can increase circulation to a given area. Cold will reduce inflammation.
30	Use clay packs.	Will reduce pain and swelling.
30	Use castor oil packs on painful joints.	The heat and castor oil will reduce pain.
30	Use herbal poultices.	Reduce inflammation, pain, and swelling.
29	Use aromatherapy.	Some essential oils have an anti-inflammatory action.
27	Consider chelation.	Can improve blood flow, which is sometimes a problem in arthritis.
33	Keep a journal regularly.	Reduces stress, which can reduce symptoms.

Asthma

The lungs are a target organ in asthma, and many toxins affect them. Because allergies play a large role in asthma, detoxification for asthmatics should emphasize allergy treatment.

RELATED CHAPTERS	WHAT TO DO	COMMENTS/CAUTIONS
See page 527.	Do the Basic Detox Measures.	Pay particular attention to chemical, dust, and mold control.
See page 529.	Do the Advanced Detox Program.	Pay attention to organ cleansing, particularly for the lungs.
23	Add specific nutrients.	Consider organic germanium, quercetin, beta-carotene, calcium, magnesium.
27	Treat all allergies and sensitivities with allergy extracts or hands-on treatments.	Wheezing is a frequent allergic symptom. Pay particular attention to inhalant allergies.
25	Exercise regularly.	Increases oxygen utilization and the function of oxygen-dependent metabolic pathways. Restores lung capacity, endurance, and strength.
22	Use hydrotherapy.	Steam baths, vapor baths, and steam inhalations clear mucous membrane congestion.
26	Have oxygen treatments.	Detoxifies and helps relieve wheezing.
28	Take homeopathic remedies.	Many remedies will help asthma. You may need the help of a trained homeopath.
29	Use herbal treatments.	Consult a trained herbalist to select the proper herb.
29	Use aromatherapy.	Has antispasmodic action.
33	Keep a journal regularly.	Reduces stress, which reduces symptoms.

Cancer

Toxic exposures play a large role in the development of cancer. Detoxification can help in the treatment, as well as the prevention, of cancer.

RELATED CHAPTERS	WHAT TO DO	COMMENTS/CAUTIONS
See page 527.	Do the Basic Detox Measures.	Emphasize chemical cleanup and avoidance.
See page 529.	Do the Advanced Detox Program.	Pay particular attention to organ cleansing, particularly the kidneys and liver.
24	Go on a macrobiotic diet.	Many people have recovered from cancer with a macrobiotic diet.
23	Add specific nutrients.	Emphasize antioxidants, particularly vitamins A, E, and beta-carotene. Organic germanium increases oxygenation of the cells, as well as pain control. CoQ_{10} is a free radical scavenger. Take enzyme therapy between meals.
27	Treat all allergies with allergy extracts or hands-on treatments.	Allergies stress the immune system, which weakens it and lowers its ability to fight cancer.
25	Exercise regularly.	Increased blood transport carries nutrients and oxygen to the cells and waste products and toxins away from cells.
28	Take homeopathic remedies.	There are many homeopathic remedies for cancer. Consult a trained homeopath for help and supervision.
29	Use herbal treatments.	There are many herbal remedies for cancer. Consult a trained herbalist for help and supervision.
31	Use coffee enemas.	Detoxify the liver, which must cleanse the waste products from cancer treatments.
32	Do light therapy.	Hemoirradiation has been helpful for cancer.
26	Have oxygen treatments.	Cancer is anaerobic and increasing oxygen to the body will help combat it.
30	Use clay packs.	Relieve pain and absorb toxins.
30	Use charcoal therapy.	Charcoal poultices applied to the affected site will draw out toxins related to the cancer and reduce pain.
33	Use laugh and hug therapy.	Laugh therapy has helped cure many serious diseases. Hugs impart caring and support for the ill individual.
32	Use sound therapy.	Sound therapy can reduce stress. Supplying missing sounds can improve health and help fight disease.
28	Take Bach Flower Remedies.	Help with emotional aspects.
33	Keep a journal regularly.	Reduces stress, which can reduce symptoms.

Chemical Problems

The following program is for people who have had some type of chemical exposure. People who have had a serious exposure to solvents, pesticides, or toxic metals will have to take more measures than those who have only been exposed to chemicals from typical daily living.

RELATED CHAPTERS	WHAT TO DO	COMMENTS/CAUTIONS
See page 527.	Do the Basic Detox Measures.	Emphasize chemical cleanup in the whole house.
See page 529.	Do the Advanced Detox Program.	Pay particular attention to organ cleansing, especially the liver. The body must be able to handle the released toxins, or damage can occur.
22	Do dry saunas.	Dry saunas cause sweating that flushes out toxins and heavy metals.
23	Add specific nutrients.	Consider L-cysteine, L-methionine, or L-gluta-thione, MSM, calcium, magnesium, organic germanium, CoQ$_{10}$, bioflavonoids, vitamin B$_{12}$.
27	Treat all allergies and sensitivities to chemicals with allergy extracts or hands-on treatments.	Blocks allergic reactions and allows release of chemicals from cells.
25	Exercise regularly.	Rapidly cleanses toxins from the blood.
25	Have bodywork.	Bodywork breaks down chemical storage and increases metabolism, which helps break down toxins.
28	Take homeopathic remedies.	Consult a trained homeopath for help and supervision.
29	Use herbal treatments.	Consult a trained herbalist for help and supervision.
27	For metal toxicity, have chelation treatments.	Chelation requires the help of a healthcare practitioner. The substances used are prescription medications.
26	Have oxygen treatments.	Oxygen is a very efficient detoxifier.
31	Use coffee enemas.	Coffee enemas are one of the best liver cleansers.
30	Use castor oil packs, charcoal therapy, or clay packs.	Castor oil can draw toxins out of the body from as deep as four inches. Charcoal adsorbs many toxins. Clay packs draw out toxins.

Children

As discussed in previous chapters, some children need detoxification procedures. However, because of their special needs, detoxification methods must be tailored for them to prevent damage to their bodies and minds.

RELATED CHAPTERS	WHAT TO DO	COMMENTS/CAUTIONS
See page 527.	Do the Basic Detox Measures.	A clean environment is particularly important for children.
See page 529.	Do the Advanced Detox Program.	Consult chapter 34 for any contraindications.
23, 34	Add specific nutrients.	Children respond well to nutrients. Adjust doses according to weight.
22, 34	Use detox baths and saunas.	Both are safe for children.
22, 34	Use hydrotherapy.	Basic hydrotherapy techniques are safe for children.
27, 34	Treat all allergies with allergy extracts or hands-on treatment.	Sublingual allergy extracts work well with children, as do hands-on treatments.
25, 34	Exercise regularly.	Do not force a child to exercise. Exercise is more important for older children.
25, 34	Have bodywork done.	Children do well with some types of bodywork. Be sure the child feels comfortable with the practitioner and the method.
28, 34	Give homeopathic remedies.	Many conditions can be helped with homeopathic remedies, which are easily given to children.
29, 34	Use herbal treatments.	Children are very responsive to herbs.
26, 34	Do breathing exercises.	Can be very effective when the child is old enough to understand the directions.
29, 34	Use aromatherapy.	Extremely effective for children.
28, 34	Give Bach Flower Remedies.	Helps with emotional problems.
27, 34	Have chelation therapy.	Effective for lead poisoning.
32, 34	Use color therapy.	A natural therapy for children.
30, 34	Use compresses, packs, and poultices.	Very helpful for children, including mustard plasters with the mounts adjusted.
26, 34	Have oxygen treatments.	Several methods can be used with children.
32, 34	Use sound therapy.	Musical sound therapy is enjoyable for children.
32, 34	Use light therapy.	Many forms of light therapy are helpful for children.
32, 34	Use electromagnetic and magnetic therapy.	Many of these techniques are easy to use and helpful for children.
33, 34	Use detoxification methods for the mind and spirit.	Reduce stress and help heal emotional toxins.

Diabetes

Detoxification procedures, particularly those related to diet and exercise, can help control diabetes, whether it is Type I or Type II. In some cases, detoxification and prevention measures can lower the blood sugar levels of a person with Type II diabetes to normal.

RELATED CHAPTERS	WHAT TO DO	COMMENTS/CAUTIONS
See page 527.	Do the Basic Detox Measures.	Give diet special emphasis, particularly lowering sugar and carbohydrate intake.
See page 529.	Do the Advanced Detox Program.	Pay particular attention to organ cleansing.
24	Follow an insulin-control diet.	Help control insulin release and carbohydrate metabolism. Type I diabetics should not fast.
22	Do detox baths.	Be particularly careful with water temperature. Decreased sensation in extremities that results from diabetes makes sensing temperature difficult.
23	Add specific nutrients.	Consider chromium, alpha-lipoic acid.
25	Exercise regularly.	Helps maintain appropriate blood sugar levels. Can reverse adult-onset diabetes.
27	Treat all allergies with allergy extracts or hands-on treatments.	Allergic reactions can cause a fluctuation in blood sugar.
28	Take homeopathic remedies.	Homeopathic remedies can help with diabetes. If you have Type I diabetes, consult a trained homeopath.
29	Use herbal treatments.	Herbal remedies can help with diabetes. If you have Type I diabetes, consult a trained herbalist.
28	Use Bach Flower Remedies.	Can help with emotional aspects.
33	Use detoxification methods for mind and spirit.	Many of these techniques reduce stress and help with emotional aspects.

Fatigue

There are many causes of fatigue and, while it is important to identify the cause of the fatigue, many symptoms can be relieved with detoxification procedures. Fatigue caused by food allergies, increased toxic load, and chronic fatigue respond favorably to detoxification.

RELATED CHAPTERS	WHAT TO DO	COMMENTS/CAUTIONS
See page 527.	Do the Basic Detox Measures.	Emphasize diet and environmental cleanup.
See page 529.	Do the Advanced Detox Program.	Pay particular attention to organ cleansing, particularly the liver.
23	Add specific nutrients.	Consider extra B vitamins, particularly B_{12}, calcium, magnesium, L-carnitine, alpha-lipoic acid, CoQ_{10}.
27	Treat all allergies with allergy extracts or hands-on techniques.	Fatigue can be a major symptom of all allergic reactions.
25	Exercise regularly.	Increases endurance, decreases inertia.
28	Take homeopathic remedies.	Consult a trained homeopath for help and supervision.
29	Use herbal treatments.	Consult a trained herbalist for help and supervision.
15	Treat all infections.	Fatigue is a symptom of all infections.
24	Consider fasting.	Can increase energy, rejuvenate cells and the body, and refresh the mind and spirit.
22	Do detox baths.	Can lower an allergic load considerably, which will increase energy.
33	Investigate emotional toxins that could be contributing to fatigue.	Counseling, NET, and journaling may be helpful techniques.
28	Take Bach Flower Remedies.	Can help with emotional aspects.

Gastrointestinal Problems

While they are not life-threatening, gastrointestinal problems are very uncomfortable and people are frequently told simply that they must learn to live with them. Many detoxification techniques will improve, if not eliminate, these problems.

RELATED CHAPTERS	WHAT TO DO	COMMENTS/CAUTIONS
See page 527.	Do the Basic Detox Measures.	Clean diet is imperative for all types of gastrointestinal problems, as is intake of sufficient water and fiber.
See page 529.	Do the Advanced Detox Program.	Emphasize organ cleansing, particularly the colon and gallbladder.
24	Consider fasting or juicing.	Cleanses the digestive tract and improves digestion and assimilation.
23	Add specific nutrients.	Consider beneficial bacteria, aloe vera, vitamins A and E, digestive enzymes.
27	Treat all allergies with allergy extracts or hands-on treatment.	Food allergies can particularly affect the gastrointestinal tract. Extracts for bowel pathogens can cleanse.
25	Exercise regularly.	Speeds up removal of toxins and waste materials from the cells and helps combat constipation.
31	Do a colon cleanse with clay and fiber.	Removes waste not ordinarily excreted.
26	Have oxygen therapy.	Improves digestion.
28	Take homeopathic remedies.	Consult a trained homeopath for help and supervision. Bowel nosodes are often helpful.
29	Use herbal treatments.	Consult a trained herbalist for help and supervision.
29	Use aromatherapy.	Strengthens peristalsis and supports digestion.
33	Get NET treatments.	Can release emotional toxins that can play a role in gastrointestinal problems.

Hormonal Problems

Hormones can be an internal toxin and play a role in toxicity when the amounts in the body are either too high or too low. Some people are sensitive to their own hormones and cannot utilize them properly. Detoxification procedures can help regulate hormone balance, and allow people to desensitize.

RELATED CHAPTERS	WHAT TO DO	COMMENTS/CAUTIONS
See page 527.	Do the Basic Detox Measures.	Emphasize a clean diet.
See page 529.	Do the Advanced Detox Program.	Pay attention to organ cleansing, particularly the liver. Hormone levels are directly affected by liver activity.
22	Use hydrotherapy.	Baths help painful ovaries or testicles, menstrual cramps, and impotence.
23	Add specific nutrients.	Consider essential fatty acids, vitamins A and E.
27	Treat allergies with allergy extracts or hands-on treatment.	In addition to treating allergies for foods, chemicals, and inhalants, treat for sensitivities to hormones.
25	Exercise regularly.	Enhances endocrine function.
25	Have bodywork.	Relieves menstrual cramps and helps PMS.
28	Take homeopathic remedies.	Remedies can treat hormonal problems for both men and women. Consult a trained homeopath for help.
29	Use herbal treatments.	Consult a trained herbalist for help.
29	Use aromatherapy.	Balances hormones.
32	Have light therapy.	Bright light therapy can help regulate hormones.

Infections

Some people tend to have frequent infections. So many people say, "I catch every-thing that comes along!" The following program will help strengthen these people so that they can better resist infections.

RELATED CHAPTERS	WHAT TO DO	COMMENTS/CAUTIONS
See page 527.	Do the Basic Detox Measures.	Clean diet and environment takes the stress off the immune system and helps prevent infections.
See page 529.	Do the Advanced Detox Program.	Bowel tolerance vitamin C plays a very important role in preventing and treating infections.
22	Take saunas.	The increased temperature of a sauna can reduce infection by inhibiting replication of bacteria and viruses. Strengthens the immune response.
24	Completely eliminate sugar from your diet.	Sugar stops the activity of white blood cells within 30 minutes of consumption. Function will not resume for 4 to 5 hours.
24	Consider a fast.	Increases resistance to disease.
23	Add specific nutrients.	Consider CoQ_{10}, organic germanium, vitamin E, zinc.
27	Treat all allergies with allergy extracts or hands-on techniques.	Allergic reactions are a stress on the immune system, weakening it and increasing susceptibility to infection. Allergic responses to organisms can play a role in symptoms of infection.
25	Exercise regularly.	Increases oxygenation to cells, which helps combat infection.
28	Take homeopathic remedies.	There are many helpful remedies for infections. Consult a qualified homeopath for help and supervision.
29	Use herbal treatments.	Echinacea and goldenseal are helpful. Consult a trained herbalist for additional help and supervision.
26	Use oxygen therapy.	Oxygen is a broad-spectrum antibiotic.
30	Use castor oil packs on the thymus.	Stimulates the thymus gland.
32	Use magnetic therapy.	Helps eliminate many different infections.
33	Keep a journal regularly.	Reduces stress, which increases immune function.

Insomnia

Toxic overload can contribute to insomnia, as can stress. Loss of sleep does not lead to long-term medical problems, but increases psychological suffering and makes people feel less healthy.

RELATED CHAPTERS	WHAT TO DO	COMMENTS/CAUTIONS
See page 527.	Do the Basic Detox Measures.	Environmental cleanup will correct situations that contribute to insomnia.
See page 529.	Do the Advanced Detox Program.	Reducing toxins in the body improves health, which can improve sleep.
22	Use hydrotherapy.	Heat treatments increase drowsiness. Can induce sleep, soothe the nervous system. Neutral baths treat insomnia.
23	Add specific nutrients.	Consider melatonin, calcium, magnesium, folic acid, B_{12}.
27	Treat all allergies with allergy extracts or hands-on treatment.	Allergies can cause nasal congestion that will interfere with sleep. Treating neurotransmitter sensitivites will help induce sleep.
25	Exercise regularly.	Reduces the perception of stress and tires the body physically.
25	Have bodywork.	Releases muscle tension, aiding relaxation.
28	Take homeopathic remedies.	Several remedies help with insomnia. Consult a qualified homeopath to help with remedy selection.
29	Use herbal treatments.	Herbal remedies can be very effective for insomnia. Consult a trained herbalist to help with remedy selection.
26	Do breathing exercises.	Reduce stress and encourage sleep and relaxation.
32	Do sound therapy.	Soothing music helps relaxation.
32	Use light therapy.	Bright light therapy normalizes delayed sleep phase syndrome.
32	Use electromagnetic/magnetic therapy.	Can reduce stress and induce sleep.
28	Take Bach Flower Remedies.	Help with emotional aspects.
33	Keep a journal regularly.	Emotional problems are one of the most common causes of insomnia.
33	Practice meditation or prayer.	Meditation can help release troubling thoughts that prevent sleep.

Medical Treatments

Many detoxification measures can reduce or eliminate the effects of standard medical treatment, including surgery, radiation diagnosis and treatment, chemotherapy, vaccinations, medications, and dental work.

RELATED CHAPTERS	WHAT TO DO	COMMENTS/CAUTIONS
See page 527.	Do the Basic Detox Measures.	Pay particular attention to diet, and avoid empty calories. The body needs nutrients to heal.
See page 529.	Do the Advanced Detox Program.	Organ cleansing, with emphasis on kidney and liver cleansing will help the body rid itself of toxins more easily.
22	Take saunas or detox baths.	Will encourage the release of fat-soluble toxins from fat cells Will help clear medications and other substances, as well as effects of radiation, either for treatment or diagnosis.
26	Have oxygen treatments.	Increasing oxygenation to tissues helps with healing and speeds detoxification.
23	Add specific nutrients.	Consider antioxidants—vitamins A and E, beta-carotene; also MSM, organic germanium, manganese, selenium, zinc, CoQ_{10}, B vitamins, NAC, cysteine, methionine, and glutathione.
27	Treat all allergies with allergy extracts or hands-on treatments.	Allergic reactions stress the immune system and slow healing. Extracts will help release toxins from medical treatments.
25	Exercise when you are able.	Speeds up the removal of toxins and waste materials from the cells; increases blood flow that carries nutrients and oxygen to every cell; increases lymph circulation.
28	Take homeopathic remedies.	There are specific remedies to help with many of the problems that can result after medical treatment. You may need to consult a trained homeopath.
29	Use herbal treatments.	Herbal remedies can speed recovery and reduce toxicity after most medical treatments. You may need to consult a trained herbalist.
30	Use packs and poultices.	Increase circulation to specific areas, help draw out toxins.
33	Use laugh and hug therapy.	Provides emotional support during healing.
28	Take Bach Flower Remedies.	Helps with emotional aspects.

Mood Disorders

Mood and emotional disorders can be affected and/or caused by toxins in the body. These problems may range from mild to severe, and many are whole body illnesses that involve the body, nervous system, moods, thoughts, and behavior.

RELATED CHAPTERS	WHAT TO DO	COMMENTS/CAUTIONS
See page 527.	Do the Basic Detox Measures.	Emphasize mold cleanup and control. Mold is a common contributor to depression and cerebral symptoms.
See page 529.	Do the Advanced Detox Program.	A toxic overload can affect neurotransmitter production, which directly controls mood.
23	Add specific nutrients.	Consider B vitamins, vitamin A, magnesium, L-carnitine, CoQ_{10}, EFA, methionine, chromium, zinc.
24	Consider a fast.	Can refresh the mind and spirit.
27	Treat allergies with allergy extracts or hands-on treatments.	Mold allergy can contribute to depressions. Extracts for neurotransmitter problems are very helpful for mood disorders.
25	Exercise regularly.	Helps emotional cleansing, reduces anxiety and tension, and alleviates depression.
28	Take homeopathic remedies.	There are many remedies that help mood disorders. Consult a trained homeopath for help with remedy selection.
29	Use herbal treatments.	Many herbs can help mood disorders. Consult a trained herbalist.
26	Do breathing exercises.	Help oxygenate the body and relieve stress.
32	Do energy balancing treatments.	Color, gem, light, and sound therapy can improve mood.
28	Take Bach Flower Remedies.	These remedies affect the emotions directly.
29	Use aromatherapy.	Reduces emotional toxicity and depression.
33	Do laugh and hug therapy.	Laugh therapy can elevate mood. Hug therapy imparts support for the individual and helps relieve anxiety.
33	Have counseling if needed.	Helps both to understand and cope with problems.
33	Keep a journal regularly.	Helps keep in touch and deal with emotions.

Obesity

Many lipid-soluble toxins can be stored in the fat cells of obese people. It is safer for a person to detoxify before beginning a weight loss program, which can result in a massive toxin release.

RELATED CHAPTERS	WHAT TO DO	COMMENTS/CAUTIONS
See page 527.	Do the Basic Detox Measures.	Emphasize chemical cleanup and clean diet.
See page 529.	Do the Advanced Detox Program.	Approach sauna or detox baths with caution because of the effects of increased temperature on high blood pressure that can accompany obesity.
24	Use diet modification techniques.	Identify the causes of obesity and follow an appropriate diet.
23	Add specific nutrients.	Consider chromium, alpha-lipoic acid, vitamins A and E, B vitamins, calcium, magnesium, zinc, L-carnitine.
27	Treat allergies with allergy extracts or hands-on treatments.	Allergies can contribute to obesity.
25	Exercise regularly.	Reduces body fat and increases muscle.
28	Take homeopathic remedies.	There are homeopathic remedies that will help. Consult a trained homeopath for help with remedy selection.
29	Use herbal treatments.	Many herbs are helpful for obesity. Consult a trained herbalist for help with remedy selection.
33	Have counseling if needed.	Emotional problems can contribute to overeating and obesity.
28	Take Bach Flower Remedies.	Can help with emotional aspects.
33	Keep a journal regularly.	Helps keep in touch and deal with emotions.

Pain

There are many different types of pain, with many different causes. Pain can be difficult to tolerate, but can often be treated without drugs. The reduction of several different types of pain can be accomplished with detoxification techniques.

RELATED CHAPTERS	WHAT TO DO	COMMENTS/CAUTIONS
See page 527.	Do the Basic Detox Measures.	Environmental cleanup helps prevent allergies, which contribute to health problems that cause pain. Clean diet helps control pain related to food allergies.
See page 529.	Do the Advanced Detox Program.	Baths and sauna treatments can reduce pain.
22	Have hydrotherapy.	Relieves pain. Hot footbath with ice on the neck can relieve a headache. Hot packs relieve pain and muscle spasms. Ice packs reduce pain and swelling.
23	Add specific nutrients.	Consider organic germanium, enzymes between meals, calcium, magnesium, EFA.
27	Treat allergies with allergy extracts or hands-on treatment.	Allergies can contribute to conditions that cause pain, such as headaches, arthritis, muscle aches, and earaches.
25	Exercise regularly.	Stimulates the production of endorphins, helping to mask pain and give a feeling of euphoria.
25	Have bodywork.	Can relieve many types of pain, including backache and headache.
28	Take homeopathic remedies.	There are many homeopathic remedies for pain. You may need the help of a trained homeopath.
29	Use herbal treatments.	Herbal remedies can help relieve pain, such as feverfew for headaches. You may need the help of a trained herbalist.
30	Use compresses, packs, and poultices.	Provides pain relief for specific areas.
30	Use charcoal therapy.	Charcoal poultices can relieve pain.
32	Use magnetic therapy.	Magnets applied to the painful area will alleviate pain.
32	Use light therapy.	Will increase neurotransmitter production and reduce pain.
33	Use meditation and prayer.	Can help reduce and relieve pain.
33	Keep a journal regularly.	Reduces stress, which can reduce symptoms.

Pregnancy Preparation

It is imperative that both parents are in good health at the time of conception. Most people tend to forget that the health of the father is just as important as the health of the mother. One of our sickest allergy patients was conceived the night her father came home from World War II, after spending a number of months in a Japanese prison camp, where nutrition was inadequate, illness was common, and stress levels were high.

RELATED CHAPTERS	WHAT TO DO	COMMENTS/CAUTIONS
See page 527.	Do the Basic Detox Measures if your health is good.*	Emphasize diet and environmental cleanup.
See page 529.	Do the Advanced Detox Program if you have health problems.*	Pay particular attention to organ cleansing, particularly the kidneys and liver.
23	Add specific nutrients.	Consider extra B vitamins, particularly folic acid (for women), as well as the antioxidant vitamins.
27	Treat allergies with allergy extracts or hands-on treatments.	Untreated and uncontrolled allergies can adversely affect health, and the tendency to develop allergies can be passed on.
25	Exercise regularly.	Speeds up removal of toxins and waste materials from the cells.
22	Take detox baths.	Will help release stored toxins quickly.
28	Take homeopathic remedies.	Consult a trained homeopath for help with remedy selection to optimize health.
29	Use herbal treatments.	Consult a trained herbalist for help with herb selection to optimize health.
15	Treat all infections.	Will strengthen the immune response and the body. Some infections can be passed to the new child.
26	Do breathing exercises.	Help oxygenate the body.
28	Take Bach Flower Remedies.	Affect any emotions that may need attention.
33	Have counseling if needed.	Will help deal with any problems that might interfere with effective parenting.
21, 28, 33	Investigate mind and spirit toxins and correct problems.	Full health requires a healthy mind and spirit. Full health makes effective parenting easier.

* Do not undertake a detoxification program if you are, or might be, pregnant.

Skin Problems

Skin problems such as rashes, eczema, and psoriasis are frequently a sign that the body is badly in need of detoxification. Toxins are emerging through the skin because the body is overloaded and there is no other way to excrete them.

RELATED CHAPTERS	WHAT TO DO	COMMENTS/CAUTIONS
See page 527.	Do the Basic Detox Measures.	Emphasize diet and chemical cleanup.
See page 529.	Do the Advanced Detox Program.	Pay particular attention to organ cleansing, especially the liver, lymph, and skin.
22	Take a wet sauna.	Steam helps many skin conditions.
24	Consider fasting or juicing.	Fasting and juicing can rapidly clear toxins that cause rashes.
23	Add specific nutrients.	Consider vitamins A, E, and D; EFA; MSM; bioflavonoids.
27	Treat allergies with allergy extracts or hands-on treatments.	Eczema and rashes are frequent symptoms of allergy.
25	Exercise regularly.	Increases elimination of toxins and oxygenation of cells.
25	Have bodywork.	Massage improves skin tone and helps releases toxins.
30	Use clay packs.	Will remove toxins from the body and help clear skin.
22	Use exfoliation or dry brushing.	Use if the skin condition will permit. Increases circulation, opens pores, and invigorates skin.
30	Use a charcoal poultice.	Will remove toxins and will treat skin ulcers.
28	Take homeopathic remedies.	Remedies will help with many different types of skin problems. You may need to consult a trained homeopath.
29	Use herbal treatment.	Consult a trained herbalist for help with herb selection.
29	Use aromatherapy.	Many aromatherapy substances treat skin problems.
32	Use light therapy.	Several types of light therapy will help skin problems.
33	Have counseling.	May be necessary for chronic skin problems.

Afterword

WITH YOUR NEW awareness of toxins, as well as treatment possibilities, you can increase your quality of health and life. Keep in mind that you want to cleanse your body, rebuild it, and maintain your new clean, healthy status. Simple precautions enable you to avoid or minimize exposures to toxins and prevent further damage to your body. Treatment methods allow you to detoxify your body of the toxins to which you have already had exposure. Armed with your new knowledge, you can regain or enhance your health. We wish you joy and success in your journey.

Glossary

Acid: Any chemical capable of releasing a hydrogen ion; it will have a pH less than 7.

Acute exposure: Short exposure to a toxin, technically an exposure of less than 14 days.

Aerobic: Organisms or metabolic processes that require oxygen.

Allergen: Substance that causes adverse symptoms, such as pollens, molds, dust, dust mites, animal dander, foods, and chemicals found in air, water, or food.

Allergic rhinitis: Runny and/or stuffy nose caused by pollen allergies.

Allergy: Attacks by the immune system on harmless or even beneficial substances entering the body. Abnormal response to substances usually well tolerated by most people.

Allergy extract: Treatment dilution of an antigen used in immunotherapy, such as a food, chemical, or pollen extract.

Amalgams: Silver-mercury fillings commonly used in teeth.

Anaerobic: Organisms or metabolic processes that do not require oxygen.

Antibody: A protein molecule produced to protect the body; made by B-lymphocytes or plasma cells in response to a perceived foreign or abnormal substance or organism.

Antigen: A substance that causes the body to produce antibodies; also refers to a concentrated solution of an allergen used for treatment.

Antioxidant: A chemical that protects against a chemical reaction known as oxidation; prevents damage from free radicals and sometimes called a free radical quencher.

Asthma: A disease of the lungs in which the airways become inflamed and produce excessive mucus, with spasm of the muscles around the small airways.

Atherosclerosis: A disease of the arterial walls that slowly causes blockages in the entire arterial system.

Autonomic nervous system: The part of the nervous system that supplies the blood vessels, heart, viscera, smooth muscles, and glands with nervous stimulation; regulates involuntary action.

Bacteria: Single-celled organisms that grow in colonies and reproduce by simple division called binary fission. Some species cause disease in humans.

Benzo[a]pyrene (BaP): A chemical emitted when tobacco, foods, garbage, wood, coal, or petroleum products are burned; a polycyclic aromatic hydrocarbon (PAH); probable human carcinogen.

Bioaccumulation: An increase in concentration of a chemical in a food chain because of the ability of one or more of the organisms in the chain to concentrate it.

Bioconcentration: The higher concentration of a substance in a plant or animal than is found in its food supply, air, or water.

Bioflavonoid: A biologically active class of compounds containing primarily pigments, and widely distributed in plants.

Biotransformation: Chemical reactions in the body that change lipid-soluble chemicals into water-soluble substances to facilitate excretion from the body.

Blood-brain barrier: A cellular barrier that prevents certain chemical substances from passing from the blood into the brain.

Bodywork: A group of therapies involving therapeutic touch, used to correct the structure and improve the function of the body.

Botanicals: Chemicals extracted from plants; can refer to herbs or insecticides extracted from plants.

Bowel dysbiosis: Imbalance in the intestinal bacteria.

Building-related illness: An illness related to an identified cause from which a group of people who work or live in the building have become ill.

Carcinogen: A substance capable of causing cancer.

Catalyst: A chemical that speeds up a chemical re-action without being consumed or permanently affected in the process.

Chelation: A therapy to restore blood flow in a person who suffers from atherosclerosis. It removes metallic irritants and allows leaky, damaged cell walls to heal; also used to treat metal poisoning.

Chi: Universal or vital energy in Chinese medicine that flows along invisible energy meridians throughout the body. Chi must be balanced for the body to be healthy. Sometimes spoken of as the breath.

Chronic exposure: A low-level exposure over a period of more than one year.

Contact dermatitis: Inflammation of the skin caused by chemicals or substances that come into contact with the skin.

Contaminants: Substances that pollute air, food, or water; includes chemicals, pesticides, microorganisms, and the toxins they produce.

Cytochrome P-450: A family of enzymes active in the Phase I metabolism of xenobiotics.

Detoxification: A process by which a toxin is changed to a harmless substance or is removed from the body.

Detoxify: To remove toxins from the body.

Ecogenetics: Genetically determined differences among people in their susceptibility to the effects of xenobiotics.

Electromagnetic: Refers to the electrical and magnetic properties of a substance.

Electromagnetic spectrum: A band of energy forms, including X-rays, light waves, heat, and radio waves, transmitted as waves of varying wavelengths.

Emotional abuse: Neglect, verbal abuse, and psychological abuse.

Endogenous toxins: Toxins originating from or caused by internal sources.

Endorphin: A natural pain-killing substance that is produced in the body.

Endotoxin: A bacterial toxin produced within a bacterial cell that is not released unless the cell is ruptured.

Enzyme: A substance, usually a protein, that is formed in living cells and stops, starts, or controls the speed of a biochemical reaction.

Epidemiology: The study of the pattern of disease in a population.

Essential oils: The oils used in aromatherapy; extracted from plants and carry the active properties, taste, and scent of the original plant.

Exogenous toxins: Toxins originating from external sources; found in food, air, and water.

Exotoxins: Toxins loosely associated with a bacterial cell.

Fatty acids: Carbon and hydrogen molecules with an acid group on one end of the molecule; occur naturally in fats and oils.

Free radicals: Chemicals (atoms, ions, or molecules) that have an unpaired electron, are highly reactive, and can cause tissue and cell membrane damage; essential in small amounts.

Fungi: A group of parasitic organisms that lack chlorophyll. Mushrooms, rusts, and smuts are macroscopic fungi; microscopic fungi are capable of infecting humans.

Generally recognized as safe (GRAS): Food additives thought to be safe, based on a history of use, rather than rigorous testing.

Genetic polymorphism: Different varieties of genes that control detoxification enzymes.

Half-life: The time it takes for a quantity of chemical to decrease by half; used to describe the length of time it takes radioactive isotopes to decay or pesticides to break down.

Hemoglobin: A red-colored protein in red blood cells that transports oxygen.

Herb: Any plant or plant part that has medicinal value.

Herbal extract: Preparation made by soaking herbs in a liquid. Vinegar, alcohol, and oil are the most common liquids used, since these media will extract the active principles from the plant during cold soaking.

Herbicide: A chemical that kills plants.

Homeostasis: A dynamic equilibrium in the body maintained by feedback and regulation.

Hormone: A biological regulator produced by the glands of the endocrine system; hormones are released into the bloodstream and carried to target cells.

Host: The species that harbors a parasite.

Hydrocarbon: An organic chemical made of hydrogen and carbon; comes from vegetable sources, petroleum, and coal tar.

Iatrogenic illness: An illness caused by the actions of a physician.

Immunoglobulins: Antibodies that are produced in the body; and include IgA, IgG, IgM, and IgE. IgE is responsible for immediate hypersensitivity and skin whealing in allergic reactions.

Immunotherapy: Treatment with allergy extracts over a period of time, with extract doses based on individual test results.

Inert ingredients: Components of a chemical product that have no intended activity; usually solvents, but can include diluents, wetting agents, or carriers; can be toxic.

Inflammation: The reaction of tissue to injury from trauma, infection, or irritating substances; the signs of inflammation are heat, redness, swelling, and tenderness.

Inhalants: Pollens, dust, dust mites, animal danders, insect parts, and molds; can be allergenic.

Insecticide: A chemical that kills insects.

Integrated pest management: A type of pest control based on management, not eradication, emphasizing maintenance of healthy plants, using natural enemies of the pests, and careful use of selected chemical pesticides when necessary.

Internal toxins: Toxins produced or stored in the body; endogenous toxins.

Isotope: An atom with the same number of protons as the normal atom but a different number of neutrons, giving the atoms slightly differing atomic weights.

Jaundice: A condition that results in a yellow color of the skin due to the pigment bilirubin, a breakdown product of hemoglobin.

Lipid: Any of numerous fats and fatlike materials that constitute the primary structural material of living cells, in addition to carbohydrates and proteins.

Lipophilic: A substance that dissolves readily in fat; lipid soluble.

Macrobiotic diet: A diet of grains, vegetables, beans, sea vegetables, and soups, with occasional fish and white meat.

Metabolism: Sum of physical and chemical changes that take place in an organism; includes material and energy changes, including transformation of foods to energy and heat. It involves anabolism (building up) and catabolism (breaking down).

Microorganisms: Bacteria, viruses, parasites (some are visible to the naked eye), fungi, or yeast.

Microsomal mixed-function oxidases: Part of the cytochrome P-450 family of enzymes that help metabolize xenobiotics.

Mold: Organisms that are part of the family *Fungi imperfecti,* found in soil and air; can grow in almost any environment.

Mycotoxins: Toxins produced by molds.

Neurotoxins: Chemicals that cause adverse effects to the nervous system.

Neurotransmitters: Chemical messengers responsible for the transmission of nerve impulses across the synapse (space) between nerve cells; produced in the nerve cells and released into the bloodstream.

Nonlipophilic: A water-soluble substance; does not dissolve in fat.

Nonpolar: A lipophilic substance that has no charge.

Nutrients: The vitamins, minerals, fatty acids, and amino acids the body needs for metabolism and repair; sometimes taken as supplements to satisfy extra demands, effect repair, and prevent degeneration of body systems.

Organic: A chemical that contains carbon and hydrogen atoms, of biologic origin.

Oxidation: The process by which an electron is removed from a molecule, which changes its chemical properties; also the process of adding oxygen to a molecule.

Oxygenation: To treat, combine, or infuse with oxygen; to increase the concentration of oxygen.

Ozone: A gas composed of three oxygen atoms to a molecule; readily removes electrons from other molecules (oxidation) and is a major ingredient in smog.

Parasite: Microscopic and macroscopic organisms that live on or within other organisms to obtain nourishment and shelter. The relationship can be temporary or permanent.

Peristalsis: An involuntary, wavelike motion that occurs in the hollow tubes of the body, especially the intestines.

Peroxidation: A chemical reaction in which free radicals destroy the fats in cell membranes, damaging the cell structure.

Pesticide: A chemical that kills unwanted insects, rodents, weeds, or other pests; includes insecticides, herbicides, and fungicides.

Phagocytosis: The ingestion of bacteria and viruses by white blood cells.

Phase I detoxification: Metabolism of a nonpolar, non–water soluble chemical into a relatively polar compound; changes the chemical so that Phase II can easily add a small molecule.

Phase II detoxification: Chemical groups are added, or conjugated, to the chemical, which becomes water-soluble and can be excreted through the kidneys.

Polycyclic aromatic hydrocarbons (PAH): Precancerous chemicals found in cigarette smoke; highly reactive chemicals composed of hydrogen and carbon.

Post-traumatic stress disorder: A disease caused by a psychologically distressing event outside the range of usual human experience; symptoms include feelings of anxiety, terror, and helplessness, as well as sleep difficulties and re-experiencing the traumatic event.

Prostaglandins: Hormone-like chemicals that regulate cell activity.

Psychoneuroimmunology: A field that studies the ways in which the mind, central nervous system, hormonal system, and immune system interact.

Radiation: The emission and transmission of waves or particles of energy, including light, heat, radio, television, microwave, ultraviolet, X-ray, and others.

Radiation therapy: The administration of radioactive substances to or in the body for therapeutic procedures.

Reduction: The process of adding electrons to a molecule, which changes its chemical properties; also the process of removing oxygen from a molecule.

Reference doses (RfDs): A dose established by the Environmental Protection Agency (EPA) for the amount of a substance that can be consumed daily without a significant lifetime risk, with a safety factor of 100% in the calculations.

Sick building syndrome: A cluster of symptoms exhibited by a large percentage of workers in a particular building, including eye, nose, and throat irritation; headaches; dizziness; and decreased concentration. The specific cause of the symptoms is usually not identified.

Susceptibility: The state of being sensitive to an external agent; alternative term for sensitivity.

Sympathetic nervous system: Part of the autonomic nervous system that controls independent reactions in the body, such as heart rate, pupil size, and gastrointestinal tract movement.

Synergism: An interaction in which the effect of two or more substances together is greater than the sum of their separate effects.

Teratogen: A substance that causes birth defects.

Terpenes: Naturally occurring chemicals that give plants their characteristic smell and taste. They are present year-round, but their concentration increases just before the plant pollinates.

Tincture: A solution in which the solvent (dissolving liquid) is an alcohol.

Toxic bioaccumulation: Accumulation of toxic lipophilic (fat-soluble) chemicals in the body.

Toxin: Any substance or condition that is harmful to the body.

Trace metals: Metals found in minute quantities in the body, which are essential for proper body functioning.

Transit time: The amount of time it takes digested food to pass through the small and large intestines.

Triglycerides: The building blocks of fat; a compound of three fatty acids and one glycerol molecule.

Vaccination: The injection of a killed or attenuated (weakened) organism as a means of producing immunity against that organism.

Virus: A microscopic organism that reproduces within a living cell and is responsible for many human diseases.

Vital force: A person's interconnected energetic and defense processes.

Volatile organic chemicals (VOCs): Substances containing carbon that produce fumes easily; a precursor to smog; many are known or suspected carcinogens.

Water soluble: Chemicals that dissolve in water, but not in fat, oils, or other solvents.

Xenobiotic: A chemical foreign to the body, including drugs, chemicals, and insecticides.

Yang: One of the two complementary qualities of Chinese philosophy; it is positive, masculine, big, light, and represents expansiveness.

Yeast: In healthcare it refers to a body yeast, usually a *Candida* species, which causes chronic infections if the balance of the body is upset and an overgrowth of the yeast occurs.

Yin: One of the two complementary qualities of Chinese philosophy; it is negative, feminine, small, dark, and represents contractiveness.

Yoga: A system of breathing movements and postures that exercises the body and coordinates breathing with posture.

Suggested Reading

Allergy Relief and Prevention (3rd ed.), Jacqueline
   A. Krohn, Frances A. Taylor, and Erla Mae
   Larson. Hartley & Marks, Point Roberts, WA,
   2000.
The full gamut of allergies, allergy treatments,
and allergy prevention is presented. This book includes a complete discussion of the body and systems in relation to allergy. Treatment, both by self
and by professionals, is discussed in detail, including nutritional and natural therapies.

Alternative Healing, Mark Kastner and Hugh Burroughs. Halcyon Publishing, La Mesa, CA, 1996.
This very informative book discusses over 160
different alternative therapies. It allows the
reader to understand other methods that help
fight disease, maintain good health, and promote
happiness, naturally.

Alternative Medicine: The Definitive Guide, com-
   piled by the Burton Goldberg Group. Future
   Medicine Publishing, Puyallup, WA, 1993.
Three hundred and fifty leading-edge physicians
explain their treatments in this very comprehensive book. It describes effective therapies, as well
as affordable self-help cures.

The Chelation Way, Morton Walker. Avery Publishing Group, Garden City Park, NY, 1990.
The full scope of chelation therapy is covered in
this easy-to-read book. Dr. Walker has been very
thorough, and a partial list of physicians using
chelation in the United States, England, Mexico,
Holland, New Zealand, and West Germany is
included.

Chemical Sensitivity, volumes 1–4, William J.
   Rea. Lewis Publishers, Boca Raton, FL,
   1992–96.
Knowledge of chemistry is helpful when reading
these very scholarly and well-researched books on
chemical sensitivity. Mechanisms of chemical
sensitivity are presented, including biochemical
pathways. Discussion includes the role of nutrients in sensitivity as well as treatment.

*Desktop Guide to Keynotes and Confirmatory Symp-
   toms*, Roger Morrison. Hahnemann Clinic
   Publishing, Albany, CA, 1993.
Keynotes and confirmatory symptoms for homeopathic remedies are presented with accuracy
and clarity, making this a very usable and helpful
reference book. Both newcomers to homeopathy,

555

as well as the experienced homeopath, will find this book valuable.

Earl Mindell's Herb Bible, Earl Mindell. Simon and Schuster, NY, 1992.
This book explains the herbal remedies available today and how they can improve the way we work, play, sleep, feel, and heal. It also covers the use of commercially prepared herbal remedies, free of synthetics and side effects.

Earl Mindell's Vitamin Bible for the 21st Century, Earl Mindell. Warner Books, New York, 1999.
Earl Mindell, a pharmacist and nutritionist, discusses the full scope of vitamins and nutritional supplements, and their effect on your health. In addition, this book contains expanded sections on nutraceuticals, homeopathy, aromatherapy, and herbal medicine.

Everybody's Guide to Homeopathic Medicine, Stephen Cummings and Dana Ullman. Jeremy P. Tarcher, CA, 1998.
Taking care of yourself and your family with safe and effective remedies is the focus. Accurate prescribing for numerous conditions is presented, along with advice on when to seek professional medical care.

Finding the Right Treatment, Jacqueline Krohn and Frances Taylor. Hartley & Marks, Point Roberts, WA, 1999.
This is a comprehensive guide to getting the best from the worlds of modern and alternative medicine. It is a handbook for becoming informed about all of your healthcare options, and a practical guide to finding the right treatment, as well as the right prevention.

Health and Healing, Andrew Weil. Dorling-Kindersley, NY, 1995.
Alternative medicine, its merits and treatments are discussed, as is traditional or standard medicine. The reader can gain a true understanding of the options for treatment of many different conditions.

Industrial Toxicology: Safety and Health, Phillip L. Williams and James L. Burson. Van Nostrand Reinhold, NY, 1989.
This book discusses various toxins, their effects on the body, and the systems affected. Toxicological cases are presented as detective stories. This book is relatively easy to read for the lay person.

The Natural Pharmacy, Skye Lininger, Jonathan Wright, Steve Austin, Donald Brown, and Alan Gaby. Prima Health, Rocklin, CA, 1998.
Covering all major ailments and conditions, these experts have included guidance on herbs, nutritional supplements, and homeopathy to treat each medical problem. Doses and timing are presented for all treatments, as well as possible side effects and interactions.

Prescription for Nutritional Healing, James F. Balch and Phyllis A. Balch. Avery Publishing Group, Garden City Park, NY, 1997.
The authors present a practical A–Z reference to drug-free remedies using vitamins, minerals, herbs, and food supplements. It provides all of the information needed for the average person to design his or her own nutritional program for better health.

Root Canal Cover-up, George Meinig. Bion Publishing, Ojai, CA, 1994.
A founder of the Association of Root Canal

Specialists discusses the damage root canals can do to your health.

Scientific Validation of Herbal Medicine, Daniel B. Mowrey. Keats Publishing, New Canaan, CT, 1990.

Herbal medicine is related to clinical medicine in this excellent book. The action of the herbs is presented, conditions for use are described, and methods for administration are discussed.

Tired or Toxic? Sherry A. Rogers. Prestige Publishing, Syracuse, NY, 1990.

Dr. Rogers discusses the effects toxins may have on the body. Many people may not be simply tired; they may be toxic. Detoxification methods for both the body and environment are presented. Although much valuable information is presented, it is difficult to find because the index is not comprehensive.

Toxicological Chemistry, Stancy E. Manahan. Lewis Publishers, Boca Raton, FL, 1992.

The chemistry of substances toxic to man are presented with simplicity and clarity. Knowledge of chemistry is helpful, but not necessary.

Vibrational Medicine, Richard Gerber. Bear & Company, Santa Fe, NM, 1988.

This excellent book on energetic medicine covers many alternative methods for diagnosis and healing. By enlightening the reader regarding these therapies, choices for treatment and health are greatly increased.

Wellness Against All Odds, Sherry A. Rogers. Prestige Publishing, Syracuse, NY, 1994.

Dr. Rogers discusses treatment and defense against toxic insults from the environment. She also includes dietary and nutritional information.

Recommended Sources and Organizations

Tʜᴇ ꜰᴏʟʟᴏᴡɪɴɢ ꜱᴏᴜʀᴄᴇꜱ and organizations represent only the products and companies with which we are familiar. Certainly, there are other sources and other products that would be of benefit in detoxification and in restoring and maintaining health.

Professional Organizations and Schools

AAEM
American Academy of
  Environmental Medicine
c/o American Finance Center
7701 East Kellog, Suite 625
Wichita, KS 67207
(316) 684-5500
Fax: (316) 684-5709

AAOA
American Academy of Otolaryngic
  Allergy
8455 Colesville Road, Suite 745
Silver Springs, MD 20910
(310) 588-1800

Acupuncture Foundation of
  Canada
2131 Lawrence Ave. E., Suite 204
Scarborough, ON M1R 5G4
(416) 752-4398

American Association of
  Acupuncture and Oriental
  Medicine
4104 Lake Boone Trail, Suite 201
Raleigh, NC 27607
(919) 787-5181

American Association of
  Naturopathic Physicians
601 Valley St., Suite 105
Seattle, WA 98109
(206) 298-0126
Fax: (206) 298-0129

American Botanical Council
P.O. Box 201660
Austin, TX 78720
(512) 331-8868

American Chiropractic
  Association
1701 Clarendon Blvd.
Arlington, VA 22209
(703) 276-8800

American College for Advancement in Medicine (ACAM)
23121 Verdugo Drive, Suite 204
Laguna Hills, CA 92653
(714) 583-7666
(800) 532-3680

American Massage Therapy
  Association
820 Davis St., Suite 100
Evanston, IL 60201
(847) 864-0123
(847) 864-1178

American Osteopathic Association
142 E. Ontario Street
Chicago, IL 60611
(800) 621-1773

American School of Ayurvedic
  Science
2115 112th Ave. NE
Bellevue, WA 98004
(425) 453-8022
Fax: (425) 451-2670

Canadian Chiropractic Association
1396 Eglinton Ave. W.
Toronto, ON M6C 2E4
(416) 781-5656
Fax: (416) 781-7344

Canadian College of Naturopathic
  Medicine
2300 Yonge St., 18th Floor
P.O. Box 2431
Toronto, ON M4P 1E4
(416) 486-8584
Fax: (416) 484-6821

Canadian Massage Therapist
  Association
365 Bloor St. E., Suite 1807
Toronto, ON M4W 3L4
(416) 968-6487
1 (800) 668-2022 (Canada only)
Fax: (416) 968-6818

Canadian Memorial Chiropractic
  College
1900 Bayview Ave.
Toronto, ON M4G 3E6
(416) 482-2340
Fax: (416) 482-9745

Canadian Network of Toxicology
  Centres
Bovey Building, Gordon Street
University of Guelph
Guelph, ON N1G 2W1
(519) 837-3320
Fax: (519) 837-3861

Institute of Chinese Herbology
5459 Shaffer Ave.
Oakland, CA 94618
(510) 428-2061
Fax: (510) 420-1039

International Institute of Chinese
  Medicine
P.O. Box 4991
Santa Fe, NM 87502
(505) 473-5233
(800) 377-4561

International Society for
  Orthomolecular Medicine
16 Florence Ave.
Toronto, ON M2N 1E9

(416) 733-2117
Fax: (416) 733-2352

National Center for Homeopathy
801 N. Fairfax Street, Suite 306
Alexandria, VA 22314
(703) 548-7790
Fax: (703) 548-7792

The Rolf Institute
205 Canyon Blvd.
Boulder, CO 80302
(800) 530-8875

Shiatsu School of Canada
547 College Street
Toronto, ON M6G 1A9
(416) 323-1818
1-800-263-1703

Detoxification Units

Center for Environmental
  Medicine
Dr. Allan Lieberman
7510 Northforest Drive
North Charleston, SC 29420
(843) 572-1600
Fax: (843) 572-1795

Environmental Health Center
Dr. William Rea
8345 Walnut Hill Lane,
  Suite 220
Dallas, TX 75231
(214) 368-4132
Fax: (214) 691-8432

Healing Naturally
Dr. Walter Crinnion
11811 NE 128th St., Suite 202
Kirkland, WA 98034
(425) 821-8118
Fax: (425) 821-4353

Preventive Medical Center of
  Marin
Dr. Elson Haas

25 Mitchell, #8
San Rafael, CA 94903
(415) 472-2343
Fax: (415) 472-7636

Robbins Environmental Medicine
  Clinic
Dr. Albert Robbins
400 S. Dixie Highway, Building 2,
  Suite 210
Boca Raton, FL 33432
(561) 395-3282
Fax: (561) 395-3304

Hands-On Techniques

BioSET™
Dr. Ellen Cutler
P.O. Box 5356
Larkspur, CA 94977
(877) 927-0741
Fax: (415) 945-0465

CRA™
Contact Reflex Analysis™ and
  Nutrition Research Foundation
Dr. D. A. Versendaal
P.O. Box 914
Jenison, MI 49429-0914
E-mail: dhoezee@i2k.com

NAET
Nambudripad's Allergy
  Elimination Technique
Dr. Devi Nambudripad
6714 Beach Blvd.
Buena Park, CA 90621
(714) 523-8900
Fax: (714) 523-3068

NET
NeuroEmotional Technique
Dr. Scott Walker
524 Second Street
Encinitas, CA 92024
(619) 944-1030
(800) 888-4638
Fax: (619) 753-7191

NRT
Nutritional Reflex Technique
Dr. Gary S. Lasneski
P.O. Box 505
Hadley, MA 01035
(413) 587-3151

TBM
Total Body Modification
Dr. Victor Frank
1907 E. Foxmoor Circle
Sandy, UT 84092
(801) 571-2411
(800) 243-4826
Fax: (801) 567-0806

Supplies

AIR CLEANERS
AllerMed Corporation
31 Steel Road
Wylie, TX 75098
(972) 442-4898
Fax: (972) 442-4897

Foust Air Purifiers
E. L. Foust Company, Inc.
P.O. Box 105
Elmhurst, IL 60126
(630) 834-4952
(800) 225-9549
Fax: (630) 834-5341

CERAMIC OXYGEN MASKS
American Environmental Health
Foundation
8345 Walnut Hill Lane, Suite 225
Dallas, TX 75231-4262
(214) 361-9515
(800) 428-2343
Fax: (214) 691-8432

ELECTROMAGNETIC
ELF Teslar
State Route 1, Box 21
St. Francisville, IL 62460
(618) 948-2393

Fax: (618) 948-2650
(watches)

Ener-G Polari-T
P.O. Box 2449
Prescott, AZ 86302-2449
(520) 778-5039
Fax: (520) 771-0611
(diodes)

EnviroTech
17171 S.E. 29th Street
Choctaw, OK 73020
(405) 390-3499
(magnets)

Essentia
100 Bronson, Suite 1001
Ottawa, ON K1R 6G8
(613) 238-4437
Fax: (613) 235-5876
(EMF meters, full-spectrum lights,
  air systems)

Radon Environmental Monitoring
3334 Commercial Ave.
Northbrook, IL 60062
(847) 205-0110
Fax: (847) 205-0114

Tachyon Energy Research
4400 186th Street
Redondo Beach, CA 90278
(800) 888-2509 (orders only)
(310) 542-3035 (direct)
Fax: (310) 542-3685
(tachyon beads)

HERBAL
Eclectic Institute
14385 S.E. Lusted Road
Sandy, OR 97055
(503) 668-4120
(800) 332-4372
Fax: (503) 668-3227

Gaia Herbs
108 Island Ford Road

Bervard, NC 28712
(828) 884-4242
(800) 831-7780
Fax: (828) 883-5960

MarcoPharma International
1857 N. 105 East Ave.
Tulsa, OK 74116
(918) 833-5060
Fax: (918) 833-5061
(Herbs and drainage remedies)

HOME SAUNAS
Heavenly Heat
1106 Second St.
Encinitas, CA 92024
(760) 942-0478
(800) 697-2862
Fax: (760) 634-1268

ENVIRONMENTAL HEALTH
SUPPLIES
N.E.E.D.S.
(National Ecological and
  Environmental Delivery System)
527 Charles Ave., Suite 12-A
Syracuse, NY 13209
(800) 634-1380
Fax: (315) 488-6336
Fax: (800) 295-6333 (orders)

HOMEOPATHIC
APEX Energetics
1701 E. Edinger Ave., Suite A-4
Santa Ana, CA 92705
(714) 973-7733
(800) 736-4381 (orders)
Fax: (714) 973-2238
Fax: (888) 286-1676 (orders)
(complex and drainage remedies)

BHI Homeopathic Products
11600 Cochiti, S.E.
Albuquerque, NM 87123
(505) 293-3843
(800) 621-7644
Fax: (505) 275-1642

(classical and complex remedies, Oscillococcinum®, Enggstol®, Traumeel®)

Boiron
East Coast:
Campus Boulevard Building A
Newtown Square, PA 19073
West Coast:
98C W. Cochran St.
Simi Valley, CA 93065
(800) 258-8823
(classical remedies)

Dolisos America
3014 Rigel Ave.
Las Vegas, NV 89102
(702) 871-7153
(800) 365-4767
Fax: (702) 871-9670
(classical remedies)

Homeopathic Educational Services
2124 Kittredge Street
Berkeley, CA 94704
(510) 649-0294
(800) 359-9051 (orders only)
(educational materials)

PHP Professional Health Products
211 Overlook Dr., Suite 5
Sewickley, PA 15143
(800) 929-4133
Fax: (412) 741-6372
(complex remedies)

Vibrant Health
150 des Grands Couteau
St-Mathieu-de-Beloeil, PQ J36 2C9
(450) 536-1295
(888) 337-8427 (orders)
Fax: (450) 536-1294
(complex remedies)

MOLD TESTING
American Environmental Health Foundation
8345 Walnut Hill Lane, Suite 225
Dallas, TX 75231-4262
(214) 361-9515
(800) 428-2343
Fax: (214) 691-8432
(mold plates)

Mold Survey Service
Dr. Sherry A. Rogers
P.O. Box 2716
Syracuse, NY 13220
(315) 488-2856
(mold plates)

NEOLIFE PRODUCTS
NeoLife
GNLD Distributor Services
3500 Gateway Blvd.
Fremont, CA 94538
(510) 651-0405
(800) 432-5848
Fax: (510) 440-2818
(NeoLife Green)

NUTRIENTS
AMNI
Advanced Medical Nutrition
600 Boyce Road
Pittsburgh, PA 15205
(800) 437-8888
Fax: (888) 245-4440
(organic germanium, hypoallergenic nutrients)

Biotics Research Corporation
6801 Biotics Research Dr.
Rosenberg, TX 77471
(281) 344-0909
(800) 231-5777
Fax: (281) 344-0725
(NutriClear, phytonutrients)

Ecological Formulas
(Cardiovascular Research/Arteria)
1061 B Shary Circle

Concord, CA 94518
(800) 351-9429
(hypoallergenic nutrients)

Ultra Balance Medical Foods
Division of Metagenics
5800 Soundview Dr.
Gig Harbor, WA 98335
(800) 843-9660
(253) 851-3943
Fax: (253) 851-9749
(UltraClear)

Klaire Laboratories (Vital Life Products)
140 Marine View Ave., Suite 110
Solana Beach, CA 92075
(760) 744-9680
Fax: (858) 350-7883
(hypoallergenic nutrients)

Nutricology/Allergy Research Group
P.O. Box 489
San Leandro, CA 94577
(800) 545-9960 (information)
(800) 782-4274 (orders)
Fax: (800) 688-7426
(570) 639-4572 (international orders)
(570) 635-6730 (international fax)
(hypoallergenic nutrients, organic germanium, BottomsUp (rectal nutrients))

Pain and Stress Therapy Center
Dr. Billie Sahley
5282 Medical Drive, Suite 160
San Antonio, TX 78229-6023
(800) 669-2256 (orders)
(210) 614-7256 (consultations)
Fax: (210) 614-4336
(specialty nutrients, Balanced Neurotransmitter Complex, Anxiety Control)

Standard Process
P.O. Box 904

1200 West Royal Lee Dr.
Palmyra, WI 53156
(414) 495-2122
(800) 848-5061 (customer service)
(800) 558-8740 (orders)
Fax: (414) 495-2512
Fax: (800) 438-3799 (orders)
(phytonutrients)

Thorne Research
P.O. Box 25
Dover, ID 83825
(208) 263-1337
Fax: (800) 747-1950
(hypoallergenic nutrients)

Twin Labs
150 Motor Parkway
Hauppauge, NY 11788
(516) 467-3140
(800) 645-5626 (outside NY)
Fax: (516) 630-3488
(hypoallergenic nutrients)

ORAL CHELATION FORMULAS
AMNI
Advanced Medical Nutrition
600 Boyce Road
Pittsburgh, PA 15205
(800) 437-8888
Fax: (888) 245-4440
(Oral Chelation Pack)

Longevity Plus
814 N. Beeline Hwy., Suite 1
Payson, AZ 85541
(800) 580-7587
Fax: (520) 474-3819
(Beyond Chelation)

SHOWER FILTERS
American Environmental Health
  Foundation
8345 Walnut Hill Lane, Suite 225
Dallas, TX 75231
(214) 361-9515
(800) 428-2343
Fax: (214) 691-8432

STABILIZED OXYGEN
Aerobic Life Industries
2916 N. 35th Ave., Suite 8
Phoenix, AZ 87017
(602) 455-6380
(800) 798-0707
(Aerobic 07, MgO_7, KO_7)

American Biologics
1180 Walnut Ave.
Chula Vista, CA 91911
(619) 429-8200
(800) 227-4473
Fax (619) 429-8004
(Dioxychlor®)

Good For You Canada Corporation
295 Midpark Way S.E., #210
Calgary, AB T2X 2A8
(403) 296-2816
(800) 661-8364
Fax (403) 254-8744
(Aerobic Oxygen)

Bibliography

Books

Ackerknecht, Erwin H. *A Short History of Medicine.* New York: The Ronald Press Company, 1968.

Anshutz, E. P. *New, Old, and Forgotten Remedies.* New Delhi, India: B. Jain Publishers Pvt., 1989.

Asai, Kazuhiko. *Miracle Cure—Organic Germanium.* Tokyo: Japan Publications, 1980.

Bailey, Janet. *Keeping Food Fresh.* Garden City, NY: The Dial Press, 1985.

Balch, James F., and Phyllis A. Balch. *Prescription for Nutritional Healing.* Garden City Park, NY: Avery Publishing Group, 1997.

Baran, R., and R.P.R. Dawber. *Diseases of the Nails and Their Management.* Boston: Blackwell Scientific Publications, 1984.

Bardswell, Frances A. *The Herb Garden.* Brattleboro, VT: Practical Press, 1987.

Beaver, Paul Chester, Rodney Clifton Jung, and Eddie Wayne Cupp. *Clinical Parasitology.* Philadelphia: Lea & Febiger, 1984.

Becker, Robert O. *Cross Currents.* Los Angeles: Jeremy P. Tarcher, 1990.

Becker, Robert O., and Gary Selden. *The Body Electric.* New York: Quill/William Morrow, 1985.

Beverly, Cal, ed. *Natural Health Secrets Encyclopedia.* Peachtree City, GA: F.C. & A. Publishing, 1991.

Bianchi, Ivo. *Principles of Homotoxicology,* vol. I. Baden-Baden, Germany: Aurelia-Verlag, 1989.

Blake, Michael. *The Natural Healer's Acupressure Handbook,* vol. I: Basic G–Jo. Fort Lauderdale: Falkynor Books, 1983.

Boericke, William. *Materia Medica with Repertory.* New Delhi, India: Homeopathic Publications, Indian ed., originally published 1927.

Boyd, Hamish. *Introduction to Homeopathic Medicine.* Beaconsfield, Bucks, England: Beaconsfield Publishers, 1981.

Braverman, Eric R., with Carl Pfeiffer. *The Healing Nutrients Within.* New Canaan, CT: Keats Publishing, 1987.

Briggs, Shirley A., and the staff of the Rachel Carson Council. *Basic Guide to Pesticides: Their Characteristics and Hazards.* Washington, D.C.: Taylor and Francis, 1992.

Brody, Jane E. *Jane Brody's Nutrition Book.* New York: W.W. Norton & Co., 1981.

Brostoff, Jonathon, and Stephen J. Challacombe, eds. *Food Allergy and Intolerance.* London: Bailliere Tindall, 1987.

Brown, Harold W., and Franklin A. Neva. *Basic Clinical Parasitology.* Norwalk, CT: Appleton-Century-Crofts, 1983.

Burger, Alfred. *Drugs and People*. Charlottesville, VA: University Press of Virginia, 1988.

Burton Goldberg Group, compilers. *Alternative Medicine: The Definitive Guide*. Puyallup, WA: Future Medicine Publishing, Inc., 1993.

Campion, Margaret Reid. *Hydrotherapy in Pediatrics*. Rockville, MD: An Aspen Publication, 1985.

Carter, Stephen K., Marie T. Bakowdki, and Kurt Hellman. *Chemotherapy of Cancer*. New York: John Wiley & Sons, 1977.

Castleman, Michael. *The Healing Herbs*. Emmaus, PA: Rodale Press, 1991.

Chabner, Bruce A., and Jerry M. Collins. *Cancer Chemotherapy*. Philadelphia: J.B. Lippincott Co., 1990.

Chaitow, Leon. *Amino Acids in Therapy*. Rochester, VT: Healing Arts Press, 1988.

Chaitow, L. *The Body/Mind Purification Program*. New York: Simon and Schuster, 1990.

Cheraskin, Emanuel, Marshall W. Ringsdorf, Jr., and Emily L. Sisley. *The Vitamin C Connection*. New York: Harper and Row, 1983.

Chopra, Deepak. *Perfect Health: The Complete Mind/Body Guide*. New York: Harmony Books, 1991.

Christopher, John R. *Dr. Christopher's Three-Day Cleansing Program, Mucusless Diet and Herbal Combinations*. Springville, UT: John R. Christopher, 1991.

Christopher, John R. *Herbal Home Health Care* (formerly *Childhood Diseases*). Springville, UT: Christopher Publications, 1976.

Clarke, John Henry. *A Dictionary of Practical Materia Medica*. New Delhi, India: Aggarwal Book Centre, originally published 1900.

Clendening, Logan. *Source Book of Medical History*. New York: Dover Publications, 1942.

Coffel, Steve, and Karyn Feiden. *Indoor Pollution*. New York: Ballantine Books, 1990.

Cooper, Kenneth H. *The Aerobics Program for Total Well-Being*. New York: Bantam Books, 1982.

Cott, Allan. *Fasting As a Way Of Life*. New York: Bantam Books, 1977.

Cridland, Marion D. *Fundamentals of Cancer Chemotherapy*. Baltimore: University Park Press, 1978.

Crompton, Paul. *The T'ai Chi Workbook*. Boston: Shambhala, 1987.

Cummings, Stephen and Dana Ullman. *Everybody's Guide to Homeopathic Medicines*. Los Angeles: Jeremy P. Tarcher, 1991.

Das, Bishamber. *Select Your Remedy*. New Delhi, India: Vishwamber Free Homeopathic Dispensary, 1991.

Davis, Jefferson C., and Thomas K. Hunt, eds. *Problem Wounds: The Role of Oxygen*. New York: Elsevier Science Publishing, 1988.

Donciger, Elizabeth. *Homeopathy: From Alchemy to Medicine*. Rochester, VT: Healing Arts Press, 1988.

Donegan, Jane B. *Hydropathic Highway to Health*. New York: Greenwood Press, 1986.

Dong, Paul, and Aristide H. Esser. *Chi Gong*. New York: Paragon House, 1990.

Dubrov, A.P. *The Geomagnetic Field and Life*. New York: Plenum Press, 1978.

Ebner, Maria. *Connective Tissue Massage*. Huntington, NY: Robert E. Krieger Publishing, 1962.

Edelstein, Ludwig. *Ancient Medicine*. Baltimore: The Johns Hopkins Press, 1967.

Editors of F, C, & A. *1,001 Home Health Remedies*. Peachtree City, GA: F, C, & A Publishing, 1993.

Evelyn, Nancy. *Herbal Medicine Chest*. Freedom, CA: Crossing Press, 1986.

Faelton, Sharon, and the editors of *Prevention Magazine*. *The Complete Book of Minerals for Health*. Emmaus, PA: Rodale Press, 1981.

Feinstein, Alice. *Training the Body to Cure Itself*. Emmaus, PA: Rodale Press, 1992.

Feltman, John, ed. *Prevention How-To Dictionary of Healing Remedies and Techniques*. Emmaus, PA: Rodale Press, 1992.

Fife, Bruce. *The Detox Book*. Colorado Springs, CO: Health Wise Publications, 1997.

Fischer, B., and others. *Handbook of Hyperbaric Oxygen Therapy*. New York: Springer-Verlag, 1988.

Foote, Clara Kroeger, and Jerald Foote. *How to Counteract Environmental Poisons*. Boulder, CO: Chapel of Miracles, 1990.

Frey, William. *Crying: The Mystery of Tears*. Minneapolis, MN: Winston Press, 1985.

Gach, Michael Reed. *Acupressure's Potent Points*. New York: Bantam Books, 1990.

Gardner, Joy. *Healing Yourself*. Seattle, WA: Healing Yourself, 1982.

Garrison, Fielding H. *An Introduction to the History of Medicine*. Philadelphia: W. B. Saunders, 1914.

Gauquelin, Michel. *How Cosmic and Atmospheric Energies Influence Your Health*. Santa Fe, NM: Aurora Press, 1984.

Gerber, Richard. *Vibrational Medicine*. Santa Fe, NM: Bear and Company, 1988.

Gerras, Charles, Joseph Golant, and E. John Hanna, eds. *The Complete Book of Vitamins*. Emmaus, PA: Rodale Press, 1977.

Goodenough, Josephus, compiler and ed. *Dr. Goodenough's Home Cures and Herbal Remedies*. New York: Avenel Books; Crown Publishers, 1982.

Gordon, Benjamin Lee. *Medicine Throughout Antiquity*. Philadelphia: F.A. Davis, 1949.

Green, James. *Herbal Medicine Maker's Handbook*. Forestville, CA: Simplers Botanical, 1990.

Green, Nancy Sokol. *Poisoning Our Children*. Chicago, IL: The Noble Press, 1991.

Grieve, Mrs. M. *A Modern Herbal*, vol. I and II. Mineola, NY: Dover Publications, 1971.

Haas, Elson M. *The Detox Diet*. Berkeley, CA: Celestial Arts, 1996.

Hallenbeck, W.H., and K.M. Cunningham-Burns. *Pesticides and Human Health*. New York: Springer-Verlag, 1985.

Harte, John, Cheryl Holdren, Richard Schneider, and Christine Shirley. *Toxics A to Z*. Berkley, CA: University of California Press, 1991.

Harvey, Clare G., and Amanda Cochrane. *The Encyclopaedia of Flower Remedies*. London: Thorsons, 1995.

Hittleman, Richard. *Yoga 28 Day Exercise Plan*. New York: Workman Publishing, 1969.

Hobbs, Christopher. *Natural Liver Therapy*. Capitola, CA: Botanica Press, 1988.

Hobbs, Christopher. *Super Immunity: Herbs and Other Natural Remedies for a Healthy Immune System*. Capitola, CA: Botanica Press, 1985.

Hobbs, Christopher. *Usnea: Herbal Antibiotic*. Capitola, CA: Botanica Press, 1984.

Hoffer, Abram. *Orthomolecular Medicine for Physicians*. New Canaan, CT: Keats Publishing, 1989.

Hoffman, David. *The Herbal Handbook: A User's Guide to Medical Herbalism*. Rochester, VT: Healing Arts Press, 1987.

Hoffman, David. *The Holistic Herbal*. Shaftesbury, Dorset, England: Element Books, 1988.

Hoffman, Matthew, William LeGro, and editors of *Prevention Magazine*. *Disease Free*. Emmaus, PA: Rodale Press, 1993.

Hoffman, Ronald L. *Tired All the Time*. New York: Poseidon Press, 1993.

Hubbard, L. Ron. *Clear Body, Clear Mind*. Los Angeles: Bridge Publications, 1990.

Huggins, Hal A., and Sharon A. Huggins. *It's All in Your Head*. Colorado Springs, CO: Huggins, 1985.

Hylton, William H., ed. *The Rodale Herb Book*. Emmaus, PA: Rodale Press Book Division, 1974.

Inlander, Charles B., and Ed Weiner. *Take This Book to the Hospital With You*. Emmaus, PA: Rodale Press, 1985.

Jensen, Bernard. *Nature Has A Remedy*. Escondido, CA: Dr. Bernard Jensen, 1978.

Joklik, Wolfgang K., et al. *Zinsser Microbiology*. Norwalk, CT: Appleton and Lange, 1988.

Jouanny, Jacques. *The Essentials of Homeopathic Materia Medica*. Boiron S.A., France: Editions Boiron, 1984.

Juhan, Deane. *Job's Body: A Handbook for Bodywork*. Barrytown, NY: Station Hill Press, 1987.

Justice, Blair. *Who Gets Sick: Thinking and Health*. Houston: Peak Press, 1987.

Kahn, Farrol S. *Why Flying Endangers Your Health: Hidden Health Hazards of Airline Travel.* Santa Fe, NM: Aurora Press, 1992.

Kale, W. S. *Your Health, Your Moods, and the Weather.* New York: Doubleday, 1982.

Kastner, Mark, and Hugh Burroughs. *Alternative Healing.* La Mesa, CA: Halcyon Publishing, 1996.

Kent, John Tyler. *Repertory of Homeopathic Materia Medica.* New Delhi, India: Homeopathic Publications, Indian ed. Reprinted from the Sixth American Edition, n.d.

Kime, Zane R. *Sunlight Could Save Your Life.* Penryn, CA: World Health Publications, 1980.

Kisner, Carolyn, and Lynn Allen Colby. *Therapeutic Exercise Foundations and Techniques.* Philadelphia: F.A. Davis Company, 1990.

Kostias, John. *The Essential Movements of T'ai Chi.* Brookline, MA: Paradigm Publications, 1989.

Krieger, Dolores. *Accepting Your Power to Heal.* Santa Fe, NM: Bear and Company, 1993.

Kroeger, Hanna. *Instant Herbal Locator.* Boulder, CO: Hanna Kroeger, 1979.

Krohn, Jacqueline, et al. *A Guide to the Identification and Treatment of Biocatalyst and Biochemical Intolerances.* Los Alamos, NM: J. Krohn, 1989.

Krohn, Jacqueline, and Frances A. Taylor. *Finding the Right Treatment.* Point Roberts, WA: Hartley & Marks, 1999.

Krohn, Jacqueline, Frances Taylor, and Erla Mae Larson. *The Whole Way To Allergy Relief and Prevention.* Point Roberts, WA: Hartley & Marks, 1996.

Kushi, Michio. *The Macrobiotic Way: The Complete Macrobiotic Diet and Exercise Book.* Wayne, NJ: Avery Publishing Group, 1985.

LaDou, Joseph. *Occupational Medicine.* Norwalk, CT: Appleton and Lange, 1990.

Lappe, Marc. *Chemical Deception.* San Francisco: Sierra Club, 1991.

Levine, Stephen, and Parris M. Kidd. *Antioxidant Adaptation.* San Leandro, CA: Biocurrents Division, Allergy Research Group, 1986.

Liberman, Jacob. *Light: Medicine of the Future.* Santa Fe, NM: Bear Publishing, 1991.

Licht, Sidney Herman, ed. *Massage, Manipulation and Traction.* New Haven, CT: Elizabeth Licht, 1960.

Lininger, Skye, Jonathan Wright, Steve Austin, Donald Brown, and Alan Gaby. *The Natural Pharmacy.* Rocklin, CA: Prima Health, 1998.

Ludlum, David M. *The Audubon Society Field Guide to North American Weather.* New York: Alfred A. Knopf, 1991.

Lust, John, and Michael Tierra. *The Natural Remedy Bible.* New York: Pocket Books, 1990.

Mairesse, Michelle. *Health Secrets of Medicinal Herbs.* New York: Arco Publishing, 1981.

Majno, Guido. *The Healing Hand: A Commonwealth Fund Book.* Cambridge, MA: Harvard University Press, 1975.

Makower, Joel. *Office Hazards: How Your Job Can Make You Sick.* Washington, D.C.: Tilden Press, 1981.

Male, David. *Immunology: An Illustrated Outline.* St. Louis, MO: The C.V. Mosby Company, 1986.

Manahan, Stanley E. *Toxicological Chemistry.* Chelsea, MI: Lewis Publishers, 1992.

Manning, Clark A., and Louis J. Vanrenen. *Bioenergetic Medicines East and West: Acupuncture and Homeopathy.* Berkeley, CA: North Atlantic Books, 1988.

Martin, Eric W. *Hazards of Medication.* Philadelphia: J.B. Lippincott, 1978.

McCann, Michael. *Artist Beware.* New York: The Lyons Press, 1992.

McGilvery, Robert W., and Gerald W. Goldstein. *Biochemistry: A Functional Approach.* Philadelphia: W. B. Saunders, 1983.

McGrew, Roderick Erle. *Encyclopedia of Medical History.* New York: McGraw Hill, 1985.

Meinig, George. *Root Canal Cover-up.* Ojai, CA: Bion Publishing, 1994.

Miller, Neil Z. *Vaccines: Are They Really Safe and Effective?* Santa Fe, NM: New Atlantean Press, 1992.

Mindell, Earl. *Earl Mindell's Herb Bible.* New York: Simon and Schuster, 1992.

▌ *Bibliography* ▌

Mindell, Earl. *Earl Mindell's Vitamin Bible*. New York: Warner Books, 1979.

Mindell, Earl. *Earl Mindell's Vitamin Bible for the 21st Century*. New York: Warner Books, 1999.

Morrison, Roger. *Desktop Companion to Physical Pathology*. Nevada City, CA: Hahnemann Clinic Publishing, 1998.

Morrison, Roger. *Desktop Guide to Keynotes and Confirmatory Symptoms*. Albany, CA: Hahnemann Clinic Publishing, 1993.

Moss, Ralph, W. *Questioning Chemotherapy*. Brooklyn: Equinox Press, 1995.

Mowrey, Daniel B. *Next Generation Herbal Medicine*. New Canaan, CT: Keats Publishing, 1990.

Mowrey, Daniel B. *The Scientific Validation of Herbal Medicine*. New Canaan, CT: Keats Publishing, 1986.

Murphy, Robin. *Homeopathic Medical Repertory*. Pagosa Springs, CO: Hahnemann Academy of North America, 1993.

Murphy, Robin. *Lotus Materia Medica*. Pagosa Springs, CO: Lotus Star Academy, 1995.

Namikoshi, Toru. *Shiatsu + Stretching*. Tokyo: Japan Publications, 1985.

Niaz, Sarfaraz K. *The Omega Connection*. Oak Brook, IL: Esquire Books, 1987.

Nuzzi, Debra. *Pocket Herbal Reference Guide*. Freedom, CA: Crossing Press, 1992.

Pangborn, Jon B. *Nutrition, Amino Acids, and Human Metabolism*. Lisle, IL: Bionostics, n.d.

Page, Linda. *Detoxification*. Carmel Valley, CA: Healthy Healing Publications, 1999.

Pauling, Linus. *Vitamin C, the Common Cold, and the Flu*. San Francisco: W.H. Freeman, 1976.

Pelletier, Kenneth R. *Holistic Medicine: From Stress to Optimum Health*. New York: Dell Publishing, 1979.

Pfeiffer, C. C. *Mental and Elemental Nutrients*. New Canaan, CT: Keats Publishing, 1975.

Philpott, William H., with Shawn Taplin. *Biomagnetic Handbook: A Guide to Medical Magnets—The Energy Medicine of Tomorrow*. Choctaw, OK: Envirotech Products, 1990.

Pischinger, Alfred. Edited by Hortmut Heine. *Matrix and Matrix Regulation: Basis for a Holistic Theory in Medicine*. Brussels, Belgium: Haug Internationals, 1991.

Purdom, Walton, ed. *Environmental Health*. San Diego, CA: Academic Press, 1980.

Rainey, Jean, in cooperation with The Consumer Advisory Committee of the National Association of Food Chains. *How to Shop for Food*. New York: Barnes and Noble, 1972.

Rea, William J. *Chemical Sensitivity*, vol. 1–4. Boca Raton, FL: Lewis Publishers, 1992–96.

Reader's Digest Magic and Medicine of Plants. Pleasantville, NY: The Reader's Digest Association, 1986.

Reckeweg, Hans-Heinrich. *Homotoxicology: Illness and Healing Through Anti-homotoxic Therapy*. Albuquerque, NM: Menaco Publishing, 1989.

Rest, Kathleen M. *Advancing the Understanding of Multiple Chemical Sensitivity*. Princeton, NJ: Princeton Scientific Publishing, 1992.

Riggs, Maribeth. *Natural Child Care: A Complete Guide to Safe and Effective Herbal Remedies and Holistic Health Strategies for Infants and Children*. New York: Harmony Books, 1989.

Rippon, John Willard. *Medical Mycology*. Philadelphia: W.B. Saunders, 1982.

Rogers, Sherry A. *Wellness Against All Odds*. Syracuse, NY: Prestige Publishing, 1994.

Rogers, Sherry A. *Tired or Toxic?* Syracuse, NY: Prestige Publishing, 1990.

Rogers, Sherry A. *You Are What You Ate. An Rx for the Resistant Diseases of the 21st Century*. Syracuse, NY: Prestige Publishing, 1988.

Ross, A.C., M.B. Gordon, and M.F. Hom. *The Amazing Healer Arnica*. Wellingborough, Northamptonshire, England: Thorsons Publishers, 1977.

Rousseau, David. *Creating a Healthy Home*. Point Roberts, WA: Hartley & Marks, 1996.

Saifer, Phyllis, and Merla Zellerbach. *Detox*. Los Angeles: Jeremy P. Tarcher, 1984.

Samet Jonathan M., and John D. Spengler. *Indoor Air Pollution: A Health Perspective*. Baltimore: The Johns Hopkins University Press, 1991.

Schause, Alexander G. *Aloe Vera*. Tacoma, WA: American Institute for Biochemical Research, 1990.

Seelig, Mildred S. *Magnesium Deficiency in the Pathogenesis of Disease*. New York: Plenum Medical Book Co., 1980.

Seelig, Mildred S. *Magnesium in Health and Disease*. New York: Medical and Scientific Books Division of Spectrum Publications, 1979.

Shandler, Nina. *Estrogen, The Natural Way*. New York: Villard, 1997.

Shaw, Non. *Bach Flower Remedies: A Step-by-Step Guide*. Boston: Element Books, 1998.

Sherris, John C., et al. *Medical Microbiology*. New York: Elsevier Science Publishing, 1984.

Siegel, Bernie S. *Peace, Love and Healing*. New York: Harper & Row, 1989.

Siegel, Bernie S. *Love, Medicine and Miracles*. New York: Harper & Row, 1986.

Sigerist, Henry E. *A History of Medicine*, vol. I and II. New York: Oxford University Press, 1951.

Smith, Cyril, and Simon Best. *Electromagnetic Man*. New York: St. Martin's Press, 1989.

Smits, Tinus. *Practical Materia Medica for the Consulting Room*. 5581 J M Waalre, Holland: Tinus Smits, 1993.

Spence, Alexander P., and Elliott B. Mason. *Human Anatomy and Physiology*. Menlo Park, CA: Benjamin/Cummings Publishing, 1987.

Stone, Irwin. *The Healing Factor: Vitamin C Against Disease*. New York: Perigee Books, 1982.

Stryer, Lubert. *Biochemistry*. New York: W.H. Freeman, 1988.

Sullivan, John B. Jr., and Gary P. Krieger. *Hazardous Materials Toxicology: Clinical Principles of Environmental Health*. Baltimore: Williams and Wilkins, 1992.

Tappan, Frances. *Healing Massage Techniques*. Norwalk, CT: Appleton & Lange, 1988.

Tarcher, Alyce Bezman, ed. *Principles and Practice of Environmental Medicine*. New York: Plenum Medical, 1992.

Tenney, Louise. *Today's Herbal Health*. Provo, UT: Woodland Books, 1983.

Thrash, Agatha, and Calvin Thrash. *Home Remedies*. Seale, AL: Thrash Publications, 1981.

Tierra, Michael. Edited and supplemented by Dr. David Frawley. *Planetary Herbology*. Santa Fe, NM: Lotus Press, 1989.

Trattler, Ross. *Better Health Through Natural Healing*. New York: McGraw-Hill, 1985.

Ullman, Dana. *Homeopathic Medicine for Children and Infants*. New York: Jeremy P. Tarcher/Perigee Books, 1992.

Ullman, Dana. *Discovering Homeopathy*. Berkeley, CA: North Atlantic Books, 1991.

Valnet, Jean. *The Practice of Aromatherapy*. Rochester, NY: Healing Arts Press, 1990.

Vander, Arthur J., James H. Sherman, and Dorothy S. Luciano. *Human Physiology*. New York: McGraw-Hill, 1998.

Vlamis, Gregory. *Bach Flower Remedies to the Rescue*. Rochester, VT: Healing Arts Press, 1990.

Wade, Carlson. *Inner Cleansing*. West Nyack, NY: Parker Publishing, 1992.

Walker, J. Frederic. *Formaldehyde*. New York: Reinhold Publishing, 1964.

Walker, Morton. *The Chelation Way*. Garden City Park, NY: Avery Publishing Group, 1990.

Walsh, James Joseph. *Medieval Medicine*. London: A.& C. Black, 1920.

Weider, Ben, and David Hapgood. *The Murder of Napoleon*. New York: Congdon & Lattes, 1982.

Weil, Andrew. *Health and Healing: Understanding Conventional and Alternative Medicine*. New York: Dorling-Kindersley, 1995.

Weil, Andrew. *Natural Health, Natural Medicine: A Comprehensive Manual for Wellness and Self-Care*. New York: Dorling-Kindersley, 1995.

Werbach, Melvyn R. *Third Line Medicine*. New York: Arkana, 1986.

Werner, David. *Where There Is No Doctor.* Palo Alto, CA: The Hesperian Foundation, 1977.

Whitney, Eleanor Noss, and Eva May Nunnelley Hamilton. *Understanding Nutrition.* St. Paul, MN: West Publishing, 1984.

Whybrow, Peter, and Robert Bahr. *The Hibernation Response.* New York: ArborHouse/Morrow, 1988.

Wildwood, Chrissie. *The Encyclopedia of Aromatherapy.* Rochester, NY: Healing Arts Press, 1996.

Wildwood, Christine. *The Aromatherapy and Massage Book.* London: Thorsons, 1994.

Williams, Phillip L., and James L. Burson, eds. *Industrial Toxicology: Safety and Health Applications in the Workplace.* New York: Van Nostrand Reinhold, 1985.

Wolf, Stewart. *Mind, Brain, and Medicine.* Piscataway, NJ: Transaction Publishers, 1993.

Journals and Periodicals

Abou-Donia, M.B., K.R. Wilmarth, et al. "Increased Neurotoxicity Following Concurrent Exposure to Pyridosigmine Bromide, DEET, and Chlorpyrifos." *Fundamental and Applied Toxicology.* 34: 201–22 (1996).

Ader, Robert, and N. Cohen. "Behaviorally-conditioned Immunosuppression and Murine Systemic Lupus Erythematosus." *Science.* 215 (4539): 1534–36 (1982).

Alvarado, Donna. "Too Much Sun May Suppress the Immune System." *Albuquerque Journal.* June 19, 1993: A-1, A-11.

Bartholomew, Anita. "Is Your Child 'Huffing'?" *Reader's Digest.* May 1996: 131–35.

Bartusiak, Marcia. "The Sunspot Syndrome." *Discover.* Nov. 1989: 45–52.

Bell, Iris R., et al. "Sensitization to Early Life Stress and Response to Chemical Odors in Older Adults." *Biol. Psychiatry* 35: 857–53 (1994).

Bland, Jeffrey S. "Food and Nutrient Effects on Detoxification." *Townsend Letter for Doctors and Patients.* Dec. 1995: 40–44.

Bland, Jeffrey S. "Managing Endo- and Exotoxicity." *Townsend Letter for Doctors and Patients.* July 1992: 590–93.

Blaylock, Russell L. "Food Additive Excitotoxins and Degenerative Brain Disorders." *Medical Sentinel.* 4: 212–15 (Nov./Dec., 1999).

Bonvie, Linda and Bill. "The Not So Friendly Skies." *Vegetarian Times.* May 1998: 16–17.

Borneman, John A. "Homeopathy and Naturopathy—Gentle Partners for Healing." *Let's Live.* April 1993: 16–25.

Branco, N. A. A. Castelo, E. Rodriguez, M. AlvePereira, and David Jones. "Vibroacoustic Disease: Some Forensic Aspects." *Aviation, Space, and Environmental Medicine.* 70(3): A145–A152 (March 1999).

Braune, S.C. Wrocklage, J. Raczek, T. Gailus, and C.H. Lucking. "Resting Blood Pressure Increase During Exposure to a Radio-frequency Electromagnetic Field." *Lancet.* 352(9119): 1857–58 (June 20, 1998).

Brien, James H. "What's Your Diagnosis?" *Infectious Diseases in Children.* 32, 50, 56 (Oct. 1999).

Brown, Michael. "Can You Detox Your Body?" *American Health.* September 1986: 53–58.

Browne, Malcolm. "High Cost of Noise." *Albuquerque Journal.* March 11, 1990: B-14.

Buttram, Harold E. "Protecting Children from Toxic Environmental Chemicals." *Townsend Letter for Doctors and Patients.* April 1993: 312–15.

Carlson, Joy E., and Birt Harvey. "Environmental Health During Childhood: Pediatrician Advocacy." *Pediatric Annals.* 24: 624–28 (Dec. 1995).

Carlson, Robert. "Aloe Vera versus Atherosclerosis." *Medical Gazette,* vol. 6 (50): 1 (Dec. 13, 1984).

Castleman, Michael. "X-ray Exposé—How to Avoid Diagnostic Mistakes." *Family Circle.* April 2000: 50–51.

Cathcart, Robert F. "The Method for Determining Proper Doses of Vitamin C by Titrating to Bowel Tolerance." *Journal of Orthomolecular Psychiatry.* 10: 125–32 (1991).

Cathcart, Robert F. "The Vitamin C Treatment of Allergy and the Normally Unprimed State of Antibodies." *Medical Hypothesis.* 21: 307–21 (1986).

Cathcart, Robert F. "Vitamin C: The Nontoxic, Non-role Limited, Antioxidant Free Radical Scavenger." *Medical Hypothesis.* 18: 61–77 (1985).

Choi, Steve. "Oxygen and Life." *Health World*. March/April 1990: 14–17.

Clark, W. W. "Noise Exposure from Leisure Activities: A review." *Journal of the Acoustical Society of America*, 90: 175–81 (1991).

Claussen, C.F. "Homotoxicology: The Basis of a Probiotic, Holistic Practice of Medicine." *Biological Therapy*. VIII (2): 37–39 (April 1989).

Clearwater, Susan. "Herbal Cleansing and Detoxification." *Enlightenments*. June 1993: 20.

Coats, Bill. "The Versatility of Whole Leaf Aloe Vera." *Dermascope Magazine*. Sept./Oct. 1991: 54, 56.

"Coenzyme Q_{10}: Animal-Vegetable-Mineral." *American Institute of Health and Nutrition News*. 1: 1–4 (1993).

Collins, Jonathan. "Carpet Toxicity." *Townsend Letter for Doctors and Patients*. April 1989: 197.

Committee on Substance Abuse and Committee on Native American Child Health. "Inhalant Abuse." *Pediatrics*. 97: 420–22 (March 1996).

Connolly, John. "Thunderstorms May Trigger Asthma Attacks, According to New Study." *Infectious Diseases in Children*. 12, n.d.

Conway, Claire. "How to Protect Your Child." *Parenting*. Sept. 1998: 41–48.

Costello, Mike, and Sarah Thurbes. "Bruised Faces and Broken Hearts: Violence in the Home." *Family Safety and Health*. 51(4): 23–27 (Winter 1992–93).

Cross, Mercer. "Lighting Up Your Life May Help Winter Depression." *Albuquerque Journal*. Feb. 14, 1988: F-6.

Debrovner, Diane. "Is Your Child's Hearing Okay?" *Parents*. March 1996: 37–40.

Dinsmoor, Robert. "The Latex Allergy Epidemic." *Asthma Magazine*. n.d.: 31–33.

Dreger, Marianne, ed. "Can Low-frequency Noise Cause Cancer, Stroke, or Epilepsy?" *ACOEM Report*. March 1999.

Engel, George. "A Life-setting Conducive to Illness: The Giving Up–Given Up Complex." *Bulletin of the Menninger Clinic*. 32: 355–65 (1968).

Epstein, Barbara. "Pollutants Clouding Up Classrooms Across U.S." *Indoor Environment Review*. 20 (August 1997).

Evans, Julie M. "The Basics of Natural Lawn Care." *The Human Ecologist*. Summer 1999: 18–20.

"Exercise is Good for the Brain." *East West*. April 1990: 13.

Fasciana, Guy S. "The E. I. Dentist—Dental Materials Part I." *The Human Ecologist* (25): 9–11 (Spring 1984).

Fasciana, Guy S. "The E. I. Dentist—Dental Materials Part II." *The Human Ecologist* (26): 11–12 (Summer 1984).

Fein, G.G., et al. "Prenatal Exposure to Polychlorinated Biphenyls: Effects on Birth Size and Gestational Age." *Journal of Pediatrics*. 105: 315–20 (1984).

Firth, Peta. "Leaving a Bad Taste." *Scientific American*. May 1999: 34–35.

Fitzgerald, Susan. "Sunlight on Winter Days Lifts Depression for Some." *Albuquerque Journal*. Dec. 11, 1986: B-8.

Flodin, Kim C. "Now Hear This." *American Health*. Jan./Feb. 1992: 59–62.

"Food Irradiation." *East West*. April 1990: 14.

Gard, Zane R., and Erma Jean Brown. "The Bio-Toxic Reduction Program: Eliminating Body Pollution." *Townsend Letter for Doctors and Patients*. April 1987: 49, 56–60.

Gard, Zane R., and Erma J. Brown. "Literature Review & Comparison Studies of the Sauna and Illness—Part II." *Townsend Letter for Doctors and Patients*. July 1992: 650–60.

Gard, Zane R., and Erma J. Brown. "Literature Review & Comparison Studies of Sauna Hyperthermia in Detoxification—Part III." *Townsend Letter for Doctors and Patients*. Oct. 1992: 844–53.

Ghen, Mitchell J. "Xenobiotics and Cellular Detoxification." *Journal of the American Medical Assoc.* 2(2): 30–32 (Summer 1999).

Gittleman, Janie L., et al. "Lead Poisoning among Battery Reclamation Workers in Alabama." *Journal of Occupational Medicine*. 36: 526–32 (May 1994).

Graham, Rex. "The Case Against Silicone." *Albuquerque Journal.* Dec. 14, 1992: A-1, A-8.

Green, Nancy Sokol. "America's Toxic Schools." *The Environmental Magazine.* n.d.: 30–37.

Hallowell, Christopher. "Clearing the Air." *Earthwise.* March 1993: 52–54.

Halpern, Steven, and Louis Savary. "Turn Up the Quiet In Your Home." *Prevention.* June 1985: 68–76.

Hebert, Lauren. "Outbreak of the Killer Potatoes." *U.S. News & World Report.* Aug. 10, 1998: 66.

Heine, Kathy. "Hearing Loss More Likely at Play Than at Work." *Albuquerque Journal.* Nov. 12, 1989: D-4.

Hodgkins, Douglas G., et al. "Influence of High Past Lead-in-Air Exposures on the Lead- in-Blood Levels of Lead-Acid Battery Workers with Continuing Exposure." *Journal of Occupational Medicine.* 33: 797–803 (July 1991).

Hoffman, David. "Herbs and Children." *Let's Live.* June 1993: 70–71.

Hoppner, K., et al. "Vitamin A Reserves of Canadians." *Canadian Medical Association Journal.* 101(12): 84–86 (Dec. 13, 1969).

Huebner, Albert L. "Protect Yourself from the Deadliest Radiation." *Let's Live.* Nov. 1996: 48–50.

Huggins, Hal A. "Root Canals." *Let's Live.* Nov. 1990: 71.

Jacobson, J.L., S.W. Jacobson, and H.E.B. Humphrey. "Effects of In Utero Exposure to Polychlorinated Biphenyls and Related Contaminants on Cognitive Functioning in Young Children." *Journal of Pediatrics.* 116(1): 38–45 (1990a).

Jacobson, J.L., S. W. Jacobson, and H.E.B. Humphrey. "Effects of Exposure to PCBs and Related Compounds on Growth and Activity in Children." *Neurotoxicol. Teratol.* 12: 319–26 (1990b).

Jacobson, S.W., et al. "The Effect of Intrauterine PCB Exposure on Visual Recognition Memory." *Child Development.* 56: 853–60 (1985).

Jancin, Bruce. "Sexually Abused Children Said to Have Lasting Changes in Hormones." *Pediatric News.* 34 (Jan. 1992).

Johnson, Barry L. "Protecting Our Children from Exposure to Hazardous Substances." *Hazardous Substances & Public Health.* 6: 1–2 (Fall 1996).

Jones, Marjorie Hurt. "Working at Wellness." *Mastering Food Allergies.* VIII(6): 1–8 (Nov.–Dec. 1993).

Jones-Smith, Jacqueline. "Safety from the Ground Up." *Home.* Feb. 1993: 27.

Khalife, Katherine. "Journaling to Health." *Delicious!— Your Guide to Natural Living.* Feb. 2000: 20–23.

Khalsa, K.P. "Herbal Enhancers for Detoxification." *Let's Live.* Nov. 1996: 78–81.

Kleiner, Susan M. "Should You Opt for Organic?" *The Physician and Sports Medicine.* Vol. 23 (12): 15–16 (Dec. 1995).

Krueger, Albert Paul. "On Air Ions—and Your Health, Moods, and Efficiency." *Executive Health.* 17(2): (Nov. 1980).

Krueger, Albert Paul, and Eddie James Reed. "Biological Impact of Small Air Ions." *Science.* 19: 1209–13 (Sept. 1976).

Lanpher, Katherine, and Kathryn Keller. "Turn Down That Noise!" *Redbook.* April 1991: 58–64.

Leviton, Richard. "How the Weather Affects Your Health." *East West.* Sept. 1989: 64–68, 112–13.

Leviton, Richard. "Can the Earth's Stress Spots Make You Sick?" *East West.* June 1989: 48–52, 83–85.

Leviton, Richard. "The Ley Lines of Seattle." *East West.* March 1989: 54–57.

Lin, David. "Antioxidants, Free Radicals, and Health." *Health Consciousness.* 14(3): 58–59 (1993).

Liska, DeAnn J. "The Detoxification Enzyme Systems." *Alternative Medicine Review.* 3(3): 187–96 (1998).

Litt, Jerome Z., ed. "Phytodermatis." *Cross Section.* 16(4): 11 (1991).

Loddeke, Leslie. "Aloe Vera to be Tried as AIDS Treatment." *The Houston Post.* Oct. 4, 1992: n.p.

Mayer, Jack L., and Sophie J. Balle. "A Pediatrician's Guide to Environmental Toxins." *Contemporary Pediatrics.* 63–76 (Aug. 1988).

McCabe, ed. "People." *Health Consciousness.* 14(3): 81–82 (1993).

Nakagawa, K. "Magnetic Field-Deficiency Syndrome and Magnetic Treatment." *Japan Medical Journal.* 2745 (Dec. 1976).

Nash, Duane D.B., Eliane Schochat, Alan A. Rozycki, and Frank E. Musie. "When Loud Noises Hurt." *Contemporary Pediatrics.* 97–109 (June 1997).

Needleman, Herbert L. "Why We Should Worry About Lead Poisoning." *Contemporary Pediatrics.* 35–36 (March 1988).

NIH Consensus Development Conference. "Noise and Hearing Loss." *Journal of the American Medical Assoc.* 263(23): 3185–90 (June 20, 1990).

Novotny, William E. "Pulmonary Hemorrhage in an Infant Following 2 Weeks of Fungal Exposure." *Archives of Pediatric and Adolescent Medicine.* 154: 271–75 (March 2000).

Osborn, Carl D. "Treatment of Spider Bites by High Voltage Direct Current." *Journal of the Oklahoma State Medical Assoc.* 84: 257–60 (June 1991).

Ott, Wayne R, and John W. Roberts. "Everyday Exposure to Toxic Pollutants." *Scientific American.* Feb. 1998: 72.

Pennisi, E. "Free-Radical Scavenger Gene Tied to ALS." *Science News.* 143: 148 (1993).

"Preliminary Evidence Points to Affective Disorder Triggered by Summer Weather." *Journal of the American Medical Assoc.* 295(7): 958 (1988).

Radetsky, Peter. "The Gulf War Within." *Discover.* August 1997: 69–75.

Rappe, Gerald C. "Your Office May Be Hazardous." *Townsend Letter for Doctors and Patients.* Feb./March 1990: 122–24.

Reigart, J. Routt. "Pesticides and Children." *Pediatric Annals.* 24: 663–68 (Dec. 1995).

Root, David, and Michael Wisner. "Detecting and Treating Chemical Exposure." *LA Weekly.* 1989.

Russell, M.A.H., and C. Feyerabend. "Blood and Urinary Nicotine in Non-smokers." *The Lancet.* 179–81 (Jan. 25, 1975).

Rynk, Peggy. "The Healing Power of Touch." *Let's Live.* April 1993: 58–59.

"Rx: Don't Mix Medications and the Sun." *Parade Magazine.* Aug. 22, 1993: 13.

"Rx for Laughter: Cancer Patients Find Fun on the Road to Recovery." *American Institute for Cancer Research Newsletter.* 41: 10 (Fall 1993).

Samet, Jonathan M., Marian C. Marbury, and John D. Spengler. "Respiratory Effects of Indoor Air Pollution." *Journal of Allergy and Clinical Immunology.* 79: 685–700 (1987).

Schechter, Steven R. "That Cad, Cadmium." *Let's Live.* Jan. 1993: 88.

Schwartz, P.M., et al. "Lake Michigan Fish Consumption as a Source of Polychlorinated Biphenyls in Human or Serum, Maternal Serum, and Milk." *American Journal of Public Health.* 73(3): 293–96 (March 1983).

Seba, Douglas B. "Thermal Chamber Depuration—A Perspective on Man in the Sauna." *Clinical Ecology.* 7(1): 1–12 (1989).

"Skin Hormone, Melatonin May Work Together." *Brain/Mind Bulletin.* Oct. 1989: 2.

"The Soils of War," *Discover.* November 1999: 26.

Spitz, Jill Jorden. "Wiping Out Mug Bugs." *Herald.* March 21, 1998.

Stauber, Camille Lee. "Managing Landscape Without Chemicals." *Our Toxic Times.* August 1996: 16–20.

Stavish, Phillip. "Irradiated Food—How Will It Impact Your Health?" *Journal of Longevity.* 4:15–17, 45–46 (1998).

Steinman, David, and R. Michael Wisner. "How to Detoxify Your Life." *Let's Live.* Nov. 1996: 45–47.

Suter, Alice H. "Noise Sources and Effects—A New Look." *Sound and Vibration.* 18–34 (Jan. 1992).

Thomson, Bill. "Rejuvenate Yourself in Three Weeks." *Natural Healing.* Jan./Feb. 1993: 2–7.

Turk, Michele. "Death Lurks Within 'High'-Inducing Products." *AAP News.* April 1996: 12–14.

Vermeer, M., et al. "Effects of Ultraviolet-B light on cutaneous immune-responses of Humans with Deeply Pigmented Skin." *Journal of Investigative Dermatology.* 97(4): 729–34 (1991).

Vimy, M.J., Takahashi, Y., and F. L. Lorscheider. "Maternal-Fetal Distribution of Mercury (203-Hg) Released from Dental Amalgam Fillings." *American Journal of Physiology.* 258: R939–R945 (1990).

Wartik, Nancy. "A Question of Abuse." *American Health.* May 1993: 62–67.

Weaver, Daniel C. "Heavy Metal." *Discover.* April 1993: 76–78.

Weisenthal, Debra Blake. "Which Peach Should You Pick?" *Natural Health.* May–June 1997: 111–26, 174–77.

Weisskopf, Michael. "Lead Astray: The Poisoning of America." *Discover.* December 1987: 68–74.

Whitaker, Julian. "Clean Up Indoor Pollution With Plants." *Health and Healing.* 3(10): 1–3 (Oct. 1993).

Whitaker, Julian. "EDTA Chelation Therapy: Your Safe Alternative to Surgery." *Health and Healing.* 2 (4): 1–4 (April 1992).

Williams, David G. "Cleaning House." *Alternatives for the Health Conscious Individual.* 4: 97–100 (1992).

Williams, Sid. "Bones of Contention." *Health.* July/Aug. 1993: 44–53.

Witlin, Barbara, and Roy Witlin. "Our Lives: Artist Finds Nontoxic Paints and Methods." *The Human Ecologist.* 13–15 (Winter 1991).

Woolf, Alan D., and Elizabeth Flynn. "Workplace Toxic Exposures Involving Adolescents Aged 14 to 19 Years." *Archives of Pediatric and Adolescent Medicine.* 154: 234–39 (March 2000).

Wooster, Sarah M. "Geopathogenic Stress and Cancer." *Townsend Letter for Doctors and Patients.* Nov. 1988: 482–86.

Yudkin, Marcia. "The Forecast for Tomorrow is Headaches." *Natural Health.* Jan./Feb. 1993: 40–41.

Zucker, Norman. "Hubbard's Purification Rundown: A Workable Detox Program." *Townsend Letter for Doctors and Patients.* Jan. 1990: 54–55.

Other

BHI. "A Modern Approach to Homeopathy." Pamphlet. Albuquerque, NM: Menaco Publishing, n.d.

Bland, Jeffrey. "Functional Testing of Detoxification Pathways in Chemical Sensitivities." Presented at the American Academy of Environmental Medicine, 28th Annual Meeting, Reno, NV, Oct. 10, 1993.

Bland, Jeffrey. "Antioxidants, Co-factors, et al. in Maximizing the Functioning of the Detoxification Pathways." Presented at the American Academy of Environmental Medicine, 28th Annual Meeting, Reno, NV, Oct. 10, 1993.

Cardiovascular Research. "Clinical Uses of Coenzyme Q_{10}." Pamphlet. Concord, CA: Cardiovascular Research, 1983.

Clark, Marler. "Outbreaks of *E. coli* Should Not Occur in Municipal Water." Accessed June 10, 2000. www.marlerclark.com

Ecological Formulas. "Intestinal Microflora and Persistent Illness." Research Perspective in Gastroenterology. Concord, CA: Ecological Formulas, n.d.

Environmental Protection Agency. "The Inside Story: A Guide to Indoor Air Quality." U.S. Environmental Protection Agency, Washington, DC, Sept. 1988.

Environmental Protection Agency. "Radon Reduction Methods: A Homeowner's Guide." U.S. Environmental Protection Agency, Washington, DC, Sept. 1987.

Environmental Working Group. "Factory Farming: Toxic Wastes Used as Fertilizer in the United States." April 21, 2000. http://www.ewg.org/pub/home/Reports/factoryfarming/fert.html

Environmental Working Group. "Factory Farming: Toxic Waste and Fertilizer in the United States, 1990–1995." Press Release. April 21, 2000. http://www.ewg.org/pub/home/Reports/factory farming/concs.html

Feng, Peter. "A Summary of Background Information and Foodborne Illness Associated with the Consumption of Sprouts." Division of Microbiological Studies, OSRS, CRSAN, FDA, Washington, DC, April 2, 2000. http://vm.cfxan.fda.gov/~mow/sprouts.html

Feingold Association. "The Feingold Program—What is it?" April 4, 2000. http://www.feingold.org/program.html

Feingold Association. "Feingold Diet—Some questions you may have." April 2, 2000. http://www.feingold.org/indexx.html

Gerba, Charles P., Ralph Meer, and Carlos E. Enriquez. "A Microbial Survey of Office Coffee Cups and Effectiveness of the FreshCup System for Reduction of Bacteria." FreshCUP System. July 7, 2000. http://www.freshcup.co.il/fc7.htm

Greenberg, Robert. "Modification of Biological Terrain in Preventive and Restorative Therapeutics." Presented at Mountain States Health Care Products Seminar, Westminster, CO, Dec. 11, 1993.

HHS News. "Consumers Advised of Risks Associated with Raw Sprouts." U.S. Department of Health and Human Services. April 2, 2000. http://vm.cfsan.fda.gov/~lrd/hhssprts.html

Jaffe, Russell. "Occurrence of Xenobiotic Hypersensitivity in an Autoimmune/ Multiple Chemical Sensitivity (AI-MCS) Cohort Compared with an Ambulatory Control Population." Presented at the American Academy of Environmental Medicine, 28th Annual Meeting, Reno, NV, Oct. 11, 1993.

Johnson, Barry L., et al. "Public Health Implications of Exposure to Polychlorinated Biphenyls (PCBs)." Agency for Toxic Substances and Disease Registry Public Health Service. April 4, 2000. http://sites.netscape.net/georgecjeffrey/Cdcpcb

Klaire Laboratories. "Vital Plex." Pamphlet. San Marcos, CA: Klaire Laboratories, n.d.

Krohn, Jacqueline. "Lead Poisoning." Presented at the American Adacemy of Environmental Medicine, 27th Annual Meeting, Lincolnshire, IL, Oct. 27, 1992.

Kroker, George F., and Leslie Peickert-Kroker. "Woodsmoke as an Environmental Hazard." Presented at the American Academy of Environmental Medicine, 18th Annual Meeting, Chicago, IL, 1984.

Laboratories. "Myths About Microbial Supplementation Dispelled." Technical bulletin. San Marcos, CA: Klaire Laboratories, 1988.

Larson, E.M., J. Krohn, and F. Taylor. "Abuse as a Contributing Factor in Environmental Illness." Presented at the American Academy of Environmental Medicine, 28th Annual Meeting, Reno, NV, Oct. 11, 1993.

Larson, E.M., J. Krohn, and F. Taylor. "Clinical Manifestations of Nutrient Deficiencies." Presented at the American Academy of Environmental Medicine, 27th Annual Meeting, Lincolnshire, IL, Oct. 27, 1992.

Larson, E.M., J. Krohn, and F. Taylor. "The Emotional and Psychological Impact of Environmental Illness." Presented at the American Academy of Environmental Medicine, 26th Annual Meeting, Jacksonville, FL, Oct. 29, 1991.

Lawrence, Ronald M. "Lignisul MSM (Methylsulfonylmethane): A Double-Blind Study of Its Use in Degenerative Arthritis." Health Benefits Scientific Studies. January 23, 2000. http://www.msm.com/trial.html

Lewis, Alan. "Coenzyme Q_{10}: A Review." Pamphlet, Karuna, n.d.

Lieberman, Allan. "The Role of Sauna Detoxification in the Treatment of Chemical Sensitivities." Presented at the American Academy of Environmental Medicine, 28th Annual Meeting, Reno, NV, Oct. 10, 1993.

Liles, Necia Dixon, and Allan Liles. "This Mercury Is Not the Gods' Messenger–II." *Let's Live*. Dec. 1992: 66–67.

Martina, Roy. Endogenous Detoxification. Seminar Notes. Los Angeles: Apex Energetics, 1992.

McEwen, L. M. "The Surprising Role of Hyperventilation in Environmentally Triggered Illness." Presented at the American Academy of Environmental Medicine, 30th Annual Meeting, Tucson, AZ, Sept. 29–Oct. 3, 1995.

McGill, Ruth C. "Pathological Fatigue: A Review of Ideas." Presented at the American Academy of Environmental Medicine, 29th Annual Meeting, Virginia Beach, VA, Oct. 15–19, 1994.

McWilliams, Charles. "Electrobiology, Homotoxicology, Overview of Homeopathy, and Today's Miasmatic Terrain." Eclectic Remedy Seminar, Nevis, West Indies, Nov. 21–24, 1992.

Metametrix Laboratory. "Liver Detoxification Functions." Pamphlet. Norcross, GA: Metametrix Laboratory, n.d.

Bibliography

Murphy, Robin. "H.A.N.A. Certificate Homeopathy Classes 1–18." Santa Fe, NM: Hahnemann Academy of North America, 1991–92.

Murphy, Robin. "H.A.N.A. Certificate Class Home Study Tapes 1–21." Santa Fe, NM: Hahnemann Academy of North America, 1991–92.

Nutritional Enzyme Support System. Ness Product Update—Ness Formula 3. Pamphlet. Forsyth, MO: Nutritional Enzyme Support System, April 1992.

Osterholm, Michael T., and S. Michael Marcy. "Food for Thought: Identifying Cases of Food-Borne Illness." *Conference Proceedings.* Annual Meeting of the American Academy of Pediatrics, Dallas, TX. Oct. 22–26, 1994: 2–8.

Phillips, Reed B. "A Brief History of Chiropractic." History of Chiropractic. May 9, 2000. http://www.chiropractor.com/Studyhistoryofchiropractic.html

Professional Health Products. "Heavy Metal Intoxication and Detoxification." Pamphlet. Sewickley, PA: Professional Health Products, 1992.

"The Purifying Program™." Booklet. Beverly Hills, CA: Eden's Secrets Corp., n.d.

Randolph, Theron G., and R. Michael Wisner. "Detoxification: Personal Survival in a Chemical World." Pamphlet. Sacramento, CA: Healthmed, 1988: n.p.

Rea, William J. "The Environmental Control Unit (ECU) as a Tool in the Diagnosis and Treatment of Chemical Sensitivities." Presented at the American Academy of Environmental Medicine, 28th Annual Meeting, Reno, NV, Oct. 10, 1993.

Rea, William. "The Non-Immunologic Mechanisms of Chemical Sensitivity." Presented at the American Academy of Environmental Medicine, 28th Annual Meeting, Reno, NV, Oct. 9, 1993.

Taylor, Frances, and Jacqueline Krohn. "Expanded Chemical Testing: Utilization of New Chemicals for More Complete Relief for the Chemically Susceptible Patient." Presented at the American Academy of Environmental Medicine, 28th Annual Meeting, Reno, NV, Oct. 11, 1993.

Taylor, Frances, Jacqueline Krohn, and Erla Mae Larson. "Allergic Implications of Viral Infections." Presented at the American Academy of Environmental Medicine, 27th Annual Meeting, Lincolnshire, IL, Oct. 27, 1992.

Vacco, Dennis C. "Integrated Pest Management: An Introduction." Brochure. New York State Department of Law. June 1998.

Answers

1. Toxins can enter the body through the skin, inhalation through the respiratory tract into the lungs, and ingestion through the mouth into the gastrointestinal tract.

2. The skin, lungs, gastrointestinal tract, and the liver are our major organs of detoxification. They try to eliminate foreign chemicals, drugs, and compounds produced by the body, such as hormones, cholesterol, and fatty acids.

3. Water flushes toxins and waste material from the cells. Nutrients must be kept in solution, available for cell nutrition and repair, and adequate fluid levels are necessary for ions in the body to flow and maintain electrical equilibrium.

4. An electromagnetic imbalance may cause electrical equipment to malfunction when you are near and may make it difficult to find a watch that keeps the correct time. Symptoms may occur when near fluorescent lights, transformers or high-powered electric lines and may worsen before a storm.

5. The most important part of any diet is chewing food well. Food should be chewed until you can feel the saliva break up the foods.

Index